Respiratory Failure

Respiratory Failure

Editor: Harvey Reid

FOSTER ACADEMICS
www.fosteracademics.com

www.fosteracademics.com

FOSTER ACADEMICS

Cataloging-in-Publication Data

Respiratory failure / edited by Harvey Reid.
p. cm.
Includes bibliographical references and index.
ISBN 978-1-63242-803-5
1. Respiratory insufficiency. 2. Lungs--Diseases. 3. Respiratory organs--Diseases.
I. Reid, Harvey.
RC776.R4 R47 2019
616.24--dc23

Foster Academics,
118-35 Queens Blvd., Suite 400,
Forest Hills, NY 11375, USA

ISBN 978-1-63242-803-5 (Hardback)

Printed and bound in China.

Contents

Preface

Respiratory failure is a serious condition associated with the respiratory tract arising from inadequate gas exchange by the respiratory system. It can broadly be categorized into hypoxemia and hypercapnia. The condition of having abnormally low level of oxygen in the blood is known as hypoxemia. Hypercapnia is a condition associated with abnormally elevated carbon dioxide levels in the blood. Respiratory failure can be classified either as Type I or Type II, on the basis of the presence of abnormal blood gases. Some of the common causes of respiratory failure include reduced breathing caused due to drug intake, reduced air flow caused due to the physical obstruction in the body by foreign masses and thromboembolic conditions. Treatment methods include mechanical ventilation, endotracheal intubation and continuous positive airway pressure. The topics included in this book on respiratory failure are of utmost significance and bound to provide incredible insights to readers. It will also provide interesting topics for research, which interested readers can take up. This book is a resource guide for experts as well as students.

The researches compiled throughout the book are authentic and of high quality, combining several disciplines and from very diverse regions from around the world. Drawing on the contributions of many researchers from diverse countries, the book's objective is to provide the readers with the latest achievements in the area of research. This book will surely be a source of knowledge to all interested and researching the field.

In the end, I would like to express my deep sense of gratitude to all the authors for meeting the set deadlines in completing and submitting their research chapters. I would also like to thank the publisher for the support offered to us throughout the course of the book. Finally, I extend my sincere thanks to my family for being a constant source of inspiration and encouragement.

Editor

Disruption of Sorting Nexin 5 Causes Respiratory Failure Associated with Undifferentiated Alveolar Epithelial Type I Cells in Mice

Sun-Kyoung Im[1,2], HyoBin Jeong[3], Hyun-Woo Jeong[1], Kyong-Tai Kim[2], Daehee Hwang[3], Machiko Ikegami[4], Young-Yun Kong[1]*

1 School of Biological Science, College of Natural Sciences, Seoul National University, Seoul, South Korea, **2** Department of Life Science, Division of Molecular and Life Science, POSTECH, Pohang, South Korea, **3** School of Interdisciplinary Biosciences and Bioengineering, POSTECH, Pohang, South Korea, **4** Division of Pulmonary Biology, Cincinnati Children's Hospital Medical Center and University of Cincinnati College of Medicine, Cincinnati, Ohio, United States of America

Abstract

Sorting nexin 5 (Snx5) has been posited to regulate the degradation of epidermal growth factor receptor and the retrograde trafficking of cation-independent mannose 6-phosphate receptor/insulin-like growth factor II receptor. Snx5 has also been suggested to interact with Mind bomb-1, an E3 ubiquitin ligase that regulates the activation of Notch signaling. However, the *in vivo* functions of Snx5 are largely unknown. Here, we report that disruption of the *Snx5* gene in mice (*Snx5*$^{-/-}$ mice) resulted in partial perinatal lethality; 40% of *Snx5*$^{-/-}$ mice died shortly after birth due to cyanosis, reduced air space in the lungs, and respiratory failure. Histological analysis revealed that *Snx5*$^{-/-}$ mice exhibited thickened alveolar walls associated with undifferentiated alveolar epithelial type I cells. In contrast, alveolar epithelial type II cells were intact, exhibiting normal surfactant synthesis and secretion. Although the expression levels of surfactant proteins and saturated phosphatidylcholine in the lungs of *Snx5*$^{-/-}$ mice were comparable to those of *Snx5*$^{+/+}$ mice, the expression levels of T1α, Aqp5, and Rage, markers for distal alveolar epithelial type I cells, were significantly decreased in *Snx5*$^{-/-}$ mice. These results demonstrate that *Snx5* is necessary for the differentiation of alveolar epithelial type I cells, which may underlie the adaptation to air breathing at birth.

Editor: You-Yang Zhao, University of Illinois College of Medicine, United States of America

Funding: This work was supported by the Basic Science Research Program through the National Research Foundation of Korea (RND no. 2012-0000121), National R&D Program for Cancer Control, Ministry of Health & Welfare, the Republic of Korea (RND no. 0920310), Bio & Medical Technology Development Program of the National Research Foundation (NRF) funded by the Korean government (MEST; RND no. 2011-0019269), and Global Frontier Project grant (RND no. 2011-0028413) of the National Research Foundation funded by the Ministry of Education, Science and Technology of Korea. The funders had no role in study design, data collection and analysis, decision to publish, or preparation of the manuscript.

Competing Interests: The authors have declared that no competing interests exist.

* E-mail: ykong@snu.ac.kr

Introduction

During lung development, the proximal-distal axis is formed by the elongation, expansion, and bifurcation of lung buds during branching morphogenesis, and the functional units for gas exchange are generated during alveologenesis. During late gestation, alveolar development occurs and type I and type II alveolar epithelial cells undergo differentiation and maturation to form functional alveoli [1,2,3,4,5,6]. Alveolar epithelial type I cells are in close contact with endothelial cells in alveolar capillaries and form an efficient gas exchange area [7]. Alveolar epithelial type II cells undergo marked biochemical and ultrastructural changes, including depletion of glycogen content, enhanced synthesis of surfactant proteins and lipids, increased numbers of lamellar bodies, and surfactant secretion. In neonates, deficiency of surfactant protein production or secretion due to pulmonary immaturity can cause clinical disorders, such as respiratory distress syndrome or bronchopulmonary dysplasia. Respiratory distress syndrome is a major cause of high morbidity and mortality in premature infants [8,9,10].

Deletion or mutation of genes encoding surfactant proteins (SP)-B, SP-C, and ATP-binding cassette (ABC) A3 (ABCA3) in mice causes respiratory failure or severe lung disease soon after birth [11,12,13,14]. In addition, recently, mutant mice with knock-in of the thyroid hormone receptor repressor silencing mediator of retinoid and thyroid hormone receptors (SMRT) have provided a novel model for alveolar epithelial type I cell-associated respiratory distress syndrome [15]. Although functional maturation of alveolar epithelial type I and II cells is critical for the adaptation of air breathing at birth, the molecular mechanisms that control the functional maturation of alveolar epithelial cells, particularly type I cells, are poorly understood [16,17].

Sorting nexins (SNXs) are a large family of proteins that contain the phosphoinositide-binding Phox homology domain. Previous studies have reported that SNX5 plays a role in endosomal trafficking of epidermal growth factor receptor (EGFR) and cation-independent mannose 6-phosphate receptor (CI-MPR)/insulin-like growth factor II receptor (IGF2R) [18,19,20,21]. Overexpression of SNX5 inhibits the degradation of EGFR, whereas the overexpression of SNX1 or SNX6 enhances EGFR degradation, suggesting that EGFR degradation may be finely regulated by SNX1, SNX5, and SNX6 [18,22,23]. Knockdown experiments of SNX5 and SNX6 using RNA interference (RNAi) show dispersed CI-MPR trafficking in HeLa cells into early endosomes [20], suggesting that CI-MPR is also regulated by SNX5 in endosome-to-trans-Golgi network (TGN) retrieval [24]. In addition, SNX5 interacts with Mind bomb-1 (Mib1), a key regulator of Notch ligands in mammalian development [25,26,27,28,29,30,31]. In zebrafish, depletion of *snx5* by morpholino leads to severe defects in vascular formation and hematopoietic cell generation [21], suggesting that *Snx5* may be involved in Notch signaling through regulation of *Mib1*. Despite a decade of studies examining the role of SNX5, the precise physiological function of SNX5 in mammals is still not known.

To study the *in vivo* functions of SNX5, we generated mice lacking the *Snx5* gene. These $Snx5^{-/-}$ mice showed partial perinatal mortality, with approximately 40% of the animals dying within a day of birth. Thirty percent of $Snx5^{-/-}$ mice survived until adulthood, but displayed severe growth inhibition. Downstream signaling of EGFR, EGFR degradation and endosome-to-TGN retrieval of CI-MPR were not affected in $Snx5^{-/-}$ murine embryonic fibroblasts (MEFs). In addition, EGFR signaling was not altered in isolated primary lung epithelial cells (PLEs). Neonatal $Snx5^{-/-}$ mice showed significant breathing defects associated with cyanosis and reduced pulmonary air space in the lungs at birth. Histological analysis revealed that $Snx5^{-/-}$ mice had reduced alveolar epithelial type I cells, while alveolar epithelial type II cells were intact. Consistently, $Snx5^{-/-}$ mice had decreased levels of the alveolar epithelial type I cell markers T1α, Aqp5, and Rage, whereas the expression levels of surfactant proteins and saturated phosphatidylcholine were comparable to wild-type mice. The results of our study indicate that *Snx5* is necessary for the differentiation of alveolar epithelial type I cells during perinatal murine lung development.

Materials and Methods

Ethics statement

Mice used in this study were housed under specific pathogen-free conditions. All animal protocols were approved by the Seoul National University Institutional Animal Care and Use committee (Approval number: SNU080623-4).

Mouse experiments

The XA155 gene-trapped ES cell line, which contained an insertion of β-geo in intron 7 of *Snx5*, was used to generate chimeric mice (BayGenomics, San Francisco, CA). Following a standard protocol (http://www.genetrap.org/info/protocols/baygenomics/blastocyst.html), XA155 ES cells were microinjected into C57BL/6 mouse blastocysts. The resultant chimeric mice were mated with C57BL/6 mice to obtain heterozygous $Snx5^{+/-}$ mice. The heterozygous mutant mice were backcrossed to C57BL/6 mice 5 times. Heterozygotes were then interbred to obtain homozygotes. Genotyping was performed using polymerase chain reaction (PCR) and confirmed with Southern blotting using tail genomic DNA as a template. Southern blotting was performed using probe-labeling with the Rediprime II DNA labeling kit (GE Healthcare, Little Chalfont, UK) and imaged with BAS-1500 (Fuji). For mouse genotyping by PCR, *Snx5*-specific forward and reverse primers were designed (common forward primer: GGA-GATGTTTGGAGGCTTTTT, wild-type reverse primer: CAG-GAATCCTTGATCCTGTTG, mutant reverse primer: GGTCGAGAGAACGGTGAGAG). Genomic DNA samples were digested with *Eco*RI and probed with a 5′external probe.

Isolation and culture of primary mouse lung epithelial cells

Lung tissues from $Snx5^{+/-}$ intercrosses were collected by caesarean section at E18.5. Primary lung epithelial cells were cultured with the methods described by Warshamana and Matsui [32,33] with slight modifications, and were used for EGF treatment experiments. Briefly, isolated lungs were removed and incubated with dispase (5 mg/mL, *STEMCELL* Technologies, Inc.) for 45 min at room temperature. The lungs were minced and transferred to Dulbecco's modified Eagle's medium (DMEM) with 0.01% DNase I (1 mg/mL, *STEMCELL* Technologies, Inc.) for 10 min at 37°C. The dissociated cells were filtered through a 40-μm nylon cell strainer and centrifuged at 1000 rpm for 10 min. The resuspended cells were plated into cell culture dishes at 37°C for 1 h in order to remove the macrophages and fibroblasts. After a 1-h incubation, nonattached cells were transferred into new cell culture dishes. This step was repeated 4 times. Final nonattached cells were filtered through a 40-μm strainer and centrifuged. The resuspended cells were plated on type-I collagen-coated 35 mm culture dishes (BD BioCoat) in DMEM/Ham's F-12 50/50 mixed medium (Cellgro) supplemented with 15 mM HEPES, 0.8 mM $CaCl_2$, 0.25% BSA, 5 μg/mL insulin, 5 μg/mL transferrin, 5 ng/mL sodium selenite, and 2% mouse serum. After 24 h, the culture medium was changed to serum-free DMEM/Ham's F-12 mixed medium supplemented as described above and maintained in the same medium. The isolated cells were almost all type II cells, as determined by qRT-PCR and immunocytochemistry analysis of T1α− and pro-SP-C.

Cell culture, EGF stimulation, and CHX treatment

Primary MEFs were isolated from embryonic day 13.5 (E13.5) $Snx5^{+/+}$ and $Snx5^{-/-}$ embryos. MEFs were maintained in Dulbecco's modified Eagle's medium (DMEM; Hyclone) containing 10% fetal bovine serum (FBS; Hyclone), antibiotic-antimycotic solution (Invitrogen, Carlsbad, CA, USA), and 2-mercaptoethanol (Invitrogen) in a humid atmosphere of 5% CO_2 at 37°C. For EGF treatments, MEFs were serum-starved for 12 h and then treated with 100 ng/mL EGF for 0, 5, 10, 20, 60, 120 and 180 min and 0, 5, 15, 30, 60 and 120 min. For CI-MPR protein detection, cells were treated with 40 μg/mL cycloheximide (CHX; Sigma, St. Louis, MO, USA) for 17 h to inhibit biosynthesis of CI-MPR protein.

RNA isolation and quantitative RT-PCR analysis

Total RNA was isolated from lung tissues using TRIzol Reagent (Invitrogen, Carlsbad, CA) and complementary DNA synthesis was performed according to the manufacturer's instructions (ImProm-II Reverse Transcription system; Promega). Quantification of cDNAs from specific mRNA transcripts was accomplished by qRT-PCR (Bio-Rad) using SYBR Green PCR mixture (Takara Bio Inc.) as described previously [25]. The relative concentration of each mRNA was normalized to the concentration of 18S rRNA in each sample. PCR primer sequences are shown in Table S2.

Western blot analysis and measurement of saturated phosphatidylcholine (Sat PC)

Protein detection in murine embryonic fibroblasts (MEFs), primary lung epithelial cells (PLEs) and total lung lysates of $Snx5^{+/+}$ and $Snx5^{-/-}$ mice by western blot has been described previously [27]. Proteins were detected using specific primary antibodies at 1:1000 dilution, including rabbit anti-epidermal growth factor receptor (EGFR), anti-cation-independent mannose 6-phosphate receptor (CI-MPR), anti-phospho-Akt, anti-Akt, anti-phospho-Erk1/2, anti-Erk1/2 (Cell Signaling Technology, Danvers, MA, USA), rabbit anti-tubulin (Abcam), rabbit anti-β-actin (Sigma), rabbit anti-Snx5, goat anti-CC-10, mouse anti-PCNA, goat anti-Pecam-1 (Santa Cruz Biotechnology, Santa Cruz, CA, USA), rabbit anti-proSP-C (Chemicon), Syrian hamster anti-T1α (1:100, Developmental Studies Hybridoma Bank), rabbit anti-pro-SP-C (1:2000, Chemicon), goat anti-CC-10 (1:2000, Santa Cruz Biotechnology), mouse anti-α-SMA (1:500, Santa Cruz Biotechnology), mouse anti-SP-B (Seven Hills Bioreagents, Cincinnati, OH, USA), mouse anti-vimentin (1:1000, Chemicon), and mouse anti-E-cadherin (1:1000, BD Biosciences). The membranes were incubated with horseradish peroxidase-conjugated secondary antibodies (goat anti-rabbit IgG, goat anti-mouse IgG, donkey anti-goat IgG or goat anti-Syrian hamster IgG, as appropriate; Promega or Santa Cruz Biotechnology). Protein bands were detected using ECL Reagent (Thermo) followed by exposure to X-ray film (Agfa) or detection in a Vilber Fusion Solo 2 chemiluminescence system (Fisher Biotec). SP-B immunoblot bands were quantified by densitometry (ImageQuant v5.2, GE Healthcare, Piscataway, NJ). Sat PC was isolated from lipid extracts of lung homogenate by using osmium tetroxide followed by phosphorus assay as described previously [34,35,36].

Histology and β-galactosidase staining

Embryonic lungs were dissected and fixed in 4% paraformaldehyde (PFA) for 24 h at 4°C. The lungs were dehydrated in a series of graded ethanol solutions and embedded in paraffin blocks. Histological analysis was performed on 5-μm sections. Hematoxylin and eosin (H&E), periodic acid Schiff (PAS), and Alcian blue staining were performed according to standard protocols [37]. For β-galactosidase staining, whole lungs were fixed in 4% PFA (pH 7.4) for 2 h at 4°C. The tissues were washed in phosphate-buffered saline (PBS) and placed in X-gal staining solution (1 M $MgCl_2$, 0.01% sodium-deoxycholate, 0.02% NP-40, 5 mM potassium ferricyanide/ferrocyanide, and 1 mg/mL X-gal in PBS) overnight at 37°C.

Floating assay

Floating assay was performed as previously described [15,38,39,40]. Briefly, as soon as *Snx5*$^{-/-}$ mice had died, the lungs were removed from newborn mice and deposited in eppendorf tubes containing PBS.

Air-breathing test

Mice were collected by caesarean section at E18.5. We cleaned the bodies and immediately removed the lung fluid. To maintain body temperature, the mice were incubated in a 37°C chamber. The mice were exposed to room air. Most mice exhibited redness and normal breathing. At this time, we set the time to zero and then observed the phenotypes of these pups for 100 min. *Snx5*$^{+/+}$ and *Snx5*$^{+/-}$ mice showed less than 10% mortality over the duration of the study, exhibiting normal breathing through the mouth.

Immunohistochemistry and immunocytochemistry

Sections were deparaffinized, rehydrated, and processed for antigen retrieval with 0.01 M citric acid solution (pH 6.0) for 15 min. Sections were then incubated with 3% H_2O_2 in methanol for 15 min to quench endogenous peroxidase activity. After blocking with blocking solution (5% horse serum, 3% bovine serum albumin, 0.1% Triton X-100 in PBS), the slides were incubated with primary antibodies in blocking solution overnight at 4°C. Antibodies used for immunohistochemistry were as follows: hamster anti-T1α (1:100, Developmental Studies Hybridoma Bank), rabbit anti-pro-SP-C (1:2000, Chemicon), goat anti-CC-10 (1:2000, Santa Cruz Biotechnology), mouse anti-α-SMA (1:500, Santa Cruz Biotechnology), rabbit anti-Ki67 (1:500, Novo Castra), and goat anti-Pecam-1 (1:100, Santa Cruz Biotechnology). The slides were washed with PBS and then incubated with Alexa 594 goat anti-rabbit IgG at a 1:200 dilution, Alexa 488 goat anti-rabbit IgG at a 1:200 dilution, Alexa 488 goat anti-mouse IgG at a 1:200 dilution, Alexa 594 goat anti-mouse IgG at a 1:200 dilution, Alexa 594 donkey anti-goat IgG at a 1:200 dilution, Alexa 488 goat anti-hamster IgG at a 1:200 dilution (Invitrogen), or reagents from a Vectastain Elite ABC kit (Vector Laboratories) for secondary detection. Immunocytochemistry was performed in *Snx5* MEF cell lines and PLEs. MEFs on gelatin-coated cover glass and PLEs on type I-coated cover glass were fixed in 4% PFA for 15 min on ice and then washed with 0.1% Triton X-100 in PBS. The samples were incubated with primary rabbit anti CI-MPR (1:100, Abcam), hamster anti-T1α (1:100, Developmental Studies Hybridoma Bank), or rabbit anti-pro-SP-C (1:2000, Chemicon) antibodies for 2 h at room temperature followed by incubation with secondary antibodies, i.e., AlexaFluor 594 goat anti-rabbit IgG (1:200, Invitrogen) and Alexa 488 goat anti-hamster IgG, for 1 h at room temperature. The cover glasses were mounted with Vectashield Mounting Medium with DAPI (VECTOR, H-1200). Images were obtained using an Axio Imager A2 microscope (Carl Zeiss, Germany) and Olympus software (Olympus micro DP71/DP70/DP30 BW Ver.03.03).

Transmission electron microscopy (TEM)

To examine the ultrastructure of E18.5 lung morphology, E18.5 lungs were collected and fixed in modified Karnovsky's fixative overnight at 4°C. Fixed tissues were washed 3 times with 0.05 M sodium cacodylate buffer (pH 7.2) and postfixed with 1% osmium tetroxide in 0.05 M sodium cacodylate buffer for 2 h. Tissues were dehydrated in graded ethanol solutions and propylene oxide and then embedded in Spurr's resin. Ultrathin sections were stained with uranyl acetate and Reynold's lead citrate. The sections were imaged with a LIBRA 120 TEM (Carl Zeiss, Germany).

Microarray analysis

Expression profiles of *Snx5*$^{+/+}$ and *Snx5*$^{-/-}$ in E18.5 mouse lungs were generated using an Illumina microarray system (Illumine Beadchip Array MouseRef-8 v2), which includes 25,697 probes corresponding to 17,214 annotated genes. Total RNA was isolated from *Snx5*$^{+/+}$ and *Snx5*$^{-/-}$ lungs using the RNeasy MiniKit (Qiagen). RNA integrity numbers (RIN) ranged from 9.3 to 9.7 when analyzed using an Agilent 2100 Bioanalyzer. RNA was reverse transcribed and amplified using Illumina Total Prep RNA amplification kit (Ambion). *In vitro* transcription was then carried out to prepare cRNA. The cRNAs were hybridized to the array and then labeled with Cy3-streptavidin (Amersham Bioscience). The fluorescent signal on the array was measured using a BeadStation 500 System (Illumina). In this study, two biological replicates of *Snx5*$^{+/+}$ and *Snx5*$^{-/-}$ lungs were analyzed. The microarray data used in this study were deposited in the GEO database (GSE37080).

Statistical analysis of gene expression data

The probe intensities from the arrays were converted to log2 intensities. The log2 intensities were then normalized using a quantile normalization method [41]. The probes were annotated using (GPL6885.annot). A gene was considered "expressed" if the probe intensity of the gene was larger than a cutoff intensity in at least one condition. The cutoff intensity (in this study, intensity = 8) was determined by mixture modeling using 2 Gaussian distributions, one for the "absent" probes and the one for the "present" (expressed) probes [42] . To identify differentially-expressed genes (DEGs) by comparing *Snx5*$^{-/-}$ vs. *Snx5*$^{+/+}$ in E18.5 lungs, the following integrative statistical hypothesis-testing was performed: (1) Student *t*-test and log2 median ratio test were performed to compute *T*-values and median ratios for all the genes [42,43]; (2) *P*-values from each test were computed using an empirical distribution of the null hypothesis (that the means of the genes were not different), which was obtained from random permutations of the samples; (3) the individual *P*-values were combined to compute the false discovery rate (FDR) using Stouffer's method [43]; and (4) the DEGs were selected as the genes with an FDR of less than 0.05 and log2-fold change larger than the cutoff of 0.3531 (1.27-fold change at the original scale). This fold-change cutoff value corresponded to the 95th percentile of the fold changes obtained from random permutation experiments using 2-tailed settings. Finally, functional enrichment analysis of DEGs was performed using DAVID software to identify cellular processes overrepresented by the DEGs governed by *Snx5*.

Statistics

In this study, all quantitative graphs are expressed as means ± standard deviations (SDs). *P*-values were calculated by Student's *t*-tests. A *P*-values ≤ 0.05 was considered statistically significant.

Results

Generation of *Snx5*$^{-/-}$ mice and expression of *Snx5*

To determine the physiological role of *Snx5*, we generated *Snx5* heterozygous mice (*Snx5*$^{+/-}$) using the gene-trapped ES cell line XA155, containing a β-galactosidase-neomycin cassette (β-geo) between exons 7 and 8 (Figure 1A). Germline transmission of the trapped allele was confirmed by Southern blot analysis with an *Snx5*-specific probe (Figure S1A). Inactivation of the *Snx5* gene was confirmed by genomic DNA PCR (Figure S1B), RT-PCR (Figure S1C), and western blotting (Figure S1D). Through β-galactosidase staining of *Snx5*$^{+/-}$ mice expressing the β-galactosidase gene, we examined the expression patterns of *Snx5*. β-galactosidase staining of E11.5 *Snx5*$^{+/-}$ tissues (Figure 1B) and adult tissues (data not shown) revealed ubiquitous expression of *Snx5*. Western blot analysis of adult tissues from *Snx5*$^{+/+}$ mice also showed that *Snx5* was expressed in various adult tissues (Figure 1C), suggesting that *Snx5* may play a role in embryonic and adult developmental stages in various tissues.

Perinatal lethality and respiratory failure in *Snx5*$^{-/-}$ mice

Examination of the survivability of *Snx5*$^{-/-}$ mice showed that 40% of mutant mice died at birth. Until E17.5, embryos from *Snx5*$^{+/-}$ intercrosses showed the expected Mendelian ratio. However, at E18.5, *Snx5*$^{-/-}$ embryos were born at a frequency of 19.4%, lower than the expected Mendelian ratio of 25% (Table 1).

Interestingly, 40% of *Snx5*$^{-/-}$ mice died within 24 h of birth (Figures 1D and 2D) and an additional 20% of *Snx5*$^{-/-}$ mice died within a month of birth (Figure 1D). The surviving *Snx5*$^{-/-}$ mice had a smaller body size compared to that of *Snx5*$^{+/-}$ and *Snx5*$^{+/+}$mice after birth (Figure S1E and F). Newborn *Snx5*$^{+/+}$ and *Snx5*$^{+/-}$ mice were pink and exhibited a normal suckling reflex and well-inflated lungs (Figure 2A–C). However, most *Snx5*$^{-/-}$ mice were cyanotic (Figure 2D and G) and had condensed lungs (Figure 2E and F), although some *Snx5*$^{-/-}$ lungs were partially inflated with air at birth (Figure 2H and I). These results suggested that *Snx5*$^{-/-}$ mice may experience respiratory failure at birth.

Table 1. Embryonic survival frequency of *Snx5*$^{+/+}$, *Snx5*$^{+/-}$ and *Snx5*$^{-/-}$ littermates.

	Genotype n (%)			
Age of embryos (day)	*Snx5*$^{+/+}$	*Snx5*$^{+/-}$	*Snx5*$^{-/-}$	*Total n*
E14.5 ~ E16.5	33 (20.3)	88(54.3)	41(25.3)	162
E17.5	18(23.3)	38(49.3)	21(27.2)	77
E18.5	124(30.2)	207(50.3)	80(19.4)*	411

Embryos from timed matings were genotyped on embryonic day 14.5~16.5, 17.5 and 18.5 day. Fourth columm shows the observed percentage of Snx5-/- mice (the Mendelian percentage is 25%).
*Caculated using χ^2 test comparing the expected and observed frequency of viable *Snx5*$^{-/-}$ mice. *(P = 0.0089)*

In order to investigate the causes of respiratory failure in *Snx5*$^{-/-}$ mice, we examined the palate, trachea, esophagus, diaphragm, intercostal muscles, and heart. In *Snx5*$^{-/-}$ mice, the palate was closed well (Figure S2A and B), and the structures of the trachea and esophagus were formed and separated properly (Figure 2C–F and 2K and L). The structure of the tracheal cartilage ring was also properly formed in mutant mice (Figure S2M and N). Histological analysis of other respiratory organs, such as the diaphragm (Figure S2G and H) and intercostal muscles (Figure S2I and J) of *Snx5*$^{-/-}$ mice showed well-formed morphologies. In addition, the heart showed the normal morphological structure in *Snx5*$^{-/-}$ mice (Figure S2O and P). Collectively, these results suggested that the respiratory failure of *Snx5*$^{-/-}$ mice was not due to malformations of the palate, trachea, esophagus, diaphragm, intercostal muscles, or heart.

Impaired alveolar formation in *Snx5*$^{-/-}$ mice

Considering that the structures of palate, trachea, esophagus, diaphragm, intercostal muscles, and heart were intact, we hypothesized that the respiratory failure observed in these mice could be due to defects in lung development. To test this possibility, we performed an air-breathing test after caesarean section at E18.5. After removing the pups from their mother, we measured the time until death from the point the pup began normal breathing in a 37°C chamber, intended to help the mouse maintain body temperature. While *Snx5*$^{+/+}$ and *Snx5*$^{+/-}$ mice survived after beginning to breathe, approximately 60% of mutant mice died within 1 h (Figure 3A and B). Moreover, while the body weights of *Snx5*$^{-/-}$ mice was similar to those of control mice at E18.5, lung weights and lung-to-body weight ratios of *Snx5*$^{-/-}$ mice were slightly lower than those of *Snx5*$^{+/+}$ and *Snx5*$^{+/-}$ mice (Figure 3C). Together with the results of the air-breathing test, these data suggested that lung defects in *Snx5*$^{-/-}$ mice could lead to the observed high mortality rate at birth.

Next, in order to investigate whether *Snx5* was expressed in the lung, we performed β-galactosidase staining on E18.5 *Snx5*$^{+/-}$ lungs. As expected, *Snx5* was expressed throughout the lung (Figure 4A), suggesting that *Snx5* may play a role in lung development. In addition, hematoxylin and eosin staining revealed that *Snx5*$^{-/-}$ lungs had thickened alveolar walls and reduced air space in the alveolar sacs at E18.5. Alveolar walls and air space were normal in E14.5 and E16.5 lungs (Figure 4B), suggesting that *Snx5* was required for alveolar formation in the saccular phase of lung development.

To examine whether the observed impaired alveolar formation was due to defective differentiation of pulmonary epithelial cells or

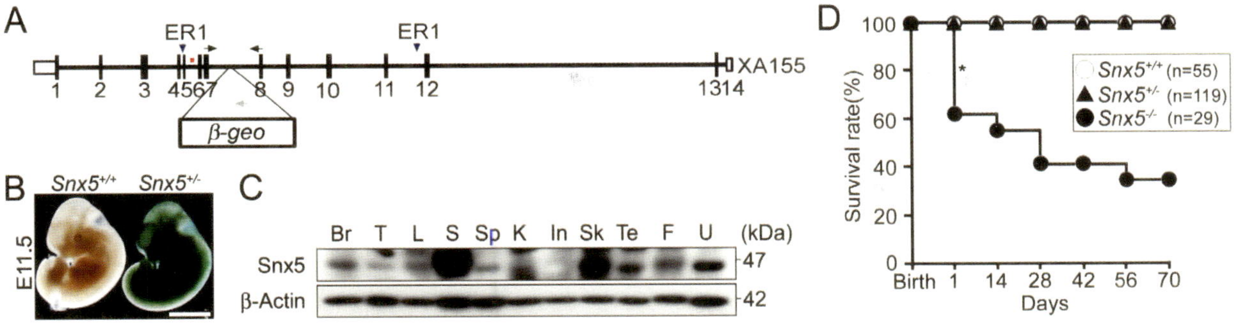

Figure 1. Generation of *Snx5*-deficient mice. (A) Schematic drawing of the *Snx5* gene-trapped (XA155) allele. Arrows indicate the genotyping primers, and the 2 arrowheads indicate the ER1 (*Eco*RI) digestion sites. The red bar represents the probe for Southern blotting. (B) Whole-embryo X-gal staining at E11.5. Scale bars: 2.5 mm. (C) Western blot analysis of the indicated mouse tissues (Br, brain; T, thymus; L, lung; S, stomach; Sp, spleen; K, kidney; In, intestine; Sk. skin; Te, testis; F, fat; U, uterus). (D) Survival rate of mice after birth. The asterisk shows the dramatic mortality observed in the neonatal stage.

defective vascular formation, we performed immunohistochemistry with specific antibodies against alveolar epithelial type II cells (proSP-C), Clara cells (CC-10), smooth muscle cells (α-SMA), and blood vessels (Pecam-1). In E18.5 *Snx5*$^{-/-}$ mice, proSP-C-expressing cells were similar to those of controls (Figure 5A and B). Western blot analysis also showed similar levels of proSP-C in *Snx5*$^{-/-}$ lungs (Figure 5I). The expression of CC-10 in mutant bronchioles was comparable to that of *Snx*$^{+/+}$ mice (Figure 5C and D), suggesting that proximal lung development was intact in mutant mice. In addition, immunohistochemical staining of α-SMA and Pecam-1 did not show significant differences between *Snx5*$^{+/+}$ and *Snx5*$^{-/-}$ lungs (Figure 5E–H and J), indicating that the terminal vascular architecture was intact in the mutant lungs. Furthermore, we also investigated whether thickened alveolar septa were correlated with increased proliferative cells in *Snx5*$^{-/-}$ lungs. At E18.5, Ki67 staining of the *Snx5*$^{-/-}$ lungs showed similar amounts of proliferating cells relative to controls (Figure S3A and B), indicating that the thickened alveolar septa of *Snx5*$^{-/-}$ lungs were not caused by increased proliferation of epithelial cells.

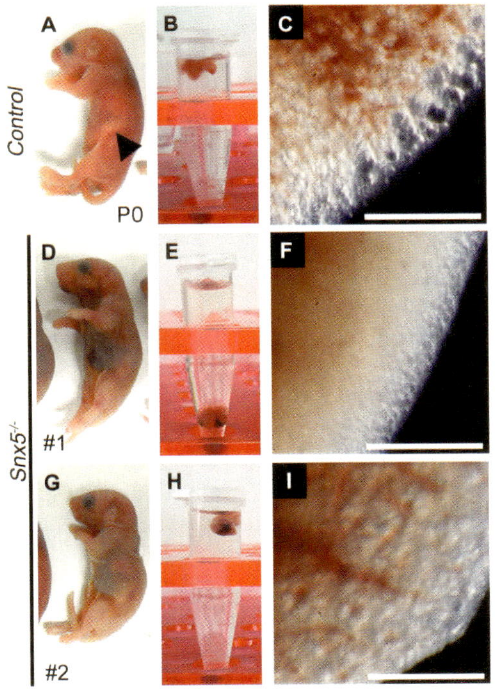

Figure 2. Perinatal lethality in *Snx5*$^{-/-}$ mice. (A, D, G) Appearance of neonates after birth. The arrowhead indicates milk in the stomach. (B, E, H) Floating assay of the lungs. (C, F, I) Appearance of the lungs. Control lungs show the inflated morphology (C). *Snx5*$^{-/-}$ lungs lack inflated morphology (F) or show partially inflated morphology (I). Scale bars: 0.5 mm.

Most lung atelectasis is caused by defective maturation of alveolar epithelial type II cells [44]. Mature alveolar epithelial type II cells secrete surfactants that reduce pulmonary surface tension and prevent atelectasis at the end of expiration [45]. These surfactants are composed of a complex mixture of proteins and lipids. To investigate whether the impaired alveolar formation was due to a maturation defect of alveolar epithelial type II cells, we compared the expression levels of surfactant proteins and lipids in *Snx5*$^{+/+}$ and *Snx5*$^{-/-}$ lungs. Alveolar epithelial type II cells expressed the surfactant proteins SP-A, -B, -C, and -D. qRT-PCR analysis showed that the mRNA expression levels of these surfactant proteins were not significantly different between *Snx5*$^{+/+}$ and *Snx5*$^{-/-}$ lungs (Figure 5K). The amount of SP-B in 15 μL of supernatant from lung homogenates (total volume 2 mL) was analyzed by western blotting (Figure S4A and B). SP-B protein/lung weight ratios were not altered by deletion of *Snx5* (Figure 5L). Levels of Sat PC, the most abundant component of surfactant lipids, were slightly lower in *Snx5*$^{-/-}$ lungs than in *Snx5*$^{+/-}$ lungs (Figure S4C). However, Sat PC content relative to lung weight was similar between groups (Figure 5M). Likewise, ultrastructure analysis by TEM revealed that *Snx5*$^{-/-}$ lungs had normal alveolar epithelial type II cells with compacted, well-organized lamellar bodies and had secreted surfactants in the alveolar air-space (Figure 5N). Taken together, it can be concluded that deletion of *Snx5* does not appear to affect the maturation of alveolar epithelial type II cells.

Impaired differentiation of alveolar epithelial type I cells in *Snx5*$^{-/-}$ lungs

In order to further investigate the causes of respiratory failure in the *Snx5*$^{-/-}$ mice, we examined whether the differentiation of alveolar epithelial type I cells was intact. Immunohistochemical analysis of T1α, a marker of typical alveolar epithelial type I cells, revealed that the expression of T1α was markedly decreased in *Snx5*$^{-/-}$ lungs, whereas T1α expression extended along the alveolar wall in control lungs (Figure 6A). Consistently, the expression levels of T1α in lung lysates from E18.5 *Snx5*$^{-/-}$ mice were dramatically decreased compared to those of controls (Figure 6B).

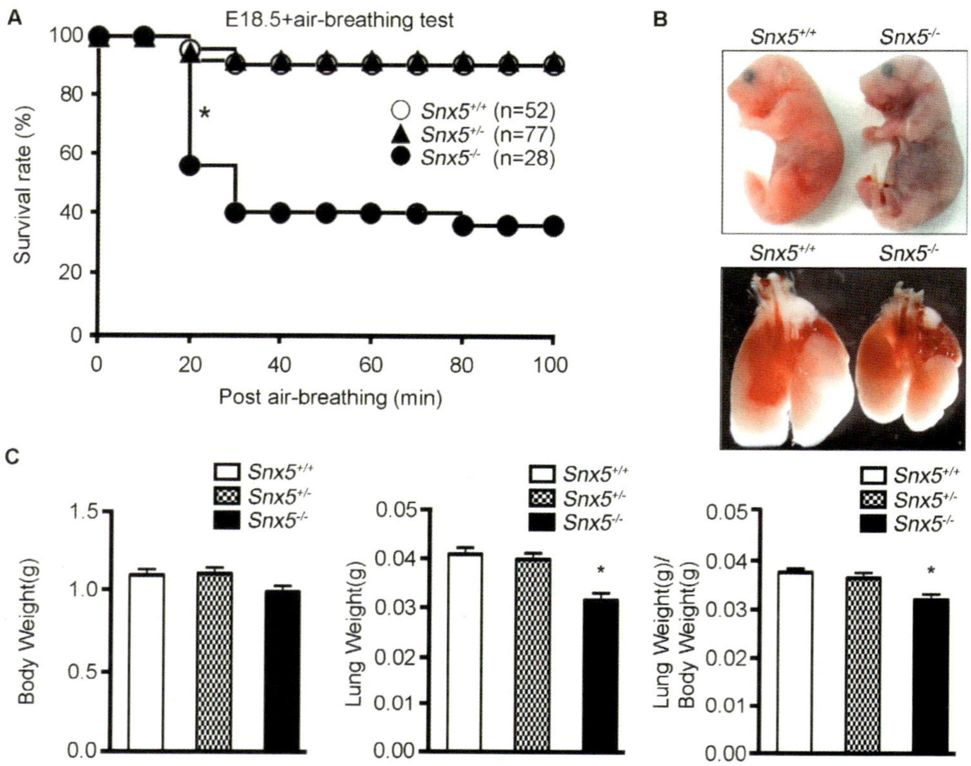

Figure 3. Respiratory failure in *Snx5*$^{-/-}$ mice. (A) Survival after air-breathing tests in *Snx5*$^{+/+}$, *Snx5*$^{+/-}$, and *Snx5*$^{-/-}$ mice. Within 30 min, nearly 60% of *Snx5*$^{-/-}$ mice had died (asterisk). (B) Appearance after air-breathing tests in E18.5 mice. Cyanotic appearance and condensed lungs in *Snx5*$^{-/-}$ mice. (C) Body and lung weights of *Snx5*$^{+/+}$, *Snx5*$^{+/-}$, and *Snx5*$^{-/-}$ mice. Lung weight and lung to body weight ratios of *Snx5*$^{-/-}$ mice were decreased by 22.9% and 14.9%, respectively, relative to *Snx5*$^{+/+}$ mice. **P* < 0.0001; data represent *Snx5*$^{+/+}$, n = 24; *Snx5*$^{+/-}$, n = 27; and *Snx5*$^{-/-}$ mice, n = 17.

Additionally, the typical markers for distal alveolar epithelial type I cells, such as T1α, AQP5, and RAGE were examined [46]. Indeed, the mRNA expression levels of *T1α*, *Aqp5*, and *Rage* were significantly decreased in E18.5 *Snx5*$^{-/-}$ lungs compared to those of controls (Figure 6C). Thus, we hypothesize that loss of *Snx5* leads to impaired differentiation of alveolar epithelial type I cells.

Reduced mRNA expression of T1α in *Snx5*$^{-/-}$ lungs was evident from E14.5 (Figure 6D). Next, we examined the expression levels

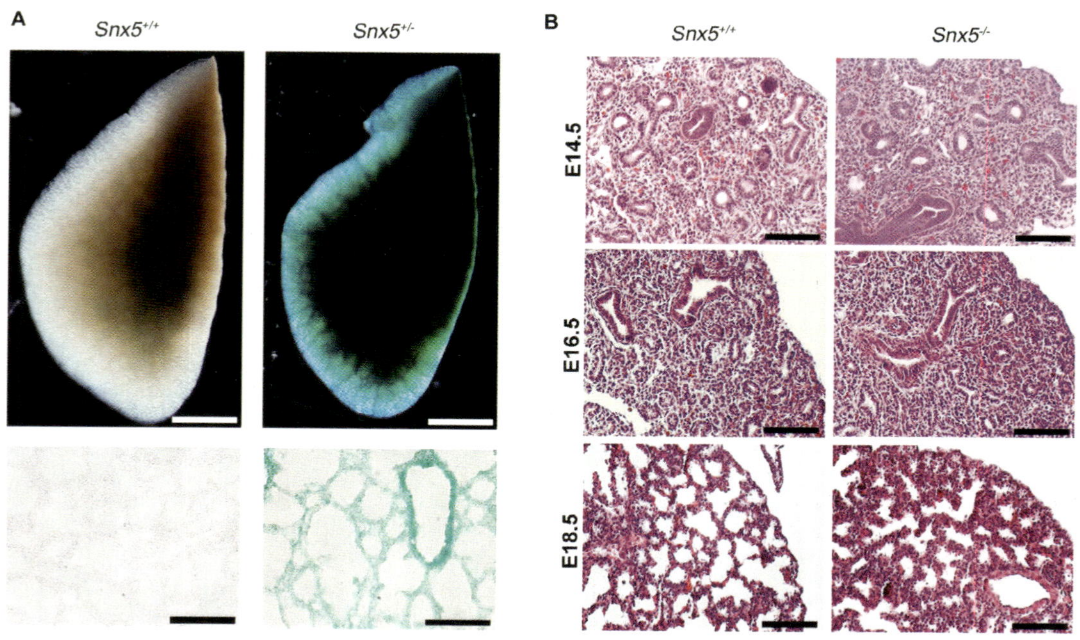

Figure 4. Expression of *Snx5* and morphological malformations in *Snx5*-deficient mice at E18.5. (A) Whole and sectional X-gal staining of E18.5 lungs. The *Snx5- βgeo* reporter gene was expressed ubiquitously in *Snx5*$^{+/-}$ lungs. Scale bars: 1 mm, 100 μm. (B) H&E staining of E14.5, E16.5, and E18.5 *Snx5*$^{+/+}$ and *Snx5*$^{-/-}$ lungs. *Snx5*$^{-/-}$ lungs exhibited thickening of the alveolar walls and reduced alveolar space at E18.5. Scale bar: 50 μm.

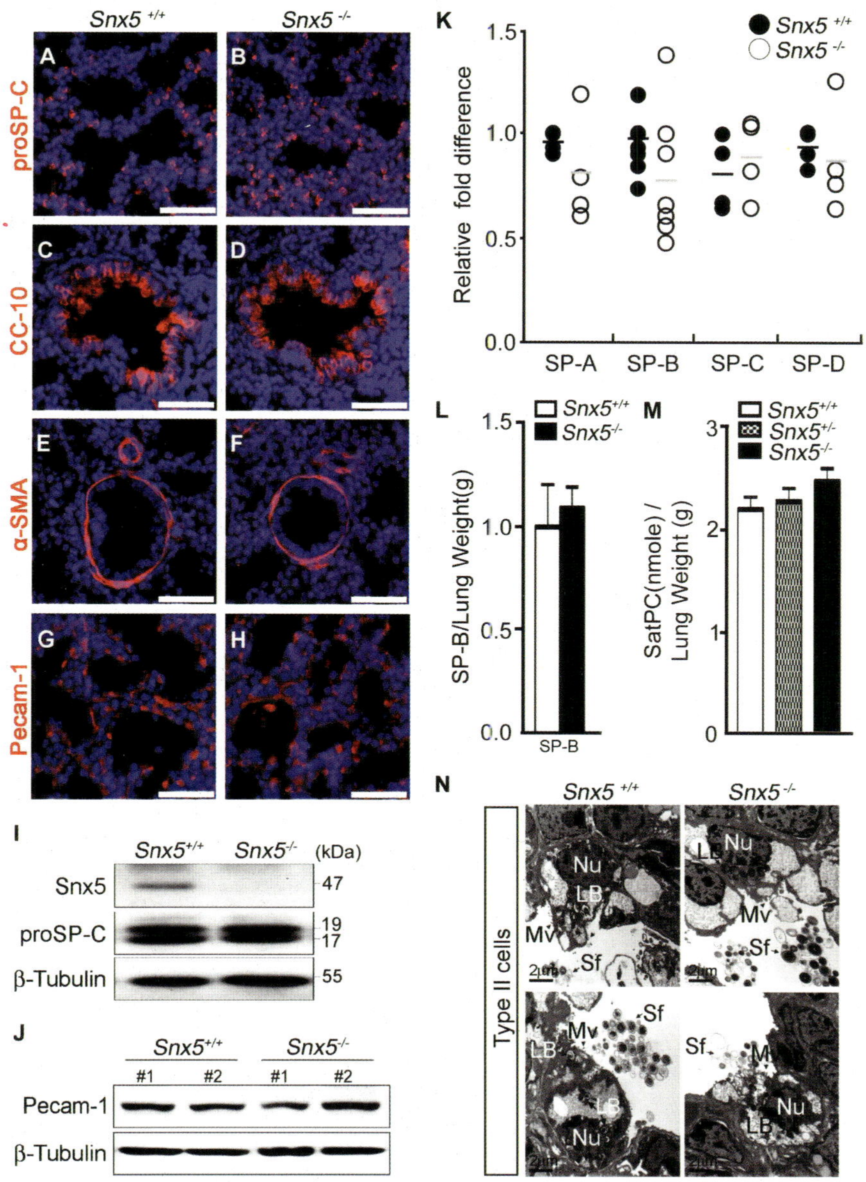

Figure 5. *Snx5* was not required for maturation of alveolar epithelial type II cells. (A–H) Immunohistochemical analysis of proSP-C, CC-10, α-SMA, and Pecam-1 in sections from *Snx5*$^{+/+}$ and *Snx5*$^{-/-}$ lungs (n = 5). Scale bars: 50 µm. (A and B) proSP-C, a marker of surfactant protein C precursor in alveolar epithelial type II cells; (C and D) CC-10, a marker of Clara cells; (E and F) α-SMA, a marker of smooth muscle cells; and (G and H) Pecam-1, a marker of blood vessels, showed similar expression levels. The nuclei were stained with Hoechst. (I and J) Western blot analysis of proSP-C (I, n = 5) and Pecam-1 (J, n = 2) proteins in E18.5 *Snx5*$^{+/+}$ and *Snx5*$^{-/-}$ lung whole lysates. (K) qRT-PCR analysis of surfactant proteins (SP-A, -B, -C, and -D) performed on RNA samples collected from total lungs (n ≥ 3). Similar expression levels of surfactants were seen. (L) Mature SP-B did not differ in *Snx5*$^{-/-}$ lungs (n = 5). (M) Sat PC were similar between *Snx5*$^{+/+}$, *Snx5*$^{+/-}$, and *Snx5*$^{-/-}$ mice (n = 6). (N) Transmission electron microscopy (TEM) of distal alveolar epithelial type II cells at E18.5. Apical microvilli (Mv; arrowhead), condensed lamellar bodies (LB), and secreted surfactants (Sf; arrow) were observed in *Snx5*$^{-/-}$ lungs. Scale bars: 2 µm.

of lectin, galactoside-binding, soluble, 3 binding protein (Lgals3bp) and indolethylamine *N*-methyltransferase (Inmt), which have been shown to be reduced in a defective type I epithelial cell-associated mouse model, SMRT^{mRID} mice [15]. Pei and colleagues reported that differentiation-defect of type I pneumocytes promoted respiratory distress syndrome at perinatal stages. In this paper, genome-wide analysis of mutant mice showed that several genes involved in Lgals3bp and Inmt signaling were reduced in mutant mice. To determine whether decreased T1α affected the expression of these genes, we performed qRT-PCR. We observed that *Lgals3bp* and *Inmt* transcripts were significantly reduced in *Snx5*$^{-/-}$ lungs (Figure 6E). Next, to further investigate the morphological differentiation of alveolar epithelial type I cells, we performed the ultrastructure analysis by using TEM. Although *Snx5*$^{-/-}$ lungs showed a less alveolar epithelial type I cells compared to *Snx5*$^{+/+}$ lungs (data not shown), The alveolar epithelial type I cells of *Snx5*$^{-/-}$ lungs represented slightly thicker nucleus and cytoplasm (Figure S5B and D) compared to *Snx5*$^{+/+}$ lungs (Figure S5A and C). However organelles enriched in alveolar epithelial type I cells, such as mitochondria (Figure S5A and B ; white arrowhead) and vesicles (Figure S5A and B ; black arrow), existed well in *Snx5*$^{-/-}$ lungs (Figure S5B). Also, extended cytoplasms were

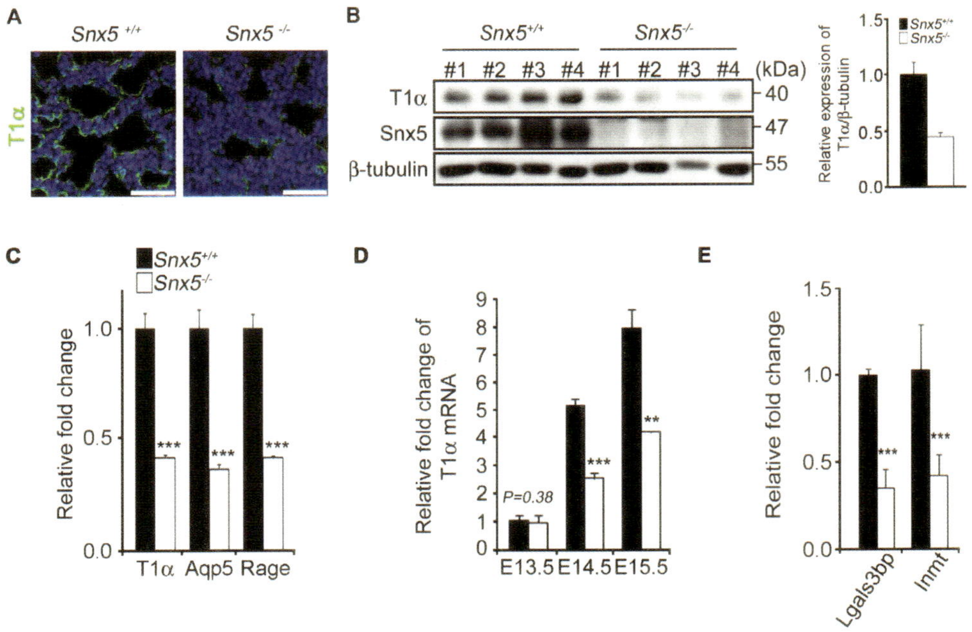

Figure 6. Impaired differentiation of alveolar epithelial type I cells in E18.5 *Snx5*$^{-/-}$ lungs. (A) Immunohistochemical analysis of T1α at E18.5. T1α, a marker of alveolar epithelial type I cells, was significantly decreased in *Snx5*$^{-/-}$ compared to *Snx5*$^{+/+}$ lung (n = 5). The nuclei were stained with Hoechst. Scale bars: 50 μm. (B) Decreased protein expression of T1α in E18.5 (n = 4). Densitometric analysis showed that average expression levels of T1α in *Snx5*$^{-/-}$ lungs were reduced compared to those in *Snx5*$^{+/+}$ lungs. (C–E) qRT-PCR analysis of type I cell-related genes from lung tissue. (C) Markers of alveolar epithelial type I cells, i.e., *T1α*, *Aqp5*, and *Rage*, were decreased in *Snx5*$^{-/-}$ lungs (n ≥ 3). (D) *T1α* mRNA during the embryonic stage. From E14.5, mRNA expression of *T1α* was decreased. (E) Decreased expression levels of *Lgals3bp* and *Inmt* (n ≥ 3). **, $P < 0.01$, ***, $P < 0.001$ using the Student's *t*-test.

observed in both groups (Figure S5C and D). It seems that there were no obvious differences in ultrastructural morphologies of alveolar epithelial type I cells. From these data, we concluded that *Snx5* was required for proper differentiation of alveolar epithelial type I cells.

Snx5 as a novel mediator required for differentiation of alveolar epithelial type I cells

Snx5 has been implicated in endosomal trafficking of EGFR and CI-MPR [18,19,20,47]. In order to investigate whether impaired differentiation of alveolar epithelial type I cells in *Snx5*$^{-/-}$ lungs was due to defective endosomal trafficking of EGFR, we examined EGFR signaling after EGF stimulation in *Snx5*$^{-/-}$ MEFs and isolated PLEs (Figure S6A-C). Expression levels of EGFR were comparable between *Snx5*$^{+/+}$ and *Snx5*$^{-/-}$ MEFs (data not shown). To further investigate the EGFR signaling, the downstream signaling molecules were measured by using immunoblot in EGF stimulated *Snx5*$^{+/+}$ and *Snx5*$^{-/-}$ MEFs. Phosphorylation of Akt and Erk1/2, the key effectors of EGFR signaling, was comparable between *Snx5*$^{+/+}$ and *Snx5*$^{-/-}$ MEFs in response to EGF treatment (Figure 7A and C). In addition, after long-term exposure to EGF, there was no difference in the downregulation of EGFR (Figure 7B and D). The *Snx5* deletion did not affect the endosomal signaling and degradation of EGFR in MEFs and PLEs and the expression levels of EGFR in the E18.5 *Snx5*$^{-/-}$ lungs were also similar between two groups (Figure S7A and B).

Next, we examined whether endosome-to-TGN retrieval of CI-MPR was affected by disruption of *Snx5*. CI-MPR has been reported to be a major retromer component in retrograde endosome-to-TGN transport [24]. Knockdown of *Snx5* using small interfering RNA inhibits trafficking of CI-MPR from endosomes to the TGN, resulting in increased degradation of CI-MPR [20,48]. To establish whether the local alteration of CI-MPR resulted from Snx5 depletion, we performed immunocytochemistry analysis of CI-MPR (Figure 7E). Additionally, to determine CI-MPR stability in *Snx5*$^{-/-}$ MEFs, we examined the degradation rate of CI-MPR (Figure 7F). Because the biosynthetic rate of CI-MPR protein varies in efficiency, we treated cells with 40 μg/mL CHX for 17 h to compare the degradation ratio of CI-MPR in *Snx5*$^{+/+}$ and *Snx5*$^{-/-}$ MEFs. Unexpectedly, however, when we examined the localization and stability of CI-MPR in *Snx5*$^{-/-}$ MEFs, there was no significant alteration in *Snx5*$^{-/-}$ MEFs compared to *Snx5*$^{+/+}$ MEFs (Figure 7E and F). This finding suggests that the loss of *Snx5* alone in a retromer complex does not affect the localization and lysosomal degradation of CI-MPR in MEFs.

No studies have reported the correlation between Snx5 and the differentiation of alveolar epithelial type I cells. Since there was no clear molecular explanation for the defective differentiation of alveolar epithelial type I cells in *Snx5*$^{-/-}$ mice, a genome-wide cRNA microarray analysis using the RNA isolated from E18.5 *Snx5*$^{+/+}$ and *Snx5*$^{-/-}$ lungs was performed. Microarray analysis data using an Agilent 2100 Bioanalyzer [49] revealed the decreased expression of more than 60 genes in *Snx5*$^{-/-}$ lungs compared to *Snx5*$^{+/+}$ lungs (data not shown). The altered genes were members of several functional categories, including genes for pulmonary epithelial cell markers, development, maturation, regulation of endocytosis and transport, serine/threonine kinases, enzyme-linked receptor signaling pathways, cell adhesion, and cell migration. Among these downregulated genes, we found that expression of the alveolar epithelial type I cell markers *T1α*, *Aqp5*, and *Rage* was significantly decreased (data not shown). In addition, several genes involved in ribosome biogenesis, RNA processing, translation and oxidative phosphorylation exhibited upregulated

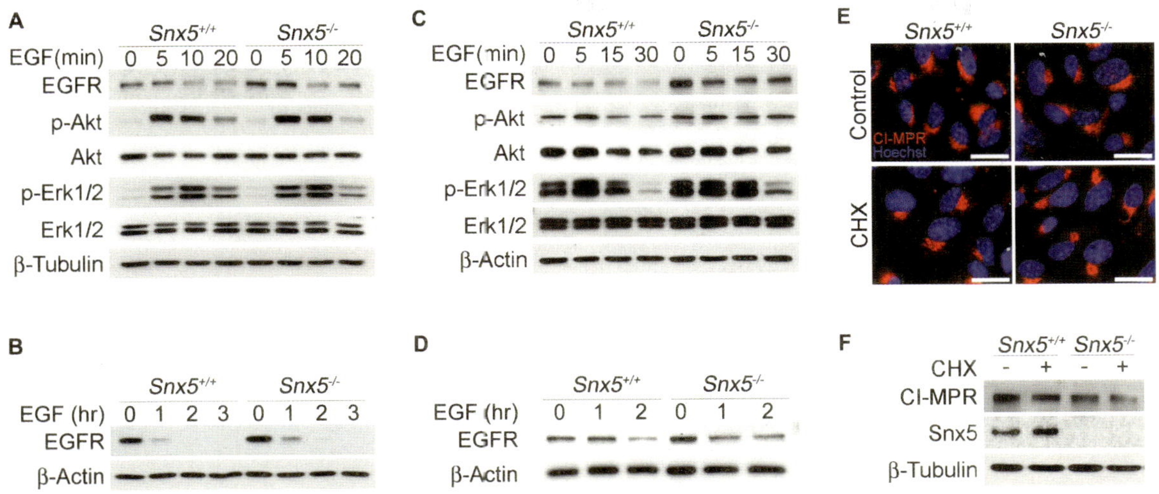

Figure 7. Regulation of EGFR signaling and CI-MPR trafficking were not altered in *Snx5*-deficient MEFs. (A–D, F) Western blotting of EGFR and CI-MPR. (A and C) Signaling downstream of EGFR and (B and D) degradation of EGFR were not altered in primary *Snx5*$^{-/-}$ MEFs (A and B) and primary lung epithelial cells (PLEs) (C and D). (E) Immunocytochemical analysis of CI-MPR. Localization of CI-MPR was not changed in *Snx5*-deficient MEFs. (F) Relative degradation ratios of CI-MPR protein in *Snx5*$^{+/+}$ and *Snx5*$^{-/-}$ MEFs.

expression (Table S1). However, from microarray analysis data and qRT-PCR, we concluded that there was no significant difference in Notch signaling-related genes, such as *Hes1*, *Hes5*, *Hey1*, *Hey2*, and *HeyL*, between groups (data not shown). Thus, these data raise the possibility that *Snx5* may be involved in other signaling pathways in addition to the Mib1-Notch signaling pathway. To address this question, we performed a literature search for previous studies on Snx5. Recently, Fei et al. reported that defective differentiation of alveolar epithelial type I cells led to a respiratory distress syndrome-like phenotype in SMRT mutant mice and that 21 genes, including *Klf2*, *Lgals3bp*, *Klf4*, *Inmt*, *Zfp36*, and *Dusp1*, were significantly decreased [15]. Interestingly, when we examined the expression levels of these genes in *Snx5*$^{-/-}$ lungs, we also found that these genes were significantly downregulated (data not shown). Taken together, although more molecular studies on Snx5 are required to determine the precise role of this protein in lung development, these finding suggest that *Snx5* could be a novel mediator for proper differentiation of alveolar epithelial type I cells.

Discussion

Here, we report that *Snx5* is necessary for the differentiation of alveolar epithelial type I cells. Targeted inactivation of the *Snx5* gene led to neonatal mortality caused by respiratory failure, in which differentiation of alveolar epithelial type I cells was impaired, while maturation of alveolar epithelial type II cells was intact. Although SNX5 has been posited to interact with Mib-1, an E3 ubiquitin ligase that regulates the activation of Notch signaling, it is unlikely that these defects are caused by Mib1-Notch signaling. In addition, other related molecules, EGFR and CI-MPR, were not affected by Snx5 depletion Collectively, our data reveal an essential role of Snx5 in the differentiation of alveolar epithelial type I cells.

Maturation defects of alveolar epithelial cells can cause neonatal respiratory failure. Thus far, various factors, such as C/EBPα, co-activator-associated arginine methyltransferase 1 (CARM1), Erk3, Foxa2, Foxm1, Fstl1, Mig6, and Pdpn (T1α), have been implicated in alveolar formation at the saccular stage of lung development. Disruption of these factors can lead to perinatal lethality caused by a respiratory distress syndrome (RDS)-like phenotype, which includes pulmonary atelectasis. This phenotype is largely caused by the excessive proliferation of immature alveolar epithelial type II cells [17,35,39,50,51,52,53]. In contrast, *Snx5*$^{-/-}$ lungs did not show a significant difference in cellular proliferation (Figure S3A and B), although cellularity was slightly increased. In addition, there were no significant differences between *Snx5*$^{+/+}$ lungs and *Snx5*$^{-/-}$ lungs in the production of surfactant proteins and Sat PC. Moreover, *Snx5*$^{-/-}$ lungs had normal alveolar epithelial type II cells with compacted, well-organized lamellar bodies and secreted surfactants in the alveolar air-space. This suggests that deletion of *Snx5* did not affect the maturation of alveolar epithelial type II cells and that the respiratory failure in the *Snx5*$^{-/-}$ mice was not due to functional defects of alveolar epithelial type II cells. However, *Snx5*$^{-/-}$ lung showed a significantly reduced expression of alveolar epithelial type I cell markers. Through these phenotypes, we could suggest that intact alveolar epithelial type II cells may reduce the severity of lung defects in *Snx5*$^{-/-}$ lung.

In present study, *Snx5*$^{-/-}$ mice showed the variability in survival rates. To determine whether leaky expression of *Snx5* could affect a different survival rates, we investigated the expression level of *Snx5* gene. In addition, we observed surviving and non-surviving *Snx5*$^{-/-}$ mice at birth and checked the expression levels of alveolar epithelial cell markers. Although we could not observed the differences between survivors and non-survivors, all mutant mice showed reduced expression of type I epithelial cell markers ; T1α, AQP5 and Rage (data not shown). So far, we did not define other causes of perinatal mortality in this study, we could suggest that the survivor mice have other complex compensatory mechanisms. Further studies will be required to address this possibility. In addition, the embryonic studies of *Snx5*$^{-/-}$ mice showed the significantly reduced numbers of mutant embryos at E18.5. Although the causes of embryonic death are ambiguous and need further studies, ubiquitous expressed of Snx5 suggests that Snx5 may play a role in various developmental contexts in embryonic stage.

Previous studies have demonstrated that EGFR-knockout mice exhibit growth retardation and epithelial immaturity, which shows partial similarity to the phenotype of *Snx5*$^{-/-}$ mice. *EGFR*$^{-/-}$ mice can be classified into 3 groups: runted, small-sized, and normal-sized pups [54]. The second group, small-sized pups, were shown to have breathing problems (gasping) and lived for up to 2 days. Dead *EGFR*$^{-/-}$ mice exhibited condensed and immature lung morphologies resembling neonatal respiratory distress syndrome. Although significant differences in EGFR signaling and degradation in MEFs after EGF stimulation were not observed in the current study, *Snx5*$^{-/-}$ and *EGFR*$^{-/-}$ mice display partially similar phenotypes such as lung immaturity, growth retardation and strain-dependent survivability. Although we did not go into details for postnatal phenotypes, we could observe that *Snx5*$^{-/-}$ mice had a longer lifespan and growth inhibition on other genetic background mice (data not shown). The inability to detect prominent differences in EGFR signaling and degradation in *Snx5*$^{-/-}$ MEFs may be due to the presence of a redundant signaling mechanism in MEFs and PLEs or the limited sensitivity of this experiment to detect subtle changes. Nevertheless, phenotypic similarities between *Snx5*$^{-/-}$ and *EGFR*$^{-/-}$ mice suggest that *Snx5* may be involved in EGFR signaling in the differentiation of alveolar epithelial type cells.

Knockdown of *Snx1* using RNA interference (RNAi) has been shown to cause dispersed cytosolic localization and degradation of CI-MPR in HeLa cells [22]. However, *Snx1/2*-deficient MEFs exhibit similar CI-MPR sublocalization and stability compared to wild-type MEFs [55,56]. Similarly, although depletion of *Snx5* and *Snx6* in HeLa cells leads to dispersed CD8-CI-MPR trafficking into early endosomes [20], no significant differences in the localization and degradation of CI-MPR were observed in *Snx5*$^{-/-}$ MEFs in the current study. The lack of consensus in these findings suggests that the retrograde activity of CI-MPR may be regulated in a context-dependent manner in different cells and tissues.

We previously reported that *Snx5* interacts with Mib1, which plays a role in Notch signaling in various contexts of mammalian development [25,26,27,28,29,30]. Snx5 morpholino injection into zebrafish embryos resulted in hematopoietic and blood vessel defects, which could be due to defective Notch signaling [21]. We hypothesized that *Snx5* could play an important role in Notch signaling and that *Snx5*$^{-/-}$ mice would exhibit Notch phenotypes; however, we did not observe Notch phenotypes, such as morphological defects of the somite, brain, vessels, intestines, kidneys, or hematopoietic cells in which Mib1-Notch signaling is required [25,26,27,28,29,30]. When we transplanted fetal liver cells from *Snx5*$^{+/+}$ and *Snx5*$^{-/-}$ mice into lethally irradiated recipient mice, we did not observe any developmental alteration of immune cells, including T and marginal zone B lymphocytes (data not shown) [26,28]. Moreover, in this experiment, E18.5 *Snx5*$^{-/-}$ lungs did not show a significant alteration in Notch signaling-related genes, such as *Hes1*, *Hes5*, *Hey1*, *Hey2*, and *HeyL*, as assessed by qRT-PCR (data not shown). Thus, we conclude that disruption of the *Snx5* gene in lungs does not alter Notch signaling.

In summary, this study demonstrated that deletion of the *Snx5* gene in mice can cause neonatal death, most likely due to saccular immaturity. Snx5 is essential for the differentiation and maturation of distal alveolar epithelial type I cells during lung development. Although the underlying mechanisms of Snx5 in lung development are unknown, it is plausible that Snx5 mediates lung maturity. Future studies of Snx5 with new binding molecules will deepen our understanding of the critical mechanisms involved in mouse lung development and provide new insight into the functions of SNXs in the cellular regulation of endocytic trafficking. Moreover, elucidation of the function of Snx5 in lung development may provide targets for novel therapeutic strategies for the prevention and treatment of respiratory distress syndrome.

Supporting Information

Figure S1 Characterization of *Snx5*-trapped mice. (A) Southern blot analysis of gene-trapped mouse tails. The wild-type (WT) allele (4.2 kb) and the mutant (MT) allele (5.8 kb) were generated by *Eco*R1 restriction enzyme digestion. (B) PCR-based genotype analysis of the progenies of *Snx5* heterozygous crosses. The WT band was detected using W-L (exon7) and W-R (exon7) primers (Figure 1A). The MT band was detected using W-L (exon7) and M-R (β-geo cassette) primers. (C) RT-PCR and (D) western blot of mouse lung tissue. Mouse *Snx5* mRNA and protein were absent in tissue derived from *Snx5*$^{-/-}$ mice. (E) A representative growth retardation phenotype in *Snx5*$^{-/-}$ mice at P30. (F) Graph shows a reduced body weight of *Snx5*$^{-/-}$ mice at P21.

Figure S2 Normal structure of the respiratory organs and heart. (A-J) Hematoxylin and Eosin (H&E) staining of respiratory organs at E18.5. (A and B) Palates, (C–F) morphology of sagittal and transverse sections of the trachea and esophagus, (G and H) diaphragm and (I and J) intercostals muscles showing similar structures in *Snx5*$^{-/-}$ mice and controls. (A and B) Scale bars: 1 mm, (C and D) scale bars: 400 μm, (E and F) scale bars: 200 μm, (G–J) scale bars: 100 μm. (K and L) Light micrograph of the separated trachea and esophagus in E18.5 *Snx5*$^{-/-}$ mice. Scale bars: 1 mm. (M and N) Alcian blue staining of tracheal cartilage at E18.5. Scale bars: 0.5 mm. (O and P) Normal morphological structure of *Snx5*$^{-/-}$ heart compared to controls. (O and P) Scale bars: 1 mm.

Figure S3 Proliferation was not altered in *Snx5*$^{-/-}$ mice. (A) Ki67 and Hoechst double staining of *Snx5*$^{+/+}$ and *Snx5*$^{-/-}$ lungs at E18.5. Scale bars: 50 μm. (B) Graph of Ki67-positive cell counts showed similar proliferation rates in *Snx5*$^{-/-}$ and *Snx5*$^{+/+}$ lungs. Ki67-positive cells were counted in 3 random 400× microscope fields. Means ± SDs were determined using 4 *Snx5*$^{+/+}$ embryos and 7 *Snx5*$^{-/-}$ embryos in each group.

Figure S4 Mature SP-B and lung Sat PC content were not decreased in *Snx5*$^{-/-}$ mice. (A) Relative density of SP-B western blotting was quantified using densitometry (n = 5). (B) Western blotting analysis of mature SP-B in 15 μl lung homogenate supernatant (n = 5). Supernatant was recovered from lung homogenate after centrifugation at 1500xg for 15 min. (C) Lung Sat PC content and Sat PC to body weight levels in *Snx5*$^{+/+}$, *Snx5*$^{+/-}$, and *Snx5*$^{-/-}$ mice (n = 6, $*P < 0.05$).

Figure S5 Ultrastructure of alveolar epithelial type I cells in *Snx5*$^{-/-}$ lungs. (A-D) Transmission electron microscopy (TEM) was used to determine ultrastructural morphology of the alveolar epithelial type I cells in *Snx5*$^{-/-}$ and *Snx5*$^{+/+}$ lungs at E18.5. (A and B) Vesicle (Vs; black arrow) and mitochondria (Mt; white arrowhead) were observed in *Snx5*$^{+/+}$ (A) and *Snx5*$^{-/-}$ (B) lungs. Scale bars: 2 μm. (C and D) Extended cytoplasm was also observed in *Snx5*$^{+/+}$ (C) and *Snx5*$^{-/-}$ (D) mice. Scale bars: 400 nm.

Figure S6 Identification of primary lung epithelial cell (PLE) characteristics. (A) Western blot analysis of lysates (10 μg) from MEFs and isolated PLEs. Isolated PLEs exhibited E-cadherin but not vimentin expression. (B) Mean relative $\log_{10}$ mRNA expression for vimentin, E-cadherin, SP-C, and T1α from MEFs and PLEs using qRT-PCR. Graphs revealed dramatic increases in E-cadherin and SP-C expression in isolated PLEs. Also, T1α was expressed at low levels in PLEs compared to the negative control, MEFs. (C) Bright-field and fluorescence images of PLEs. Bright-field images showed a type II epithelial cell-like morphology. Fluorescence images revealed partial T1α and strong proSP-C expression. Scale bars: 100 μm.

Figure S7 EGFR expression in E18.5 *Snx5*$^{-/-}$ lungs was not altered. (A) Western blotting of EGFR protein in whole-lung lysates from E18.5 *Snx5*$^{+/+}$ and *Snx5*$^{-/-}$ mice (n = 10 each). (B) Densitometric analysis showed that the ratio of EGFR to β-tubulin was similar between E18.5 *Snx5*$^{-/-}$ and *Snx5*$^{+/+}$ lungs.

Table S1 Biological processes enriched with up or down-regulated DEGs of E18.5 *Snx5*$^{-/-}$ lungs. Genome-wide analysis of E18.5 *Snx5*$^{-/-}$ lungs showed the biological processes enriched with up or down-regulated DEGs.

Table S2 Used primers for qRT-PCR in lungs. The qRT-PCR primers for analysis of changed mRNA expression levels in *Snx5*$^{-/-}$ compared to *Snx5*$^{+/+}$ lung.

Acknowledgments

We would like to thank Min Soo Park at Yonsei University College of Medicine and Suk Chul Bae at Chungbuk National University for providing us with antibodies, as well as Dr. Brigid L.M. Hogan at Duke University Medical Center for critical comments.

Author Contributions

Conceived and designed the experiments: SKI YYK. Performed the experiments: SKI HBJ HWJ MI. Analyzed the data: SKI HBJ HWJ DH MI YYK. Contributed reagents/materials/analysis tools: SKI HBJ DH MI YYK. Wrote the paper: SKI KTK YYK.

References

1. Morrisey EE, Hogan BL (2010) Preparing for the first breath: genetic and cellular mechanisms in lung development. Dev Cell 18: 8–23.
2. Hogan BL (1999) Morphogenesis. Cell 96: 225–233.
3. Costa RH, Kalinichenko VV, Lim L (2001) Transcription factors in mouse lung development and function. Am J Physiol Lung Cell Mol Physiol 280: L823–838.
4. Kumar VH, Lakshminrusimha S, El Abiad MT, Chess PR, Ryan RM (2005) Growth factors in lung development. Adv Clin Chem 40: 261–316.
5. Rawlins EL (2011) The building blocks of mammalian lung development. Dev Dyn 240: 463–476.
6. Warburton D, Wuenschell C, Flores-Delgado G, Anderson K (1998) Commitment and differentiation of lung cell lineages. Biochem Cell Biol 76: 971–995.
7. Williams MC (2003) Alveolar type I cells: molecular phenotype and development. Annu Rev Physiol 65: 669–695.
8. Cole FS, Hamvas A, Nogee LM (2001) Genetic disorders of neonatal respiratory function. Pediatr Res 50: 157–162.
9. Glasser SW, Nogee LM (2006) Genetically engineered mice in understanding the basis of neonatal lung disease. Semin Perinatol 30: 341–349.
10. Lyra PP, Diniz EM (2007) The importance of surfactant on the development of neonatal pulmonary diseases. Clinics (Sao Paulo) 62: 181–190.
11. Clark JC, Wert SE, Bachurski CJ, Stahlman MT, Stripp BR, et al. (1995) Targeted disruption of the surfactant protein B gene disrupts surfactant homeostasis, causing respiratory failure in newborn mice. Proc Natl Acad Sci U S A 92: 7794–7798.
12. deMello DE, Heyman S, Phelps DS, Hamvas A, Nogee L, et al. (1994) Ultrastructure of lung in surfactant protein B deficiency. Am J Respir Cell Mol Biol 11: 230–239.
13. Glasser SW, Burhans MS, Korfhagen TR, Na CL, Sly PD, et al. (2001) Altered stability of pulmonary surfactant in SP-C-deficient mice. Proc Natl Acad Sci U S A 98: 6366–6371.
14. Ban N, Matsumura Y, Sakai H, Takanezawa Y, Sasaki M, et al. (2007) ABCA3 as a lipid transporter in pulmonary surfactant biogenesis. J Biol Chem 282: 9628–9634.
15. Pei L, Leblanc M, Barish G, Atkins A, Nofsinger R, et al. (2011) Thyroid hormone receptor repression is linked to type I pneumocyte-associated respiratory distress syndrome. Nat Med 17: 1466–1472.
16. Galambos C, Ng YS, Ali A, Noguchi A, Lovejoy S, et al. (2002) Defective pulmonary development in the absence of heparin-binding vascular endothelial growth factor isoforms. Am J Respir Cell Mol Biol 27: 194–203.
17. Wan H, Xu Y, Ikegami M, Stahlman MT, Kaestner KH, et al. (2004) Foxa2 is required for transition to air breathing at birth. Proc Natl Acad Sci U S A 101: 14449–14454.
18. Liu H, Liu ZQ, Chen CX, Magill S, Jiang Y, et al. (2006) Inhibitory regulation of EGF receptor degradation by sorting nexin 5. Biochem Biophys Res Commun 342: 537–546.
19. Merino-Trigo A, Kerr MC, Houghton F, Lindberg A, Mitchell C, et al. (2004) Sorting nexin 5 is localized to a subdomain of the early endosomes and is recruited to the plasma membrane following EGF stimulation. J Cell Sci 117: 6413–6424.
20. Wassmer T, Attar N, Bujny MV, Oakley J, Traer CJ, et al. (2007) A loss-of-function screen reveals SNX5 and SNX6 as potential components of the mammalian retromer. J Cell Sci 120: 45–54.
21. Yoo KW, Kim EH, Jung SH, Rhee M, Koo BK, et al. (2006) Snx5, as a Mind bomb-binding protein, is expressed in hematopoietic and endothelial precursor cells in zebrafish. FEBS Lett 580: 4409–4416.
22. Carlton J, Bujny M, Peter BJ, Oorschot VM, Rutherford A, et al. (2004) Sorting nexin-1 mediates tubular endosome-to-TGN transport through coincidence sensing of high- curvature membranes and 3-phosphoinositides. Curr Biol 14: 1791–1800.
23. Cavet ME, Pang J, Yin G, Berk BC (2008) An epidermal growth factor (EGF) -dependent interaction between GIT1 and sorting nexin 6 promotes degradation of the EGF receptor. FASEB J 22: 3607–3616.
24. McGough IJ, Cullen PJ (2011) Recent advances in retromer biology. Traffic 12: 963–971.
25. Jeong HW, Jeon US, Koo BK, Kim WY, Im SK, et al. (2009) Inactivation of Notch signaling in the renal collecting duct causes nephrogenic diabetes insipidus in mice. J Clin Invest 119: 3290–3300.
26. Kim YW, Koo BK, Jeong HW, Yoon MJ, Song R, et al. (2008) Defective Notch activation in microenvironment leads to myeloproliferative disease. Blood 112: 4628–4638.
27. Koo BK, Lim HS, Song R, Yoon MJ, Yoon KJ, et al. (2005) Mind bomb 1 is essential for generating functional Notch ligands to activate Notch. Development 132: 3459–3470.
28. Song R, Kim YW, Koo BK, Jeong HW, Yoon MJ, et al. (2008) Mind bomb 1 in the lymphopoietic niches is essential for T and marginal zone B cell development. J Exp Med 205: 2525–2536.
29. Yoon KJ, Koo BK, Im SK, Jeong HW, Ghim J, et al. (2008) Mind bomb 1-expressing intermediate progenitors generate notch signaling to maintain radial glial cells. Neuron 58: 519–531.
30. Yoon MJ, Koo BK, Song R, Jeong HW, Shin J, et al. (2008) Mind bomb-1 is essential for intraembryonic hematopoiesis in the aortic endothelium and the subaortic patches. Mol Cell Biol 28: 4794–4804.
31. Weinmaster G, Fischer JA (2011) Notch ligand ubiquitylation: what is it good for? Dev Cell 21: 134–144.
32. Warshamana GS, Corti M, Brody AR (2001) TNF-alpha, PDGF, and TGF-beta(1) expression by primary mouse bronchiolar-alveolar epithelial and mesenchymal cells: tnf-alpha induces TGF-beta(1). Exp Mol Pathol 71: 13–33.
33. Matsui R, Brody JS, Yu Q (1999) FGF-2 induces surfactant protein gene expression in foetal rat lung epithelial cells through a MAPK-independent pathway. Cell Signal 11: 221–228.
34. Mason RJ, Nellenbogen J, Clements JA (1976) Isolation of disaturated phosphatidylcholine with osmium tetroxide. J Lipid Res 17: 281–284.
35. Martis PC, Whitsett JA, Xu Y, Perl AK, Wan H, et al. (2006) C/EBPalpha is required for lung maturation at birth. Development 133: 1155–1164.
36. Bartlett GR (1959) Phosphorus assay in column chromatography. J Biol Chem 234: 466–468.
37. Geng Y, Dong Y, Yu M, Zhang L, Yan X, et al. (2011) Follistatin-like 1 (Fstl1) is a bone morphogenetic protein (BMP) 4 signaling antagonist in controlling mouse lung development. Proc Natl Acad Sci U S A 108: 7058–7063.
38. Matzke A, Sargsyan V, Holtmann B, Aramuni G, Asan E, et al. (2007) Haploinsufficiency of c-Met in cd44-/- mice identifies a collaboration of CD44 and c-Met in vivo. Mol Cell Biol 27: 8797–8806.
39. Jin N, Cho SN, Raso MG, Wistuba I, Smith Y, et al. (2009) Mig-6 is required for appropriate lung development and to ensure normal adult lung homeostasis. Development 136: 3347–3356.
40. Compernolle V, Brusselmans K, Acker T, Hoet P, Tjwa M, et al. (2002) Loss of HIF-2alpha and inhibition of VEGF impair fetal lung maturation, whereas treatment with VEGF prevents fatal respiratory distress in premature mice. Nat Med 8: 702–710.
41. Bolstad BM, Irizarry RA, Astrand M, Speed TP (2003) A comparison of normalization methods for high density oligonucleotide array data based on variance and bias. Bioinformatics 19: 185–193.
42. Lee JS, Kim Y, Kim IS, Kim B, Choi HJ, et al. (2010) Negative regulation of hypoxic responses via induced Reptin methylation. Mol Cell 39: 71–85.

43. Hwang D, Smith JJ, Leslie DM, Weston AD, Rust AG, et al. (2005) A data integration methodology for systems biology: experimental verification. Proc Natl Acad Sci U S A 102: 17302–17307.
44. Wert SE, Whitsett JA, Nogee LM (2009) Genetic disorders of surfactant dysfunction. Pediatr Dev Pathol 12: 253–274.
45. Andreeva AV, Kutuzov MA, Voyno-Yasenetskaya TA (2007) Regulation of surfactant secretion in alveolar type II cells. Am J Physiol Lung Cell Mol Physiol 293: L259–271.
46. McElroy MC, Kasper M (2004) The use of alveolar epithelial type I cell-selective markers to investigate lung injury and repair. Eur Respir J 24: 664–673.
47. Hara S, Kiyokawa E, Iemura S, Natsume T, Wassmer T, et al. (2008) The DHR1 domain of DOCK180 binds to SNX5 and regulates cation-independent mannose 6-phosphate receptor transport. Mol Biol Cell 19: 3823–3835.
48. Seaman MN (2004) Cargo-selective endosomal sorting for retrieval to the Golgi requires retromer. J Cell Biol 165: 111–122.
49. Panaro NJ, Yuen PK, Sakazume T, Fortina P, Kricka LJ, et al. (2000) Evaluation of DNA fragment sizing and quantification by the agilent 2100 bioanalyzer. Clin Chem 46: 1851–1853.
50. Kalin TV, Wang IC, Meliton L, Zhang Y, Wert SE, et al. (2008) Forkhead Box m1 transcription factor is required for perinatal lung function. Proc Natl Acad Sci U S A 105: 19330–19335.
51. Klinger S, Turgeon B, Levesque K, Wood GA, Aagaard-Tillery KM, et al. (2009) Loss of Erk3 function in mice leads to intrauterine growth restriction, pulmonary immaturity, and neonatal lethality. Proc Natl Acad Sci U S A 106: 16710–16715.
52. O'Brien KB, Alberich-Jorda M, Yadav N, Kocher O, Diruscio A, et al. (2010) CARM1 is required for proper control of proliferation and differentiation of pulmonary epithelial cells. Development 137: 2147–2156.
53. Schacht V, Ramirez MI, Hong YK, Hirakawa S, Feng D, et al. (2003) T1alpha/podoplanin deficiency disrupts normal lymphatic vasculature formation and causes lymphedema. EMBO J 22: 3546–3556.
54. Miettinen PJ, Berger JE, Meneses J, Phung Y, Pedersen RA, et al. (1995) Epithelial immaturity and multiorgan failure in mice lacking epidermal growth factor receptor. Nature 376: 337–341.
55. Griffin CT, Trejo J, Magnuson T (2005) Genetic evidence for a mammalian retromer complex containing sorting nexins 1 and 2. Proc Natl Acad Sci U S A 102: 15173–15177.
56. Verges M (2007) Retromer and sorting nexins in development. Front Biosci 12: 3825–3851.

2

Comorbidities and Mortality in Hypercapnic Obese under Domiciliary Noninvasive Ventilation

Jean-Christian Borel[1,3*], Benoit Burel[2], Renaud Tamisier[1,2], Sonia Dias-Domingos[1,2], Jean-Philippe Baguet[4], Patrick Levy[1,2], Jean-Louis Pepin[1,2*]

1 INSERM U 1042, HP2 Laboratory, Université Joseph Fourier, Faculté de Médecine, Grenoble, France, **2** CHU, Hôpital A. Michallon, Pôle Locomotion, Rééducation et Physiologie, Grenoble, France, **3** AGIRadom, Research and Development department, Meylan, France, **4** CHU, Hôpital A. Michallon, Département de cardiologie, Grenoble, France

Abstract

Background: The higher mortality rate in untreated patients with obesity-associated hypoventilation is a strong rationale for long-term noninvasive ventilation (NIV). The impacts of comorbidities, medications and NIV compliance on survival of these patients remain largely unexplored.

Methods: Observational cohort of hypercapnic obese patients initiated on NIV between March 2003 and July 2008. Survival curves were estimated by the Kaplan–Meier method. Anthropometric measurements, pulmonary function, blood gases, nocturnal SpO_2 indices, comorbidities, medications, conditions of NIV initiation and NIV compliance were used as covariates. Univariate and multivariate Cox models allowed to assess predictive factors of mortality.

Results: One hundred and seven patients (56% women), in whom NIV was initiated in acute (36%) or chronic conditions, were followed during 43±14 months. The 1, 2, 3 years survival rates were 99%, 94%, and 89%, respectively. In univariate analysis, death was associated with older age (>61 years), low FEV1 (<66% predicted value), male gender, BMI×time, concomitant COPD, NIV initiation in acute condition, use of inhaled corticosteroids, ß-blockers, nonthiazide diuretics, angiotensin-converting enzyme inhibitors and combination of cardiovascular drugs (one diuretic and at least one other cardiovascular agent). In multivariate analysis, combination of cardiovascular agents was the only factor independently associated with higher risk of death (HR = 5.3; 95% CI 1.18; 23.9). Female gender was associated with lower risk of death.

Conclusion: Cardiovascular comorbidities represent the main factor predicting mortality in patient with obesity-associated hypoventilation treated by NIV. In this population, NIV should be associated with a combination of treatment modalities to reduce cardiovascular risk.

Editor: Xin-Liang Ma, Thomas Jefferson University, United States of America

Funding: The authors have no support or funding to report.

Competing Interests: The authors have read the journal's policy and have the following conflicts: Jean-Christian Borel is employed by AGIR a` dom.

* E-mail: jpepin@chu-grenoble.fr (JLP); j.borel@agiradom.com (JCB)

These authors contributed equally to this work.

Introduction

Obesity is a chronic condition associated with metabolic, hormonal, cardiovascular and respiratory impairments causing an increase in death rate [1]. Obstructive sleep apnea syndrome (OSAS), commonly associated with obesity [2], is also a risk factor for cardio-metabolic morbidity [3,4]. Beyond OSAS, a subgroup of obese patients is affected by chronic respiratory failure, characterized by diurnal hypercapnia [5]. Two main syndromes can be encountered in obesity-associated chronic hypercapnia. Firstly, the obesity hypoventilation syndrome (OHS), defined as a combination of obesity (BMI $\geq$30 kg/m^2), daytime hypercapnia ($PaCO_2 \geq 45$ mmHg) and various types of sleep-disordered breathing after ruling out other disorders that may cause alveolar hypoventilation [6]. Secondly, the overlap syndrome defined as the combination of OSAS and chronic obstructive pulmonary disease (COPD) [7,8,9]. Indeed, COPD, OSAS and obesity acted synergistically to increase the risk of sleep hypoxemia and hypercapnia [9], and therefore causes chronic respiratory failure [7,10]. Both OHS and overlap syndrome are characterized by a high rate of cardiovascular morbimortality [5,11,12].

Noninvasive ventilation (NIV) effectively improves some characteristics of obesity-associated hypoventilation [13]. Particularly, sleep-related breathing disorders encountered in obese patients are a modifiable obesity-related cardio-vascular risk factor. In observational cohorts [14,15,16] NIV seems to be effective in reducing mortality in obese patients suffering from sleep breathing disorders but the overall mortality rate remains higher than long-term mortality rates observed in large cohorts of obese patients submitted to bariatric surgery [17]. It is possible that some key factors predicting mortality in obese patients treated with NIV have not been yet identified. The main objective of this study was to assess the factors related to risk of death in a cohort of patients with obesity-associated hypoventilation treated with home-based long term NIV. We included a full description of comorbidities and medications as covariates of mortality, which have never been included in previous mortality studies.

Materials and Methods

Study Design and Patients' Selection

Observational cohort study of patients with obesity (BMI $\geq$30 kg.m^{-2}) and hypercapnia ($PaCO_2 \geq 45$ mmHg) treated after hospital discharge with at-home, long-term, noninvasive ventilation (NIV). Patients who started NIV between March 2003 and July 2008 were identified through a regional home-care database. NIV was initiated during hospitalization for acute or chronic hypoventilation in five different medical facilities (one tertiary university hospital, one general hospital and three private practice centers). The standard definition for inclusion was "patients in whom obesity was the main explanation for hypoventilation". Patients suffering from neuromuscular disorders, untreated hypothyroidism, progressive restrictive parenchymal lung diseases (such as fibrosis) were not included. The presence of any other respiratory disease (history of COPD [when 30%<FEV1/VC <70%], asthma, moderate thoracic restrictive diseases) that could participate to hypoventilation was not an exclusion criterion.

Ethical committee approval was obtained by "Le Comité consultatif sur le traitement de l'information en matière de recherche en santé" (C.C.T.I.R.S 11.371) and authorization from the "Commission Nationale Informatique et Liberté" (C.N.I.L), the French information technology and personal data protection authority. According to the C.N.I.L and C.C.T.I.R.S's recommendations for this retrospective study, an information letter was mailed to each patient but a written consent was not required. The information letter mentioned that the patients could refuse that their information to be used for the study. Regarding the patients who had died, an exemption for the requirement of information was obtained by the CNIL.

Data Collection

Patients' medical charts were retrospectively analyzed in each of the five centers by the same investigator (B.B.). Medical and smoking history, anthropometric data, daytime and sleep respiratory parameters and usual medical treatment before NIV initiation were extracted. The condition of NIV initiation (acute respiratory failure or chronic respiratory failure) was also reported. Baseline reference arterial blood gases (ABG) should have been drawn maximum one day before NIV initiation. In acute hypercapnic respiratory failure condition, ABG values were considered as acceptable even though they were performed under supplemental O_2. Pulmonary function tests must have been performed within a month preceding NIV initiation in order to be considered as valid data.

Follow-up and Outcomes

After hospital discharge, patients were systematically followed every three months by the same home care provider until death or NIV discontinuation. Health authorities, in France, require visits by home care nurses or technicians before providing reimbursement for the ventilatory support. Vital status was ascertained by home care provider or in case of NIV discontinuation by patient's general practitioner. The analysis was censored on October 1, 2010. Adherence to NIV was assessed via the time counter of the ventilator. NIV adherence was considered at 0 hour/day in patients who discontinued NIV during the survey. During follow up, patients who were switched to continuous positive airway pressure therapy (CPAP) were considered and analyzed as pursuing NIV.

Data Management and Statistical Analysis

Data were analyzed using Statistical Analysis System (SAS®) software version 9.1.3 (SAS Institute, Cary, NC, USA). Continuous data were expressed as mean ± standard deviation (SD), and categorical data as percentage. Baseline variables were compared according to conditions of NIV initiation using Kruskal-Wallis rank sum test or ANOVA.

Univariate Cox proportional hazards regression models were used to determine baseline parameters (i.e. at NIV initiation) that were associated with survival. Continuous data were converted to dichotomous data (> or<to the median value). Since BMI did not respect proportional risks hypothesis (time-dependent variable), it was converted to a new variable: BMI x time. To describe the frequency and outcomes according to baseline variables, all- cause mortality were constructed according to the Kaplan-Meier analysis.

Variables associated with survival in univariate analysis with $p<0.2$ were included in a multivariable Cox proportional hazards regression model (backward selection). Co-linearity between variables (defined as $p<0.2$ and $r>0.4$) was assessed by Pearson's or Spearman's coefficient or Cramer's V2. Variables which had more than 15% of missing values were discarded. For other variables, the missing values were replaced by the variable's median for continuous data and for categorical data by the most frequent value. Only a p-value <0.05 was considered statistically significant.

Results

Flow Chart

As depicted in Figure 1, a total of 107 patients who started NIV between March 2003 and July 2008 were included in the study. NIV was initiated in either acute hypercapnic respiratory failure (AHRF) (26.4% in respiratory ward or 9.3% in intensive care unit [ICU], respectively) or in a chronic stable state of hypercapnic respiratory failure (64.4%).

Baseline Assessment

Table 1 shows the baseline characteristics according to patient's NIV initiation conditions. As expected, $PaCO_2$, pH and respiratory function were more severely affected in patients referred for acute respiratory failure. Medical history revealed high rates of cardiovascular comorbidities regardless of NIV initiation conditions. However, patients referred in acute respiratory failure were significantly more likely to have a previous diagnosis of heart failure. Accordingly, these patients were more frequently treated with cardiovascular medications (antiplatelets agents, anticoagulants, non-thiazidic diuretics). Moreover, AHRF patients exhibited a higher rate of COPD and were more often former smokers. Before the inclusion in the study, seven patients (6,5%) had been previously treated by CPAP but were no longer treated at the time of inclusion; sixteen patients (15%) had been treated by CPAP until the inclusion and were then switched to NIV owing to persistent hypercapnia.

Follow-up (Figure 1 and Table 2)

For the group as a whole, the mean observation time was 43±14 months. Thirteen patients (12%) died after a mean duration of 25±12 months. The 1, 2, 3 years survival probabilities were 99%, 94% and 89%, respectively. Fourteen patients (14%)

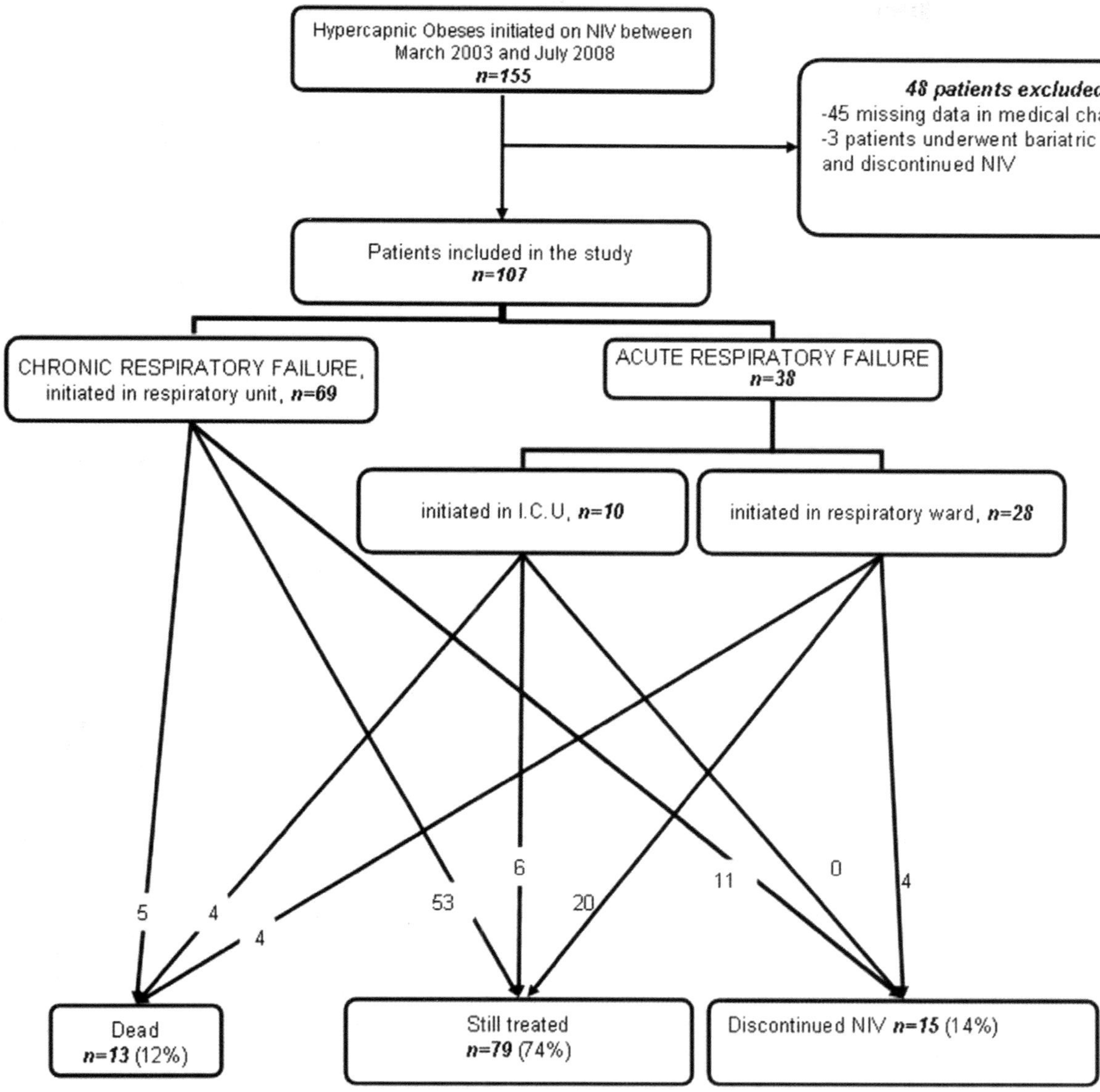

Figure 1. Flow chart of the survey. CRF: Chronic Respiratory Failure; AHRF: Acute Hypercapnic Respiratory Failure; I.C.U: Intensive Care Unit.

with persistent non adherence discontinued NIV. Seven patients were switched to CPAP therapy. The mean daily use for NIV was 5.4±3.5 hours/day. The mean follow-up duration as well as the mean NIV adherence was similar whatever NIV initiation conditions. Nevertheless, patients with AHRF exhibited higher rates of death and they were more likely to receive additional long term oxygen therapy to NIV.

Factors Associated with Risk of All-cause Mortality

Figure 2 shows the Kaplan-Meier survival curves of factors which were significantly associated with risk of all-cause mortality in univariate analysis. Table 3 displays baseline characteristics associated with the risk of death with a p-value <0.2 in univariate analysis. The choice between collinear variables was based on clinical considerations. The following were included in a multivariate Cox proportional hazards regression model: Age, gender, BMI×time, NIV initiation conditions, vital capacity, FEV1/VC (reflecting COPD history and intake of inhaled corticosteroids), Combination of cardiovascular agents, history of diabetes, former smoker status, additional long-term O_2, psycho-active drugs. Combination of cardiovascular agents was the only factor independently associated with higher risk of death in multivariate analysis. Female gender was associated with lower risk of death (Figure 3).

Discussion

The main objective of this study was to assess the factors associated with risk of death in a cohort of obese hypercapnic patients treated with home-based long-term NIV. The results can be summarized as follows: (i) A third of obese hypercapnic patients with the most severe comorbidities were diagnosed on the occasion of an acute respiratory failure and were then initiated on NIV in the ICU or in respiratory ward. (ii) Beyond the condition of NIV initiation, gender, age, BMI, history of COPD, and cardiovascular comorbidities (recognized by the use of a combination of cardiovascular medications) were associated with higher risk of death when treated by NIV. (iii) In multivariate analysis,

Table 1. Baseline Characteristics according to NIV initiation conditions.

	Chronic/respiratory ward, n = 69	Acute/respiratory ward, n = 28	Acute/I.C.U, n = 10	p-value
Age, *years*	59±13	63±10	65±8	ns
Gender, *% male*	42	39	70	ns
BMI, *kg/m*^{2}	40.2±6.7	41.4±7.3	37.9±5.5	ns
PaO_2, *kPa* (n of ABG with O_2)	9.7±1.5 (0)	8.9±2.4 (10)	9.1±2.7 (7)	ns
$PaCO_2$, *kPa*	6.1±0.7*#	6.7±1.3 #	8.5±2.3*	<0.001
pH	7.40±0.03 *	7.39±0.04	7.32±0.07 *	0.001
VC, *% predicted value*	76±21 *	65±20*	62±22	0.03
FEV_1/VC, %	77±14	81±14	70±16	ns
Apnea-Hyponea index, *n/h* (n of missing data)	42±32 (9)	44±32 (11)	37±36 (6)	ns
Mean nocturnal SpO2, *% h* (n of missing data)	91±4 (10)	89±7 (5)	89±4 (6)	ns
SpO2<90%, *%recording time h* (n of missing data)	27±30 (12)	37±31 (8)	44±29 (6)	ns
Medical History				
Former smoker, %	46.4	50.0*	90.0*	0.04
Hypertension, %	81.2	82.1	80.0	ns
Heart Failure,%	34.8*	60.7*	70.0	0.02
coronary heart disease, %	14.5	10.7	40.0	<0.1
Pulmonary Hypertension,%	8.7 #	28.6 #	30.0	0.02
Thrombo-embolism, %	5.8	14.3	10.0	ns
Stroke, %	5.8	14.3	10.0	ns
Type 2 diabetes, %	34.8	39.3	40.0	ns
Dyslipidemia, %	42.0	39.3	40.0	ns
COPD, %	21.7	35.7	60.0	0.03
Asthma, %	13.0	7.1	30.0	ns
Sleep apnea, %	72.5	57.1	60.0	ns
Depression, %	29.0	32.1	40.0	ns
Medications				
ß-blokers, %	29.0	28.6	20.0	ns
Diuretics, %	52.2	60.7	80.0	ns
Non-thiazide diuretics, %	24.6*#	57.1*	80.0#	<0.001
Calcium antagonists, %	17.4	39.3	30.0	<0.1
CEI, %	24.6	28.6	50.0	ns
ARBs, %	34.8%	25.0	30.0	ns
Anti-platelet drugs, %	18.8#	35.7	60.0#	0.01
Anticoagulants, %	4.3*	25.0*	20.0	0.01
Statins, %	34.8	42.9	50.0	ns
Insulin, %	11.6	3.6	20.0	ns
Inhaled corticoids, %	27.5	21.4	60.0	<0.1
Oral antidiabetics, %	31.9	39.3	40.0	ns
Psychoacticve drugs, %	71.0	57.1	70.0	ns
NIV settings				
Inspiratory pressure* *(cmH$_2$O)*	18.9±3.0	19.4±3.7	20.8±5.0	ns
Expiratory pressure *(cmH$_2$O)*	9.6±1.9	10.0±2.2	9.1±2.6	ns
Back-up frequency *(/min)*	12.7±2.6	13.0±3.6	14.1±1.7	ns

Chronic = Chronic Respiratory Failure; Acute: Acute Respiratory Failure; I.C.U: Intensive Care Unit; BMI: Body Mass Index; n of ABG with O2: number of arterial blood gases realized with additional O_2; VC: Vital Capacity expressed as percentage of predicted value; FEV1/VC: Forced Expiratory Volume in one second/Vital Capacity ratio; Heart failure included (ischemic, hypertrophic or dilated); COPD: Chronic Obstructive Pulmonary Disease; OSAS: Obstructive Sleep Apnea Syndrome; CEI: Angiotensin Converting Enzyme Inhhnibitors; ARBs: Angiotensin II Receptor Blockers.

*#: represent significant difference between pairwise comparisons.

Table 2. Follow-up data according to the condition of NIV initiation.

	Chronic/respiratory ward, n = 69	Acute/respiratory ward, n = 28	Acute/I.C.U, n = 10	p-value
Mean daily use of NIV, *h/day*	5.2±3.4	5.3±3.9	5.7±3.3	ns
Mean follow-up duration, *months*	45±13	41±15	39±1	ns
Rate of death, %	7.2*	14.3	40.0*	0.01
Additonal long term O_2, %	13.0 #*	32.1 *	60.0 #	0.001

cardiovascular comorbidities remained the only factor independently associated with a higher risk of death.

Obesity-associated Hypoventilation Remains a Largely Undiagnosed Syndrome

The finding that NIV was initiated in acute respiratory failure in a third of the patients of the present cohort is in accordance with previous studies [18,19]. However, these studies were including patients initiated on NIV in the 1990s. Our study underscores that there is always –within current knowledge- a lack of screening for hypoventilation in obese patients and that initiation of NIV is dramatically delayed [20]. Moreover, patients initiated under NIV in acute conditions were more likely to have previously developed cardiovascular complications favoring multiple organ failure and a higher rate of death. When initiated early, there is growing evidence to suggest that NIV would be efficient in reducing requirement of intensive care, general health care resources [21]as well as improving survival [14,15]. Taken together these results reinforce the need for better screening for hypercapnia in patients with obesity-associated hypoventilation, particularly in primary care resources. In obese patients, serum bicarbonate level >27 mMol/L is associated with a high prevalence of OHS. This marker would be sensitive - low cost – and easily available to better screen obesity-related hypoventilation and thus anticipate patient's referral to respiratory physicians [22].

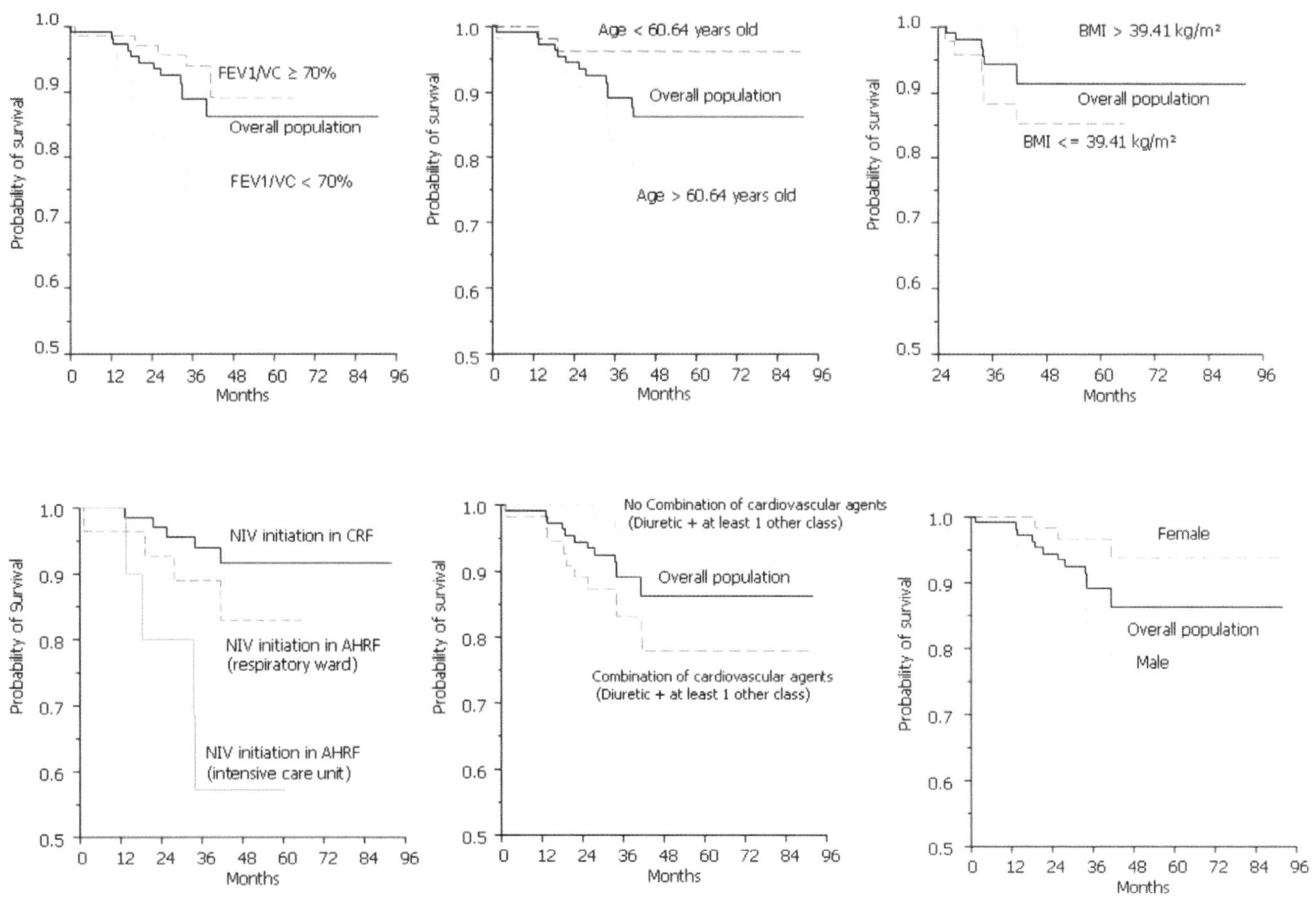

Figure 2. Kaplan-Meier survival curves referring to BMI, gender, FEV1/VC, use of combination of cardiovascular agents and condition of NIV initiation.

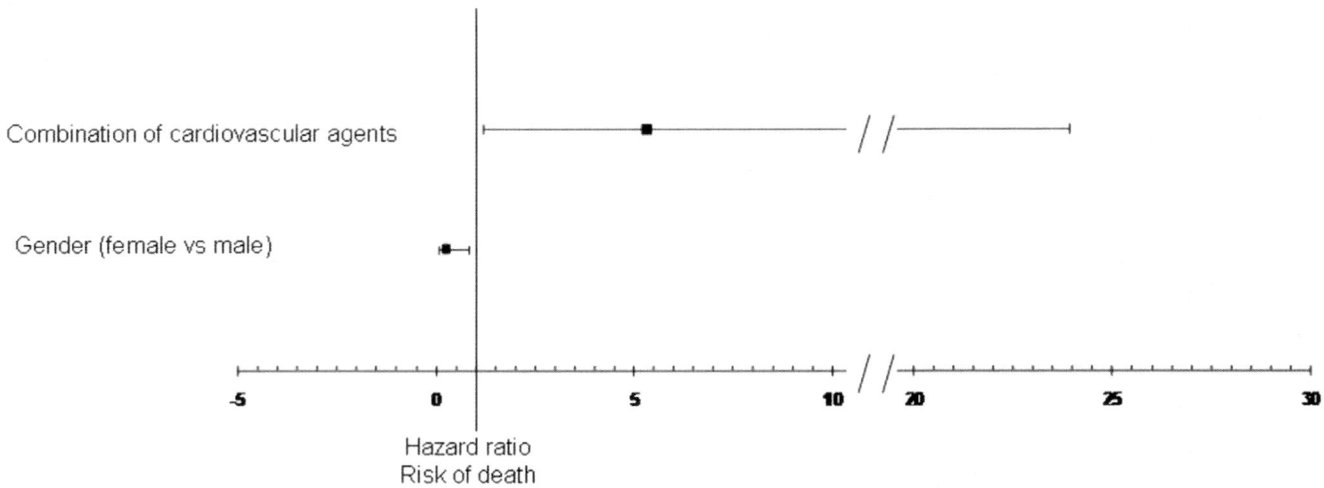

	Hazard Ratio	Confidence Interval		P-value
Combination of cardiovascular agents	5.301	1.18	23.9	0.030
Gender (female vs male)	0.226	0.06	0.82	0.024

Figure 3. Independent factors associated with risk of all-cause mortality (multivariate Cox model). Combination of cardiovascular agents: Combination of a diuretic and at least one other cardiovascular agent among ß-Blokers, Calcium antagonists, Converting Enzime Inhibitors, Antagiotensin II receptor blockers.

Survival Rates in Patients Treated by NIV for Obesity-associated Hypoventilation

The two and three years mortality rates were comparable in the present study with those of previous published reports [14,19]. Priou et al [19] and Budweiser et al [14] reported survival rates of 93 and 92% at two years of follow-up compared to 94% in the present study. However, in their studies, Budweiser et al [14] and Priou et al [19] applied tighter inclusion criteria for COPD patients and excluded subjects with FEV1/VC<50% and FEV1/IC <60%, respectively. In the present study, exclusion criteria were less restrictive (FEV1>30% of predicted value) to better document the association between obesity-associated hypoventilation and COPD in terms of mortality. Indeed, the association between untreated sleep breathing disorders and COPD is known to increase the risk of death. This has been demonstrated for patients with mild to moderate COPD (average BMI = 30.5±5.1 $kg.m^{-2}$) [12] as well as for GOLD IV hypercapnic COPD (mean BMI = 32.3±5.4 $kg.m^{-2}$) already established on long-term oxygen therapy [8]. Marin et al.[12] showed that CPAP improved survival in patients with a mild to moderate overlap syndrome. In the Marin's study, significant limitation was that $PaCO_2$ values were not available and only a limited number of patients were treated by NIV.

Overlap syndrome and obesity hypoventilation syndrome are linked by sleep apnea, episodes of REM hypoventilation and a high frequency of cardiovascular comorbidities. We firmly believe that a clear cut distinction between these two syndromes is arbitrary and does not reflect the reality of clinical practice. Accordingly, Nowbar et al [5] in their paper on obesity-associated hypoventilation reported that 38% of patients had previously received a diagnosis of COPD. In the field of COPD, Garcia-Aymerich et al [23] described the cluster of *"systemic COPD"* characterized by obesity, a mild respiratory impairment and a high prevalence of cardiovascular diseases.

Cardiovascular Comorbidities: The Best Predictor of Mortality in Obese Patients Treated with Noninvasive Ventilation

Our study extends knowledge by demonstrating that cardiovascular comorbidities are the major determinants of death in patients with obesity-associated hypoventilation treated by NIV. The use of a combination of cardiovascular agents as a marker of cardiovascular comorbidities probably underestimates the prevalence of comorbidities as the use of secondary prevention medications remains low [24]. However, even with a lack of sensitivity, the use of two or more cardiovascular agents represented a consistent surrogate marker of cardiovascular comorbidities. Indeed, in a recent study, Weber et al. [25] compared patients at heightened cardiovascular risk that are using a monotherapy versus a combination therapy. The two groups of patients had similar histories of stroke or coronary events and the comparison between the two groups was adjusted for prior cardiovascular disease and left ventricular hypertrophy (other major clinical characteristics, including the prevalence of diabetes mellitus, were not different in these two groups). These authors demonstrated a clear increase in mortality rate and a higher proportion of cardiovascular events in patients with a combination therapy. The hypothesis was that a combination of cardiovascular medications reflected a more severe history of previous cardiovascular disease. Another study [26] raised the same conclusions. Accordingly, we strongly believe that a combination of cardiovascular agents is a reliable marker of risk in our hypercapnic obese

Table 3. Factors associated with risk of all-cause mortality (univariate Cox model).

	Hazard ratio	95% confidence interval	p-value
Age (>60.6 years)	5.464	1.2; 24.6	0.03
Gender (female vs male)	0.221	0.06; 0.8	0.02
Time *BMI (≥39.4 kg.m^{-2} after 24 months)	0.079	0.01; 0.6	0.01
NIV initiation (Acute versus Chronic)	3.24	1.1; 9.9	0.04
VC (>72% predicted value)	0.228	0.05; 1.0	<0.1
FEV_1 (>66% of predicted value)	0.2	0.04; 0.9	0.04
FEV_1/VC (>77.5%)	0.332	0.09; 1.2	<0.1
AIH (>33/h)	3.098	0.6; 15.3	<0.2
Mean nocturnal SpO_2 (>91.4%)	0.264	0.06; 1.2	<0.1
Medical History			
Former smoker	3.226	0.9; 11.7	<0.1
Type 2 Diabetes	2.224	0.7; 6.6	<0.2
COPD	3.112	1.0; 9.7	0.05
Dyslipidemia	1.218	0.4; 3.6	>0.7
Stroke	1.964	0.4; 8.9	0.3801
Sleep apnea	1.648	0.4; 6.0	>0.4
Hypertension	–	–	>0.9
Heart Failure	2.36	0.8; 7.0	<0.2
coronary heart disease	1.47	0.4; 5.4	>0.5
Pulmonary Hypertension	1.986	0.5; 7.2	>0.2
Thrombo-embolism	2.166	0.5; 9.8	>0.3
Asthma	1.269	0.3; 5.7	>0.7
Depression	0.686	0.2; 2.5	>0.5
Usual Medical treatment			
ß-blokers, %	3.418	1.1; 10.2	0.03
Diuretics, %	4.274	0.9; 19.3	<0.1
Non-thiazide diuretics, %	6.257	1.7; 22.8	0.005
CEI, %	3.022	1.0; 9.0	0.05
Combination of cardiovascular agents, %	5.429	1.02; 24.5	0.03
Oral antidiabetics, %	2.568	0.9; 7.7	<0.1
Psychoacticve drugs, %	0.368	0.1; 1.7	<0.2
Inhaled corticoids	4.507	1.5; 13.8	0.01
Calcium antagonists	0.936	0.26; 3.4	>0.9
ARBs	0.599	0.17; 2.2	>0.4
Anti-platelet drugs	1.639	0.54; 5.0	>0.3
Anticoagulants	0.682	0.09; 5.2	>0.7
Statins	0.947	0.3; 2.9	>0.9
Insulin	1.86	0.4; 8.4	>0.4
Follow-up			
Additonal long term O_2	2.208	0.7; 6.8	<0.2

Time*BMI: Body Mass Index; VC: Vital Capacity expressed as percentage of predicted value; FEV1: Forced Expiratory Volume in one second; AIH: Apnea Hypopnea index expressed as number of events per hour of sleep; Combination of cardiovascular agents: Combination of a diuretic and at least one other cardiovascular agent among ß-Blokers, Calcium antagonists, Converting Enzime Inhibitors, Antagiotensin II receptor blockers; COPD: Chronic Obstructive Pulmonary Disease. Continuous data were converted to dichotomous data (> or< to the median value); Since BMI did not respect proportional risks hypothesis (time-dependant variable), it was converted to a new variable: BMI x time. This variable should be interpreted as follows: After 24 months, BMI above 39.4 kg m^{-2} is associated with lower risk of death than BMI bellow 39.4 kg.m^{-2}.

patients. There is an important and simple clinical message behind this: Hypercapnic obese patients treated at home with long term NIV and requiring combination of cardiovascular agents are at higher risk of mortality and justify a closer follow-up.

We have recently demonstrated in a randomized control trial that one-month NIV clearly improved diurnal and nocturnal respiratory outcomes in patients suffering from OHS, but cardiovascular parameters such as blood pressure, endothelial dysfunction as well as arterial stiffness remained unchanged [27]. Interestingly, low-grade inflammation was not influenced by NIV probably because in these morbidly obese patients, obesity per-se is the major explanation for persistent chronic inflammation. In severe COPD, chronic inflammation probably also persist even after treatment of sleep disordered breathing. Although NIV has been shown to be effective in reducing mortality in patients with obesity-associated hypoventilation, the long-term mortality rate for these patients remains higher when compared to data observed in large cohorts of obese patients who underwent bariatric surgery which treats obesity-related complications more entirely than NIV [17].

Methodological Considerations

We acknowledge that we could not provide evidence of long term NIV effectiveness such as follow-up arterial blood gases, nocturnal oxymetry, polygraphy and clinical outcomes (dyspnea severity score, sleepiness, quality of life). Future prospective studies should specifically address the question oflong term variations in NIV efficacy and mortality.

Conclusion and Perspectives

This study shows that better screening for patients with obesity-associated hypoventilation is necessary in order to reduce the delay of NIV initiation and avoid acute respiratory failure. Cardiovascular comorbidities remain the major determinant of death in these patients who are treated by NIV for sleep breathing abnormalities. Thus, NIV should be combined with other modalities of treatment such as rehabilitation programs including physical training, weight loss, lifestyle changes and appropriate medication to further improve cardiovascular risk factors in patients with obesity-associated hypoventilation.

Author Contributions

Conceived and designed the experiments: JCB BB JLP. Performed the experiments: BB. Analyzed the data: SDD. Contributed reagents/materials/analysis tools: BB. Wrote the paper: JCB BB RT JPB PL JLP.

References

1. Whitlock G, Lewington S, Sherliker P, Clarke R, Emberson J, et al. (2009) Body-mass index and cause-specific mortality in 900 000 adults: collaborative analyses of 57 prospective studies. Lancet 373: 1083–1096.
2. Young T, Shahar E, Nieto FJ, Redline S, Newman AB, et al. (2002) Predictors of sleep-disordered breathing in community-dwelling adults: the Sleep Heart Health Study. Arch Intern Med 162: 893–900.
3. Peppard PE, Young T, Palta M, Skatrud J (2000) Prospective study of the association between sleep-disordered breathing and hypertension. N Engl J Med 342: 1378–1384.
4. Sharma SK, Agrawal S, Damodaran D, Sreenivas V, Kadhiravan T, et al. (2011) CPAP for the metabolic syndrome in patients with obstructive sleep apnea. N Engl J Med 365: 2277–2286.
5. Nowbar S, Burkart KM, Gonzales R, Fedorowicz A, Gozansky WS, et al. (2004) Obesity-associated hypoventilation in hospitalized patients: prevalence, effects, and outcome. Am J Med 116: 1–7.
6. Mokhlesi B (2010) Obesity hypoventilation syndrome: a state-of-the-art review. Respir Care 55: 1347–1362; discussion 1363–1345.
7. Chaouat A, Weitzenblum E, Kessler R, Schott R, Charpentier C, et al. (2001) Outcome of COPD patients with mild daytime hypoxaemia with or without sleep-related oxygen desaturation. Eur Respir J 17: 848–855.
8. Machado MC, Vollmer WM, Togeiro SM, Bilderback AL, Oliveira MV, et al. (2010) CPAP and survival in moderate-to-severe obstructive sleep apnoea syndrome and hypoxaemic COPD. Eur Respir J 35: 132–137.
9. Sanders MH, Newman AB, Haggerty CL, Redline S, Lebowitz M, et al. (2003) Sleep and sleep-disordered breathing in adults with predominantly mild obstructive airway disease. Am J Respir Crit Care Med 167: 7–14.
10. Lee R, McNicholas WT (2011) Obstructive sleep apnea in chronic obstructive pulmonary disease patients. Curr Opin Pulm Med 17: 79–83.
11. Chaouat A, Weitzenblum E, Krieger J, Sforza E, Hammad H, et al. (1999) Prognostic value of lung function and pulmonary haemodynamics in OSA patients treated with CPAP. Eur Respir J 13: 1091–1096.
12. Marin JM, Soriano JB, Carrizo SJ, Boldova A, Celli BR (2010) Outcomes in patients with chronic obstructive pulmonary disease and obstructive sleep apnea: the overlap syndrome. Am J Respir Crit Care Med 182: 325–331.
13. Borel JC, Borel AL, Monneret D, Tamisier R, Levy P, et al. (2011) Obesity Hypoventilation Syndrome: From Sleep Disordered Breathing to Systemic Comorbidities and the Need to Offer Combined Treatment Strategies. Respirology.
14. Budweiser S, Riedl SG, Jorres RA, Heinemann F, Pfeifer M (2007) Mortality and prognostic factors in patients with obesity-hypoventilation syndrome undergoing noninvasive ventilation. J Intern Med 261: 375–383.
15. Heinemann F, Budweiser S, Dobroschke J, Pfeifer M (2007) Non-invasive positive pressure ventilation improves lung volumes in the obesity hypoventilation syndrome. Respir Med 101: 1229–1235.
16. Kessler R, Chaouat A, Schinkewitch P, Faller M, Casel S, et al. (2001) The obesity-hypoventilation syndrome revisited: a prospective study of 34 consecutive cases. Chest 120: 369–376.
17. Adams TD, Gress RE, Smith SC, Halverson RC, Simper SC, et al. (2007) Long-term mortality after gastric bypass surgery. N Engl J Med 357: 753–761.
18. Laub M, Midgren B (2007) Survival of patients on home mechanical ventilation: a nationwide prospective study. Respir Med 101: 1074–1078.
19. Priou P, Hamel JF, Person C, Meslier N, Racineux JL, et al. (2010) Long-term outcome of noninvasive positive pressure ventilation for obesity hypoventilation syndrome. Chest 138: 84–90.
20. Quint JK, Ward L, Davison AG (2007) Previously undiagnosed obesity hypoventilation syndrome. Thorax 62: 462–463.
21. Berg G, Delaive K, Manfreda J, Walld R, Kryger MH (2001) The use of health-care resources in obesity-hypoventilation syndrome. Chest 120: 377–383.
22. Mokhlesi B, Tulaimat A, Faibussowitsch I, Wang Y, Evans AT (2007) Obesity hypoventilation syndrome: prevalence and predictors in patients with obstructive sleep apnea. Sleep Breath 11: 117–124.
23. Garcia-Aymerich J, Gomez FP, Benet M, Farrero E, Basagana X, et al. (2011) Identification and prospective validation of clinically relevant chronic obstructive pulmonary disease (COPD) subtypes. Thorax 66: 430–437.
24. Yusuf S, Islam S, Chow CK, Rangarajan S, Dagenais G, et al. (2011) Use of secondary prevention drugs for cardiovascular disease in the community in high-income, middle-income, and low-income countries (the PURE Study): a prospective epidemiological survey. Lancet 378: 1231–1243.
25. Weber MA, Julius S, Kjeldsen SE, Jia Y, Brunner HR, et al. (2012) Cardiovascular outcomes in hypertensive patients: comparing single-agent therapy with combination therapy. J Hypertens 30: 2213–2222.
26. Zhang Y, Zhang X, Liu L, Wang Y, Tang X, et al. (2012) Higher cardiovascular risk and impaired benefit of antihypertensive treatment in hypertensive patients requiring additional drugs on top of randomized therapy: is adding drugs always beneficial? J Hypertens 30: 2202–2212.
27. Borel JC, Tamisier R, Gonzalez-Bermejo J, Baguet JP, Monneret D, et al. (2011) Noninvasive Ventilation in Mild obesity hypoventilation syndrome: A randomized controlled trial. Chest.

Acute Respiratory Distress Syndrome Induced by a Swine 2009 H1N1 Variant in Mice

Yi Zhang[1]❡, Honglei Sun[1]❡, Lihong Fan[1], Yuan Ma[1], Yipeng Sun[1], Juan Pu[1], Jun Yang[1], Jian Qiao[1], Guangpeng Ma[2]*, Jinhua Liu[1,3]*

1 Key Laboratory of Animal Epidemiology and Zoonosis, College of Veterinary Medicine, China Agricultural University, Ministry of Agriculture, Beijing, China, **2** China Rural Technology Development Center, Beijing, China, **3** Shandong Animal Disease Control Center, Shandong, China

Abstract

Background: Acute respiratory distress syndrome (ARDS) induced by pandemic 2009 H1N1 influenza virus has been widely reported and was considered the main cause of death in critically ill patients with 2009 H1N1 infection. However, no animal model has been developed for ARDS caused by infection with 2009 H1N1 virus. Here, we present a mouse model of ARDS induced by 2009 H1N1 virus.

Methodology Principal Findings: Mice were inoculated with A/swine/Shandong/731/2009 (SD/09), which was a 2009 H1N1 influenza variant with a G222D mutation in the hemagglutinin. Clinical symptoms were recorded every day. Lung injury was assessed by lung water content and histopathological observation. Arterial blood gas, leukocyte count in the bronchial alveolar lavage fluid and blood, virus titers, and cytokine levels in the lung were measured at various times post-inoculation. Mice infected with SD/09 virus showed typical ARDS symptoms characterized by 60% lethality on days 8–10 post-inoculation, highly edematous lungs, inflammatory cellular infiltration, alveolar and interstitial edema, lung hemorrhage, progressive and severe hypoxemia, and elevated levels of proinflammatory cytokines and chemokines.

Conclusions/Significance: These results suggested that we successfully established an ARDS mouse model induced by a virulent 2009 H1N1 variant without previous adaptation, which may be of benefit for evaluating the pathogenesis or therapy of human ARDS caused by 2009 H1N1 virus.

Editor: Rory Edward Morty, University of Giessen Lung Center, Germany

Funding: This work was supported by the National Natural Science Foundation of China (No. 31172324, 31172323), the National Basic Research Program (973 Program) (No. 2011CB504702), the National Key Technologies Research and Development Program (2010BAD04B01), China Postdoctoral Science Foundation funded project (2011M500456), and Chinese Universities Scientific Fund (2011BH041). Dr. Liu was funded by the Taishan Scholar Foundation. The funders had no role in study design, data collection and analysis, decision to publish, or preparation of the manuscript.

Competing Interests: The authors have declared that no competing interests exist.

* E-mail: ljh@cau.edu.cn. (JL); maguangpeng1977@163.com (GM)

❡ These authors contributed equally to this work.

Introduction

A novel influenza A (H1N1) virus of swine origin emerged among humans in Mexico during the spring of 2009 and rapidly spread worldwide [1]. The pandemic prompted the World Health Organization (WHO) to raise the alert level to the highest rating of six, the pandemic phase, within 2 months [2]. In August 2010, WHO officially declared that the disease was in the post-pandemic period [3]; however, it is still circulating among humans, together with seasonal viruses. Although most influenza cases caused by 2009 H1N1 virus infection typically display mild upper respiratory tract syndrome, some cases progress to severe pneumonia and acute respiratory distress syndrome (ARDS) [4,5]. Many studies have shown that ARDS caused by 2009 H1N1 virus results in 17.3–56% mortality [4,6,7,8], which was regarded as the major cause of death by 2009 H1N1 virus infection [9]. ARDS is the result of acute injury to lung tissue, commonly resulting from sepsis, trauma, and severe pulmonary infections [10]. Infectious factors, most of which are viruses, have become one of the most important causes of ARDS in humans [11,12,13]. Clinical cases and established animal models have revealed that the pathogenesis and pathological features of ARDS induced by different viral pathogens are distinct [14,15]. However, knowledge of the pathogenesis of 2009 H1N1 virus, especially ARDS induced by 2009 H1N1 virus, is still limited and hinders therapeutic strategies. Therefore, it is necessary to evaluate the pathogenesis of ARDS caused by 2009 H1N1 virus infection in an appropriate animal model to assess potential therapies.

Mice are a good model for evaluating the pathogenesis and antiviral therapy of influenza pneumonia, due to the general fidelity of the illness in mice to the human disease [16]. Moreover, a mouse model of ARDS caused by highly pathogenic H5N1 avian influenza virus infection has been well established [13]. The typical 2009 H1N1 virus, such as A/California/04/2009 (CA/04), can efficiently replicate in mouse lungs without prior host adaptation. However, it only causes moderate lung lesions and no mortality, even when inoculated at a high dose of 10^6 pfu [17,18]. Thus, such typical 2009 H1N1 viruses may not be able to induce ARDS in a mouse model.

In the present study, we used a virulent variant 2009 H1N1 virus, which was isolated from a pig and possessed a virulence-associated HA-D222G mutation, to establish an ARDS mouse model. The model established here provides a useful tool to explore the mechanism of ARDS, as well as screening and therapeutic options.

Results

Clinical and gross pathologic observation

Six-week-old female mice were infected intranasally (i.n.) with $10^{2.5}$ pfu SD/09 virus. Some of the infected mice showed signs of illness, such as altered gait, inactivity, ruffled fur, and anorexia on day 2 post-infection (p.i.). From day 2 p.i., the body weight of most mice significantly decreased (Figure S1). By day 6 p.i., most mice presented with more severe clinical signs of respiratory disease, including labored respiration and respiratory distress, and most mice lost almost 20% of their initial body weight. On day 8 p.i., most mice were nearly unable to respond to exterior stimuli, and acute respiratory rates and labored respiration were observed (Video S1, and Video S2 for control). Approximately 60% of mice died between days 8 and 10 p.i. Gross observation of infected mice showed that the lungs were highly edematous, with profuse areas of hemorrhage and consolidation. No obvious gross lesions were observed in the kidneys, liver, spleen or brain of infected mice.

Replication kinetics of SD/09 virus in mouse tissues

Mice were infected i.n. with $10^{2.5}$ pfu SD/09 virus, and three mice were euthanized on days 2, 4, 6, 8, 10 and 14 p.i., and the virus titers in viscera were determined. As shown in Figure 1A, the virus titer in the lung gradually increased between days 2 and 6 p.i., and reached a peak on day 6 p.i. The virus titers in the lung gradually decreased from day 6 p.i., and only one of three mice possessed detectable virus in the lungs on day 10 p.i. No viruses were detected in other organs, including heart, spleen, liver, kidneys, blood and brain, at the indicated time. These results indicate that SD/09 virus could replicate efficiently in mouse lung but did not cause systemic infection.

Lung edema induced by SD/09 virus

As shown in Figure 1B, the effect of SD/09 viral infection on lung wet:dry weight ratio did not change significantly within 2 days p.i. However, a dramatic increase was observed from day 4 p.i., and reached a peak on day 8 p.i., which was nearly twice that observed in control group lungs ($p<0.01$). The change in lung wet weight:body weight ratio was similar to the change in lung wet:dry weight ratio (Figure 1C). The results indicated that the SD/09 virus could induce acute lung edema in mice.

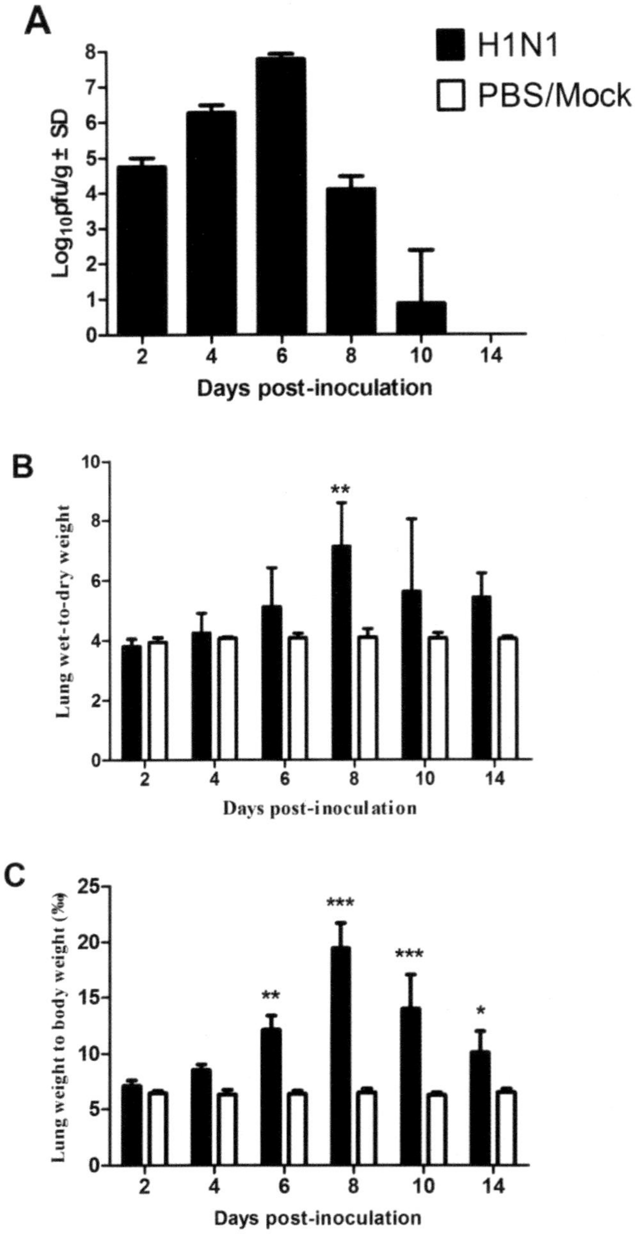

Figure 1. Virus titers in lung (A), wet:dry weight ratio (B) and wet weight:body weight ratios (C) of SD/09-infected mice. Mice were inoculated i.n. with $10^{2.5}$ pfu SD/09 viruses; tissues were collected at indicated times p.i. and viruses were titrated in MDCK cells. Body weight, lung wet and dry weight were determined and recorded. The lung wet weight:body weight ratio and lung wet:dry weight ratio were calculated and used as an indicator of lung edema. *$p<0.05$, **$p<0.01$, ***$p<0.001$, comparison between ratios obtained from the virus-infected and control groups. Bars represent means ± SD of data from three mice.

Histopathology and immunohistochemistry

Kinetic observation of lung lesions of SD/09-virus-infected mice is shown in Figure 2. On day 4 p.i., lung lesions were characterized by dropout of mucous epithelium and inflammatory cells adhering to the bronchiolar surface (Figure 2C, D). On day 6 p.i., severe edema could be seen around blood vessels (Figure 2E); interstitial pneumonia was also observed that showed interstitial edema and thickening of the alveolar walls; and the alveolar lumen was flooded with detached alveolar cells, erythrocytes, and inflammatory cells (Figure 2E, F). On day 8 p.i., the virus caused more severe interstitial pneumonia and peribronchiolitis, characterized by edema and extensive of lymphocytes, neutrophils and plasma cells around the area of bronchiolitis (Figure 2G, H). Lesions in the lungs of infected mice were still severe on day 14 p.i., with extensive alveolar collapse, and remaining alveoli were filled with fibrin, desquamated alveolar cells, and inflammatory cells. Lymphocytes and alveolar macrophages were the predominant inflammatory cells observed at high magnification (Figure 2J). Masson's stain revealed that alveolar walls and spaces were filled with collagen fibers (Figure 3A, B), indicating that proliferative fibroblastic lesions may develop. In comparison, lungs from mock-infected control mice had no apparent histological changes (Figure 2A, 2B, 3C).

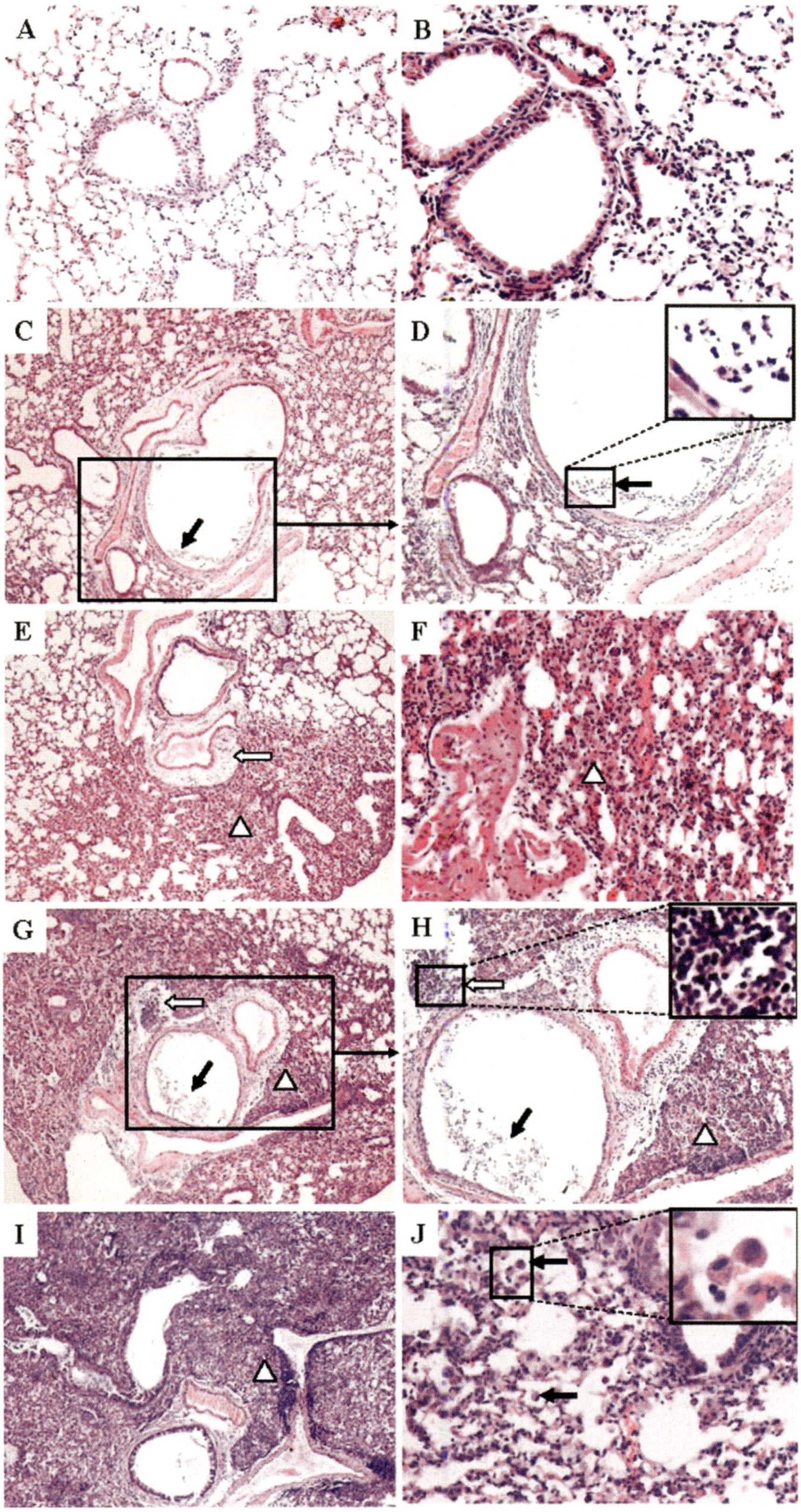

Figure 2. Hematoxylin-eosin stained sections from lung tissues of SD/09-infected mice. Normal mouse lungs (A, B). On day 4 p.i., dropout of mucous epithelium and inflammatory cells adhered to the surface of bronchioles (C, D, solid arrows). On day 6 p.i., severe edema around blood vessels (E, open arrows); dropout of alveolar epithelial, erythrocytes, and inflammatory cells within alveolar spaces (E, F, Δ). On day 8 p.i., the virus caused more severe interstitial pneumonia (G, H, Δ), bronchiolitis (G, H, solid arrows) and peribronchiolitis (G, H, open arrows). On day 14 p.i., the interstitial tissue was thickened with fibrin exudation and organization (I, Δ). Lymphocytes and alveolar macrophages were the predominant inflammatory cells observed (J, solid arrows). Magnification: C, E, G, and I, ×100; A, D and H, ×200; B, F and J, ×400.

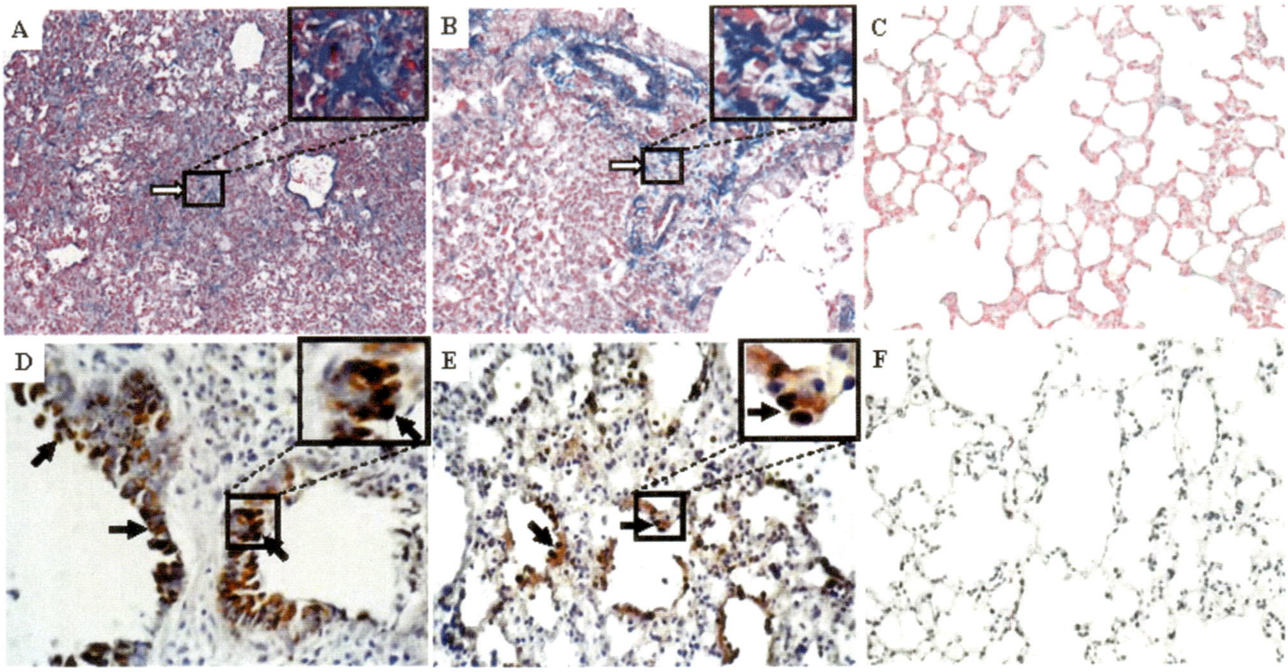

Figure 3. Masson's trichrome stained sections (A–C) and immunohistochemical staining for influenza A nucleoprotein (D–F) of the SD/09-infected mouse lung. Alveoli were collapsed and filled with collagen fibers (A, B, open arrows); normal mouse lungs (C). Influenza A nucleoprotein (brown) in the epithelial cells of the bronchioles (D, solid arrows); viral nucleoprotein in abundant terminal bronchioles epithelial cells and few alveolar epithelial cells (E, solid arrows); normal mouse lungs (F). Magnification: A, ×100; B, C, D, E and F, ×400.

Immunohistochemistry revealed viral antigens in the epithelial cells of the bronchioles (Figure 3D), terminal bronchioles, and alveolar epithelial cells (Figure 3E). These data indicated that SD/09 virus could infect the epithelia of the lower airway and cause viral pneumonia in mice.

Arterial blood gas analysis

As shown in Table 1, virus-infected mice showed a slightly decreased partial pressure of arterial oxygen (Pa_{O2}), saturation of arterial oxygen (Sa_{O2}), and slightly increased partial pressure of arterial carbon dioxide (Pa_{CO2}) from days 4 to 6 p.i. Most infected mice presented with severe clinical signs of respiratory distress on day 8 p.i., and blood gas analysis also showed that Pa_{O2} and Sa_{O2} dramatically decreased compared with the controls ($p<0.05$). These results suggested acute respiratory dysfunction and severe hypoxemia in virus-infected mice.

Leukocyte counts in Bronchial Alveolar Lavage Fluid (BALF)

The number of leukocytes in BALF from SD/09-infected mice showed an increase from day 4 p.i. (Table 2). The BALF of virus-infected mice on day 6 p.i contained 1.1×10^6 cells/ml and was significantly different from the 1.6×10^5 cells/ml observed for PBS-inoculated mice ($p<0.001$). These data indicate a dramatic increase in inflammatory cells in the lungs of SD/09-infected mice. To quantify the immune cell subpopulations responding to viral infection, we next determined cell differential counts in the infected lungs by Wright staining. Compared with PBS-inoculated animals, mice infected with SD/09 virus exhibited an increase of neutrophils from 4 days p.i., and the peak was 18-fold greater than that of the control group on day 8 p.i.

Peripheral blood leukocyte counts

Figure 4A shows a progressive reduction in the number of leukocytes observed on days 4–10 p.i. in virus-infected mice.

Table 1. Arterial blood gas analysis.

Time (d)	PaO_2 (mmHg)		$PaCO_2$ (mmHg)		SaO_2 (%)	
	H1N1	Control	H1N1	Control	H1N1	Control
4	82.00±1.41	93.00±9.65	35.00±5.65	29.50±3.54	91.00±1.41	91.50±2.12
6	74.50±2.12	91.00±1.41	41.00±5.65	30.75±3.18	86.50±2.12	91.00±2.83
8	57.50±3.54*	90.50±3.54	52.50±4.95*	28.50±2.83	78.50±3.54**	91.50±0.71
10	73.00±12.72	89.50±2.12	43.00±4.24	29.25±2.47	83.50±3.54	89.00±4.24
14	71.50±12.02	91.50±3.54	39.50±13.44	31.50±6.36	85.50±3.54	91.50±2.12

Mice were inoculated i.n. with $10^{2.5}$ pfu SD/09 viruses. Arterial blood samples were collected at indicated times p.i.
Values are expressed as mean ± SD.
*$p<0.05$,
**$p<0.01$, comparison between virus-infected and control groups.

Table 2. White blood cell (WBC) summary and differential counts in BALF.

Time (d)		WBC Summary (1×10^5)	WBC count %		
			Macrophages	Lymphocytes	Neutrophils
4	H1N1	3.92±0.14	55.16±6.80*	38.26±5.60*	3.69±0.89**
	Control	1.57±0.26	89.38±6.21	8.62±1.25	0.68±0.21
6	H1N1	10.75±5.62***	31.66±2.39**	49.44±6.26**	12.72±2.77***
	Control	1.49±0.29	90.65±2.71	6.97±2.25	0.69±0.35
8	H1N1	9.16±2.21**	26.63±2.19**	40.4±3.22**	28.93±1.98***
	Control	1.85±0.59	88.66±4.34	7.65±1.20	1.58±0.48
10	H1N1	8.59±2.81**	33.23±2.70**	42.25±4.42**	21.62±7.90***
	Control	1.69±0.48	89.32±4.8	6.93±1.2	0.99±0.37

Mice were inoculated i.n. with $10^{2.5}$ pfu SD/09 viruses, and BALF was prepared at indicated times p.i.
Values are expressed as mean ± SD.
*p<0.05.
**, p<0.01,
***p<0.001, comparison between virus-infected and control groups.

Leukopenia was detected on day 4 p.i., and was statistically significant on day 6 p.i. ($p<0.05$); the lowest value appeared on day 8 p.i. ($p<0.001$). Furthermore, differential blood counts revealed that the number of lymphocytes sharply decreased in infected mice. The lowest number of lymphocytes observed occurred on day 8 p.i. (Figure 4B), which dropped to <20% of the control group number ($p<0.001$).

Cytokine production following SD/09 infection

To determine the cytokine responses that occur after SD/09 virus infection, we measured the levels of five cytokines and chemokines in lungs of infected mice on days 2, 4, 6, 8 and 10 p.i. As shown in Figure 5, all five were significantly different between virus-infected and control mice. Interleukin (IL)-6 and IL-10 in the virus-infected mice reached peak levels as early as day 2 p.i. and were significantly higher than those of the control group ($p<0.001$). Interferon (IFN)-γ, monocyte chemotactic protein (MCP)-1, and tumor necrosis factor (TNF) dramatically increased in mouse lungs on days 6–8 p.i. ($p<0.001$), consistent with the appearance of pulmonary lesions. These results showed that infection with SD/09 viruses resulted in elevated amounts of proinflammatory chemokines and cytokines in the lungs of mice.

Discussion

In the spring of 2009, a novel influenza A(H1N1) virus rapidly spread worldwide, resulting in the first influenza pandemic of the 21st century [1]. Critically ill cases caused by 2009 H1N1 virus retrospectively showed that most had progressed or died due to ARDS [4,6]. However, the pathogenesis and therapeutic intervention of ARDS caused by 2009 H1N1 infection have still not been elucidated. Animal models of disease are important for characterizing pathogenesis and developing the preclinical evidence for revised approaches to ventilating patients with ARDS [19]. Here, we present a mouse model for the study of ARDS induced by SD/09 virus, a virulent 2009 H1N1 variant.

Previous studies have indicated that typical 2009 H1N1 viruses such as CA/04 bind only to α-2,6-linked sialic acid (SA) receptor

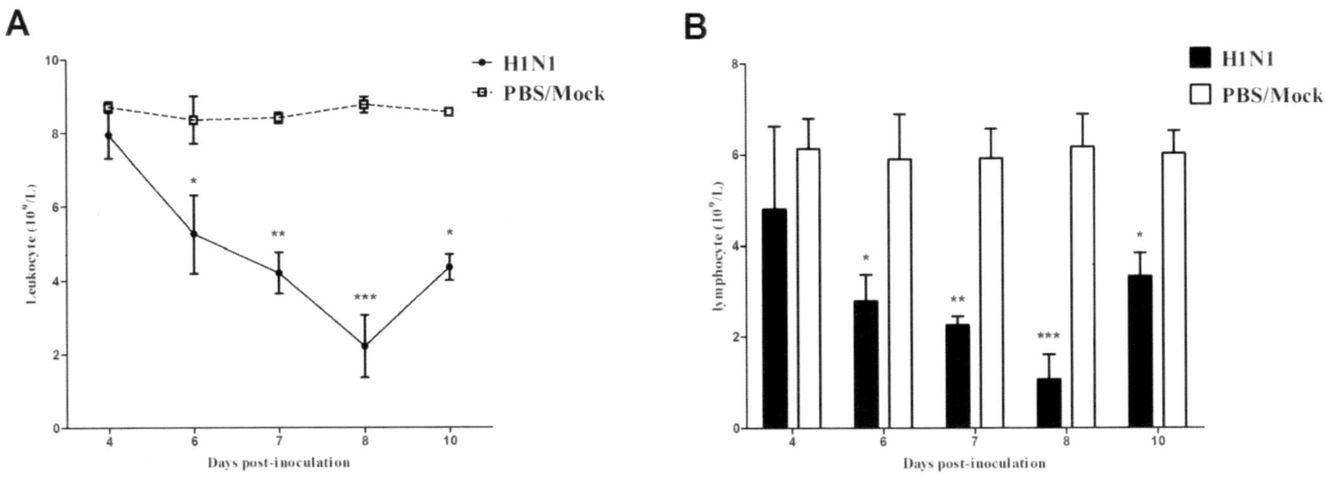

Figure 4. Kinetic analysis of circulating leukocytes (A) and lymphocyte (B) following SD/09 virus infection. Peripheral blood samples were collected at indicated times p.i. The total number of leukocytes and differential blood counts for three individual mice were analyzed. *p<0.05 **, p<0.01, ***p<0.001, comparison between virus-infected and control groups.

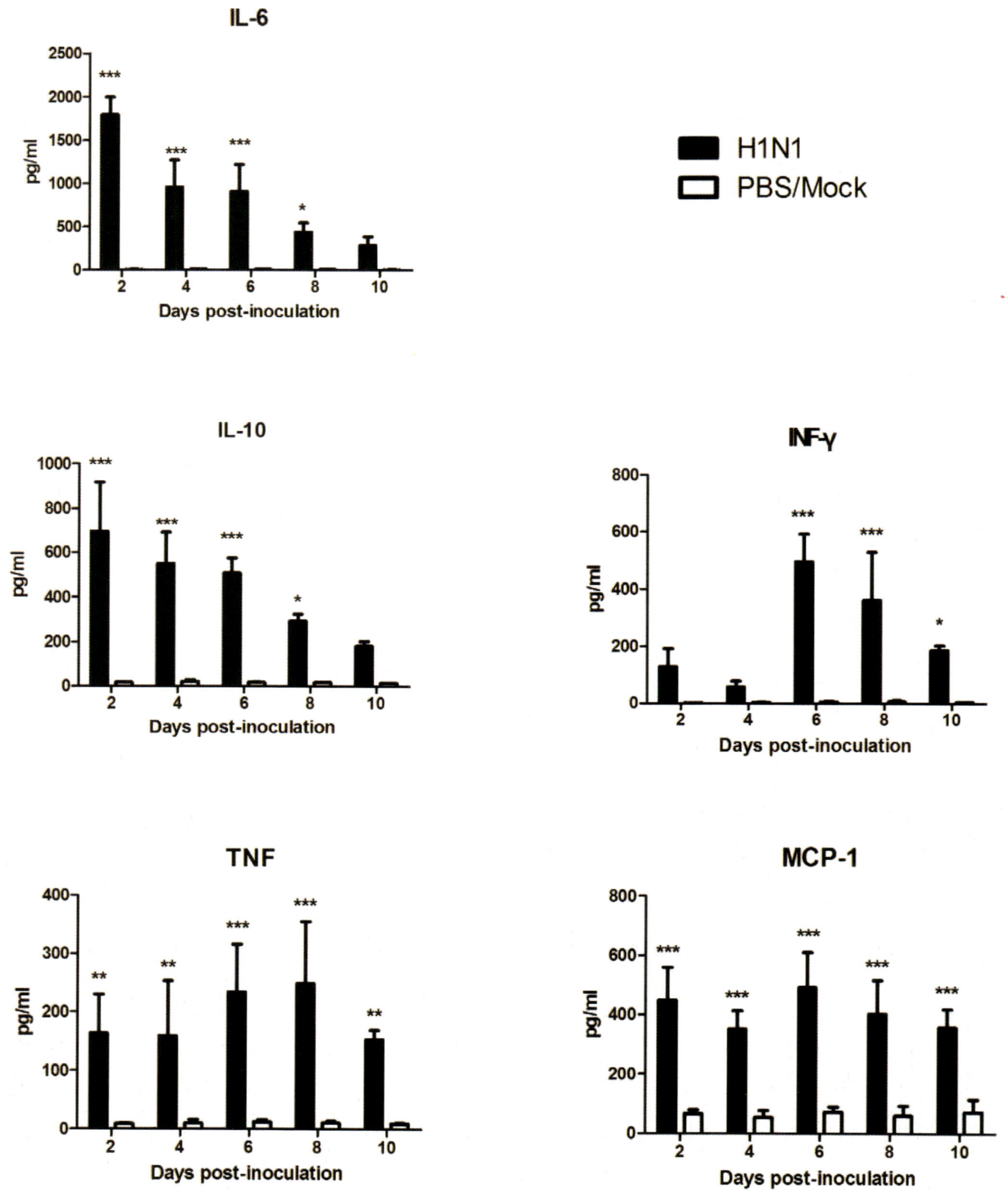

Figure 5. Cytokine levels in virus-infected mouse lungs. Mice were euthanized at indicated times p.i. The collected lungs were weighed, and 10% homogenates were prepared in cold PBS. Cytokine levels from lung homogenates were measured using the Cytokine Bead Array system. *$p<0.05$, **$p<0.01$, ***$p<0.001$, comparison between virus-infected and control groups.

[17], but only the α-2,3-linked SA receptor is found in the mouse respiratory tract [20]. Therefore, such a typical 2009 H1N1 virus may not be able to induce ARDS in mice. In fact, we used CA/04 virus to induce ARDS in mice; however, animals inoculated with a high dose of CA/04 virus ($10^{6.5}$ pfu) only showed moderate respiratory symptoms, and no lethality was observed (unpublished

data). It has been shown that 2009 H1N1 virus possessing a D222G mutation in hemagglutinin (HA) could increase the pathogenicity in mice [21,22] and binding to the α-2,3 SA receptor [23]. Moreover, clinical data indicate that such variants are only associated with severe H1N1 human infection [24]. Therefore, we suggest that the variant possessing the D222G mutation in HA can induce ARDS in a mouse model. The virus used in the present study was isolated from swine in 2009, and sequence analysis revealed that all the eight genes of the isolate had a close relationship with the 2009 H1N1 influenza virus circulating in humans. Notably, the swine isolate, SD/09, had a D222G mutation in HA. Compared with CA/04 virus ($LD_{50}>10^6$ pfu), SD/09 showed significantly increased virulence in mice, with an LD_{50} of $10^{2.25}$ pfu, which was nearly identical to that of the mouse-adapted strain A/Hong Kong/415742Md/09 ($LD_{50}=10^{2.2}$pfu) [17,21]. Mice infected i.n. with $10^{2.5}$ pfu SD/09 virus showed obvious respiratory symptoms, including visually prominent signs of respiratory distress and abdominal respiration, with approximately 60% mortality between days 8 and 10 p.i. The lungs of virus-infected mice were highly edematous, which was also demonstrated by dramatically increased lung wet:dry weight ratio. Pathological changes presented a progressive pattern, typically diffuse alveolar damage, interstitial and alveolar edema, neutrophil and macrophage-dominant inflammatory cellular infiltration, and areas of hemorrhage and necrotizing bronchiolitis. Arterial blood gas saturation is a key parameter of ARDS in humans [25]. In the present mouse model, Pao_2 and Sao_2 of infected mice were significantly lower than in the control group from day 2 p.i., especially on day 8 p.i., where these parameters sharply decreased, and most virus-infected mice began to die. These changes in arterial blood gas demonstrated that most infected mice developed severe hypoxemia consistent with of the appearance of clinical signs and lung lesions of ARDS.

Previous studies showed that mice infected with typical 2009 H1N1 virus only exhibited mild interstitial inflammatory infiltration and limited alveolitis [18,21], whereas severe lung damage was found in the SD/09-infected mice, including severe edema around the blood vessels and bronchiolitis, and extensive inflammatory accumulation from 4 to 8 days p.i. At 10 days p.i., the surviving mice developed an irreversible fibrosis involving collagen deposition in alveolar walls and spaces, which was similar to that observed in human ARDS patients with 2009 H1N1 infection [26]. Our histopathological results were consistent with ARDS induced by other influenza viruses. Mice infected with mouse-adapted virus of the A/Puerto Rico/8/34 (H1N1), or high pathogenic H5N1 virus also showed a progressive series of pathological changes from interstitial pneumonia to diffuse alveolar damage [13,27]. However, in contrast to highly pathogenic H5N1 virus, mice infected with SD/09 virus did not show viral spread to extrapulmonary organs.

Immunohistochemical examination revealed the presence of viral antigens in the bronchioles, terminal bronchiolar epithelium, and alveolar epithelial cells. Perhaps SD/09 virus infection of the alveoli, particularly type II pneumocytes, rather than bronchioles, is a key to the development of ARDS. Type II pneumocytes are responsible for the production and secretion of surfactant to lower the surface tension of water and allow membrane separation, and insufficient pulmonary surfactant in the alveoli may result in alveolar collapse [28,29]. The 1918 pandemic H1N1 and high pathogenic H5N1 viruses preferentially infect type II pneumocytes and alveolar macrophage in mice [15,30]. Alveolar macrophages may play a critical role in disease pathogenesis, not through production of infectious virus but rather through the upregulation of proinflammatory cytokines that may further damage alveolar pneumocytes [31]. These phenomena suggest that viral cell tropism may determine the processes of ARDS.

Pulmonary aberrant immune response is considered a significant feature of ARDS induced by 2009 H1N1 virus [19,32]. In the present mouse model, the number of leukocytes observed in the BALF of virus-infected mice significantly increased compared with the control mice on day 8 p.i. Different counts in BALF showed that the proportion of neutrophils dramatically increased. These innate immune cells were capable of reducing the virus load in the lung [33]; however, they could cause lung injury through direct or indirect mechanisms. Neutrophil oxidants and proteases can cause direct injury of cells in the alveolar-capillary membrane [34]. Neutrophils and macrophages can secrete copious amounts of chemokines and cytokines that can recruit more immune cells into lung tissues, and produce a "cytokine storm", one of the most important factors in the production of ARDS [35].

A retrospective cohort study of 74 2009 H1N1 patients found that higher levels of proinflammatory cytokines and chemokines in plasma were observed in the ARDS-death group compared with the survived-without-ARDS or the mild-disease groups [5]. Another study in critically ill patients with ARDS caused by 2009 H1N1 virus infection has shown that the hallmarks of disease severity were elevated levels of IL-6, IL-15, IL-8 and TNF-α [36]. We examined the levels of five cytokines and chemokines in infected mouse lungs and found significant differences between the virus-infected and mock groups. It has proved that high levels of IL-6 were able to mediate acute lung injury [37], and had a negative correlation with the Pa_{O2}:Fi_{O2} ratio in severely affected patients with 2009 H1N1 virus infection [36]. Our data showed SD/09 viral infection induced high levels of IL-6 in mouse lung, which may also play an important role in the course of ARDS. Hagau etc. found the levels of TNF-α increased significantly in the 2009 H1N1-related ARDS patients [36]. In present study, TNF levels also dramatically increased in the lungs of virus-infected mice, and were consistent with the clinical symptoms and reached peak levels when mice began to die. In addition, high levels of IL-10, IFN-γ and MCP-1 were also present in the virus-infected mouse lungs, similar to observations found in severely affected humans with 2009 H1N1 infection [38].

In summary, we successfully established an ARDS mouse model induced by a virulent 2009 H1N1 variant, which demonstrated key human ARDS clinical and pathological features, such as respiratory distress, low Pa_{O2}, exudative, proliferative and fibrotic lung, and high levels of inflammatory cells and cytokines. The mouse model may contribute to the study of the pathogenesis and therapy of ARDS induced by 2009 H1N1 virus.

Materials and Methods

Ethics statement

All animal research was approved by the Beijing Association for Science and Technology (approval ID SYXK (Beijing) 2007-0023) and complied with the guidelines of Beijing Laboratory Animal Welfare and Ethics of the Beijing Administration Committee of Laboratory Animals.

Viruses

The pandemic 2009 H1N1 virus, A/swine/Shandong/731/2009 (SD/09), was isolated from swine in Shandong Province, China, in December 2009. The complete genomic sequences for this virus are available in the GenBank database under accession numbers FJ951848–FJ951855. All the eight gene segments from the swine isolate have a close relationship to 2009 H1N1 influenza virus circulating in the human population and possess homologies of 99.3–99.9% to those of a human representative 2009 H1N1 strain A/California/04/2009. Virus stock was propagated in the Madin–Darby canine kidney (MDCK) cells at 37°C for 48 h and stored at −80°C for use in all the experiments. The titers of stock viruses were determined by plaque assays in MDCK cells. To determine LD_{50} of SD/09 virus, eight 6-week-old female BALB/c mice per group were inoculated i.n. with 10^1–10^6 pfu (50 μl) viruses and monitored for 14 days. The value of MLD50 was calculated using the Spearman–Karber method and expressed by pfu per MLD_{50} [39].

Experimental infections

We evaluated the pathogenicity of the virus in mice and found that it could efficiently replicate in the lungs of mice with high lethality ($10^{2.25}$ pfu per MLD_{50}). To determine the optimal dose of inoculation, 10 mice in each group were infected i.n. with $10^{1.5}$, $10^{2.5}$ or $10^{3.5}$ pfu viruses, and the signs, body weight, and mortality were monitored daily for each group for 14 days. Pilot experiments indicated that a dose of $10^{2.5}$ pfu was optimal, because the course of the disease was prolonged and the mice presented with obvious signs of respiratory illness.

BALB/c mice were lightly anesthetized and inoculated i.n. with 50 μl $10^{2.5}$ pfu SD/09 virus in PBS. Mock-infected animals were inoculated i.n. with 50 μl PBS. At the indicated time, infected mice were sacrificed, and the parameters that present the course of the disease were determined. Twenty mice (10 infected with SD/09 virus and 10 inoculated with PBS) were used to investigate clinical signs and mortality for 14 days.

Virus titration

Three mice were euthanized on days 2, 4, 6, 8, 10 and 14 p.i. and their organs were collected. The collected tissues were weighed, and 10% homogenates were prepared in cold PBS. The homogenates were centrifuged at 3000 rpm for 10 min to remove cell debris, and then the supernatants were 10-fold serially diluted for viral titer determination by plaque assay in MDCK cells. Virus titers were expressed as mean log pfu/g ± standard deviation (SD).

Assessment of lung water content

Three mice were euthanized on days 2, 4, 6, 8, 10 and 14 p.i., and the lungs were removed and weighed and then desiccated in an oven at 60°C for 72 h. The lung wet weight:body weight ratio and lung wet:dry weight ratio were calculated and used as an indicator of lung edema, as previously described [40].

Histopathological examination

Three mice were euthanized on days 4, 6, 8 and 14 p.i. The lungs were fixed in 10% buffered formalin, embedded in paraffin, sectioned, and stained with hematoxylin and eosin. Lungs on day 14 p.i. were also stained with Masson's trichrome.

Immunohistochemistry

Lung tissue sections taken on day 6 p.i. were stained for influenza A virus antigens. An anti-influenza nucleoprotein monoclonal antibody (AA5H; Abcam, Hong Kong) was used to identify influenza A virus nucleoprotein in sections. Secondary antibody (Millipore, Billerica, MA, USA) against the primary antibody was labeled with horseradish peroxidase, and the color reaction was developed with a horseradish peroxidase reaction kit (diaminobenzidine- tetrahydrochloride; Sigma, St. Louis, MO, USA).

Arterial blood gas analysis

Blood gas analysis was performed as previously described [13,41]. Three mice were anesthetized with Zoletil (tiletamine-zolazepam; Virbac; 20 μg/g) on days 4, 6, 8, 10 and 14 p.i. Arterial blood samples were withdrawn into a heparinized syringe by percutaneous left ventricular sampling of lightly anesthetized mice that were spontaneously breathing room air. Blood gas analysis was immediately performed using a Vetstat Electrolyte and Blood Gas Analyzer (Idexx laboratories, Westbrook, MA, USA).

Leukocyte counts in BALF

Leukocyte counts in BALF were performed as previously described [42,43]. Briefly, three mice were euthanized on days 4, 6, 8 and 10 p.i., and the lungs were lavaged twice *in situ* with the chest cavity opened by midline incision with a total volume of 1.0 ml saline (4°C) inserted through an endotracheal tube. The rate of recovery of BALF was not less than 90% for all animals tested. After the amount of fluid recovered was recorded, an aliquot of BALF was diluted 1:1 with 0.01% crystal violet and 2.7% acetic acid for leukocyte staining and erythrocyte hemolysis. The number of leukocytes in the BALF was counted with a hemacytometer under a microscope. For differential counts, the BALF samples from each mouse were stained with Wright stain, and the numbers of monocytes, neutrophil and lymphocytes were determined, on the basis of morphologic criteria, under a light microscope, with evaluation of at least 200 cells per slide. All slides were counted twice by different observers blinded to the status of the animal.

Peripheral blood leukocyte counts

Heparinized blood samples were collected on days 4, 6, 8 and 10 p.i. The total numbers of leukocytes and differential blood counts for three individual mice were analyzed using an automated hematology analyzer.

Cytokine analysis in mouse lung

IL-6, IL-10, TNF, IFN-γ and MCP-1 levels were determined in lung homogenates using a cytometric bead array technique (BD Cytometric BEAD Array Mouse Inflammation Kit; BD Bioscience, San Diego, CA, USA) according to the manufacturer's instructions. Briefly, 50 μl mouse inflammation capture bead suspension and 50 μl PE detection reagent were added to an equal amount of sample standard dilution and incubated for 2 h at room temperature in the dark. Subsequently, samples were washed by adding 1 ml wash buffer and centrifugation at 200× g at room temperature for 5 min. Supernatants were discarded and 300 μl wash buffer was added. Samples were analyzed on a BD FACSArray bioanalyzer (BD Bioscience) according to the manufacturer's instructions. Standard curves were prepared similar to the method above. Data were analyzed using BD CBA Software (BD Bioscience). Finally, the chemokine or cytokine levels were recorded as pg/ml homogenate.

Statistics

Data were analyzed by two-way analysis of variance using GraphPad Prism version 5.00 (GraphPad Software, San Diego, CA, USA). When a significant effect was observed, pairwise comparisons were performed using the Bonferroni post-hoc test. All data are reported as mean ± SD.

Supporting Information

Figure S1 Body weight changes p.i. Mice were inoculated i.n. with indicated doses of SD/09 viruses or PBS. Body weights were recorded every day p.i. The percentage of the body weight p.i. to the initial weight is shown. Bars represent means ± SD.

Video S1 Clinical symptoms of the mice infected with SD/09 virus on day 8 p.i.

Video S2 Normal appearance of the mice inoculated with PBS on day 8 p.i.

Acknowledgments

The authors thank Dr. Yanxin Hu and Dr. Deping Han for technical assistance in histopathologic observation.

Author Contributions

Conceived and designed the experiments: JL GM YZ HS. Performed the experiments: YZ HS YM JY JP. Analyzed the data: YZ HS YS LF GM JP. Wrote the paper: YZ HS YS JQ JL.

References

1. Writing Committee of the WHO Consultation on Clinical Aspects of Pandemic (H1N1) 2009 Influenza (2010) Clinical Aspects of Pandemic 2009 Influenza A (H1N1) Virus Infection. New Engl J Med 362: 1708–1719.
2. World Health Organization. World now at the start of 2009 influenza pandemic. In: Statement to the press by WHO director June 11 2009. Available: http://www.who.int/mediacentre/news/statements/2009/h1n1_pandemic_phase6_20090611/en/index.html. [Accessed 3 September 2010].
3. World Health Organization. H1N1 now in the post-pandemic period. Available: http://www.who.int/csr/disease/swineflu/en/. [Accessed 10 August 2010].
4. Estenssoro E, Rios FG, Apezteguia C, Reina R, Neira J, et al. (2010) Pandemic 2009 influenza A (H1N1) in Argentina: a study of 337 patients on mechanical ventilation. Am J Resp Crit Care Med 182: 41–48.
5. To Kelvin KW, Hung Ivan FN, Li Iris WS, Lee KL, Koo CK, et al. (2010) Delayed Clearance of Viral Load and Marked Cytokine Activation in Severe Cases of Pandemic H1N1 2009 Influenza Virus Infection. Clin Infect Dis 50: 850–859.
6. The ANZIC Influenza Investigators (2009) Critical Care Services and 2009 H1N1 Influenza in Australia and New Zealand. New Engl J Med 361: 1925–1934.
7. Kumar A, Zarychanski R, Pinto R, Cook DJ, Marshall J, et al. (2009) Critically ill patients with 2009 influenza A (H1N1) infection in Canada. JAMA 302: 1872.
8. Roch A, Lepaul-Ercole R, Grisoli D, Bessereau J, Brissy O, et al. (2010) Extracorporeal membrane oxygenation for severe influenza A (H1N1) acute respiratory distress syndrome: a prospective observational comparative study. Intensive Care Med 36: 1899–1905.
9. Centers for Disease Control and Prevention (CDC) (2009) Update: swine influenza A (H1N1) infections–California and Texas, April 2009. MMWR Morb Mortal Wkly Rep 58: 435–437.
10. Udobi KF, Childs E, Touijer K (2003) Acute respiratory distress syndrome. Am Fam Physician 67: 315–322.
11. Levy MM, Baylor MS, Bernard GR, Fowler R, Franks TJ, et al. (2005) Clinical issues and research in respiratory failure from severe acute respiratory syndrome. Am J Resp Crit Care Med 171: 518.
12. Chen CY, Lee CH, Liu CY, Wang JH, Wang LM, et al. (2005) Clinical features and outcomes of severe acute respiratory syndrome and predictive factors for acute respiratory distress syndrome. J Chin Med Assoc 68: 4–10.
13. Xu T, Qiao J, Zhao L, Wang G, He G, et al. (2006) Acute Respiratory Distress Syndrome Induced by Avian Influenza A (H5N1) Virus in Mice. Am J Resp Crit Care Med 174: 1011–1017.
14. Peiris M (2008) Pathogenesis of Avian Flu H5N1 and SARS. In: Derek J. Chadwick, Organizer JG, eds. Innate Immunity to Pulmonary Infection John Wiley & Sons, Ltd. pp 56–65.
15. Garigliany M-M (2010) Influenza A Strain-Dependent Pathogenesis in Fatal H1N1 and H5N1 Subtype Infections of Mice. Emerg Infect Dis 16: 595–603.
16. Barnard DL (2009) Animal models for the study of influenza pathogenesis and therapy. Antivir Res 82: A110–A122.
17. Maines TR, Jayaraman A, Belser JA, Wadford DA, Pappas C, et al. (2009) Transmission and pathogenesis of swine-origin 2009 A (H1N1) influenza viruses in ferrets and mice. Science 325: 484.
18. Ye J, Sorrell EM, Cai Y, Shao H, Xu K, et al. (2010) Variations in the Hemagglutinin of the 2009 H1N1 Pandemic Virus: Potential for Strains with Altered Virulence Phenotype? PLoS Pathog 6: e1001145.
19. Matthay MA (2005) Acute Lung Injury and the Acute Respiratory Distress Syndrome: Four Decades of Inquiry into Pathogenesis and Rational Management. Am J Resp Cell Mol 33: 319–327.
20. Ibricevic A, Pekosz A, Walter MJ, Newby C, Battaile JT, et al. (2006) Influenza Virus Receptor Specificity and Cell Tropism in Mouse and Human Airway Epithelial Cells. J Virol 80: 7469–7480.
21. Zheng B, Chan KH, Zhang AJ, Zhou J, Chan CC, et al. (2010) D225G mutation in hemagglutinin of pandemic influenza H1N1 (2009) virus enhances virulence in mice. Exp Biol Med (Maywood) 235: 981–988.
22. Xu L, Bao L, Lv Q, Deng W, Ma Y, et al. (2010) A single-amino-acid substitution in the HA protein changes the replication and pathogenicity of the 2009 pandemic A (H1N1) influenza viruses in vitro and in vivo. Virol J 7: 325.
23. Chutinimitkul S, Herfst S, Steel J, Lowen AC, Ye J, et al. (2010) Virulence-Associated Substitution D222G in the Hemagglutinin of 2009 Pandemic Influenza A (H1N1) Virus Affects Receptor Binding. J Virol 84: 11802–11813.
24. Kilander A, Rykkvin R, Dudman SG, Hungnes O (2010) Observed association between the HA1 mutation D222G in the 2009 pandemic influenza A(H1N1) virus and severe clinical outcome, Norway 2009–2010. Euro Surveill 15: 1–3.
25. Connelly KG, Repine JE (1997) Markers for predicting the development of acute respiratory distress syndrome. Annu Rev Med 48: 429–445.
26. Pinilla I, Martí de Gracia M, Quintana-Díaz M, Figueira J (2011) Radiological prognostic factors in patients with pandemic H1N1 (pH1N1) infection requiring hospital admission. Emergency Radiology 18: 313–319.
27. Fukushi M, Ito T, Oka T, Kitazawa T, Miyoshi-Akiyama T, et al. (2011) Serial Histopathological Examination of the Lungs of Mice Infected with Influenza A Virus PR8 Strain. PloS one 6: e21207.
28. Griese M (1999) Pulmonary surfactant in health and human lung diseases: state of the art. Eur Respir J 13: 1455–1476.
29. Greene KE, Wright JR, Steinberg KP, Ruzinski JT, Caldwell E, et al. (1999) Serial changes in surfactant-associated proteins in lung and serum before and after onset of ARDS. Am J Resp Crit Care Med 160: 1843.
30. Kash JC, Tumpey TM, Proll SC, Carter V, Perwitasari O, et al. (2006) Genomic analysis of increased host immune and cell death responses induced by 1918 influenza virus. Nature 443: 578.
31. Cheung C, Poon L, Lau A, Luk W, Lau Y, et al. (2002) Induction of proinflammatory cytokines in human macrophages by influenza A (H5N1) viruses: a mechanism for the unusual severity of human disease? The Lancet 360: 1831–1837.
32. Mauad T, Hajjar LA, Callegari GD, da Silva LFF, Schout D, et al. (2010) Lung Pathology in Fatal Novel Human Influenza A (H1N1) Infection. Am J Resp Crit Care Med 181: 72–79.
33. Tumpey TM, Garcia-Sastre A, Taubenberger JK, Palese P, Swayne DE, et al. (2005) Pathogenicity of influenza viruses with genes from the 1918 pandemic virus: functional roles of alveolar macrophages and neutrophils in limiting virus replication and mortality in mice. J Virol 79: 14933–14944.
34. Cochrane C, Spragg R, Revak S (1983) Pathogenesis of the adult respiratory distress syndrome. Evidence of oxidant activity in bronchoalveolar lavage fluid. J Clin Invest 71: 754–761.
35. Osterholm MT (2005) Preparing for the Next Pandemic. New Engl J Med 352: 1839–1842.
36. Hagau N, Slavcovici A, Gonganau DN, Oltean S, Dirzu DS, et al. (2010) Clinical aspects and cytokine response in severe H1N1 influenza A virus infection. Crit Care 14: R203.
37. Imai Y, Kuba K, Neely G, Yaghubian-Malhami R, Perkmann T, et al. (2008) Identification of oxidative stress and Toll-like receptor 4 signaling as a key pathway of acute lung injury. Cell 133: 235–249.
38. Bermejo-Martin JF, Ortiz de Lejarazu R, Pumarola T, Rello J, Almansa R, et al. (2009) Th1 and Th17 hypercytokinemia as early host response signature in severe pandemic influenza. Crit Care 13: R201.
39. Hamilton MA, Russo RC, Thurston RV (1977) Trimmed Spearman-Karber method for estimating median lethal concentrations in toxicity bioassays. Environ Sci Technol 11: 714–719.
40. Lang JD, Figueroa M, Sanders KD, Aslan M, Liu Y, et al. (2005) Hypercapnia via Reduced Rate and Tidal Volume Contributes to Lipopolysaccharide-induced Lung Injury. Am J Resp Crit Care Med 171: 147–157.
41. Fagan K, Fouty B, Tyler R, Morris K, Jr., Hepler L, et al. (1999) The pulmonary circulation of homozygous or heterozygous eNOS-null mice is hyperresponsive to mild hypoxia. J Clin Invest 103: 291–299.
42. Majeski EI, Paintlia MK, Lopez AD, Harley RA, London SD, et al. (2003) Respiratory reovirus 1/L induction of intraluminal fibrosis, a model of bronchiolitis obliterans organizing pneumonia, is dependent on T lymphocytes. Am J Pathol 163: 1467–1479.
43. Nick JA, Young SK, Brown KK, Avdi NJ, Arndt PG, et al. (2000) Role of p38 Mitogen-Activated Protein Kinase in a Murine Model of Pulmonary Inflammation. J Immunol 164: 2151–2159.

4

Adiponectin Gene Polymorphisms and Acute Respiratory Distress Syndrome Susceptibility and Mortality

Amy M. Ahasic[1]*, Yang Zhao[2], Li Su[3], Chau-Chyun Sheu[4], B. Taylor Thompson[5], David C. Christiani[3,5]

1 Section of Pulmonary, Critical Care and Sleep Medicine, Department of Medicine, Yale School of Medicine, New Haven, Connecticut, United States of America, **2** Department of Epidemiology and Biostatistics, School of Public Health, Nanjing Medical University, Nanjing, China, **3** Environmental and Occupational Medicine and Epidemiology Program, Department of Environmental Health, Harvard School of Public Health, Boston, Massachusetts, United States of America, **4** Division of Pulmonary and Critical Care Medicine, Kaohsiung Medical University Hospital, Kaohsiung Medical University, Kaohsiung, Taiwan, **5** Pulmonary and Critical Care Unit, Department of Medicine, Massachusetts General Hospital, Boston, Massachusetts, United States of America

Abstract

Rationale: Adiponectin is an anti-inflammatory adipokine that is the most abundant gene product of adipose tissue. Lower levels have been observed in obesity, insulin resistance, and in critical illness. However, elevated levels early in acute respiratory failure have been associated with mortality. Polymorphisms in adiponectin-related genes (*ADIPOQ*, *ADIPOR1*, *ADIPOR2*) have been examined for relationships with obesity, insulin resistance and diabetes, cardiovascular disease, and to circulating adipokine levels, but many gaps in knowledge remain. The current study aims to assess the association between potentially functional polymorphisms in adiponectin-related genes with acute respiratory distress syndrome (ARDS) risk and mortality.

Methods: Consecutive patients with risk factors for ARDS admitted to the ICU were enrolled and followed prospectively for development of ARDS. ARDS cases were followed through day 60 for all-cause mortality. 2067 patients were successfully genotyped using the Illumina CVD BeadChip high-density platform. Of these, 567 patients developed ARDS. Forty-four single nucleotide polymorphisms (SNPs) on *ADIPOQ*, *ADIPOR1* and *ADIPOR2* were successfully genotyped. Of these, 9 SNPs were hypothesized to be functional based on their location (promoter, exon, or 3′ untranslated region). These 9 SNPs were analyzed for association with ARDS case status and mortality among ARDS cases.

Results: After multivariable analysis and adjustment for multiple comparisons, no SNPs were significantly associated with ARDS case status. Among ARDS cases, homozygotes for the minor allele of rs2082940 (*ADIPOQ*) had increased mortality (hazard ratio 2.61, 95% confidence interval 1.36–5.00, $p = 0.0039$) after adjustment for significant covariates. The significance of this association persisted after adjustment for multiple comparisons ($FDR\_q = 0.029$).

Conclusions: A common and potentially functional polymorphism in *ADIPOQ* may impact survival in ARDS. Further studies are required to replicate these results and to correlate genotype with circulating adiponectin levels.

Editor: Xiaoping Miao, MOE Key Laboratory of Environment and Health, School of Public Health, Tongji Medical College, Huazhong University of Science and Technology, China

Funding: This study was funded in part by the following grants: American Heart Association (www.heart.org) 10FTF3440007 (PI: Ahasic); National Institutes of Health/NIH Heart, Lung and Blood Institute (www.nhlbi.nih.gov) R01 HL60710 (PI: Christiani). The funders had no role in study design, data collection and analysis, decision to publish, or preparation of the manuscript.

Competing Interests: The authors have declared that no competing interests exist.

* E-mail: amy.ahasic@yale.edu

Introduction

Adipose tissue is now recognized as an active endocrine organ. Adipocytes, the primary cells making up adipose, secrete adipokines that have been studied as phenotypic markers for obesity. Adipokines are involved in vascular and generalized inflammation, as well as insulin resistance and atherogenesis [1–5]. They have also been studied in animal models of sepsis [6,7].

Adiponectin is an anti-inflammatory, anti-diabetic, and anti-atherogenic adipokine that is the most abundant gene product of adipose tissue [1–4,8]. Adiponectin is encoded by *ADIPOQ*, located on chr3q27. Adiponectin binds to the AdipoR1 and AdipoR2 receptors, encoded by *ADIPOR1* (chr1q32) and *ADIPOR2* (chr12p13) respectively. AdipoR1 is ubiquitously expressed, particularly in skeletal muscle, while AdipoR2 is primarily expressed in liver as well as skeletal muscle [9,10]. These receptors mediate the biologic effects of adiponectin, and they have strong similarities to G-protein-coupled receptors although they are distinct from this class of receptors. Binding of adiponectin to its receptors results in activation of unique signaling molecules such as AMPK, p38 MAPK, and PPAR-α [10].

Adiponectin has been studied widely in obesity and diabetes, and it is a key suppressor of the metabolic derangements leading to insulin resistance, type 2 diabetes mellitus, metabolic syndrome, and cardiovascular disease [11]. For instance, lower plasma levels of plasma adiponectin have been observed in obesity, insulin resistance, and type 2 diabetes mellitus [12–15]. Adiponectin is also inversely correlated with body mass index (BMI) [9,16]. Genetic studies have investigated the association between adiponectin-related genes and a wide variety of health outcomes, including obesity, diabetes, cardio- and cerebrovascular disease and dyslipidemia, nonalcoholic fatty liver disease, and a variety of cancers including breast, colon and prostate [17].

Adiponectin acts through multiple pathways: it enhances glucose utilization through AMPK phosphorylation; it antagonizes TNF-alpha by negatively regulating its expression in various tissues such as liver and macrophages; and it inhibits endothelial NF-kappa-B signaling through a cAMP-dependent pathway [1,2,4]. It may exert its anti-inflammatory effects by limiting aberrant leukocyte-endothelial interactions and augmenting nitric oxide availability [16]. Lower adiponectin levels have been associated with inflammation, oxidative stress, and glucocorticoids, and the link with insulin signaling suggests that adiponectin secretion is highly affected by the insulin sensitivity of adipocytes [1]. It has been postulated that adiponectin may be associated with development of insulin resistance during critical illness [18].

Because of its links to inflammation and insulin sensitivity, adiponectin has been investigated in a few critical care studies in humans [16,18–21]. In general, these studies observed lower levels of adiponectin at the onset of critical illness, with a rise during recovery [16,18,19,21]. In one study of acute respiratory failure patients, higher levels of adiponectin were associated with fewer ventilator-free days and higher mortality [16]. This limited literature on adiponectin in critical illness has not included studies of genetic variations of the genes encoding adiponectin and its receptors. Thus, the current study aims to investigate the association between genetic variations in adiponectin-related genes and the development of and survival in acute respiratory distress syndrome (ARDS) in a large intensive care unit (ICU) cohort.

Materials and Methods

The Human Subjects Committees (HSC) at the Massachusetts General Hospital (MGH) and the Harvard School of Public Health approved this study, and all participants or appropriate surrogates provided informed consent and signed HSC-approved consent forms.

Study Population and Design

This study is part of the ongoing Molecular Epidemiology of ARDS Study of which study design and exclusion criteria have been described in depth previously [22]. Adult ICU admissions to MGH (Boston, MA) from January 1999 to March 2009, and at Beth Israel-Deaconess Medical Center (BIDMC, Boston, MA) from January 2007 to February 2009 were screened daily for study-defined clinical risk factors for ARDS: pneumonia, sepsis or septic shock, aspiration, massive transfusions, pulmonary contusion or multiple fractures. Eligible patients were approached and enrolled in the prospective cohort after consent was obtained. Patients were followed daily until ICU discharge or death. They were defined as having ARDS if they developed respiratory failure requiring intubation and mechanical ventilation, and if they met the North American-European Consensus Conference (AECC) criteria for ARDS: arterial oxygen tension/fraction of inspired oxygen ratio (PaO_2/FiO_2) of $\leq$200 mm Hg; bilateral infiltrates on chest radiograph; and pulmonary arterial occlusion pressure $\leq$18 mm Hg, or no clinical evidence of left atrial hypertension. In the parent study, ARDS patients are cases, and patients with ARDS risk factors who did not develop ARDS are controls. Day 0 of ARDS was defined as the day on which the case patient first met all AECC criteria simultaneously. ARDS cases were followed until Day 60 for all-cause mortality; controls were not followed for mortality. The primary outcomes of the current substudy are (1) development of ARDS in the at-risk cohort, and (2) death among ARDS cases.

Genotyping

Genotyping of the parent cohort has been described in detail previously [23,24]. Briefly, genomic DNA was extracted from whole blood drawn during the first 48 hours of admission using the Autopure LS robotic workstation (Gentra Systems, Minneapolis, MN) and DNA Purification Reagent Kits (Qiagen, Valencia, CA). Genotyping was done at the Center for Applied Genomics, Children's Hospital of Philadelphia (Philadelphia, PA), using the Illumina Human-CVD BeadChip (Illumina, San Diego, CA). The Human-CVD BeadChip is a high-density genotyping platform covering 48,742 markers across roughly 2100 genes associated with cardiovascular, metabolic, and inflammatory pathways [25]. Genotyping personnel were blinded to ARDS case status, and samples were processed according to Illumina's protocols. Quality control has also been described previously [23,24].

Forty-four single nucleotide polymorphisms (SNPs) on *ADIPOQ*, *ADIPOR1* and *ADIPOR2* are included in the CVD BeadChip platform. Of these, we hypothesized 9 SNPs *a priori* as functional based on location, and as common with MAF>5% (Table 1). These 9 SNPs were then analyzed for association with ARDS case status, and mortality among ARDS cases.

Statistical Analysis

Demographic and clinical characteristics between various groups were compared using chi-square tests for categorical variables, and by Wilcoxon tests for continuous variables. Correlations between genotypes and BMI or diabetes were tested by calculating Spearman correlation coefficients. Diabetes status

Table 1. Selected Adiponectin and Receptor SNPs and Genotype Frequencies in the Total Cohort.

			Genotype, N (%)			
Gene	**Polymorphism**	**Location**	**AA***	**AB**	**BB**	**MAF****
ADIPOQ	rs266729	Promoter	1151 (56)	790 (38)	120 (6)	25.0%
ADIPOQ	rs822387	5′ of Promoter	1699 (82)	349 (17)	17 (1)	9.3%
ADIPOQ	rs864265	5′ of Promoter	1531 (74)	496 (24)	40 (2)	13.3%
ADIPOQ	rs2082940	3′ UTR	1562 (76)	453 (22)	49 (2)	13.4%
ADIPOQ	rs16861194	Promoter	1738 (84)	496 (24)	40 (2)	8.3%
ADIPOR1	rs7539542	3′ UTR	929 (45)	914 (44)	224 (11)	32.9%
ADIPOR2	rs1029629	5′ of Promoter	999 (48)	865 (42)	203 (10)	30.7%
ADIPOR2	rs1044471	3′ UTR	536 (26)	1076 (52)	455 (22)	48.1%
ADIPOR2	rs16928751	Coding exon	1626 (79)	409 (20)	30 (1)	11.4%

*A denotes major allele; B denotes minor allele;
**MAF = minor allele frequency.

was abstracted from the medical record with any physician-recorded documentation of type 1 or type 2 diabetes mellitus defining positive diabetes status.

Logistic regression models were used to test the association of SNP genotypes with ARDS case status. Cox proportional hazards models were used to assess the association between SNP genotypes and mortality. A multivariable model for each outcome without genotypes was used to select significant predictors. A backward elimination algorithm with $p \leq 0.2$ for entry into the model was used to test significance of the following clinically relevant covariates: age, gender, Acute Physiology and Chronic Health Evaluation (APACHE) III score, risk factor for ARDS (eg. sepsis, pneumonia, trauma), massive transfusion (defined as requiring ≥8 units of red blood cells in 24 hours), and current history of cirrhosis. Diabetes status and BMI were also included *a priori* given the known biology of adiponectin. In multivariable analyses, the APACHE III score was revised to exclude age and PaO_2/FiO_2 to avoid collinearity [26]. BMI was considered as a 4-category variable using the National Heart, Lung, and Blood Institute's cutoffs for underweight, normal weight, overweight, and obese (<18.5, 18.5–24.9, 25–29.9, and ≥30 respectively) [27]. The significant variables were then used in multivariable models that included genotypes for each SNP. Given no preexisting knowledge of mode of inheritance, additive, recessive, and dominant modes were considered for all SNPs. Correction for multiple comparisons was done using positive false discovery rate (FDR) statistics. The *FDR_q* values were calculated using multivariable models with the significant variables as above. All statistical analyses were performed using SAS Version 9.3 (SAS Inc., Cary, North Carolina).

Results

Patient population

From September 1999 to April 2009, consecutive ICU admissions were screened for possible inclusion. In total, 4244 patients were eligible, of whom 2786 patients were successfully consented, enrolled and followed for development of ARDS. Of those enrolled, 387 had no or poor quality DNA samples, and an additional 101 patients had genotyping call rates ≤95%. Also excluded were 22 patients with incomplete clinical data, previous enrollment, or previous history of ARDS, and 209 patients who were not of European descent. Racial and ethnic categorization was abstracted from hospital registration information with self-report from patients or their surrogates. No genetic determination of ancestry was attempted in this cohort. Thus, 2067 white patients were successfully genotyped using the BeadChip at the loci of interest. Of these, 567 patients developed ARDS.

Cases and control patients differed significantly in age, APACHE III, and sepsis, septic shock, or direct pulmonary injury as the risk factor ARDS (Table 2). Among ARDS cases, survivors and nonsurvivors also differed significantly in age, APACHE III, and septic shock or trauma as the risk factor ARDS (Table 3). BMI was also significantly higher in ARDS cases than controls, although BMI among survivors with ARDS was higher than in nonsurvivors (Tables 2 and 3). Of note, the median for all groups fell in the overweight range.

Genotype analysis

Genotype frequencies in this cohort for the 9 polymorphisms from *ADIPOQ*, *ADIPOR1* and *ADIPOR2* are displayed in Table 1. Our genotype frequencies are similar to publicly available databases of European samples. Overall genotyping success rate was 99.9% among the 2067 successfully genotyped with the chip.

Spearman correlation coefficients were calculated for genotype at each SNP by BMI and by diabetes status. There were no significant correlations between BMI and any SNP. There was a statistically significant but weak positive correlation between rs16861194 genotype (increasing number of variant alleles from 0 to 2) and diabetes status ($\rho = 0.060$, $p = 0.0068$).

Significant predictors of primary outcomes

As described above, multivariable logistic regression and Cox proportional hazards regression were used to select relevant covariates for inclusion in models with genotypes, with a conservative $p<0.2$ for inclusion in the model. Significant predictors for development of ARDS were: age [odds ratio (OR) 0.98, 95% confidence interval (CI) 0.98–0.99, $p<0.0001$]; BMI (OR 1.20, 95% CI 1.08–1.33, $p = 0.0005$); septic shock (OR 1.86, 95% CI 1.50–2.32, $p<0.0001$); direct pulmonary injury (OR 3.64, 95% CI 2.92–4.54, $p<0.0001$); diabetes (OR 0.56, 95% CI 0.44–0.73, $p<0.0001$); and need for RBC transfusions (OR 1.57, 95% CI 1.28–1.94, $p<0.0001$). Among ARDS cases, significant predictors of mortality were: age [hazard ratio (HR) 1.03, 95% CI 1.02–1.04, $p<0.0001$]; BMI (HR 0.89, 95% CI 0.79–1.01, $p = 0.075$); cirrhosis (HR 2.40, 95% CI 1.54–3.72, $p<0.0001$); APACHE III (HR 1.02, 95% CI 1.02–1.03, $p<0.0001$); and trauma (HR 0.21, 95% CI 0.067–0.67, $p<0.0078$). As mentioned, BMI and diabetes status were chosen *a priori* to be included in all models based on known biology of adiponectin.

Adiponectin-related genes and development of ARDS

The presence of the variant allele of rs1029629 on *ADIPOR2* was significantly associated with development of ARDS in the unadjusted model (OR 0.81, 95% CI 0.66–0.98, $p = 0.03$). This did not persist, however, after adjustment for significant covariates ($p = 0.05$), and adjustment for multiple testing (*FDR_q* = 0.20). The presence of the variant allele of rs16928571, also on *ADIPOR2*, was associated with development of ARDS in both unadjusted and multivariable models (OR 1.28, 95% CI 1.00–1.64, $p = 0.05$; OR 1.39, 95% CI 1.06–1.83, $p = 0.02$). When adjusting for multiple comparisons, however, the result was not significant (*FDR_q* = 0.13). No other SNPs showed any significant association with development of ARDS.

Adiponectin-related genes and mortality among ARDS cases

Genotype frequencies in ARDS cases, including those in survivors and nonsurvivors, are shown in Table 4. In unadjusted analysis, homozygous variants of rs2082940 on *ADIPOQ* had a highly significant increase in mortality (Table 5). This association remained significant after adjusting for both relevant covariates and for multiple comparisons. Hazard ratios for the other variables included in the model are as follows: age (HR 1.03, 95% CI 1.02–1.04, $p<0.0001$); APACHE III (HR 1.02, 95% CI 1.01–1.03, $p<0.0001$); BMI (HR 0.87, 95% CI 0.75–1.00, $p = 0.05$); cirrhosis (HR 2.37, 95% CI 1.48–3.81, $p = 0.0004$); diabetes (HR 1.19, 95% CI 0.83–1.69, $p = 0.34$); and trauma (HR 0.25, 95% CI 0.079–0.79, $p = 0.018$). No other SNPs were associated with mortality in the ARDS cases. Results were similar when modeling survival using logistic regression.

Among the 11 homozygous variants of rs2082940, 9 of the 10 nonsurivors died between 0 and 15 days after ARDS onset, and one patient died after a prolonged hospital and ICU course, 57 days after onset of ARDS. The one survivor also had a protracted hospital and ICU course. Among all 11 patients, there were no major outliers in basic demographics or clinical features. Of note,

Table 2. Baseline Cohort Characteristics.

	Total Cohort (n = 2067)	Controls (n = 1500)	Cases (n = 567)	*P**
Age, mean ± SD	61.5±17.4	62.5±17.1	58.8±18.0	<0.0001
Female gender, n (%)	785 (38)	577 (38)	208 (37)	0.46
BMI, median (IQR)	26.5 (8.0)	26.4 (7.8)	27.4 (9.0)	0.017
APACHE III score, mean ± SD	60.4±21.5	58.7±20.9	65.3±22.2	<0.0001
Sepsis syndrome, n (%)	644 (31)	510 (34)	134 (24)	<0.0001
Pulmonary source	363 (56)	260 (51)	103 (77)	
Septic shock, n (%)	1035 (50)	672 (45)	363 (64)	<0.0001
Pulmonary source	561 (54)	302 (45)	259 (71)	
Trauma, n (%)	174 (8)	130 (9)	44 (8)	0.51
Massive transfusion, n (%)	215 (10)	161 (11)	54 (10)	0.42
Aspiration, n (%)	143 (7)	95 (6)	48 (9)	0.09
Direct pulmonary injury, n (%)	1153 (56)	730 (49)	423 (75)	<0.0001

**P*-value reflects comparison between cases and controls.
SD = standard deviation; IQR = interquartile range; NS = not significant.

however, 9 patients were overweight or obese, and 10 had sepsis or septic shock, higher percentages than in our total cohort. The sole survivor was also the only underweight patient of the 11, with an ICU admission BMI of 18.0. An unadjusted Kaplan-Meier survival plot is shown in Figure 1.

Discussion

This is the first study in the literature to report on variants of *ADIPOQ*, *ADIPOR1* and *ADIPOR2* in association with mortality in critically ill adults. Specifically, our results show a significant increase in mortality for ARDS patients homozygous for the rs2082940 variant. The rs2082940 polymorphism has also been associated with increased risk of developing Type 2 diabetes mellitus [28] and decreased risk of prostate cancer [29]. This SNP is common (MAF 13.4%) and is located in the 3′ UTR of *ADIPOQ*. It has been shown in other studies to affect circulating levels of adiponectin with the variant allele associated with increased levels of adiponectin [28,29]. Thus, inference would suggest that the higher mortality seen in our ARDS patients may be associated with higher levels of adiponectin. Although we do not have corresponding plasma adiponectin measurements in this cohort, this inference would be consistent with previous human studies showing lower adiponectin levels at ICU admission are associated with improved survival [16,20].

Having said this, we know from previous genetic studies that while adiponectin levels are highly heritable, SNPs in *ADIPOQ* account for only a small percent of variability in circulating adiponectin, ranging from <2% to 8% across studies [30–32]. Thus, there are likely other important factors such as epigenetic and environmental factors, interactions between loci, copy number variations, and genetic polymorphisms outside of *ADIPOQ* [30,31]. For instance, the GEMS study identified a locus within *CDH13* that was strongly associated with adiponectin levels [31]. This was reiterated in a genome-wide association study (GWAS) of adiponectin levels in Korean adults in which polymorphisms in

Table 3. Cohort Characteristics of ARDS Cases by Mortality.

	Survivors (n = 355)	Nonsurvivors (n = 212)	*P**
Age, mean ± SD	54.5±18.1	66.1±15.4	<0.0001
Female gender, n (%)	124 (35)	84 (40)	0.26
BMI, median (IQR)	27.8 (9.7)	26.1 (6.8)	0.005
APACHE III score, mean ± SD	58.1±19.6	77.5±20.9	<0.0001
Sepsis syndrome, n (%)	88 (25)	46 (22)	0.40
Pulmonary source	65 (74)	38 (83)	
Septic shock, n (%)	214 (60)	149 (70)	0.02
Pulmonary source	151 (75)	98 (66)	
Trauma, n (%)	41 (12)	3 (1)	<0.0001
Massive transfusion, n (%)	35 (10)	19 (9)	0.72
Aspiration, n (%)	23 (8)	20 (9)	0.52
Direct pulmonary injury, n (%)	257 (75)	156 (74)	0.67

**P*-value reflects comparison between survivors and nonsurvivors.
SD = standard deviation; IQR = interquartile range; NS = not significant.

Table 4. Genotype Frequencies in ARDS Cases.

	ARDS Cases, N (%)			Survivors N (%)			Nonsurvivors N (%)		
	AA*	AB	BB	AA	AB	BB	AA	AB	BB
rs266729	312 (55)	220 (39)	33 (6)	192 (54)	138 (39)	25 (7)	120 (57)	82 (39)	8 (4)
rs822387	464 (82)	99 (17)	4 (1)	292 (82)	61 (17)	2 (1)	172 (81)	38 (18)	2 (1)
rs864265	422 (74)	137 (24)	8 (2)	267 (75)	81 (23)	7 (2)	155 (73)	56 (26)	1 (1)
rs2082940	435 (77)	120 (21)	11 (2)	285 (80)	69 (20)	1 (<1)	150 (71)	51 (24)	10 (5)
rs16861194	477 (84)	88 (16)	2 (<1)	302 (85)	51 (14)	2 (1)	175 (83)	37 (17)	0 (0)
rs7539542	247 (44)	260 (46)	60 (11)	159 (45)	161 (45)	35 (10)	88 (42)	99 (47)	25 (12)
rs1029629	252 (44)	257 (45)	58 (10)	159 (45)	157 (44)	39 (11)	93 (44)	100 (47)	19 (9)
rs1044471	157 (28)	276 (49)	134 (24)	102 (29)	167 (47)	86 (24)	55 (26)	109 (51)	48 (23)
rs16928751	463 (82)	95 (17)	9 (1)	286 (80)	66 (19)	3 (1)	177 (83)	29 (14)	6 (3)

*A denotes major allele; B denotes minor allele.

the cadherin 13 gene (*CDH13*) made up 6 of the top 20 hits, and *ADIPOQ* polymorphisms were not even represented among the top 20 [33]. This may also explain why we did not see any significant results for rs822387, a polymorphism in the *ADIPOQ* promoter that has been significantly associated with plasma adiponectin levels in several studies [30,32]. This finding was not replicated, however, in a whole genome analysis within the GEMS study [31], or in a multiethnic meta-analysis [34]. Thus the functions of *ADIPOQ* clearly go beyond just expression of adiponectin.

There have also been several previous genome-wide association studies that have identified expression quantitative trait loci (eQTLs) for plasma adiponectin [30,31,34]. These include rs6810075, rs17300539/rs822387, rs17366568, and rs6773957. Using the SNP Annotation and Proxy Search database (SNAP, http://www.broadinstitute.org/mpg/snap/), pairwise linkage analysis reveals that both rs6773957 and rs17366568 are in complete linkage disequilibrium with rs2082940 (D′ = 1.0) [35]. However, r^2 for both eQTLs is low (0.19 and 0.02 respectively), likely reflecting differences in allele (and thus haplotype) frequencies. Still, the high D′ suggests a strong coinheritance of rs2082940 with these eQTLs. In pairwise analysis with the remaining eQTLs and rs2082940, linkage disequilibrium was extremely low (D′≤0.007).

Table 5. Cox Proportional Hazards Models of Mortality by Genotype in ARDS Cases (n = 566).±

	Crude HR (95% CI)	*P*	Adjusted HR*(95% CI)	*P*	*FDR_q*
ADIPOQ					
rs266729	0.60 (0.30–1.21)	0.16	0.71 (0.34–1.45)	0.34	0.37
rs822387	1.07 (0.27–4.30)	0.93	1.95 (0.48–7.91)	0.35	0.37
rs864265	0.27 (0.038–1.92)	0.19	0.23 (0.032–1.64)	0.14	0.27
rs2082940	4.09 (2.16–7.74)	<0.0001	2.61 (1.36–5.00)	0.004	0.02
rs16861194	—**	0.97	—**	0.98	0.68
ADIPOR1					
rs7539542	1.18 (0.78–1.79)	0.44	1.46 (0.94–2.27)	0.09	0.27
ADIPOR2					
rs1029629	0.87 (0.54–1.39)	0.56	0.96 (0.59–1.57)	0.87	0.68
rs1044471	0.98 (0.71–1.36)	0.91	0.92 (0.66–1.29)	0.64	0.57
rs16928751	2.12 (0.94–4.78)	0.07	1.78 (0.77–4.09)	0.17	0.27

±Models shown represent recessive inheritance pattern.
*Also included in the model: age, BMI, APACHE, trauma, cirrhosis, diabetes.
**HR could not be calculated because only 0.7% of subjects genotyped at this locus had the homozygous variant genotype.
HR = hazard ratio; CI = confidence interval; *FDR_q* = false discovery rate q-value.

Since adiponectin is anti-inflammatory in nature, it is somewhat unintuitive that lower adiponectin levels on ICU admission would be associated with better survival, but this has been show in at least two studies [16,20]. One hypothesis is that lower adiponectin acutely allows the proinflammatory response to predominate, but that as critical illness progresses into a more subacute or chronic phase, adiponectin rises or normalizes as the anti-inflammatory response becomes more important [36], and this biphasic response has been described by several authors [16,18,21,36]. It is later in critical illness when production of anti-inflammatory cytokines such as IL-10 increases, and macrophages shift to their M2 form which has local anti-inflammatory and insulin-sensitizing features [36]. This biphasic theory of adiponectin in critical illness may partly explain why animal models have shown hypoadiponectinemia to be associated with worsened survival in sepsis and acute lung injury [6,7]. Although not entirely analogous to human studies, these studies used adiponectin knockout mice, and thus the animals would not have the ability to increase adiponectin levels during the evolution of their critical illness.

Of the 10 ARDS case patients who were homozygous variant at rs2082940, only one died outside the first 2 weeks after onset of ARDS. This would suggest that patients generally died of multiorgan failure, overwhelming infection, and/or severe hypoxemic respiratory failure. Even the lone survivor had a prolonged hospital course lasting nearly 2 months from ARDS onset, and that case was the only underweight patient among the homozygous recessive group. The only salient features of nonsurvivors, as noted above, were a high percentage of BMI≥25 and sepsis/septic shock. Overall, this would support the hypothesis that blunting of the pro-inflammatory response in acute critical illness is detrimental, if indeed adiponectin levels are increased in these patients.

In one respect, we would not necessarily expect adiponectin to act differently in ARDS patients than in other critically ill subjects with acute inflammation of various etiologies. ARDS respresents an intense inflammatory syndrome localized in the lung but with

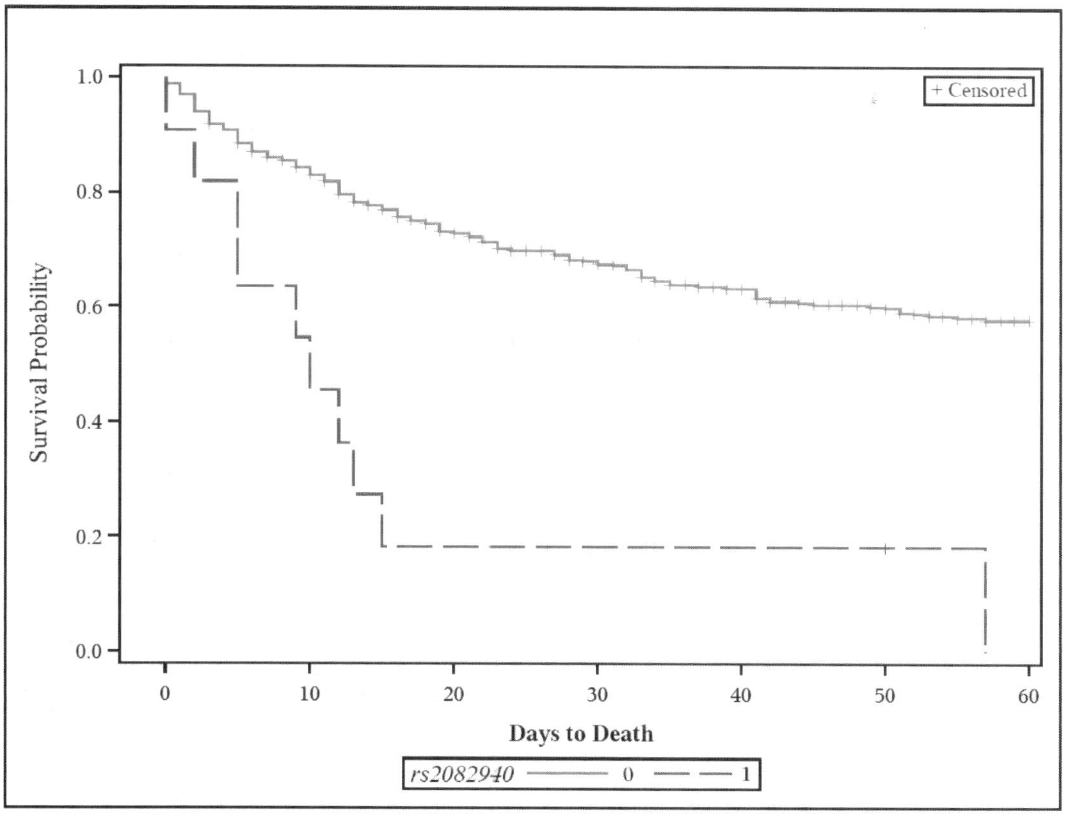

Figure 1. Kaplan-Meier survival plot for rs2082940 among ARDS case patients. All case patients were followed out to 60 days from enrollment. Note: 0 = non-homozygous variant genoypte; 1 = homozygous variant genotype.

systemic effects. Sepsis and septic shock also represent intense systemic inflammation, and such patients make up a large subset of our cohort developing ARDS. The observation that plasma cortisol and plasma adiponectin are highly correlated in healthy subjects may support that adiponectin is a marker for severity of illness [19], although we adjusted our results for APACHE III scores. In another respect, however, adiponectin may act differently in that obesity has been implicated as a risk factor for developing acute lung injury [37–39], yet diabetes has been well-described as a protective factor against developing ARDS [40]. Given adiponectin's link to both of these risk factors with quite opposite effects on ARDS susceptibility, there has been specific interest in adiponectin in ARDS [7].

We found no relationship between SNPs and BMI, and weak correlation between diabetes status and rs16861194. BMI is an imperfect measure in the ICU where weight can reflect the effects of acute illness or of fluid resuscitation. And although many studies have shown an inverse correlation between BMI and adiponectin, plasma levels are certainly affected by many genetic and nongenetic factors, and we examined only a small number of SNPs. BMI has also been associated with an increased risk of ARDS in a weight-dependent manner as mentioned above, [37] and BMI was significant in our multivariable models of outcomes.

We acknowledge limitations in this study. No measurements of adipokine levels are available for this cohort, and thus we cannot specifically link a genotype to a phenotypic correlate. We were also not able to control for insulin dosing or serum glucose levels throughout the ICU stay. This study is an exploratory analysis of available SNPs, several without known function. However, the most significant finding was in a SNP that has been studied, as above, although there were few homozygous recessive patients at this locus.

There are many strengths in this study. Perhaps most importantly, this is a large, prospective, well-characterized cohort with minimal misclassification. DNA quality was excellent with high genotyping success rates. This cohort also has a high percentage of patients with sepsis and septic shock, and along with ARDS itself, the cohort thus represents well the inflammatory sequelae of severe infection and critical illness. We controlled for diabetes and weight (BMI) as these are known to be associated with variations in adiponectin levels. This study also represents an addition to limited existing literature on the role of these genes and their polymorphisms in the critically ill.

Conclusion

A common and potentially functional polymorphism in *ADIPOQ* may impact survival in ARDS. In general, adipokine-related genes may be relevant in survival from critical illness, possibly via insulin resistance and endothelial reactivity and inflammatory pathways.

Acknowledgments

We thank Kezia Ellison, Hanae Fujii-Rios, Ian Taggart and Yael Tarshish for patient recruitment; Marcia Chertok, Julie DelPrato and Janna Frelich for data management; and Andrea Shafer for research assistance.

Author Contributions

Conceived and designed the experiments: AMA DCC. Performed the experiments: LS CCS. Analyzed the data: AMA YZ. Wrote the paper: AMA. Critical revision of manuscript for important intellectual content: YZ CCS BTT DCC.

References

1. Swarbrick MM, Havel PJ (2008) Physiological, pharmacological, and nutritional regulation of circulating adiponectin concentrations in humans. Metab Syndr Relat Disord 6:87–102.
2. Garaulet M, Hernandez-Morante JJ, Perez de Heredia F, Tebar FJ (2007). Adiponectin, the controversial hormone. Public Health Nutr 10(10A)1145–1150.
3. Vendrell J, Broch M, Vilarrasa N, Molina A, Gomez JM, et al. (2004) Resistin, adiponectin, ghrelin, leptin, and proinflammatory cytokines: relationships in obesity. Obes Res 12(6):962–971.
4. Tilg H, Moschen AR (2008) Role of adiponectin and PBEF/visfatin as regulators of inflammation: involvement in obesity-associated diseases. Clin Sci 114:275–288.
5. Matsumoto M, Ishikawa S, Kajii E (2008) Adiponectin and noncardiovascular death: a nested case-control study. Metabolism 57:811–818.
6. Teoh H, Quan A, Bang KW, Wang G, Lovren F, et al. (2008) Adiponectin deficiency promotes endothelial activation and profoundly exacerbates sepsis-related mortality. Am J Physiol Endocrinol Metab 295(3):E658–664.
7. Konter JM, Parker JL, Baez E, Li SZ, Ranscht B, et al. (2012) Adiponectin attenuates lipopolysaccharide-induced acute lung injury through suppression of endothelial cell activation. J Immunol 188:854–863.
8. Maeda K, Okubo K, Shimomura I, Funahashi T, Matsuzawa Y, et al. (1996) cDNA cloning and expression of a novel adipose specific collagen-like factor, apM1 (AdiPose Most abundant Gene transcript 1). Biochem Biophys Res Commun 221:286–289.
9. Potapov VA, Chistiakov DA, Dubinina A, Shamkhalova MS, Shestakova MV, et al. (2008) Adiponectin and adiponectin receptor gene variants in relation to type 2 diabetes and insulin resistance-related phenotypes. Rev Diabet Stud 5:28–37.
10. Yamauchi T, Kamon J, Ito Y, Tsuchida A, Yokomizo T, et al. (2003) Cloning of adiponectin receptors that mediate antidiabetic metabolic effects. Nature 423:762–769.
11. Lau C, Muniandy S (2011) Adiponectin and resistin gene polymorphisms in association with their respective adipokine levels. Ann Hum Genet 75:370–382.
12. Hotta K, Funahashi T, Arita Y, Takahashi M, Matsuda M, et al. (2000) Plasma concentrations of a novel, adipose-specific protein, adiponectin, in type 2 diabetic patients. Arterioscler Thromb Vasc Biol 20:1595–1599
13. Weyer C, Funahashi T, Tanaka S, Hotta K, Matsuzawa Y, et al. (2001) Hypoadiponectinemia in obesity and type 2 diabetes: close association with insulin resistance and hyperinsulinemia. J Clin Endocrinol Metab 86:1930–1935.
14. Diez JJ, Iglesias P (2003) The role of novel adipocyte-derived hormone adiponectin in human disease. Eur J Endocrinol 148:293–300.
15. Chandran M, Phillips SA, Ciaraldi T, Henry RR (2003) Adiponectin: more than just another fat cell hormone? Diabetes Care 26:2442–50.
16. Walkey AJ, Rice TW, Konter J, Ouchi N, Shibata R, et al. (2010) Plasma adiponectin in critically ill subjects with acute respiratory failure. Crit Care Med 38:2329–2334.
17. Shehzad A, Iqbal W, Shehzad O, Lee YS (2012) Adiponectin: regulation of its production and its role in human diseases. Hormones (Athens) 11(1):8–20.
18. Jernas M, Olsson B, Sjoholm K, Sjogren A, Rudemo M, et al. (2009) Changes in adipose tissue gene expression and plasma levels of adipokines and acute-phase proteins in patients with critical illness. Metabolism 58:102–108.
19. Venkatesh B, Hickman I, Nisbet J, Cohen J, Prins J (2009) Changes in serum adiponectin concentrations in critical illness: a preliminary investigation. Crit Care 13:R105.
20. Koch A, Sanson E, Voigt S, Helm A, Trautwein C, et al. (2011) Serum adiponectin upon admission to the intensive care unit may predict mortality in critically ill patients. J Crit Care 26:166–174
21. Langouche L, Vander Perre S, Frystyk J, Flyvbjerg A, Hansen TK, et al. (2009) Adiponectin, retinol-binding protein 4, and leptin in protracted critical illness of pulmonary origin. Crit Care 13:R112.
22. Gong MN, Thompson BT, Williams P, Pothier L, Boyce PD, et al. (2005) Clinical predictors of mortality in acute respiratory distress syndrome: potential role of red cell transfusion. Crit Care Med 33(6): 1191–1198.
23. Frank AJ, Sheu CC, Zhao Y, Chen F, Su L, et al. (2012) *BCL2* genetic variants are associated with acute kidney injury in septic shock. Crit Care Med 40:2116–2123.
24. Tejera P, Meyer N, Chen F, Feng R, Zhao Y, et al. (2012) Distinct and replicable genetic risk factors for acute respiratory distress syndrome of pulmonary or extrapulmonary origin. J Med Genet 49:671–680.
25. Keating BJ, Tischfield S, Murray SS, Bhangale T, Price TS, et al. (2008) Concept, design and implementation of a cardiovascular gene-centric 50k SNP array for large-scale genomic association studies. PloS ONE 3:e3583.
26. Knaus WA, Wagner DP, Draper EA, Zimmerman JE, Bergner M, et al. (1991) The APACHE III prognostic system. Risk prediction of hospital mortality for critically ill hospitalized adults. Chest 100(6): 1619–1636.
27. NIH/NHLBI (1998) Clinical guidelines on the identification, evaluation, and treatment of overweight and obesity in adults: the evidence report. Rockville (MD): NIH publication no. 98-4083.
28. Siitonen N, Pulkkinen L, Lindstrom J, Kolehmainen M, Eriksson JG, et al. (2011) Association of ADIPOQ gene variants with body weight, type 2 diabetes and serum adiponectin concentrations: the Finnish Diabetes Prevention Study. BMC Med Genet 12:5.
29. Dhillon PK, Penney KL, Schumacher F, Rider JR, Sesso HD, et al. (2011) Cancer Epidemiol Biomarkers Prev 20:2618–2627.
30. Heid IM, Henneman P, Hicks A, Coassin S, Winkler T, et al. (2010) Clear detection of ADIPOQ locus as the major gene for plasma adiponectin: results of genome-wide association analyses including 4659 European individuals. Atherosclerosis 208:412–420.
31. Ling H, Waterworth DM, Stirnadel HA, Pollin TA, Barter PJ, et al. (2009) Genome-wide linkage and association analyses to identify genes influencing adiponectin levels: the GEMS study. Obesity 17:737–744.
32. Dastani Z, Johnson T, Kronenberg F, Nelson CP, Assimes TL, et al. (2013) The shared allelic architecture of adiponectin levels and coronary artery disease. Atherosclerosis 229:145–148.
33. Jee SH, Sull JW, Lee J, Shin C, Park J, et al. (2010) Adiponectin concentrations: a genome-wide association study. Am J Hum Genet 87:545–552.
34. Dastani Z, Hivert M, Timpson N, Perry JRB, Yuan X, et al. (2012) Novel loci for adiponectin levels and their influence on type 2 diabetes and metabolic traits: a multi-ethnic meta-analysis of 45,891 individuals. PLoS Genet 8(3):e1002607.
35. Johnson AD, Handsaker RE, Pulit S, Nizzari MM, O'Donnell CJ, et al. (2008) SNAP: a web-based tool for identification and annotation of proxy SNPs using HapMap. Bioinformatics 24(24):2938–2939.
36. Marques MB, Langouche L (2013) Endocrine, metabolic, and morphologic alterations of adipose tissue during critical illness. Crit Care Med 41:317–325.
37. Gong MN, Bajwa E, Thompson BT, Christiani DC (2010) Body mass index is associated with the development of acute respiratory distress syndrome. Thorax 65(1): 44–50.
38. Gajic O, Dabbagh O, Park PK, Adesanya A, Chang SY, et al. (2011) Early identification of patients at risk of acute lung injury: evaluation of lung injury prediction score in a multicenter cohort study. Am J Respir Crit Care Med 183:462–270.
39. Stapleton RD, Dixon AE, Parsons PE, Ware LB, Suratt BT; NHLBI Acute Respiratory Distress Syndrome Network (2010) The association between BMI and plasma cytokine levels in patients with acute lung injury. Chest 138:568–577.
40. Yu S, Christiani DC, Thompson BT, Bajwa EK, Gong MN (2013) Role of diabetes in the development of acute respiratory distress syndrome. Crit Care Med 41(12):2720–2732.

5

Inflammation and Immune-Related Candidate Gene Associations with Acute Lung Injury Susceptibility and Severity

D. Shane O'Mahony[1], Bradford J. Glavan[1], Tarah D. Holden[1], Christie Fong[1], R. Anthony Black[3], Gail Rona[1], Paula Tejera[2], David C. Christiani[2], Mark M. Wurfel[1]*

1 Division of Pulmonary and Critical Care Medicine, Harborview Medical Center, University of Washington, Seattle, Washington, United States of America, **2** Harvard School of Public Health, Harvard University, Boston, Massachusetts, United States of America, **3** Institute of Translational Health Sciences (ITHS), University of Washington, Seattle, Washington, United States of America

Abstract

Introduction: Common variants in genes related to inflammation, innate immunity, epithelial cell function, and angiogenesis have been reported to be associated with risks for Acute Lung Injury (ALI) and related outcomes. We tested whether previously-reported associations can be validated in an independent cohort at risk for ALI.

Methods: We identified 37 genetic variants in 27 genes previously associated with ALI and related outcomes. We prepared allelic discrimination assays for 12 SNPs from 11 genes with MAF>0.05 and genotyped these SNPs in Caucasian subjects from a cohort of critically ill patients meeting criteria for the systemic inflammatory response syndrome (SIRS) followed for development of ALI, duration of mechanical ventilation, and in-hospital death. We tested for associations using additive and recessive genetic models.

Results: Among Caucasian subjects with SIRS (n = 750), we identified a nominal association between rs2069832 in *IL6* and ALI susceptibility (OR_{adj} 1.61; 95% confidence interval [CI], 1.04–2.48, $P = 0.03$). In a sensitivity analysis limiting ALI cases to those who qualified for the Acute Respiratory Distress Syndrome (ARDS), rs61330082 in *NAMPT* was nominally associated with risk for ARDS. In terms of ALI outcomes, SNPs in *MBL2* (rs1800450) and *IL8* (rs4073) were nominally associated with fewer ventilator-free days (VFDs), and SNPs in *NFE2L2* (rs6721961) and *NAMPT* (rs61330082) were nominally associated with 28-day mortality. The directions of effect for these nominal associations were in the same direction as previously reported but none of the associations survived correction for multiple hypothesis testing.

Conclusion: Although our primary analyses failed to statistically validate prior associations, our results provide some support for associations between SNPs in *IL6 and NAMPT* and risk for development of lung injury and for SNPs in *IL8, MBL2, NFE2L2* and *NAMPT* with severity in ALI outcomes. These associations provide further evidence that genetic factors in genes related to immunity and inflammation contribute to ALI pathogenesis.

Editor: Yong-Gang Yao, Kunming Institute of Zoology, Chinese Academy of Sciences, China

Funding: This work was supported by National Institutes of Health grants 5RC2HL101779-02 and UL1RR025014. The funders had no role in study design, data collection and analysis, decision to publish, or preparation of the manuscript.

* E-mail: mmwurfel@u.washington.edu

Introduction

Acute Lung Injury (ALI) and it's more severe manifestation, Acute Respiratory Distress Syndrome (ARDS) are associated with high mortality rates among intensive care unit patients [1–4]. Despite multiple clinical trials, no pharmacological agent has been shown to improve ALI-related outcomes [5]. Failure of these trials is due, in part, to an incomplete understanding of the key biologic pathways involved in the development and persistence of ALI in humans. One approach to identification of the key biologic pathways in ALI pathogenesis is gene-association studies.

Candidate gene studies in ALI have focused on variation within pathways thought to be important in ALI pathogenesis including genes involved in inflammation, immunity, oxidation, coagulation, angiogenesis, cell growth, endothelial barrier, surfactant function, and transcription regulation [6]. However, only a subset of putative ALI risk alleles have been validated in independent populations [7–11]. Robust associations between candidate gene polymorphisms and ALI validated in independent populations could support the development of more accurate models predicting risk for ALI and provide additional rationale for novel therapeutic interventions.

In this study, we sought to determine whether previously-reported associations between variants in genes of immunity, inflammation, angiogenesis and oxidative stress and risk for development of ALI or related outcomes, are robust. We used a nested case-control study design in a prospective cohort of critically ill patients with SIRS followed for development of ALI. Secondary analyses looked at ALI related outcomes in a case-only design.

Methods

SNP selection

We searched PubMed (www.ncbi.nlm.nih.gov/pubmed/) for publications reporting associations between genetic variants and development of ALI and/or ALI related outcomes as of August 2010. A panel of ALI investigators (DSO, BJG, MMW) selected variants based on strength of prior studies, biological relevance, and HapMap [12] minor allele frequencies (MAF) of >0.05 in Caucasians. Variants were then further narrowed to those for which Taqman™ allelic discrimination assays could be designed or that were in high linkage disequilibrium (LD) with another SNP for which an assay could be prepared. As we were unable to design a Taqman assay for rs1800795, we used a surrogate SNP, rs2069832 (pairwise $r^2 = 0.97$).

Study population

The cohort used for this study has been previously described [13]. Briefly, patients admitted to the intensive care unit at Harborview Medical Center, Seattle, WA (Dec 2006–Dec 2010) with systemic inflammatory response syndrome (SIRS) were followed prospectively for development of ALI and related outcomes such as death and other organ dysfunction. Patients were categorized as having SIRS if they had three or more of the following concurrently within a 24 hour period; a) body temperature (<36°C or >38°C) b) HR>90/min, c) RR>20/min or were on the vent and had PCO2<32 mmHg, and d) WBC<4,000/mm^3 or >12,000/mm^3. Exclusion criteria included trauma, HIV or immunosuppression, neurological injury, current diagnosis of cancer, and presence of a "do not resuscitate" order. ALI cases were as defined as per the American-European Consensus Committee (AECC) criteria for ARDS; presence of a proximal risk factor for ALI, presence of a PaO2/FiO2 (ratio of partial pressure of oxygen in arterial blood/fraction of oxygen in gas delivered) <300, absence of overt congestive heart failure, and a chest radiograph with bilateral parenchymal opacities as adjudicated by three critical care physicians [13]. We further subclassified cases as ARDS if the PaO2/FiO2 <200. According to the recently published Berlin Definition for Acute Respiratory Distress Syndrome, our definition of ALI would equate to mild, moderate, or severe ARDS while our definition of ARDS would equate to moderate and severe ARDS [14]. At-risk patients who did not meet criteria for development of ALI during the ICU hospitalization were classified as control subjects. This study was approved by the University of Washington, Division of Human Subjects Research.

Genotyping

Genomic DNA was extracted from whole blood samples using the Puregene DNA Isolation Kit (Qiagen, CA). All SNPs were genotyped using Taqman-based allelic discrimination assays, (Applied Biosystems, CA), on a multichannel microfluidics chip (Fluidigm, CA). Genotyping was carried out per the vendor's protocol in a blinded fashion.

Statistical Analysis

We identified differences in demographic variables between ALI and control subjects using Fisher's exact test for categorical variables and Student's *t*-test for continuous variables. Observed genotype frequencies were compared with expected frequencies to test for deviations from Hardy-Weinberg equilibrium using Fisher's exact test. To reduce possible confounding from population-stratification and racial differences, all analyses were restricted to Caucasian subjects. As a screen for major population substructure, we performed principal component analysis (PCA) using SNP genotypes from 67 SNPs available on our samples and which were also publically available for HapMap 3 subjects [12]. None of the first 5 PCs associated with case/control status.

We used multivariate logistic regression to estimate the genotype-specific odds ratio (OR) and 95% confidence interval (CI) for ALI susceptibility. The genotype associations were analyzed in both additive and recessive models. Covariates were chosen *a priori* based on known effects on risk for ALI development and mortality and included age, sex, APACHE III score, comorbidities, smoking status and alcohol abuse. A two sided P value <0.05 was considered to be nominally significant in all analyses. To control for type I error from multiple hypotheses testing, we used a false discovery rate (FDR) approach setting a threshold of 0.1 as indicative of corrected significance. FDR was calculated separately for each association test using the total number of SNPs tested.

We conducted a sensitivity analysis restricting case and control subjects to avoid phenotype misclassification. We restricted cases of ALI to only those qualifying for moderate and severe ARDS by oxygenation criteria (PaO2/FiO2 <200) and we restricted at-risk controls to only subjects who did not have an episode of hypoxemia (PaO2/FiO2 <300).

In secondary analyses we tested for associations between genotypes and ventilator free days (VFDs) using linear regression and mortality within 28 days using logistic regression, adjusting for covariates as above.

In a post hoc analysis, and for SNPs with adequate genotyping data available in prior publications, we completed unadjusted meta-analyses for genotype associations with ALI risk or mortality in ALI subjects by combining our results with the published data.

We estimated that, under an additive model, our study would have adequate statistical power ($1-\beta>0.8$) to detect associations of moderate strength with ALI (relative risk (RR) >1.5) for SNPs with MAF>0.2. Assuming a recessive model, we would have adequate power to detect a strong association (RR greater than or equal to 3) with SNPs having a MAF>0.25. See Figure S2 for a description of power calculations and the range of power over varying models, allele frequencies and genotype effect strengths.

Statistical analyses were run using the R statistical package and SNP and Variation Suite 7™ (Golden Helix™, Bozeman, MT).

Results

Characteristics of the Study Population

We genotyped 879 subjects; 238 subjects who developed ALI and 641 at-risk control subjects (See Figure 1 for the subject exclusion flow chart diagram). For analyses, we restricted only to subjects that met 3 criteria for SIRS (Figure 1). These subjects had a mean age of 54 (StdDev ±16) years, were predominantly male (63.1%), and were moderately ill with a mean APACHEIII score of 64.7 (StdDev ±25). The baseline characteristics for the study population and comparisons of co-morbidities and clinical risk factors for ALI between groups are shown in Table 1. Compared with subjects who did not develop ALI, ALI cases were of similar age, more likely to be male, and had higher APACHE III scores. The proportion of subjects with coexisting end-stage renal disease, liver failure, alcohol abuse, and shock was greater in the ALI group. Hospital mortality for subjects with ALI was 24.6% which

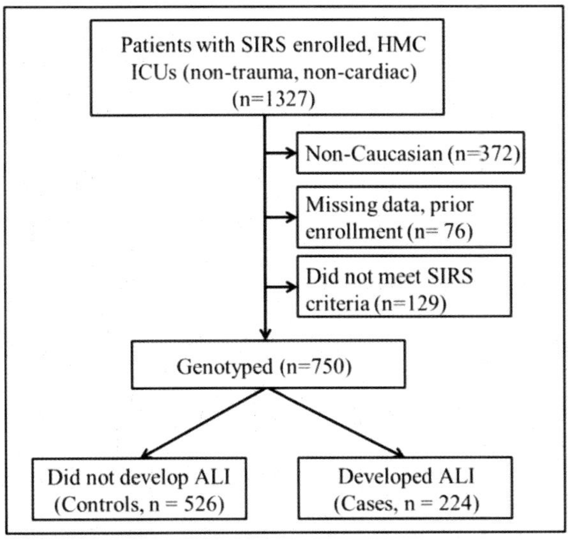

Figure 1. Flow diagram for Study design. Subjects with suspected systemic inflammatory response syndrome (SIRS), n = 1327, were enrolled at Harborview Medical Center (HMC), Seattle, WA during the period December 2006–December 2010. In this study, we excluded non-Caucasian subjects, subjects who were found to have previous enrollment or missing data, and subjects that did not meet 3 SIRS criteria present concurrently within a 24 hour period.

is similar to observed rates in recent ARDSNet studies [15,16]. As would be expected, ALI cases were more likely to have acute kidney injury, sepsis, shock and fewer VFDs.

SNPs selected for validation

We searched PubMed for gene association studies of ALI and ARDS susceptibility and related outcomes. At the time of the search (August, 2010), we identified 37 genetic variants in 27 genes including SNPs, insertion/deletions, and SNP haplotypes (Table S1). The set of SNPs selected for this validation study tagged unique linkage disequilibrium bins that have been associated with ALI risk and/or ALI related outcomes and were located in or near the candidate genes. See Table 2 for the list of SNPs used in this study.

Genotyping results

We achieved genotype call rates across all subjects of over 99% for each of the 12 SNPs. One of the SNPs, rs4444903, had genotype frequencies for the control subjects that deviated from predicted frequency under Hardy Weinberg equilibrium (HWE). The remaining SNPs had genotype results for the control subjects that were not significantly different from HWE predictions using the χ^2 test.

We did not observe strong evidence of population stratification by PCA comparing 67 shared genotypes among our subjects and HapMap3 subjects. When plotting PC1 vs. PC2, our subjects clustered with HapMap CEU and TSI subjects but not with Asian or African clusters as expected. No subject outliers or associations between phenotype and eigenvalue were observed See Figure S1.

Association between SNPs and development of ALI

Genotype frequencies for control and case subjects are presented in Table 3. The A allele of rs4444903 in EGF was over-represented in cases but genotype frequencies for this SNP in controls deviated from HWE.

Table 1. HMC SIRS cohort population characteristics.

	All subjects	*ALI Cases*	*At risk Controls*	*P value*
Subjects n	750	224	526	
Age, yrs, (IQR)	54 (45–64)	55 (44–66)	54 (44–64)	0.381
Male (%)	480 (64)	159 (71)	321 (61)	0.007
Caucasian, %	100	100	100	
ARDS	126 (16.8)	126 (56.3)	0	
APACHE III*	64.7±25	79±25	63±24	<0.001
ALI risk factor				
Sepsis	533 (71)	195 (87)	342 (65)	<0.001
Pneumonia	180 (24)	87 (39)	89 (17)	<0.001
Aspiration	90 (12)	49 (22)	42 (8)	<0.001
Transfusion	16 (2.1)	8 (3.6)	8 (1.5)	0.096
Comorbidities				
Diabetes	203 (27)	56 (25)	142 (27)	0.65
ESRD	18 (2.4)	3 (1.3)	15 (2.9)	0.30
Liver failure	90 (10.2)	35 (14.7)	55 (8.6)	0.08
Alcohol	263 (35)	94 (42)	168 (32)	0.015
COPD	143 (19)	40 (18)	100 (19)	0.75
CHF	83 (11)	31 (14)	47 (9)	0.06
Smoking	450 (60)	146 (65)	300 (57)	0.062
Outcomes				
VFD	19.3±10	13±11	22±10	<0.001
Death	120 (16)	56 (25)	63 (12)	<0.001
AKI	632 (84)	204 (91)	428 (81)	<0.001
Hemodialysis	53 (7)	25 (11)	32 (6)	0.013

Data is presented as mean ± SD for continuous variables and n (%) for categorical variables. P values represent results of t test comparison for difference of means for continuous variables and Fisher's exact test for frequency counts for categorical variables. IQR, interquartile range; VFD, ventilator free days; AKI, presence of acute kidney injury by AKIN score >/= 1 with lowest creatinine during hospitalization used as baseline; Death, subject death within 28 days of admission.

In analyses adjusted for age, gender, APACHEIII score, presence of diabetes mellitus, end stage renal disease, chronic alcohol use, cirrhosis and smoking status, we identified a nominal association between the A allele of rs2069832 in *IL6* by recessive modeling (OR_{adj} 1.61; 95% confidence interval [CI], 1.04–2.48, $P = 0.03$) (Table 4). The direction of effect and magnitude of the odds ratio result was consistent with the prior publication [17]. However, this association result did not meet our predetermined threshold for FDR (FDR<0.1). We did not observe any other significant associations with ALI susceptibility for any of the remaining SNPs in adjusted (Table 4) or unadjusted analyses (Table 3).

We evaluated whether we could complete meta-analyses by combining our genotype results with the previously published results but found that the many of the publications lacked adequate genotyping results details. However, we were able to complete meta-analyses for several of the SNPs including in *NAMPT*, *VEGF*, *IL8*, *MBL2* and *TNF*. In unadjusted genotype association meta-analyses using additive modeling, we observed an association between rs59744560 in *NAMPT* and increased risk for ALI (OR 1.33 (95% CI 1.14–1.56) p value <0.0003) and an association between rs61330082 in *NAMPT* and decreased risk for

Table 2. Genetic variants studied.

GENE	SNP	MAF*	Effect	Case**	Control**	Reference
ANGPT2 (Angiopoietin-2)	rs2515475	0.14	↑ risk ARDS	EA 449	1080 at risk	Su et al, 2009 [33]
EGF (Epidermal growth factor)	rs4444903	0.39	↑ risk ARDS	EA 416	1052 at risk	Shue et al, 2009 [34]
IL6 (Interleukin-6)	rs1800795	0.47	↑ mortality in ARDS	EA; 96	88 at risk; 174 healthy	Marshall et al, 2002 [17]
IL6 (Interleukin-6)	rs1800795 haplotypes		↑ risk ARDS			[11,29,30]
IL8 (Interleukin-8)	rs4073	0.40	↑ days on MV, ↑ IL8 levels	EA; 23	74 at risk	Hildebrand et al, 2007 [20]
IL10 (Interleukin-10)	rs1800896	0.47	↑ risk ARDS	EA; 211	429 at risk	Gong et al, 2006 [35]
MBL2 (Mannose-binding Lectin 2)	rs1800450	0.15	↑ risk ARDS	EA; 212	412 at risk	Gong et al, 2007 [36]
NFE2L2 (Nuclear factor, erythroid-derived, 2-like 2)	rs6721961	0.06	↑ risk ARDS	EA,AA; 30	60, matched case control	Marzec et al, 2007 [8]
NAMPT (Pre-B cell Colony-enhancing factor 1)	rs59744560, rs61330082	0.16, 0.33	↑ risk ARDS; ↓ risk ARDS	EA; 87	100 at risk	Ye et al, 2005 [19]
SFTPB (Surfactant. protein B)	rs1130866	0.43	↑ risk ARDS	EA,AA; 12	390 at risk	Quasney et al, 2004 [37]
TNF (Tumor necrosis factor α)	rs1800629	0.17	↑ mortality in ARDS	EA 237	476 at risk	Gong et al, 2005 [21]
VEGFA (vascular endothelial growth factor A)	rs3025039	0.19	↑ risk ARDS	EA 117	137 at risk; 103 healthy	Medford et al, 2005 [38]

*MAF, minor allele frequency in the HapMap;
**CEU population; EA, European American; AA, African American; Number refers to number of subjects in group of the referenced study.

ALI (OR 0.86 (95% CI 0.74–1.0) p value 0.049). We did not observe associations between SNPs in *VEGF, IL8, MBL2* or *TNF* and ALI risk in this meta-analysis. See Table S3.

Association between SNPs and development of moderate or severe ARDS

We performed a sensitivity analysis excluding subjects with a higher likelihood for phenotypic misclassification as suggested by prior reports [13,18]. We compared controls (n = 288) without hypoxemic respiratory failure and cases with the more severe lung injury phenotypes, moderate and severe ARDS, n = 126. We identified a nominal association between rs61330082 in *NAMPT* and reduced ARDS susceptibility (OR_{adj} 0.61; 95% confidence interval [CI], 0.40–0.95, $P = 0.02$) which replicates the direction of effect seen previously for this SNP [19]. We observed trends toward increased ARDS risk for homozygous carriers of rs6721961 in *NFE2L2* (OR_{adj} 3.83; 95% confidence interval [CI], 0.93–15.7), and rs2069832 in *IL6* (OR_{adj} 1.91; 95% confidence interval [CI], 0.96–3.40) (Table 5). None of the other SNPs were associated with ARDS risk in this sensitivity analysis.

Associations with mortality and ventilator free-days

Several of the SNPs selected for this study were previously associated with ALI-related outcomes [17,20,21]. In secondary analyses, we tested the 12 SNPs for associations with 28 day mortality and VFD among subjects with ALI. Genotype frequencies for survivors and non-survivors of ALI are presented in Table S2. We observed nominal associations between rs4073 in *IL8* and rs1800450 in *MBL2* and decreased VFD in adjusted analyses (Table 6). We also observed nominal associations between rs61330082 in *NAMPT* and rs6721961 in *NFE2L2* and increased risk for mortality when using a recessive model (Table 7). Neither of these associations met our pre-test threshold for significance by FDR. Using genotype data included in published studies, we combined our data and the published data to complete meta-analyses for the SNPs in *TNF* and *MBL2*. In an unadjusted genotype association meta-analysis using recessive modeling, rs1800629 in *TNF* was associated with increased mortality (OR 4.6 (95% CI 1.4–14.9), p value 0.001) and rs1800450 in*MBL2* displayed a trend toward increased risk (OR 3.07 (95% CI 0.99–9.5), p value 0.07). See Table S4.

Discussion

At the time of our study, candidate gene association studies had identified more than 30 genetic variants in over 27 genes that associate with risk for ALI or ALI-related outcomes. These associations provide evidence that genetic factors contribute to ALI and strengthen the link between these specific genes in disease pathogenesis. In this study, we sought to identify robust associations between previously-associated genetic variants and risk for ALI and related outcomes. Using a nested case-control study in a well-phenotyped ICU cohort, we compared SIRS subjects who remained at-risk for ALI to those who developed ALI. Although, in the primary multivariable analyses, the significance levels for the associations with ALI did not survive correction for multiple comparisons, our nominal association results provide some support for prior findings. We observed a nominal association between a SNP in *IL6* (rs2069832, surrogate for rs1800795) and risk for ALI. In analyses restricting case and control definitions to minimize misclassification, we observed a nominal association between rs61330082 in *NAMPT* and reduced risk for moderate and severe ARDS consistent with previous reports [19]. In terms of ALI-related outcomes, we observed nominal associations between rs4073 in *IL8* and rs1800450 in *MBL2* and decreased VFDs. We observed nominal associations between rs61330082 in *NAMPT* and rs6721961 in *NFE2L2* and increased 28-day mortality. None of the associations observed in the secondary analyses survived correction for multiple hypothesis testing.

IL6 and *IL8* have been extensively studied as important proinflammatory mediators in ALI. Elevated levels of IL-6 and IL-8 are associated with development of ALI, and persistence of

Table 3. Genotype frequencies in at-risk controls versus ALI cases.

Gene	SNP rs#	At Risk Controls (%) (n = 526)			χ^2 p-value for HWE in at-risk control	ALI cases (%) (n = 224)			Fisher's Exact test genotype freq. (p-value)[a]
SFTPB	rs1130866	TT 134 (25)	TC 257 (49)	CC 135 (26)	0.60	TT 57 (25)	TC 116 (52)	CC 51 (23)	0.66
MBL2	rs1800450	CC 370 (70)	CT 142 (27)	TT 14 (3)	0.93	CC 162 (72)	CT 56 (25)	TT 6 (3)	0.64
TNF	rs1800629	GG 383 (71)	GA 131 (25)	AA 12 (2)	0.84	GG 160 (71)	GA 56 (27)	AA 4 (2)	0.82
IL10	rs1800896	TT 144 (27)	TC 256 (49)	CC 126 (24)	0.56	TT 51 (23)	TC 114 (51)	CC 59 (26)	0.22
IL6	rs2069832	GG 173 (33)	GA 273 (52)	AA 80 (15)	0.10	GG 78 (35)	GA 99(44)	AA 47 (21)	0.49
ANGPT2	rs2515475	CC 410 (78)	CT 102 (19)	TT 14 (3)	0.016	CC 178 (79)	CT 42 (19)	TT 4 (2)	0.53
VEGF	rs3025039	CC 381 (72)	CT 133 (25)	TT 12 (2)	0.92	CC 168 (75)	CT 52 (23)	TT 4 (2)	0.44
IL8	rs4073	TT 163 (31)	TA 252 (48)	AA 110 (21)	0.49	TT 61 (27)	TA 108 (48)	AA 55 (25)	0.19
EGF	rs4444903	AA 143 (27)	AG 301 (57)	GG 81 (15)	0.0002	AA 91 (41)	93 (42)	40 (18)	0.041
NAMPT	rs59744560	GG 398 (76)	GT 114 (22)	TT 14 (3)	0.10	GG 159 (71)	GT 59 (26)	TT 6 (3)	0.25
NAMPT	rs61330082	CC 300 (57)	CT 185 (35)	TT 40 (8)	0.13	CC 141 (63)	CT 67 (30)	TT 16 (7)	0.21
NFE2L2	rs6721961	GG 409 (78)	GT 109 (21)	TT 8 (2)	0.81	GG 175 (78)	GT 44 (20)	TT 5 (2)	0.93

HWE Hardy-Weinberg equilibrium;
[a]p value for the Fisher's exact test comparing genotypes for at risk controls and ALI cases.

Table 4. Associations with ALI susceptibility.

		ADDITIVE				RECESSIVE			
	Predictor	Odds Ratio	OR Conf. Interval	P-Value	FDR	Odds Ratio	OR Conf. Interval	P-Value	FDR
SFTPB	rs1130866	0.93	0.73–1.18	0.55	0.72	0.83	0.56–1.23	0.35	0.90
MBL2	rs1800450	0.98	0.71–1.36	0.90	0.98	1.20	0.43–3.34	0.73	1.00
TNF	rs1800629	0.99	0.71–1.38	0.95	0.95	0.56	0.16–2.03	0.36	0.79
IL10	rs1800896	1.09	0.86–1.38	0.49	0.80	1.03	0.70–1.53	0.87	1.00
IL6	**rs2069832**	1.08	0.85–1.38	0.53	0.76	**1.61**	**1.04–2.48**	**0.03**	**0.43**
ANGPT2	rs2515475	0.85	0.59–1.38	0.38	0.70	0.66	0.18–2.43	0.52	0.85
VEGF	rs3025039	0.84	0.60–1.19	0.34	0.73	0.84	0.24–2.89	0.78	1.00
IL8	rs4073	1.13	0.90–1.43	0.30	0.79	1.29	0.87–1.92	0.21	0.90
EGF	rs4444903	0.80	0.62–1.03	0.08	0.55	1.33	0.85–2.07	0.21	0.70
PBEF1	rs59744560	1.26	0.91–1.74	0.17	0.57	1.08	0.39–3.02	0.89	0.96
PBEF1	rs61330082	0.82	0.62–1.07	0.14	0.62	0.99	0.52–1.89	0.99	0.99
NFE2L2	rs6721961	1.11	0.77–1.58	0.58	0.69	2.22	0.68–7.25	0.20	1.00

Multivariate logistic regression adjusted for age, sex, APACHE III score, alcohol abuse, smoking status, and history of chronic renal failure and diabetes mellitus.

elevated levels has been associated with poor outcomes [22–24]. rs1800795 is a promoter SNP that results in decreased expression of IL-6, and multiple disease associations have been reported for this SNP [25]. Similarly, rs4073 in *IL8* is a promoter SNP that affects gene transcription and has multiple published disease associations [26–28]. Our study employed a larger carefully-phenotyped ICU population as compared to the prior published studies for genetic risk associations between these genes and ALI. The CC genotype of rs1800795 in *IL6* which results in lower promoter activity was previously associated with reduced mortality in ARDS but not with risk for ALI [17]. Nonas et al. observed that a 3-SNP haplotype in *IL6* that included the C allele of rs1800795 was actually associated with reduced risk of ALI [29]. In a subsequent publication, Flores et al. tested 14 SNPs across *IL6* tagging all common linkage disequilibrium bins and found that none of these SNPs demonstrated an association with ALI. However, they did find that carriage of two copies of a 6-SNP haplotype that included the G allele at rs1800795 was associated with an OR of 2.73 (95% CI, 2.39–5.37) for development of ALI [11]. Finally, Sutherland et al. reported that carriage of 2 copies of an *IL6* haplotype clade that included the G allele of rs1800795 was associated with increased risk of death and fewer days alive and free of ALI [30]. Here we now report that a surrogate for rs1800795 (rs2069832, $r^2 = 0.98$), is associated with increased risk for ALI and, similar to the studies by Flores and Sutherland, the effect was best modeled assuming a recessive effect. The SNP in *IL8* was previously associated with increased days on mechanical ventilation [20]; in our study, rs4073 in *IL8* was similarly

Table 5. Associations with moderate or severe ARDS susceptibility.

		ADDITIVE				RECESSIVE			
	Predictor	Odds Ratio	OR Conf. Interval	P-Value	FDR	Odds Ratio	OR Conf. Interval	P-Value	FDR
SFTPB	rs1130866	1.05	0.73–1.51	0.80	0.87	0.85	0.46–1.55	0.59	0.70
MBL2	rs1800450	0.86	0.54–1.37	0.52	0.75	0.69	0.17–2.79	0.60	0.64
TNF	rs1800629	0.87	0.53–1.43	0.58	0.76	0.49	0.09–2.63	0.40	0.74
IL10	rs1800896	1.29	0.92–1.8	0.14	0.94	1.23	0.70–2.16	0.47	0.77
IL6	**rs2069832**	1.22	0.85–1.74	0.28	0.90	**1.81**	**0.96–3.40**	**0.068**	**0.44**
ANGPT2	rs2515475	0.92	0.56–1.50	0.74	0.87	0.65	0.13–3.15	0.58	0.75
VEGF	rs3025039	0.74	0.45–1.23	0.24	1.00	1.01	0.21–4.87	0.99	0.99
IL8	rs4073	1.20	0.85–1.68	0.29	0.76	1.57	0.88–2.80	0.13	0.41
EGF	rs4444903	0.87	0.61–1.25	0.45	0.74	1.36	0.71–2.60	0.35	0.77
NAMPT	rs59744560	1.06	0.65–1.74	0.81	0.81	0.24	0.04–1.67	0.11	0.49
NAMPT	**rs61330082**	**0.62**	**0.40–0.95**	**0.02**	**0.30**	0.71	0.24–2.08	0.52	0.75
NFE2L2	**rs6721961**	1.27	0.79–2.06	0.33	0.72	**3.83**	**0.94–15.6**	**0.066**	**0.86**

Multivariate logistic regression adjusted for age, sex, APACHE III score, alcohol abuse, smoking status, and history of chronic renal failure and diabetes mellitus. n = 414 (126 with ARDS).

Table 6. Associations with VFDs.

		ADDITIVE			RECESSIVE		
	Predictor	**Slope**	**P-value**	**FDR**	**Slope**	**P-value**	**FDR**
SFTPB	rs1130866	0.07	0.94	0.94	0.09	0.96	0.96
MBL2	**rs1800450**	−0.43	0.75	0.97	**−10.25**	**0.0149**	**0.19**
TNF	rs1800629	−1.00	0.48	1.00	−2.07	0.70	0.91
IL10	rs1800896	−0.32	0.75	1.00	−1.03	0.52	0.96
IL6	rs2069832	0.78	0.41	1.00	1.03	0.55	0.89
ANGPT2	rs2515475	−0.73	0.64	1.00	4.32	0.47	1.00
VEGF	rs3025039	−1.53	0.28	1.00	−1.95	0.70	0.83
IL8	**rs4073**	−0.70	0.47	1.00	**−3.73**	**0.0196**	**0.13**
EGF	rs4444903	−0.82	0.38	1.00	−2.93	0.10	0.43
NAMPT	rs59744560	0.46	0.73	1.00	1.11	0.79	0.86
NAMPT	rs61330082	−0.22	0.84	0.91	−2.25	0.39	1.00
NFE2L2	rs6721961	0.36	0.80	0.95	−3.16	0.50	1.00

Multivariate linear regression adjusted for age, sex, APACHE III score, alcohol abuse, smoking status, and history of chronic renal failure and diabetes mellitus. n = 224.

associated with reduced days alive and free of ventilation. These data suggest that common variants in inflammatory cytokines contribute to disease pathogenesis among subjects at risk for or who have ALI.

NAMPT (PBEF1) has been associated with lung injury pathogenesis in recent translational and genetic association studies. Pre-B-cell colony-enhancing factor (PBEF) is a cytokine encoded by the gene *NAMPT* and that has been shown to be present at higher concentrations in serum and BALF from patients with ALI [19]. Two studies have reported associations between SNPs in *NAMPT* and development of ALI. Ye et al. identified 11 SNPs in *NAMPT* and, in a comparison between ALI cases and healthy controls, demonstrated that two of the SNPs in the promoter region, T-1001G (rs59744560) and C-1543T (rs61330082) were associated with risk for sepsis and ALI [19]. A second study using a nested case-control design in a larger population replicated the association with the −1001G allele and increased risk for ALI while the −1543T allele was associated with decreased risk for ARDS [9]. In our study, we observed the same effect of reduced risk of ALI for carriers of the −1543T genotype in sensitivity analyses restricting to cases with ARDS and controls without hypoxemia. On the other hand, we did not replicate the risk association for the −1001G SNP (rs59744560) in our primary adjusted analysis. In a post hoc meta-analysis combining our data and published genotype data for rs59744560, we did observe a strongly significant association with risk for ALI. Taken together, these findings support a role for *NAMPT* in ALI pathogenesis and suggest that *NAMPT* promoter variants are associated with risk for disease development.

NFE2L2 is a gene that has been identified as a potential mediator of hyperoxia-induced lung damage via linkage analysis and positional cloning in mice [31]. *NFE2L2* is a transcription factor that targets antioxidant response elements (AREs) leading to gene regulation that is protective in the setting of oxidative stress. Resequencing of *NFE2L2* identified a variant (rs6721961) that resulted in diminished promoter activity in an *in vitro* transfection experiment [8]. The authors also reported that rs6721961 was associated with increased risk for development of trauma-associated acute lung injury. We observed a trend for association of this variant with increased risk for ALI among subjects with SIRS, with a stronger trend in the sensitivity analysis with ARDS as the outcome. Our analysis resulted in a strong odds ratio for increased risk for developing ALI similar to the prior report [8].

Misclassification of ALI, particularly the inclusion of subjects without true ALI among cases, can lead to significant reductions in statistical power to detect true genetic associations [32]. For example, a recent study found that removal of subjects with equivocal CXR results from a set of patients classified with ALI resulted in an improvement in the strength of associations observed [18]. We undertook a sensitivity analysis to determine

Table 7. Associations with 28-day ALI-related mortality.

		ADDITIVE				RECESSIVE			
	Predictor	**Odds Ratio**	**OR Conf. Interval**	**P-Value**	**FDR**	**Odds Ratio**	**OR Conf. Interval**	**P-Value**	**FDR**
SFTPB	rs1130866	0.91	0.55–1.50	0.71	1.00	0.73	0.30–1.73	0.46	0.80
MBL2	rs1800450	1.02	0.52–2.01	0.96	0.96	1.74	0.27–11.3	0.57	0.76
TNF	rs1800629	0.65	0.31–1.34	0.23	0.76	6.00	0.41–87.2	0.17	0.67
IL10	rs1800896	0.81	0.48–1.35	0.42	0.78	0.80	0.35–1.83	0.60	0.72
IL6	rs2069832	0.96	0.59–1.58	0.88	1.00	0.94	0.39–2.26	0.89	0.97
ANGPT2	rs2515475	1.12	0.50–2.5	0.78	1.00				
VEGF	rs3025039	1.27	0.62–2.60	0.52	0.84	1.11	0.09–14.5	0.93	0.93
IL8	rs4073	1.01	0.62–1.66	0.95	1.00	1.49	0.67–3.31	0.33	0.79
EGF	rs4444903	1.36	0.84–2.21	0.21	1.00	1.79	0.75–4.26	0.19	0.58
NAMPT	rs59744560	1.46	0.77–2.80	0.25	0.66	2.26	0.32–15.8	0.43	0.85
NAMPT	**rs61330082**	1.42	0.82–2.45	0.22	0.94	**4.37**	**1.36–14.1**	**0.016**	**0.20**
NEF2L2	**rs6721961**	1.40	0.68–2.88	0.37	0.80	**9.73**	**1.27–74.8**	**0.030**	**0.18**

Multivariate logistic regression adjusted for age, sex, APACHE III score, alcohol abuse, smoking status, and history of chronic renal failure and diabetes mellitus. n = 224 (49 non-survivors at 28 days).

if we would observe stronger associations following reduction of potential misclassification of ALI cases and at-risk controls. We restricted cases to only those ALI cases qualifying for ARDS (PF<200) while also restricting control subjects to those who did not have hypoxemia. This approach reduced the analysis sample size but resulted in associations with effects that were farther from the null for the SNPs in *IL6*, *NAMPT* and *NFE2L2*. While these findings did not achieve statistical significance after correction for type I error they provide support for the contention that phenotypic misclassification is a major issue reducing power and precision in case-control studies of ALI.

Overall, our study failed to demonstrate robust associations between the SNPs studied and risk for ALI and related outcomes. Reasons for lack of validation include inadequate statistical power, misclassification of subject phenotypes, sample population differences compared to the prior studies, population substructure, and absence of true association with ALI. As power was limiting to identify small effect sizes, especially in the recessive model, we cannot exclude the possibility that we failed to observe true associations between the SNPs and ALI susceptibility and related outcomes. A limited analysis on 67 genotypes demonstrated that subjects from our cohort clustered with HapMap CEU and TSI subjects suggesting that there was not obvious evidence for cryptic admixture. However, more subtle differences in population substructure could have also have affected our ability to detect true associations. Finally, most of the SNPs included in this study have not been definitively shown to have functional significance and may merely serve as markers for causal variants. Future work will require more dense genotyping or sequencing at these loci to gain further insight into potential mechanisms.

This study used a well-phenotyped cohort of ICU subjects with SIRS and a nested-case control design to replicate ALI risk associations for several previously identified genetic variants. We observed nominal associations for between SNPS in *IL6* and *NAMPT*, and risk for ALI and ARDS, but these associations failed to meet significance after adjusting for multiple comparisons. Nominal associations were also identified between SNPs in *IL8*, *MBL2*, *NAMPT* and *NFE2L2* and ALI severity outcomes, namely VFDs and 28-day mortality. The failure to replicate the majority of ALI risk and outcome associations with statistical significance emphasizes the challenges of genetic association studies in critical care populations including sample size and disease classification. Our results also highlight the importance of independent confirmatory studies of associations with ALI susceptibility and related outcomes in order to support a better understanding of ALI pathogenesis and prognosis.

Supporting Information

Figure S1 Genotype principal component analysis plot demonstrating overlap of our subjects with HapMap ethnic populations. Population stratification was assessed by PCA for 67 shared genotypes among our subjects and HapMap 3 subjects [12]. Our subjects overlapped with CEU and TSI HapMap subjects but separated from subjects of African or Asian ethnicity when plotting eigenvalues 1 versus 2.

Figure S2 Plot of power estimates based on minor allele frequency and genotype effect size. Using CaTS [39], we generated results for estimated statistical power (1-b>0.8) to detect additive and recessive model associations over varying allele frequencies and genotype relative risks, using our known sample size and case frequency and an alpha error rate of 0.05. Each line represents a genotype relative risk: A, power estimates for the additive model for genotype relative risks of 1.25, 1.5, 1.75 and 2; B, power estimates for the recessive model for genotype relative risks of 1.5, 2, 2.5 and 3.

Table S1 Genetic variants associated with acute lung injury and associated outcomes in peer reviewed publications.

Table S2 Genotype frequencies and unadjusted frequency analysis for ALI survivors vs. non-survivors at 28 days.

Table S3 Meta-analysis for ALI risk: genotype frequencies used in meta-analysis calculations. Results for Fisher exact test.

Table S4 Meta-analysis for ALI-related mortality: genotype frequencies used in meta-analysis calculations. Results for Fisher exact test.

Acknowledgments

We would like to acknowledge all contributors to data collection for the SIRS repository and the clinical lab at Harborview Medical Center for providing blood samples for DNA collection.

Author Contributions

Conceived and designed the experiments: DSO BJG PT DCC MMW. Performed the experiments: DSO TDH GR. Analyzed the data: DSO CF RAB MMW. Contributed reagents/materials/analysis tools: DCC MMW RAB. Wrote the paper: DSO CF PT DCC MMW.

References

1. Luhr OR, Antonsen K, Karlsson M, Aardal S, Thorsteinsson A, et al. (1999) Incidence and mortality after acute respiratory failure and acute respiratory distress syndrome in Sweden, Denmark, and Iceland. The ARF Study Group. Am J Respir Crit Care Med 159: 1849–1861.
2. Roupie E, Lepage E, Wysocki M, Fagon JY, Chastre J, et al. (1999) Prevalence, etiologies and outcome of the acute respiratory distress syndrome among hypoxemic ventilated patients. SRLF Collaborative Group on Mechanical Ventilation. Société de Réanimation de Langue Française. Intensive Care Med 25: 920–929.
3. Goss CH, Brower RG, Hudson LD, Rubenfeld GD (2003) Incidence of acute lung injury in the United States. Crit Care Med 31: 1607–1611. doi:10.1097/01.CCM.0000063475.65751.1D.
4. Bersten AD, Edibam C, Hunt T, Moran J (2002) Incidence and mortality of acute lung injury and the acute respiratory distress syndrome in three Australian States. Am J Respir Crit Care Med 165: 443–448.
5. Rubenfeld GD, Caldwell E, Peabody E, Weaver J, Martin DP, et al. (2005) Incidence and outcomes of acute lung injury. N Engl J Med 353: 1685–1693. doi:10.1056/NEJMoa050333.
6. Gao L, Barnes KC (2009) Recent advances in genetic predisposition to clinical acute lung injury. American Journal of Physiology - Lung Cellular and Molecular Physiology 296: L713–L725. doi:10.1152/ajplung.90269.2008.
7. Christie JD, Ma S-F, Aplenc R, Li M, Lanken PN, et al. (2008) Variation in the MYLK gene is associated with development of acute lung injury after major trauma. Crit Care Med. Available: http://www.ncbi.nlm.nih.gov/pubmed/18766098. Accessed 6 June 2011.

8. Marzec JM, Christie JD, Reddy SP, Jedlicka AE, Vuong H, et al. (2007) Functional polymorphisms in the transcription factor NRF2 in humans increase the risk of acute lung injury. FASEB J 21: 2237–2246. doi:10.1096/fj.06-7759com.
9. Bajwa EK, Yu C-L, Gong MN, Thompson BT, Christiani DC (2007) Pre-B-cell colony-enhancing factor gene polymorphisms and risk of acute respiratory distress syndrome. Crit Care Med 35: 1290–1295. doi:10.1097/01.CCM.0000260243.22758.4F.
10. Christie JD (2006) Interleukin-10, age and acute lung injury genetics: the action is in the interaction. Eur Respir J 27: 669–670. doi:10.1183/09031936.06.00017306.
11. Flores C, Ma S-F, Maresso K, Wade MS, Villar J, et al. (2008) IL6 gene-wide haplotype is associated with susceptibility to acute lung injury. Transl Res 152: 11–17. doi:10.1016/j.trsl.2008.05.006.
12. The International HapMap Project (2003) Nature 426: 789–796. doi:10.1038/nature02168.
13. Glavan BJ, Holden TD, Goss CH, Black RA, Neff MJ, et al. (2011) Genetic variation in the FAS gene and associations with acute lung injury. Am J Respir Crit Care Med 183: 356–363. doi:10.1164/rccm.201003-0351OC.
14. Ranieri VM, Rubenfeld GD, Thompson BT, Ferguson ND, Caldwell E, et al. (2012) Acute respiratory distress syndrome: the Berlin Definition. JAMA 307: 2526–2533. doi:10.1001/jama.2012.5669.
15. Stapleton RD, Martin TR, Weiss NS, Crowley JJ, Gundel SJ, et al. (2011) A phase II randomized placebo-controlled trial of omega-3 fatty acids for the treatment of acute lung injury. Crit Care Med 39: 1655–1662. doi:10.1097/CCM.0b013e318218669d.
16. Wiedemann HP, Wheeler AP, Bernard GR, Thompson BT, Hayden D, et al. (2006) Comparison of two fluid-management strategies in acute lung injury. N Engl J Med 354: 2564–2575. doi:10.1056/NEJMoa062200.
17. Marshall RP, Webb S, Hill MR, Humphries SE, Laurent GJ (2002) Genetic polymorphisms associated with susceptibility and outcome in ARDS. Chest 121: 68S–69S.
18. Shah CV, Lanken PN, Localio AR, Gallop R, Bellamy S, et al. (2010) An alternative method of acute lung injury classification for use in observational studies. Chest 138: 1054–1061. doi:10.1378/chest.09-2697.
19. Ye SQ, Simon BA, Maloney JP, Zambelli-Weiner A, Gao L, et al. (2005) Pre-B-cell colony-enhancing factor as a potential novel biomarker in acute lung injury. Am J Respir Crit Care Med 171: 361–370. doi:10.1164/rccm.200404-563OC.
20. Hildebrand F, Stuhrmann M, van Griensven M, Meier S, Hasenkamp S, et al. (2007) Association of IL-8-251A/T polymorphism with incidence of Acute Respiratory Distress Syndrome (ARDS) and IL-8 synthesis after multiple trauma. Cytokine 37: 192–199. doi:10.1016/j.cyto.2007.03.008.
21. Gong MN, Zhou W, Williams PL, Thompson BT, Pothier L, et al. (2005) −308GA and TNFB polymorphisms in acute respiratory distress syndrome. Eur Respir J 26: 382–389. doi:10.1183/09031936.05.00000505.
22. Bouros D, Alexandrakis MG, Antoniou KM, Agouridakis P, Pneumatikos I, et al. (2004) The clinical significance of serum and bronchoalveolar lavage inflammatory cytokines in patients at risk for Acute Respiratory Distress Syndrome. BMC Pulm Med 4: 6. doi:10.1186/1471-2466-4-6.
23. Meduri GU, Headley S, Kohler G, Stentz F, Tolley E, et al. (1995) Persistent elevation of inflammatory cytokines predicts a poor outcome in ARDS. Plasma IL-1 beta and IL-6 levels are consistent and efficient predictors of outcome over time. Chest 107: 1062–1073.
24. Parsons PE, Eisner MD, Thompson BT, Matthay MA, Ancukiewicz M, et al. (2005) Lower tidal volume ventilation and plasma cytokine markers of inflammation in patients with acute lung injury. Crit Care Med 33: 1–6; discussion 230–232.
25. Fishman D, Faulds G, Jeffery R, Mohamed-Ali V, Yudkin JS, et al. (1998) The effect of novel polymorphisms in the interleukin-6 (IL-6) gene on IL-6 transcription and plasma IL-6 levels, and an association with systemic-onset juvenile chronic arthritis. J Clin Invest 102: 1369–1376. doi:10.1172/JCI2629.
26. Wang N, Zhou R, Wang C, Guo X, Chen Z, et al. (2012) −251 T/A polymorphism of the interleukin-8 gene and cancer risk: a HuGE review and meta-analysis based on 42 case-control studies. Mol Biol Rep 39: 2831–2841. doi:10.1007/s11033-011-1042-5.
27. Ahn M-H, Park B-L, Lee S-H, Park S-W, Park J-S, et al. (2011) A promoter SNP rs4073T>A in the common allele of the interleukin 8 gene is associated with the development of idiopathic pulmonary fibrosis via the IL-8 protein enhancing mode. Respir Res 12: 73. doi:10.1186/1465-9921-12-73.
28. Andia DC, Letra A, Casarin RCV, Casati MZ, Line SRP, et al. (2012) Genetic analysis of the IL8 gene polymorphism (rs4073) in generalized aggressive periodontitis. Archives of oral biology. Available: http://www.ncbi.nlm.nih.gov/pubmed/22727395. Accessed 10 July 2012.
29. Nonas SA, Finigan JH, Gao L, Garcia JGN (2005) Functional genomic insights into acute lung injury: role of ventilators and mechanical stress. Proc Am Thorac Soc 2: 188–194. doi:10.1513/pats.200501-005AC.
30. Sutherland AM, Walley KR, Manocha S, Russell JA (2005) The association of interleukin 6 haplotype clades with mortality in critically ill adults. Arch Intern Med 165: 75–82. doi:10.1001/archinte.165.1.75.
31. Cho H-Y, Jedlicka AE, Reddy SPM, Zhang L-Y, Kensler TW, et al. (2002) Linkage analysis of susceptibility to hyperoxia. Nrf2 is a candidate gene. Am J Respir Cell Mol Biol 26: 42–51.
32. Edwards BJ, Haynes C, Levenstien MA, Finch SJ, Gordon D (2005) Power and sample size calculations in the presence of phenotype errors for case/control genetic association studies. BMC Genet 6: 18. doi:10.1186/1471-2156-6-18.
33. Su L, Zhai R, Sheu C-C, Gallagher DC, Gong MN, et al. (2009) Genetic variants in the angiopoietin-2 gene are associated with increased risk of ARDS. Intensive Care Med 35: 1024–1030. doi:10.1007/s00134-009-1413-8.
34. Sheu CC, Zhai R, Su L, Tejera P, Gong MN, et al. (2009) Sex-specific association of epidermal growth factor gene polymorphisms with acute respiratory distress syndrome. Eur Respir J 33: 543–550. doi:10.1183/09031936.00091308.
35. Gong MN, Thompson BT, Williams PL, Zhou W, Wang MZ, et al. (2006) Interleukin-10 polymorphism in position −1082 and acute respiratory distress syndrome. Eur Respir J 27: 674–681. doi:10.1183/09031936.06.00046405.
36. Gong MN, Zhou W, Williams PL, Thompson BT, Pothier L, et al. (2007) Polymorphisms in the mannose binding lectin-2 gene and acute respiratory distress syndrome. Crit Care Med 35: 48–56. doi:10.1097/01.CCM.0000251132.10689.F3.
37. Quasney MW, Waterer GW, Dahmer MK, Kron GK, Zhang Q, et al. (2004) Association between surfactant protein B+1580 polymorphism and the risk of respiratory failure in adults with community-acquired pneumonia. Crit Care Med 32: 1115–1119.
38. Medford ARL, Keen LJ, Bidwell JL, Millar AB (2005) Vascular endothelial growth factor gene polymorphism and acute respiratory distress syndrome. Thorax 60: 244–248. doi:10.1136/thx.2004.034785.
39. Skol AD, Scott LJ, Abecasis GR, Boehnke M (2006) Joint analysis is more efficient than replication-based analysis for two-stage genome-wide association studies. Nat Genet 38: 209–213. doi:10.1038/ng1706.

6

Clinical Study of Critical Patients with Hemorrhagic Fever with Renal Syndrome Complicated by Acute Respiratory Distress Syndrome

Hong Du[9], Jing Li[9], Wei Jiang, Haitao Yu, Ye Zhang, Junning Wang, Pingzhong Wang*, Xuefan Bai*

Center for Infectious Diseases, Tangdu Hospital, Fourth Military Medical University, Xi'an, Shaanxi, China

Abstract

Objectives: The aim of this study was to investigate the clinical characteristics and outcomes of critical patients with hemorrhagic fever with renal syndrome (HFRS) complicated by acute respiratory distress syndrome (ARDS).

Materials and Methods: To observe the demographic, epidemiological and clinical characteristics, and to explore the predictive effects for prognosis in laboratory findings, we conducted a detailed retrospective analysis of clinical records for critical patients with HFRS complicated by ARDS, treated at the center for infectious diseases, Tangdu Hospital, between January 2008 and December 2012.

Results: A total of 48 critical patients with laboratory confirmed HFRS accompanied by ARDS were enrolled in the study, including 27 survivors and 21 non-survivors, with a fatality rate of 43.75%. Thirty-one individuals (64.6%) contracted HFRS between the months of September and December. The non-survivors tended to have lower incidence of overlapping phase ($P = 0.025$). There were no obvious differences in the needs for mechanical ventilation (MV) and renal replacement therapy (RRT), except for the need for vasoactive drugs between the survivors and non-survivors ($P = 0.001$). The non-survivors were found to have higher frequencies of encephalopathy, refractory shock and multiple organ dysfunction syndrome (MODS), lower incidences of acute renal failure (ARF) and secondary hypertension ($P < 0.05$). The non-survivors tended to have lower levels of serum creatinine (Scr) ($P < 0.001$) and fibrinogen (Fib) ($P = 0.003$), higher incidences of prolonged prothrombin time (PT) ($P = 0.006$) and activated partial thromboplastin time (APTT) ($P = 0.020$) and higher levels of aspartate aminotransferase (AST) ($P = 0.015$), and the laboratory parameters mentioned above reached statistical significance for predicting prognosis ($P < 0.05$).

Conclusion: The high mortality rate of critical patients with HFRS complicated by ARDS emphasizes the importance of clinicians' alertness and timely initiation of systemic supportive therapy.

Editor: Xia Jin, University of Rochester, United States of America

Funding: Funding provided by National Basic Research Program of China (973 Program) (No.2012CB518905) and the National Natural Science Foundation of China (No.30901346, No.81071370). The funders had no role in study design, data collection and analysis, decision to publish, or preparation of the manuscript.

Competing Interests: The authors have declared that no competing interests exist.

* E-mail: wangpz63@126.com (PW); xfbai2011@163.com (XB)

[9] These authors contributed equally to this work.

Introduction

Hantaviruses are enveloped RNA viruses of the family *Bunyaviridae* [1]. These emerging zoonotic pathogens cause two distinct syndromes in humans: hemorrhagic fever with renal syndrome (HFRS) in Europe and Asia and hantavirus pulmonary syndrome (HPS) in the Americas [2,3]. China is the most severe endemic area of HFRS in the world, with 30,000–50,000 cases reported annually, which account for > 90% of the total number of cases worldwide [4,5]. The Shaanxi province is one of the most severely affected provinces in China, and Xi'an city is the central district of the Shaanxi province, with an increasing incidence and mortality rate in the last three years [6].

A hallmark of HFRS is capillary leak syndrome, causing edema and hemorrhage, which suggests that the vascular endothelium may be the prime target of the virus infection [7,8,9].Typical cases of HFRS progress through five successive phases: febrile, hypotensive, oliguric, diuretic and convalescent [10,11,12]. In some grave cases, the febrile, hypotensive and oliguric phases can overlap, resulting in acute progressive noncardiogenic pulmonary edema, appearing as acute respiratory distress syndrome (ARDS) and leading to greatly increased fatality rate. As far as we know, ARDS has become a major cause of death on severe sepsis patients treated in the intensive care unit (ICU) [13].

In the last five years, more than 1,200 cases of symptomatic patients with laboratory confirmed HFRS were treated at the Center for Infectious Diseases, Tangdu Hospital, a 300-bed primary care and tertiary referral medical center in the northeast district of China. In view of the higher incidence and hospital mortality rate of critical patients with HFRS complicated by ARDS, it is essential to gain a better, more comprehensive understanding of the clinical characteristics and outcomes of the patients, and to help clinicians provide timely monitoring and effective supportive therapy during the early stage of this disease.

Materials and Methods

Ethics Statement

This retrospective study was reviewed and approved by the Institutional Review Board of Tangdu Hospital. The patients' medical records were anonymized and de-identified prior to analysis.

Study Participants

The records of 432 typical patients with laboratory confirmed HFRS, treated at the Center for Infectious Diseases, Tangdu Hospital, between January 2008 and December 2012 were reviewed. The medical records of the selected patients were reviewed for analysis of the demographic, epidemiologic and clinical conditions, complications, outcomes and major supportive therapies. Patients who had other kidney diseases, diabetes, cardiovascular disease, hematological disease, autoimmune disease, viral hepatitis, and other liver diseases were excluded from this study.

Based upon the degree of hypotension, renal function, effusion, hemorrhage, and edema of the patients, the severity of HFRS was classified into four types [14]: (1) mild, defined as patients who had kidney injury without oliguria and hypotension; (2) moderate, defined as patients who had uremia, effusion (bulbar conjunctiva), hypotension, hemorrhage (skin and mucous membranes), and AKI with typical oliguria; (3) severe, defined as patients who had severe uremia, effusion (bulbar conjunctiva and either peritoneum or pleura), hemorrhage (skin and mucous membranes), hypotension and AKI with oliguria (urine output of 50–500 mL/day) for ≤ 5 days or anuria (urine output of <100 mL/day) for ≤ 2 days;(4) critical, defined as patients who usually had one or more of the following complications compared with the severe patients: refractory shock (≥ 2 days), visceral hemorrhage, heart failure, pulmonary edema, brain edema, severe secondary infection, and severe AKI with oliguria (urine output of 50–500 mL/day) for >5 days or anuria (urine output of <100 mL/day) for >2 days. Commonly, the so-called acute stage of the disease is defined as the period of febrile, hypotensive and oliguric phases; overlapping phases are defined as periods with overlapping febrile, hypotensive and oliguric phase. Overall, eighty-six of the cases were classified as of the critical type. According to the Berlin Definition of ARDS [15], forty-eight of the 86 critical patients exhibited ARDS during the clinical course and were eventually enrolled in this study.

Laboratory and Imaging Studies

Laboratory and imaging results that documented the clinical presentations and outcomes of the critical patients with HFRS complicated by ARDS were analyzed and compared Biochemical tests of blood samples were performed using an autoanalyzer (Sysmex, XT-4000i, Japan), including basic metabolic,liver and renal function and glucose tests. Blood clotting functions were tested using hematology analyzers (CA7000, Sysmex, Japan; ACL, TOP700, United States). Chest and abdomen organs were visualized using X-ray radiography (PLOYMOBIL 2.5, Siemens, Germany) and ultrasonography (DC-6, MINDRAY, China). Computed tomography (CT) (CTTM64, Siemens, Germany) was performed in some patients. Cardiac function was measured using Cardiofax (1350p, NIHON KOHDEN, Japan) and ultrasonography (DC-7, MINDRAY, China). Arterial blood gases were measured using an automatic blood gas system (ABL80, Denmark). Hemo cultures were tested using an autoanalyzer (BD9120, United States).

The diagnosis of HFRS was made based upon the detection of specific IgM and IgG antibodies to Hantaan virus (HTNV) in acute phase serum specimens by enzyme-linked immunosorbent (ELISA) assay. The assay was performed using IgG/IgM capture ELISA kits, which were analyzed using a multifunctional autoanalyzer(BIORAD-680, United States).

Renal replacement therapy (RRT)

There were two major patterns of RRT used in the study patients in our center: continuous renal replacement therapy (CRRT) and intermittent hematodialysis (IHD). According to the Chinese Medical Association's guide for blood purification in the ICU [16], critical patients with evidence of unstable hemodynamic status accompanied by multiple organ injury, pulmonary edema, fluid overload,severe electrolyte disturbances,encephalopathy and AKI were started with CRRT. For patients with stable hemodynamic status and less potentially fatal complications during their clinical course, IHD was chosen by clinicians as the first choice. However, over the period of treatment, a minority of critical patients may have lost the option of CRRT because of their critical condition on admission, and some of them even signed informed consents to withdraw RRT due to poor economic status.

Patients treated with CRRT were catheterized in the femoral vein with a double-lumen catheter. Replacement of catheters was performed in some patients with critical condition. The median duration of catheterization was 12 days (range of 3–28 days), and AN69 Hemofilters were used for patients treated with a PRISMA machine with an M100 extra-corporeal circuit. Substitution fluid: port prescription was used in all patients, and a bicarbonate buffer solution and other fluids were added separately. CRRT (24 h) was provided for most patients during the acute stage, particularly during the hypotensive overlapping oliguric phase. The main modality of CRRT was continuous venovenous hemodiafiltration (CVVHDF). Fluids were exchanged at a rate of 25–35 ml/(kg·h). To prevent coagulation, the filter and circuit were primed with heparinized saline. Heparin was given at an initial dose of 5–10 iu/kg and was maintained at a dose of 5–10 iu/kg/h in patients without bleeding tendency. No anticoagulant was used in patients with bleeding tendency, and frequent washing of the filter with substitution fluid was performed.

Patients treated with IHD were catheterized in the femoral vein with a double-lumen catheter. Ployflux 17L Capillary Dialyzers were used on patients treated with a hemodialyzer (AK96S, Gambro, Sweden). The dialysate flow rate was 400–600 ml/min with bagged fluid. All patients were treated with bicarbonate dialysate at a sodium concentration of 140 mmol/L. All patients were heparinized with low dose heparin or administered no anticoagulant and dialyzed for 3.0–4.0 hours, depending on the patient's condition.

Mechanical ventilation

According to the guidelines for the diagnosis and treatment of ALI/ARDS [13], the majority of the critical patients were treated with invasive mechanical ventilation (MV) (PB760, Tyco, United States) or noninvasive MV (SMARTAIR ST, AIROX, France) during the acute stage. However, for a minority of the critical patients, who eventually died because of their critical conditions or apparent respiratory and cardiac arrest on admission, family members provided informed consents to withdraw any invasive supporting treatments, including MV and hemodynamic monitoring due to poor economic status.

Definition of HFRS-related complications

Acute renal failure (ARF) was defined as the third stage of AKI according to the criteria of the Acute Kidney Injury Network (AKIN) [17]. Patients who manifested altered mental status (drowsiness, spasm, lethargy, agitation, or coma) were defined as having encephalopathy. Patients who manifested acute respiratory distress within a duration of one week including dyspnea, shortness of breath, cyanosis, pleural effusions on X-ray, and hypoxemia accompanied by oxygenation index (PaO_2/FiO_2) ≤200 mmHg that could not be explained by cardiac dysfunction and fluid overload were defined as having ARDS [15]. Gastrointestinal hemorrhage was defined as hematemesis or dark stools with hemodynamic instability and rapid decline of hemoglobin level to ≤7.0 g/dL. Secondary hyperglycemia was defined as an increase of fasting blood sugar ≥7.1 mmol/L without primary diabetes. Concurrent bacteremia was defined as a positive bacterial growth from blood culture within 72 h of hospital admission. Secondary hypertension was defined as systolic blood pressure (SBP) ≥140 mmHg during the hospital course without primary hypertension. Arrhythmia, including atrial premature beat, ventricular premature contraction, atrial fibrillation, ventricular fibrillation, supraventricular tachycardia, ventricular tachycardia and atrial ventricular block was confirmed by electrocardiography (ECG). Refractory shock was defined as shock of ≥ 24 h duration, which could not be resolved by fluid resuscitation or vasoactive drugs. In this study, MODS was defined as organ dysfunction involving two or more organs, with the exception of the lungs, during the acute stage after hospitalization, according to the current definition of MODS [18,19]. Patients who had upper gastrointestinal tract symptoms, including abdominal distension,nausea, vomiting and upper abdominal pain accompanied by elevated blood and urinary amylase and adrenomegaly on imaging were defined as having acute pancreatitis (AP) [20,21].

Statistical Analyses

Statistical analyses were performed using the SPSS 17.0 software (SPSS Inc, Chicago, IL, USA). The tables were prepared using Excel 2003 (Microsoft), and the figure was drawn using GraphPad Prism 5 (GraphPad Software, SanDiego CA). The demographic, clinical, laboratorial and imaging data between the survivors and non-survivors were compared using univariate analysis. Continuous variables were presented as means ± SD and analyzed using the Kolmogorov-Smirnov test for distribution normality and Levene's test for the homogeneity of variance. For normally distributed variables, the data were compared using Student's t-test. For variables with non-Gaussian distribution, the nonparametric Mann-Whitney U-test was used. The frequencies and percentages of qualitative variables were calculated. Significant differences between the survivors and non-survivors were tested by the chi-square test, and Fisher's exact test was used when numbers were too small to perform the chi-square test. Spearman's correlation coefficient was used to determine the correlation between laboratory values, complications and survival outcomes. Predictive value for the prognosis of the laboratory results were tested using receiver operating characteristic (ROC) curves and calculated by measuring the area under the curve (AUC) and 95% confidence interval (CI). A two-tailed $P < 0.05$ was considered statistically significant.

Results

Clinical, demographic and epidemiologic characteristics of the critical patients with HFRS complicated by ARDS

Of the 48 critical patients with laboratory confirmed HFRS accompanied by ARDS, 27 patients survived and 21 died, with a fatality rate of 43.75%. Of the 21 non-survivors, 16 cases died during the overlapping phase within the first week from the onset of the illness. 38 patients (79.2%) were male, and 35 cases (72.9%) reported 'farmer' as their occupation. The mean age and sex of the survivors and non-survivors were not significantly different ($P = 0.078$ and $P = 0.929$, respectively). There were also no significant differences in the seasonal incidence (September to December), occupation, interval from symptom onset to patients' hospital arrival and duration of febrile phase ($P = 0.732$, $P = 0.653$, $P = 0.936$, $P = 0.385$, respectively) (Table 1). The incidence of the overlapping phase in the non-survivors was greater than that of the survivors ($P = 0.025$) (Table 1). Of the main supportive treatments, there were no significant differences in the frequencies of MV and RRT, except for the need for vasoactive drugs ($P = 0.001$) (Table 1).

Complication related to HFRS in critical patients with ARDS

Among HFRS-related complications, the incidences of encephalopathy, refractory shock and MODS in the non-survivors were significantly higher than that of the survivors($P<0.001$), while the incidences of ARF and secondary hypertension in the survivors were significantly higher than that of the non-survivors ($P = 0.011$ and $P = 0.003$, respectively) (Table 2). No significant differences in the frequencies of arrhythmia, gastrointestinal hemorrhage, hyperglycemia, concurrent bacteremia and acute pancreatitis were identified ($P>0.05$) (Table 2).

Laboratory findings in critical patients with HFRS complicated by ARDS during the acute stage

Of the critical study patients, the mean levels of the maximum leukocyte counts, alanine aminotransferase (ALT), aspartate aminotransferase (AST), serum creatinine (Scr) and glucose during the acute stage were higher than the reference values; the prothrombin time (PT), activated partial thromboplastin time (APTT) and thrombin time (TT) during the acute stage were more prolonged than the reference values. Except for the levels of the maximum mahemoglobin (HGB) and uric acid (UA) in the non-survivors; the means levels of the nadir platelet (PLT), serum albumin (ALB) and minimum fibrinogen (Fib) were lower or shorter than the reference values ($P<0.001$) (Table 3). Compared with the survivors, the non-survivors were found to have lower Scr ($P<0.001$) and Fib ($P = 0.003$), and to have higher incidences of prolonged PT ($P = 0.006$), and APTT ($P = 0.020$), as well as higher levels of AST ($P = 0.015$) (Table 3).

Spearman correlation and ROC analysis

Of the laboratory data, Spearman correlation analysis revealed that the levels of AST, PT and APTT were negatively correlated with survival outcome, while Scr and Fib were positively correlated with survival outcome ($P<0.05$) (Table 4).

To explore the predictive value of the laboratory data for prognosis, the ROC and AUC were analyzed. The results for Scr, Fib, AST, PT and APTT were all found to be statistically significant for predicting prognosis ($P<0.05$), with AUCs of 0.878, 0.744, 0.764, 0.742 and 0.690, respectively (Figure 1,Table 5).

Discussion

As far as we know, this is the first clinical investigation of critical patients with HFRS complicated by ARDS in China. In this study, we compared the demographic, epidemiological, clinical and laboratory characteristics of the survivor and non-survivors, and

Table 1. Clinical, epidemiological and demographic characteristics of critical patients with HFRS complicated by ARDS

Variables	Survivors (n = 27)	Non-survivors (n = 21)	p value*
Mean age, years	46.41±13.36	52.71±11.82	0.078
Male/Female, n	22/5	16/5	0.929
Occupation (farmer), n (%)	19 (70.4)	16 (76.2)	0.653
Seasonal incidence (September to December), n (%)	18 (66.7)	13 (62.9)	0.732
Frequency of MV (n/%), n (%)	24 (88.9)	18 (85.7)	1.000
Single invasive MV, n (%)	18 (66.7)	13 (62.9)	0.732
Single noninvasive MV, n (%)	3 (11.1)	2 (9.5)	1.000
Combination, n (%)	3 (11.1)	3 (14.3)	1.000
Incidence of overlapping phase, n (%)	15 (55.6)	18 (85.7)	0.025
Frequency of RRT, n (%)	26 (95.3)	16 (76.2)	0.099
CRRT initiated, n (%)	18 (66.7)	13 (61.9)	0.732
Frequency of vasoactive drugs, n (%)	8 (29.6)	16 (76.2)	0.001
Interval from onset to admission, days	4.04±1.72	4.00±1.34	0.936
Duration of febrile phase, days	5.04±1.87	4.62±1.43	0.385

Mean ± SD for continuous variables, n (%) for categorical variables.
MV, mechanical ventilation; RRT, renal replacement therapy; CRRT, continuous renal replacement therapy.
* Survivors vs. non-survivors.

identified the predictive value of laboratory finding on patients' survival.

In this study, forty-eight of the 86 critical patients with HFRS reviewed exhibited ARDS during the acute stage with an incidence of 55.81%, which indicates that ARDS is a common clinical complication in critical patients infected by HTNV in Xi'an city [6]. Of the 48 critical patients with HFRS enrolled, 21 patients died, representing a high fatality rate of 43.75%, which was similar with that of patients with severe septic or septic shock in the ICU [22,23]. The pathophysiologic mechanism of ARDS is thought to involve continuous fluid leakage from the intravascular lumen to the extravascular compartment and the lung alveolar space [24,25]. Analogous to several reports of patients with HFRS infected by Puumala virus (PUUV) in the Europe [26–28], this study also revealed that more critical HFRS patients in the northwest region of China can manifest pulmonary-renal syndrome during the clinical course, leading to high permeability pulmonary edema and hypoxic respiratory failure associated with high mortality rate. Not only the hantavirus pulmonary syndrome (HPS) prevailed in the America continent [29], hantavirus infection should also be considered as a cause of acute respiratory distress in all endemic areas worldwide.

HFRS is widely accepted as having the basic clinical characteristics of systemic inflammatory response syndrome (SIRS), and the patient's pathophysiologic manifestations of the hypotensive phase are similar to those of typical distributive shock [5]. Acute progressive noncardiogenic pulmonary edema is a main cause of ARDS in critical patients with HFRS, which is commonly accompanied by a concurrent marked hemoconcentration during the acute stage, especially the hypotensive phase. Generally, the hypotensive phase of HFRS (e.g., low blood pressure and circulatory collapse) occurs between day 3 and day 7 of the

Table 2. HFRS-related complications in critical patients with ARDS.

Variables	Survivors (n = 27)	Non-survivors (n = 21)	p value*
Arrhythmia, n (%)	6 (22.2)	4 (19.0)	1.000
Gastrointestinal hemorrhage, n (%)	10 (37.0)	12 (57.1)	0.165
Hyperglycemia, n (%)	22 (81.5)	18 (85.7)	1.000
Encephalopathy, n (%)	6 (22.2)	20 (95.2)	<0.001
Concurrent bacteremia, n (%)	11 (40.7)	5 (23.8)	0.217
Secondary hypertension, n (%)	18 (66.7)	5 (23.8)	0.003
Refractory shock, n (%)	2 (7.4)	13 (61.9)	<0.001
MODS, n (%)	4 (14.8)	13 (61.9)	0.001
AP, n (%)	8 (29.6)	3 (14.3)	0.364
ARF, n (%)	25 (92.6)	12 (57.1)	0.011

n (%) for categorical variables.
MODS, multiple organ dysfunction syndrome; AP, acute pancreatitis; ARF, acute renal failure.
* Survivors vs. non-survivors.

Table 3. Laboratory findings in critical patients with HFRS complicated by ARDS during the acute stage.

Variables	Survivors (n = 27)	Non-survivors (n = 21)	p value'
Maximum leukocyte counts, $\times 10^9$/L	35.95±15.49*	46.93±22.45*	0.051
Nadir PLT, $\times 10^9$/L	11.81±12.93**	15.29±10.94**	0.330
Maximum HGB, g/L	170.96±22.29*	162.48±19.94	0.178
Maximum ALT, U/L	208.07±256.04*	350.33±324.42*	0.096
Nadir serum ALB, g/L	22.74±5.14**	21.31±5.16**	0.344
Maximum Scr, μmol/L	788.95±236.27*	411.88±197.49*	<0.001
Maximum UA, μmol/L	543.20±213.00*	433.76±154.57	0.054
Maximum glucose, mmol/L	13.58±6.30*	14.52±8.30*	0.656
Longest PT, sec	15.95±3.87*	23.73±11.32*	0.006
Longest APTT, sec	50.92±16.16*	63.58±20.13*	0.020
Longest TT, sec	25.19±6.79*	26.44±7.49*	0.554
Minimum Fib, g/L	1.63±0.64**	1.13±0.40**	0.003
Maximum AST, U/L	370.33±406.15*	1271.9±1531.14*	0.015

Reference values: Leukocyte count (3.2–9.7)×109/L; PLT (100–300)×109/L; HGB (120–160) g/L (male), (110–150) g/L (female); ALT (4–44) U/L; AST (8–38) U/L; serum ALB (35–55) g/L; serum Cr (53–97) μmol/L (male), (35–71) μmol/L (female); UA (210–430) μmol/L (male), (150–360) μmol/L (female); glucose (3.89–6.11) mmol/L; PT (8.8–13.8) sec; APTT (25.1–36.5) sec; TT (10.3–16.6) sec, and Fib (2.38–4.98) g/L.

PLT, platelet; HGB, hemoglobin; ALT, alanine aminotransferase; ALB, albumin; Scr, serum creatinine; UA, uric acid; PT, prothrombin time; APTT, activated partial thromboplastin time; TT, thrombin time; Fib, fibrinogen;AST, aspartate aminotransferase.

'Survivors vs. non-survivors.

* Higher or longer than the reference value, P<0.05.

** Lower than the reference value, P<0.05.

clinical course. Some critical patients even have overlapping phases combined with various fatal complications such as refractory shock, encephalopathy and MODS except for ARDS, which was demonstrated in the present study (Table 2). Our study revealed that the frequency of administration of vasoactive drugs in non-survivors was higher, while the frequencies of MV and RRT were not significantly different between the survivors and non-survivors (Table 1). This result appears to indicate that the invasive supportive treatments mentioned above were not capable of altering the final prognosis. We acknowledge that a minority of patients in the non-survivors were treated conservatively without the use of MV and RRT because of their critical condition on admission and their poor financial means, which may have influenced the statistical significance of the result to some degree. Although no specific antiviral therapy for HFRS is currently available, earlier diagnosis, earlier monitoring, earlier admission to the ICU, and timely and systematically supportive therapy would be necessary to ensure patients' survival during the acute stage and significantly reduce the mortality rate compared to critical patients with HFRS treated conservatively [4,30].

Of the 48 critical patients with HFRS complicated by ARDS, 38 patients (79.2%) were male and the occupation of 35 patients (79.2%) was farming. A total of 31 patients (64.6%) contracted the disease between September and December. Until now, the hantavirus strains from host rodents and patients in Xi'an only belong to the HTNV, and SEOV strains have not been found [6]. The high incidence and seasonal distribution (Table 1) are consistent with the known biological and epidemical characteristics of the predominant natural host of HTNV, *Apodemus agrarius*, and the susceptibility of patients working in surroundings that are the natural habitats of rodents in Xi'an city [5,6]. Furthermore, the incidence of the overlapping phase in non-survivors was higher

Table 4. Spearman correlation analysis of laboratory data and patient outcome.

Variables	Outcome		Variables	Outcome	
	r	p value		r	p value
Scr	0.650	<0.001	Fib	0.420	0.003
PT	–0.416	0.003	AST	–0.453	0.001
APTT	–0.327	0.023			

r, correlation coefficient; Scr, serum creatinine; PT, prothrombin time; APTT, activated partial thromboplastin time; Fib, fibrinogen;AST, aspartate aminotransferase.

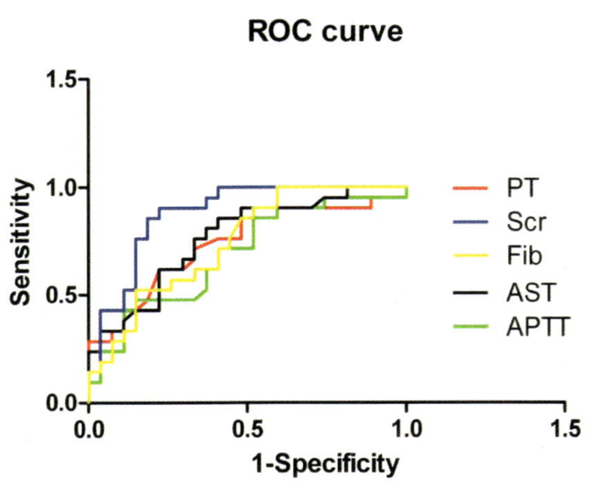

Figure 1. ROC analysis of laboratory data in predicting death in critical patients with HFRS complicated by ARDS.

Table 5. Predictive values for prognosis of laboratory data in critical patients with HFRS accompanied by ARDS.

Variables	AUC	P value[a]	Cut-off value[b]	Sensitivity[c]	Specificity[c]	95% CI[c]	
						Lower	Upper
Scr[c]	0.878	<0.001	650.85	90.5	77.8	78.1	97.6
PT	0.742	0.004	13.15	61.9	77.8	59.6	88.7
APTT	0.690	0.025	43.2	85.7	48.1	53.8	84.3
			66.6	47.6	85.2		
Fib[d]	0.744	0.004	1.106	52.4	85.2	60.7	88.1
			1.429	85.7	51.9		
AST	0.764	0.002	310	76.2	66.7	62.9	89.9

AUC, area under the curve; CI, confidence interval.
[a]P value for calculated AUC in predicting death (ROC analysis).
[b]Units of measure of the cut-off values are μmol/L, sec, sec, g/L and U/L, respectively.
[c]Sensitivity, specificity and 95% confidence interval are presented as percentages.
[d]Test direction: lower test result indicates a more positive test.

than that of the survivors (Table 1), which was consistent with the clinical course of critical HFRS. After all, some critical patients died of fatal clinical complications during the acute stage, particularly during the hypotensive phase or overlapping phases. Almost all the critical patients who survived the overlapping phases manifested obvious oliguria with AKI. Because of the reasonable utilization of RRT, including CRRT and IHD [31], only a minority of the patients would have died of AKI.

Kidney is a major organ damaged during HFRS, and previous research had demonstrated that the most prominent pathological presentation was acute tubulointerstitial nephritis following the infiltration of inflammatory cells [32]. In this study, 37 critical patients with HFRS complicated by ARDS (77.1%) developed ARF, the third stage of AKI [17] (Table 2). Interestingly, we observed that the incidence of ARF in the survivors was significantly higher than that of the non-survivors (Table 2). We also observed that Scr levels were positively correlated with the survival outcome by correlation analysis (Table 4). Non-survivors were also found to have lower Scr levels (Table 3), and a low level of Scr was statistically associated with increased mortality, with an AUC of 0.878 (Table 4, Figure 1). As it mentioned above, the overlapping phase usually occurs within the first week of the clinical course, and some critical patients may have died of fatal complications during the phase when ARF was not detected. Once the patients pass through the overlapping phase, severe AKI and secondary hypertension will become the major clinical complications accompanied with the occurrence of single oliguric and diuretic phase. Given that a majority of the critical patients would survive the oliguric and diuretic phase because of the reasonable application of RRT and vasoactive agents, the stage of AKI and secondary hypertension have not been the direct influential factors for prognosis.

In our study, univariate analysis demonstrated that non-survivors had lower levels of Scr and Fib, and higher incidences of prolonged PT, APTT and higher levels of AST (Table 3). Spearman correlation analysis revealed that AST, PT and APTT were negatively correlated with survival outcome, whereas Fib was positively correlated with survivor outcome (Table 4). ROC analysis also revealed that Fib, AST, PT and APTT were all statistically significant for predicting patient prognosis, with AUC of 0.744, 0.764, 0.742 and 0.690, respectively (Figure 1,Table 5). This observation indicated that critical patients with HFRS complicated by ARDS often experienced hepatic, cardiac and kidney injuries. Stress hyperglycemia and hypermetabolism were also common during the acute stage. Severe plasma leakage, massive bleeding and profound shock are known to lead to tissue hypoperfusion, potentially triggering AKI and hepatic injury. Furthermore, the non-survivors appeared to be in more critical condition, with a higher degree of inflammation and coagulation abnormality compared with the survivors. The high concentration of HGB was closely related to the degree of pachyemia; the low level of PLT may reflect decreased platelet production or increased platelet consumption, which may be associated with the severity of the underlying hemorrhage [33,34]. Furthermore, the low level of ALB correlated with degree of the loss of vascular integrity, enhanced vascular permeability and liver dysfunction [35]. Overall, all the laboratory parameters discussed above reflected the severity of the disease, and clinicians should pay attention to their dynamic changes that occur during the acute stage, by close monitoring and initiation of timely management, as indicated.

Being a retrospective study, some limitations must be addressed. First, our study was conducted at the largest center for infectious diseases in the northwest region of China. Most patients with severe clinical conditions come to our medical center, but a significant number of critical patients may still have been admitted to local hospitals. Therefore, the demographic and epidemiological characteristics and mortality rate of the critical patients with HFRS complicated by ARDS in our study may have been biased. Second, we were unable to calculate the acute physiology, age, chronic health evaluation (APACHE II) score [36], sepsis related organ failure assessment (SOFA) [37] and simplified acute physiology score (SAPS II) [38] of the patients on admission in this study because of the loss of detailed clinical data on central nervous system dysfunction. These data may be very important for predicting the prognosis and the diagnosis of these clinical conditions may have been biased based upon clinicians' personal recognition of the clinical severity of this disease. Third, the relatively small number of cases limited the statistical power of our study. Finally, the clinical outcomes and classifications of patients with HFRS might be biased due to the lack of a more standardized protocol for the management of patients with HFRS. For example, the choice of resuscitation fluid (i.e., crystal or colloid solution), optimal dose of vasoactive agents, optimal timing and modality of MV, which are each important in the treatment of HFRS, were not standardized in this study.

In summary, the high mortality rate of critical patients with HFRS complicated by ARDS underscores the importance of clinicians' alertness and timely initiation of systematic supportive therapy.

Author Contributions

Conceived and designed the experiments: HD PW XB. Analyzed the data: HD WJ YZ. Wrote the paper: HD. Reviewed and collected the data: HD JL JW HY. Reviewed the manuscript: PW XB. Approved the final manuscript: HD JL WJ HY YZ JW PW XB.

References

1. Jonsson CB, Figueiredo LT, Vapalahti O (2010) A global perspective on hantavirus ecology, epidemiology, and disease. Clin Microbiol Rev 23: 412–41.
2. Schmaljohn CS, Hasty SE, Dalrymple JM, LeDuc JW, Lee HW, et al. (1985) Antigenic and genetic properties of viruses linked to hemorrhagic fever with renal syndrome. Science 227: 1041–4.
3. Muranyi W, Bahr U, Zeier M, van der Woude FJ (2005) Hantavirus infection. J Am Soc Nephro 16: 3669–79.
4. Song G (1998) Manual for prevention and cure of hemorrhagic fever with renal syndrome. Beijing: People's Health Press. P316.
5. Luo CW, Chen HX (2008) Epidemiological characteristics and the strategy of vaccination on hemorrhagic fever with renal syndrome in the last 10 years, in China. Zhonghua Liu Xing Bing Xue Za Zhi 29: 1017–9.
6. Ma C, Yu P, Nawaz M, Zuo S, Jin T, et al. (2012) Hantaviruses in rodents and humans, Xi'an, PR China. J Gen Virol 93: 2227–2236.
7. Schmaljohn C, Hjelle B (1997) Hantaviruses: a global disease problem. Emerg Infect Dis 3: 95–104.
8. Gavrilovskaya IN, Brown EJ, Ginsberg MH, Mackow ER (1999) Cellular entry of hantaviruses which cause hemorrhagic fever with renal syndrome is mediated by β3 integrins. J Virol 73: 3951–9.
9. Hayasaka D, Maeda K, Ennis FA, Terajima M (2007) Increased permeability of human endothelial cell line EA.hy926 induced by hantavirus-specific cytotoxic T lymphocytes. Virus Res 123: 120–7.
10. World Health Organization (1983) Hemorrhagic fever with renal syndrome: memorandum from a WHO meeting. Bull World Health Organ 61: 269–275.
11. Ministry of Health, People's Republic of China (1987) Prevention and Treatment Program of Epidemic Hemorrhagic Fever. Categorization number 2360028701. China.
12. Ma Y, Liu B, Yuan B, Wang J, Yu H, et al. (2012) Sustained high level of serum VEGF at convalescent stage contributes to the renal recovery after HTNV Infection in patients with hemorrhagic fever with renal syndrome. Clin Dev Immuno 2012: 812386. doi: 10.1155/2012/812386. Epub 2012 Oct
13. Chinese Medical Association to severe medicine branch (2006) Guidelines for the diagnosis and treatment of acute lung injury/acute respiratory distress syndrome. Available: http://www.cscem.org/cn/news.asp?id = 115.html. Accessed 15 November 2011.
14. Bai XF, Xu ZK (2013) Hemorrhagic Fever with Renal Syndrome. Beijing: People's Medical Publishing House. P722.
15. Ranieri VM, Rubenfeld GD, Thompson BT, Ferguson ND, Caldwell E, et al. (2012) Acute respiratory distress syndrome (ARDS): The Berlin Definition. JAMA 307: 2526–33.
16. Chinese Medical Association to severe medicine branch (2009) Guidelines for blood purification in ICU. Available: http://www.cscem.org/cn/news.asp?id = 121.html. Accessed 15 November 2011.
17. Mehta RL, Kellum JA, Shah SV, Molitoris BA, Ronco C, et al. (2007) Acute Kidney Injury Network: report of an initiative to improve outcomes in acute kidney injury. Critical Care 11: R31.
18. Johnson D, Mayers I (2001) Multiple organ dysfunction syndrome: a narrative review. Can J Anaesth 48: 502–9.
19. Wheeler AP (2007) Recent developments in the diagnosis and management of severe sepsis. Chest 132: 1967–76.
20. Sarr MG (2013) 2012 revision of the Atlanta classification of acute pancreatitis. Pol Arch Med Wewn 123: 118–24.
21. Greer SE, Burchard KW (2009) Acute pancreatitis and critical illness: a tale of hypoperfusion and inflammation. Chest 136: 1413–9.
22. Chen WC (2012) Possible interventional therapies in severe sepsis or septic shock. Acta Anaesthesiol Taiwan 50: 74–7.
23. Liu DV (2010) Practical Critical Care Medicine. Beijing: People's Medical Publishing House. P1054.
24. Bhargava M, Wendt CH (2012) Biomarkers in acute lung injury. Transl Res 159: 205–17.
25. Launay D, Thomas CH, Fleury D, Roueff S, Line ML, et al. (2003) Pulmonary-renal syndrome due to hemorrhagic fever with renal syndrome: an unusual manifestation of puumala virus infection in France. Clin Nephrol 59: 297–300.
26. Brackett LE, Rotenberg J, Sherman CB (1994) Hantavirus pulmonary syndrome in New England and Europe. N Engl J Med 331: 545; author reply 547–8.
27. Clement J, Maes P, Lagrou K, Van Ranst M, Lameire N (2012) A unifying hypothesis and a single name for a complex globally emerging infection: hantavirus disease. Eur J Clin Microbiol Infect Dis 31: 1–5.
28. Rasmuson J, Adnersson C, Norrman E, Haney M, Evander M, et al. (2011) Time to revise the paradigm of hantavirus syndromes? Hantavirus pulmonary syndrome caused by European hantavirus. Eur J Clin Microbiol Infect Dis 30: 685–90.
29. Duchin JS, Koster FT, Peters CJ, Simpson GL, Tempest B, et al. (1994) Hantavirus pulmonary syndrome: a clinical description of 17 patients with a newly recognized disease. The Hantavirus Study Group. N Engl J Med 330: 949–55.
30. Huggins JW, Hsiang CM, Cosgriff TM, Guang MY, Smith JI, et al. (1991) Prospective, double-blind, concurrent, placebo-controlled clinical trial of intravenous ribavirin therapy of hemorrhagic fever with renal syndrome. J Infect Dis 164: 1119–27.
31. Ghahramani N, Shadrou S, Hollenbeak C (2008) A systematic review of continuous renal replacement therapy and intermittent haemodialysis in management of patients with acute renal failure. Nephrology (Carlton) 13: 570–8.
32. Kim S, Sung SH, An HR, Jun YH, Yu M, et al. (2010) A case report of crescentic glomerulonephritis associated with hantaan virus infection. Nephrol Dial Transplant 25: 2790–2.
33. Levi M, Löwenberg EC (2008) Thrombocytopenia in critically ill patients. Semin Thromb Hemost 34: 417–24.
34. Vanderschueren S, De Weerdt A, Malbrain M, Vankersschaever D, Frans E, et al. (2000) Thrombocytopenia and prognosis in intensive care. Crit Care Med 28: 1871–6.
35. Kim YO, Yoon SA, Ku YM, Yang CW, Kim YS, et al. (2003) Serum albumin level correlates with disease severity in patients with hemorrhagic fever with renal syndrome. J Korean Med Sci 18: 696–700.
36. Knaus WA, Draper EA, Wagner DB, Zimmerman JE (1985) Apache II: A severity of disease classification system. Crit Care Med 13: 818–29.
37. Vincent J-L, De Mendonca A, Cantraine F, Moreno R, Takala J, et al. (1998) Use of the SOFA score to assess the incidence of organ dysfunction/failure in intensive care units: Results of a multicenter, prospective study. Working group on "sepsis-related problems" of the European Society of Intensive Care Medicine. Crit Care Med 26: 1793–800.
38. Le Gall JR, Lemeshow S, Saulnier F (1993) A new simplified acute physiology score (SAPS II) based on a European/North American multicenter study. JAMA 270: 2957–63.

Heart Rate-Corrected QT Interval Helps Predict Mortality after Intentional Organophosphate Poisoning

Shou-Hsuan Liu, Ja-Liang Lin, Cheng-Hao Weng, Huang-Yu Yang, Ching-Wei Hsu, Kuan-Hsing Chen, Wen-Hung Huang, Tzung-Hai Yen*

Division of Clinical Toxicology, Department of Nephrology, Chang Gung Memorial Hospital and College of Medicine, Chang Gung University, Taipei, Taiwan

Abstract

Introduction: In this study, we investigated the outcomes for patients with intentional organophosphate poisoning. Previous reports indicate that in contrast to normal heart rate-corrected QT intervals (QTc), QTc prolongation might be indicative of a poor prognosis for patients exposed to organophosphates.

Methods: We analyzed the records of 118 patients who were referred to Chang Gung Memorial Hospital for management of organophosphate poisoning between 2000 and 2011. Patients were grouped according to their initial QTc interval, i.e., normal (<0.44 s) or prolonged (>0.44 s). Demographic, clinical, laboratory, and mortality data were obtained for analysis.

Results: The incidence of hypotension in patients with prolonged QTc intervals was higher than that in the patients with normal QTc intervals (P = 0.019). By the end of the study, 18 of 118 (15.2%) patients had died, including 3 of 75 (4.0%) patients with normal QTc intervals and 15 of 43 (34.9%) patients with prolonged QTc intervals. Using multivariate-Cox-regression analysis, we found that hypotension (OR = 10.930, 95% CI = 2.961–40.345, P = 0.000), respiratory failure (OR = 4.867, 95% CI = 1.062–22.301, P = 0.042), coma (OR = 3.482, 95% CI = 1.184–10.238, P = 0.023), and QTc prolongation (OR = 7.459, 95% CI = 2.053–27.099, P = 0.002) were significant risk factors for mortality. Furthermore, it was revealed that non-survivors not only had longer QTc interval (503.00±41.56 versus 432.71±51.21 ms, P = 0.002), but also suffered higher incidences of hypotension (83.3 versus 12.0%, P = 0.000), shortness of breath (64 versus 94.4%, P = 0.010), bronchorrhea (55 versus 94.4%, P = 0.002), bronchospasm (50.0 versus 94.4%, P = 0.000), respiratory failure (94.4 versus 43.0%, P = 0.000) and coma (66.7 versus 11.0%, P = 0.000) than survivors. Finally, Kaplan-Meier analysis demonstrated that cumulative mortality was higher among patients with prolonged QTc intervals than among those with normal QTc intervals (Log-rank test, Chi-square test = 20.36, P<0.001).

Conclusions: QTc interval helps predict mortality after intentional organophosphate poisoning.

Editor: Loren E. Wold, Ohio State University, United States of America

Funding: The authors have no support or funding to report.

Competing Interests: The authors have declared that no competing interests exist.

* E-mail: m19570@adm.cgmh.org.tw

Introduction

Accidental or intentional ingestion of pesticides or herbicides is common in Taiwan because these poisons are easily accessible [1]. In a nationwide study [2], all 4799 organophosphate poisonings reported to Taiwan's Poison Control Centers between July 1985 and December 2006 were reviewed. Most organophosphate exposures were to a single organophosphate (80.37%) and nearly all were acute (98.37%). Ingestion was the most common route of exposure (74.50%), and attempted suicide (64.72%) was the most common reason given for exposure. Most of the reported exposure occurred in adults (93.25%) and males were more commonly exposed than females (64.95%). Most patients (61.97%) received atropine and/or pralidoxime. The mortality rate for all 4799 organophosphate poisonings was 12.71% [2].

There are 3 distinct clinical syndromes after acute organophosphate poisoning [3]: (1) acute cholinergic crisis (<0.5 d) as a result of acetylcholinesterase inhibition, (2) an intermediate syndrome (0.5–7 d) that has an underlying mechanism that is still unclear, and (3) delayed neuropathy (6–21 d) that is explained by the inhibition of neuropathy-target esterase. Acute cholinergic crisis [3] includes signs and symptoms resulting from hyperstimulation of muscarinic receptors (e.g., bradycardia, bronchoconstriction, bronchorrhea, hypotension, increased gastrointestinal motility, abdominal cramps, miosis, hypersalivation), nicotinic receptors (e.g., hypertension, tachycardia, fibrillation, fasciculation, necrosis of striated muscles), and both central muscarinic and nicotinic receptors (e.g., tremor, movement incoordination, seizures, central depression of respiration, coma, death). The intermediate syndrome [4] is characterized by the onset of proximal muscle weakness and cranial nerve palsies. Difficulty in breathing may progress to respiratory failure due to paralysis of the diaphragm and other muscles of respiration. Delayed polyneuropathy [4] predominantly affects the long nerves or tracts in the nervous system, causing symmetrical weakness of peripheral muscles in the hands and feet, and resulting in variable degrees of sensory impairment.

The cardiac complications associated with organophosphate poisoning are not fully appreciated by many medical practitioners. Organophosphate poisoning may precipitate complex ventricular arrhythmias, a frequently overlooked and potentially lethal aspect of this condition [5]. The mechanism by which organophosphates induce cardiotoxicity is still uncertain. In 1982, Ludomirsky et al [6] described 3 phases of cardiac toxicity after organophosphate poisoning: phase 1, a brief period of increased sympathetic tone; phase 2, a prolonged period of parasympathetic activity; and phase 3, in which QT prolongation is followed by torsade de pointes ventricular tachycardia and ventricular fibrillation [6]. The long QT-interval syndrome is believed to originate from intense and unequal sympathetic stimulation of myocardial fibers. QT-interval prolongation has been observed in some cases of severe bradycardia or disease of the central nervous system. Therefore, both sympathetic and parasympathetic overactivity may cause QT-interval prolongation, and it is not surprising to find QT-interval prolongation in cases of severe organophosphate poisoning.

In a preliminary study at Chang Gung Memorial Hospital [7], Chuang et al reported that patients with QTc prolongation had a higher mortality rate (19.6% vs. 4.8%, $P<0.001$) and a higher incidence of respiratory failure (56.7% vs. 20.6%, $P<0.001$) than patients without QTc prolongation. However, the data was not examined using Cox proportional hazard models, so analysis of multiple risk factors was not possible. Therefore, in this study, we investigated the clinical features, QTc interval, physiological markers, and clinical outcomes of Taiwanese patients after intentional organophosphate poisoning. We determined what association, if any, exists between these variables. Most importantly, we evaluated QTc interval prolongation as a predictor of mortality after organophosphate poisoning.

Materials and Methods

This retrospective observational study complied with the guidelines of the Declaration of Helsinki and approved by the Medical Ethics Committee of Chang Gung Memorial Hospital, a tertiary referral center located in the northern part of Taiwan. Since this study involved retrospective review of existing data, the Institutional Review Board approval was obtained, but without specific informed consent from patients. However, the informed consent of risk of acute organophosphate poisoning and all treatment modalities (including cardiopulmonary cerebral resuscitation, etc) were obtained from all patients on their initial admission. In addition, all individual information was securely protected (by delinking identifying information from main data set) and available to investigators only. Furthermore, all the data were analyzed anonymously. On the other hand, if this study involved retrospective review of existing data plus retrospective analysis of remaining biological samples, both Institutional Review Board approval and specific informed consent must be obtained from all patients. The Institutional Review Board of Chang Gung Memorial Hospital has specifically waived the need for consent. Finally, all primary data were collected according to strengthening the reporting of observational studies in epidemiology guidelines.

Patients

We analyzed the records of 118 patients with intentional organophosphate poisoning who were examined at Chang Gung Memorial Hospital between 2000 and 2011. Diagnosis of organophosphate poisoning was based on history of exposure, clinical effects, and serum cholinesterase activity. Blood cholinesterase activity was determined using an enzymatic method (normal values, 7–19 U/mL) immediately after patient arrival at the hospital. The pesticide involved was determined by history, container label, or product information provided by the patient. A complete clinical profile of each patient was recorded using a standardized form. We obtained the following data for each patient: age, sex, blood pressure, heart rate, type and toxicity classification of organophosphate, underlying diseases, smoking habits, alcohol consumption, use of medications that might be associated with QTc-prolongation, time elapsed between poisoning and arrival at the hospital, duration of follow-up, clinical manifestations, electrocardiogram results, blood cholinesterase level, hemogram, biochemistry, detoxification protocol used, and mortality. The electrocardiogram recordings were obtained upon arrival at the emergency department. Of the 118 patients, there were 75 patients with normal (<0.44 s) QTc intervals, and 43 patients with prolonged (>0.44 s) QTc intervals.

Inclusion and exclusion criteria

All patients older than 18 years of age who were diagnosed with organophosphate poisoning at Chang Gung Memorial Hospital between 2000 and 2011 were eligible for inclusion in this study. Patients were excluded from this study if they were younger than 18 years of age or did not have low blood cholinesterase levels despite suspicions of exposure.

Detoxification protocols

The protocols used to treat patients included gastric lavage with large amounts of normal saline, followed by infusion of 1 g/kg activated charcoal and 250 mL magnesium citrate via nasogastric tube. Magnesium citrate was used to prevent constipation after charcoal administration. Patients were also treated with specific antidotes that included atropine and oximes. Intravenous atropine was administered at a starting dose of 2 mg every 1–2 h, and dosing was titrated to the clearing of respiratory secretions and cessation of bronchoconstriction. Pralidoxime therapy (1 g every 4 h, intravenous) was also given to all patients with evidence of cholinergic toxicity.

Definition of clinical events

Classification of organophosphate toxicity followed formal World Health Organization recommendations: Ia, extremely hazardous; Ib, highly hazardous; II, moderately hazardous; III, slightly hazardous; and U, unlikely to present acute hazard [8]. Acute renal failure was diagnosed if serum creatinine level increased to greater than 1.27 mg/dL in males or 1.03 mg/dL in females. Acute respiratory failure was defined as a condition of respiratory insufficiency requiring intubation and mechanical ventilation for more than 24 h, regardless of the fraction of inspired oxygen [9]. Hypotension was defined as a systolic blood pressure of less than 90 mmHg [10]. Structural heart disease was defined as non-coronary cardiovascular disease processes and related interventions [11]. Uses of medications that might be associated with QTc-prolongation were recorded. In this regard, the anti-arrhythmic agents included class Ia, class Ic, and class III agents [12]. The anti-microbials include macrolides/ketolides, certain fluoroquinolones, certain anti-malarials, pentamidine and azole anti-fungals [13]. The anti-psychotics and antidepressants included a) typical anti-psychotics such as chlorpromazine, pimozide, thioridazine, perphenazine, trifluoperazine, haloperidol, and droperidol; b) atypical anti-psychotics such clozapine, quetiapine, risperidone, sultopride, ziprasidone, and loxapine; c) tricyclic anti-depressants such as amitryptyline, amoxapine,

Table 1. Baseline characteristics of patients with organophosphate poisoning (N = 118).

Variable	Normal QTc (N = 75)	Prolonged QTc (N = 43)	P
QT interval, ms	323.26±42.32	390.65±51.15	0.000
QTc interval, ms	411.13±16.76	500.35±35.52	0.000
Age, years	52.04±16.94	56.37±14.65	0.163
Male, n (%)	52 (69.3)	25 (58.1)	0.219
Organophosphate type, n (%)			0.466
Mevinphos	6 (8.0)	4 (9.3)	
Parathion	3 (4.0)	1 (2.3)	
Phorate	1 (1.3)	0 (0.0)	
Terbufos	1 (1.3)	1 (2.3)	
Dichlorvos	1 (1.3)	0 (0.0)	
Fenamiphos	1 (1.3)	0 (0.0)	
Methamidophos	10 (13.3)	4 (9.3)	
Chlorpyrifos	31 (41.3)	17 (39.5)	
Dimethoate	3 (4.0)	6 (14.0)	
Profenofos	8 (10.7)	8 (18.6)	
Trichlorfon	3 (4.0)	0 (0.0)	
Acephate	2 (2.7)	1 (2.3)	
Malathion	5 (6.7)	1 (2.3)	
Organophosphate toxicity, n (%)			0.509
Ia Extremely hazardous	11 (14.7)	6 (14.0)	
Ib Highly hazardous	12 (16.0)	4 (9.3)	
II Moderately hazardous	45 (60.0)	31 (72.1)	
III Slightly hazardous	7 (9.3)	2 (4.7)	
U Unlikely to present acute hazard	0 (0)	0 (0)	
Hypertension, n (%)	14 (18.7)	7 (16.3)	0.744
Old stroke, n (%)	7 (9.3)	3 (7.0)	0.658
Coronary artery disease, n (%)	1 (1.3)	2 (4.7)	0.270
Structural heart disease, n (%)	5 (6.7)	6 (14.0)	0.190
Chronic obstructive pulmonary disease, n (%)	4 (5.3)	5 (11.6)	0.215
Malignancy, n (%)	1 (1.3)	2 (4.7)	0.270
Mental disorder, n (%)	34 (45.3)	17 (39.5)	0.541
Smoking habit, n (%)	31 (41.3)	21 (48.8)	0.429
Alcohol consumption, n (%)	30 (40.0)	19 (44.2)	0.657
Use of medications that might be associated with QTc-prolongation			
Anti-arrhythmic agents, n (%)	13 (17.63)	7 (16.3)	0.883
Anti-psychotics and anti-depressants, n (%)	20 (25.7)	10 (23.3)	0.682
Anti-microbials, n (%)	6 (8.0)	4 (9.3)	0.807
Time from poisoning to hospital, hour	6.29±14.05	4.48±4.70	0.413
Duration of follow-up, months	18.43±33.21	7.76±21.27	0.061

clomipramine, desipramine, citalopram, doxepin, imipramine, nortryptyline, and trimipramine; and d) other anti-depressants such as fluoxetine, sertraline, and venlafaxine [14].

Statistical analysis

Continuous variables are expressed as means and standard deviations and categorical variables as numbers with percentages in brackets. All data were tested for normality of distribution and equality of standard deviations before analysis. For comparisons between patient groups, we used Student's t test for quantitative variables and Chi-square or Fisher's exact tests for categorical variables. Mortality data were compared using the Kaplan-Meier method and significance was tested using a log-rank test. An initial univariate Cox regression analysis was performed to compare the frequency of possible risk factors associated with mortality. To control for possible confounding factors, a multivariate Cox regression analysis (stepwise backward approach) was performed to analyze those factors that were significant in univariate models

Table 2. Clinical manifestations of patients with organophosphate poisoning (N = 118).

Variable	Normal QTc (N = 75)	Prolonged QTc (N = 43)	P
1. Cholinergic crisis			
Cardiovascular system:			
Systolic blood pressure, mmHg	122.40±18.54	107.05±27.23	0.000
Diastolic blood pressure, mmHg	84.01±14.57	72.12±21.47	0.001
Heart rate, beats per minute	77.15±9.40	85.28±41.77	0.108
Hypotension, n (%)	12 (16.0)	15 (34.9)	0.019
Gastrointestinal system:			
Diarrhea, n (%)	21 (28.0)	14 (32.6)	0.602
Emesis, n (%)	22 (29.3)	20 (46.5)	0.061
Respiratory system:			
Shortness of breath	47 (62.7)	34 (79.1)	0.065
Bronchorrhea	41 (54.7)	31 (72.1)	0.062
Bronchospasm	38 (50.7)	29 (67.4)	0.077
Respiratory failure, n (%)	34 (45.3)	26 (60.5)	0.114
Genitourinary system:			
Acute renal failure, n (%)	5 (6.7)	6 (14.0)	0.190
Central nervous system:			
Seizure, n (%)	6 (8.0)	4 (9.3)	0.807
Coma, n (%)	11 (14.7)	12 (27.9)	0.081
2. Intermediate syndrome, n (%)	6 (8.0)	4 (9.3)	0.807
3. Delay neuropathy, n (%)	1 (1.3)	2 (4.7)	0.270

($P<0.05$) and met the assumptions of a proportional hazard model. We considered results that rejected the null hypothesis with 95% confidence to be significant. All analyses were performed using SPSS 12.0 for Windows (SPSS Inc., Chicago, Illinois, USA).

Results

Baseline characteristics

Table 1 shows the baseline characteristics of the 118 patients with organophosphate poisoning, grouped according to QTc

Table 3. Laboratory analysis of blood from patients with organophosphate poisoning (N = 118).

Variable	Normal QTc (N = 75)	Prolonged QTc (N = 43)	P
Hemoglobin, g/dL	14.24±2.06	14.34±1.63	0.770
Blood urea nitrogen, mg/dL	17.07±20.12	15.89±6.09	0.775
Creatinine, mg/dL	1.06±0.83	1.02±0.40	0.811
Sodium, mEq/L	140.88±3.11	141.21±4.31	0.644
Potassium, mEq/L	3.60±0.54	3.41±0.49	0.071
Calcium, mg/dL	8.78±0.60	8.53±0.57	0.342
Cholinesterase, initial, U/mL	3.58±3.37	2.90±3.59	0.299
Cholinesterase, lowest, U/mL	2.95±2.90	2.35±3.20	0.298
C-reactive protein, mg/dL	9.30±20.31	6.17±5.90	0.700
Amylase, U/L	147.62±126.05	276.18±245.99	0.113
Lipase, U/L	117.00±95.11	105.00±60.03	0.780
CK-MB, ng/mL	11.37±6.75	28.89±60.65	0.376
Troponin-I, ng/mL	0.09±0.11	0.06±0.09	0.411

Table 4. Detoxification protocol and outcome for patients with organophosphate poisoning (N = 118).

Variable	Normal QTc (N = 75)	Prolonged QTc (N = 43)	P
Gastric lavage, n (%)	58 (77.3)	37 (86.0)	0.250
Active charcoal and magnesium citrate, n (%)	55 (73.3)	33 (76.7)	0.682
Atropine, n (%)	74 (98.7)	42 (97.7)	0.688
Pralidoxime, n (%)	73 (97.3)	42 (97.7)	0.910
Mortality, n (%)	3 (4.0)	15 (34.9)	0.000
Causes of mortality, n (%)			0.383
Cardiac arrhythmia	1 (33.3)	9 (60.0)	
Respiratory failure	1 (33.3)	5 (33.3)	
Sepsis	1 (33.3)	1 (6.7)	

interval. There were no significant differences in baseline variables between groups.

Respiratory symptoms were common after organophosphate poisoning (Table 2). Further, there were more cases of hypotension among these patients than among those with normal QTc interval (P = 0.019). Patients with prolonged QTc interval had lower systolic (P = 0.000) and diastolic (P = 0.001) blood pressure than patients with normal QTc interval. No other clinical (Table 2) or laboratory (Table 3) variables differed between groups.

As shown in Table 4, most patients were treated aggressively with gastric lavage of large amounts of normal saline, followed by an infusion of 1 g/kg activated charcoal and 250 mL magnesium citrate. In addition, nearly all patients were treated with systemic atropine and pralidoxime injections. There was no difference in treatment modality between groups.

By the end of this study, 18 of 118 (15.2%) patients had died, including 3 of 75 (4.0%) patients with normal QTc interval and 15 of 43 (34.9%) patients with prolonged QTc interval. Regarding the causes of mortality (Table 4), one patient from normal QTc interval died of cardiac arrhythmia, one died of respiratory failure, and one died of sepsis. On the other hand, 9 patients from prolonged QTc interval died of cardiac arrhythmia, 5 died of respiratory failure, and one died of sepsis. This difference was not significant (P = 0.383), probably due to the small sample size. Multivariate Cox regression analysis revealed that hypotension (odds ratio (OR) = 10.930, 95% confidence interval (CI) = 2.961–40.345, P = 0.000), respiratory failure (OR = 4.867, 95% CI = 1.062–22.301, P = 0.042), coma (OR = 3.482, 95% CI = 1.184–10.238, P = 0.023), and QTc prolongation (OR = 7.459, 95% CI = 2.053–27.099, P = 0.002) were significant risk factors for mortality (Table 5). Finally, Kaplan-Meier analysis demonstrated that cumulative mortality was higher among patients with prolonged QTc intervals than among those with normal QTc intervals (Figure 1, Log-rank test, Chi-square test = 20.36, P<0.001).

A direct comparison between non-survivors and survivors (Table S1) revealed that non-survivors not only had longer QTc interval (503.00±41.56 versus 432.71±51.21 ms, P = 0.002), but also suffered higher incidences of hypotension (83.3 versus 12.0%, P = 0.000), shortness of breath (64 versus 94.4%, P = 0.010), bronchorrhea (55 versus 94.4%, P = 0.002), bronchospasm (50.0 versus 94.4%, P = 0.000), respiratory failure (94.4 versus 43.0%, P = 0.000) and coma (66.7 versus 11.0%, P = 0.000) than survivors. Furthermore, the systolic (P = 0.000) and diastolic (P = 0.000) blood pressure was lower, but heart rate (P = 0.005) was higher in non-survivors than survivors.

Discussion

It has been well demonstrated that QT-interval prolongation affects mortality rate in the general population [15]. QT-interval prolongation also affects the mortality rates of patients with a variety of diseases, including end-stage renal disease [16], coronary artery disease, congestive heart failure [17], diabetes mellitus [18], acute ischemic stroke [19], chronic liver disease [20], and chronic obstructive pulmonary disease [21]. Using a multivariate Cox regression model, we have demonstrated in this study that QTc interval prolongation might be an important risk factor for mortality after intentional organophosphate poisoning.

The relationship between QTc interval prolongation and subsequent mortality after organophosphate poisoning remains uncertain (Table 6). Baydin et al [22] reported that 35.4% of the 20 Turkish patients studied presented with prolonged QTc

Table 5. Univariate and multivariate Cox regression analysis for mortality (N = 118).

Variable	Univariate analysis OR (95% CI)	P	Multivariate analysis OR (95% CI)	P
Hypotension	21.596 (6.237–74.780)	0.000	10.930 (2.961–40.345)	0.000
Respiratory failure	8.504 (1.955–36.997)	0.004	4.867 (1.062–22.301)	0.042
Coma	10.317 (3.857–27.595)	0.000	3.482 (1.184–10.238)	0.023
QTc prolongation	9.974 (2.885–34.478)	0.000	7.459 (2.053–27.099)	0.002

Note: OR odds ratio, CI confidence interval.

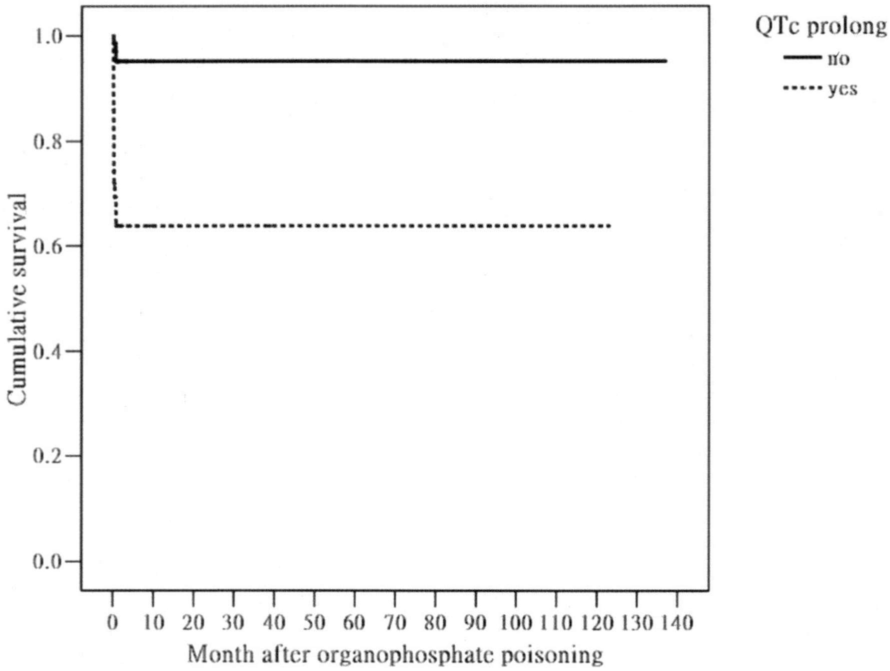

Figure 1. Kaplan-Meier analysis of data from patients with organophosphate poisoning, grouped according to the duration of the QTc interval. Patients with prolonged QTc intervals suffered higher cumulative mortality than patients with normal QTc intervals (Log-rank test, Chi-square test = 20.36, P<0.001).

intervals. Further, there was a negative correlation between QTc interval and blood cholinesterase level. In a study of 13 Indian patients who died of organophosphate poisoning, Annad et al [23] found 4 with episodic tachycardia and ST-T changes, 3 with QT prolongation, and 2 with episodic bradycardia. On autopsy, all 13 patients had myocardial interstitial edema and vascular congestion, while 8 had patchy interstitial inflammation, 2 had patchy myocarditis, and 6 had a mural thrombus. Yurumez et al [24] analyzed the records of 85 Turkish patients with organophosphate poisoning and found that 47 patients (55.5%) had a prolonged QTc interval. Only 2 patients died in this study (2.4%), and no QTc prolongation was found in either patient (QTc intervals: 0.44 s and 0.40 s). The authors therefore concluded that QTc interval prolongation could not be used as a unique predictive factor in determining short-term mortality in their study [24]. In contrast, Shadnia et al [25] reported that the mortality rate of Iranian patients with long QTc intervals was significantly higher than that of those with normal QTc intervals. In a subsequent study, Akdur et al [26] found that 26 of 54 (53.7%) Turkish patients had prolonged QTc intervals. However, no significant correlation was found between poisoning severity and QTc interval. More recently [27], Vijayakumar evaluated 20 Indian patients with organophosphate poisoning and discovered that 12 patients (60.0%) had prolonged QTc intervals. However, the predictive power of QTc interval prolongation on subsequent mortality was not explored.

In this study, we found that patients with QTc-interval prolongation were slightly older than those with normal QTc intervals despite not reaching the level of statistical significance (56.37 ± 14.65 versus 52.04 ± 16.94, $P = 0.163$). In a longitudinal

Table 6. Summary of published studies reporting a possible association between QTc and mortality rate after organophosphate poisoning.

Year	Study	Area	Sample size, n	Mortality rate, n (%)	QTc prolongation rate, %	Statistical association between QTc and mortality rate
1996	[7]	Taiwan	223	25 (11.2)	43.5	Yes
2007	[22]	Turkey	20	2 (10)	35.4	
2009	[23]	India	36	13 (36.1)	23.1	
2009	[24]	Turkey	85	2 (2.4)	55.5	No
2009	[25]	Iran	42	15 (37.5)	59.5	Yes
2010	[26]	Turkey	54	3 (5.6)	48.1	No
2011	[27]	India	20		60.0	
2012	Current study	Taiwan	118	18 (15.2)	36.4	Yes

study [28], Su et al reported that QTc interval increased significantly with age in a population of healthy elderly subjects. Elderly hearts tend to have relative midmyocardial myocyte hypertrophy and a distinct increase in connective tissue as compared to younger hearts [29]. Myocyte hypertrophy may be associated with a significant prolongation of the transmembrane action potential, explaining the prolongation of the QTc interval [30] with age. There are also reports of an exaggerated shift towards sympathetic activity in the elderly [31], and such sympathetic overactivity might be an important factor in the prolongation of the QT interval. Therefore, it is not surprising to find longer QT intervals among elderly patients with organophosphate poisoning than among younger organophosphate poisoning patients.

As shown in Table 1 and 2, there was a trend that the patients in the group with prolonged QTc were older (P = 0.163). It is possible that the increased mortality in this group might due to the age and or age-related diseases like chronic obstructive pulmonary disease and coronary artery disease. The data in the present study also showed a trend of higher percentage of patients with chronic obstructive pulmonary disease (P = 0.215), structural heart disease (P = 0.190), and coronary artery disease (P = 0.270) in the group with prolonged QTc although not reaching the level of statistical significance due to the small numbers. This group of patient also had a trend of increased frequencies in developing hypotension (P = 0.019), and respiratory distress like shortness of breath (P = 0.065), bronchorrhea (P = 0.062), bronchospasm (P = 0.077), and respiratory failure (P = 0.114). The patients in prolonged QTc group also had a trend of increased renal failure (P = 0.190) as well. Nevertheless, a direct comparison between non-survivors and survivors (Supporting Information Table S1) revealed that non-survivors not only had longer QTc interval (P = 0.002), but also suffered higher incidences of hypotension (P = 0.000), shortness of breath (P = 0.010), bronchorrhea (P = 0.002), bronchospasm (P = 0.000), respiratory failure (P = 0.000) and coma (P = 0.000) than survivors. Therefore, further large-scale study is necessary to delineate the associations between the clinical features, QTc interval, physiological markers, and clinical outcomes of patients with organophosphate poisoning.

Finally, multivariate Cox regression analysis confirmed that hypotension (P = 0.000), respiratory failure (P = 0.042), coma (P = 0.023), and QTc prolongation (P = 0.002) were significant risk factors for mortality after organophosphate poisoning. The associations between both hypotension [32] and coma with mortality are not surprising, because both are important vital signs, irrespective of the cause of disease. Similarly, it is not surprising to find an association between respiratory failure and mortality because respiratory failure is a prominent feature of acute organophosphate poisoning with an early central apnea followed by later pulmonary effects [33]. Laboratory studies also support the idea that organophosphate-induced respiratory failure results from local effects of organophosphates acting on brainstem circuits underlying respiratory rhythmogenesis, and on lung tissues underlying pulmonary secretory, airway and vascular function [33]. Furthermore, Chuang et al [7] also confirmed in their study that patients with QTc prolongation had a higher mortality rate and a higher incidence of respiratory failure than patients without QTc prolongation.

In summary, QTc interval helps predict mortality after intentional organophosphate poisoning. However, the retrospective nature of the study, small patient population, absence of routine serum magnesium measurement, and lack of serial electrocardiogram recordings limit the certainty of our conclusions.

Author Contributions

Analyzed the data: S-HL. Wrote the paper: S-HL. Performed the study: S-HL. Supervised the study: J-LL. Contributed to patient care and management: J-LL C-HW H-YY C-WH K-HC W-HH T-HY. Conceived and designed the study: T-HY. Helped in data analysis and manuscript writing: T-HY.

References

1. Lin JL, Lin-Tan DT, Chen KH, Huang WH, Hsu CW, et al. (2011) Improved survival in severe paraquat poisoning with repeated pulse therapy of cyclophosphamide and steroids. Intensive Care Med 37: 1006–1013.
2. Lin TJ, Walter FG, Hung DZ, Tsai JL, Hu SC, et al. (2008) Epidemiology of organophosphate pesticide poisoning in Taiwan. Clin Toxicol 46: 794–801.
3. Antonijevic B, Stojiljkovic MP (2007) Unequal efficacy of pyridinium oximes in acute organophosphate poisoning. Clin Med Res 5: 71–82.
4. Kamanyire R, Karalliedde L (2004) Organophosphate toxicity and occupational exposure. Occup Med (Lond) 54: 69–75.
5. Bar-Meir E, Schein O, Eisenkraft A, Rubinshtein R, Grubstein A, et al. (2007) Guidelines for treating cardiac manifestations of organophosphates poisoning with special emphasis on long QT and Torsades De Pointes. Crit Rev Toxicol 37: 279–285.
6. Ludomirsky A, Klein HO, Sarelli P, Becker B, Hoffman S, et al. (1982) Q-T prolongation and polymorphous ("torsade de pointes") ventricular arrhythmias associated with organophosphorus insecticide poisoning. Am J Cardiol 49: 1654–1658.
7. Chuang FR, Jang SW, Lin JL, Chern MS, Chen JB, et al. (1996) QTc prolongation indicates a poor prognosis in patients with organophosphate poisoning. Am J Emer Med 14: 451–453.
8. (World Health Organization) () The WHO Recommended Classification of Pesticides by Hazard and Guidelines to Classification 2009. Web address http://www.who.int/ipcs/publications/pesticides_hazard_2009.pdf (Accessed on 17 March 2012).
9. Luhr OR, Antonsen K, Karlsson M, Aardal S, Thorsteinsson A, et al. (1999) Incidence and mortality after acute respiratory failure and acute respiratory distress syndrome in Sweden, Denmark, and Iceland. The ARF Study Group. Am J Respir Crit Care Med 159: 1849–1861.
10. Victorino GP, Battistella FD, Wisner DH (2003) Does tachycardia correlate with hypotension after trauma? J Am Coll Surg 196: 679–684.
11. Steinberg DHSS, Franke J, Sievert H (2010) Defining structural heart disease in the adult patient: current scope, inherent challenges and future directions. Eur Heart J Suppl 12: E2–E9.
12. Shantsila E, Watson T, Lip GY (2007) Drug-induced QT-interval prolongation and proarrhythmic risk in the treatment of atrial arrhythmias. Europace 9 Suppl 4: iv37–44.
13. Owens RC, Jr., Nolin TD (2006) Antimicrobial-associated QT interval prolongation: pointes of interest. Clin Infect Dis 43: 1603–1611.
14. Sicouri S, Antzelevitch C (2008) Sudden cardiac death secondary to antidepressant and antipsychotic drugs. Expert Opin Drug Saf 7: 181–194.
15. Zhang Y, Post WS, Dalal D, Blasco-Colmenares E, Tomaselli GF, et al. (2011) QT-Interval Duration and Mortality Rate: Results From the Third National Health and Nutrition Examination Survey. Arch Intern Med 171: 1727–1733.
16. Hage FG, de Mattos AM, Khamash H, Mehta S, Warnock D, et al. (2010) QT prolongation is an independent predictor of mortality in end-stage renal disease. Clin Cardiol 33: 361–366.
17. Foroughi M, Karkhaneh Yousefi Z, Majidi Tehrani M, Noori Foroutaghe A, Ghanavati A, et al. (2009) Prolonged QT interval and coronary artery bypass mortality due to heart failure. Asian Cardiovasc Thorac Ann 17: 604–607.
18. Rossing P, Breum L, Major-Pedersen A, Sato A, Winding H, et al. (2001) Prolonged QTc interval predicts mortality in patients with Type 1 diabetes mellitus. Diabet Med 18: 199–205.
19. Stead LG, Gilmore RM, Bellolio MF, Vaidyanathan L, Weaver AL, et al. (2009) Prolonged QTc as a predictor of mortality in acute ischemic stroke. J Stroke Cerebrovasc Dis 18: 469–474.

20. Kosar F, Ates F, Sahin I, Karincaoglu M, Yildirim B (2007) QT interval analysis in patients with chronic liver disease: a prospective study. Angiology 58: 218–224.
21. Zulli R, Donati P, Nicosia F, De Vecchi M, Tantucci C, et al. (2006) Increased QT dispersion: a negative prognostic finding in chronic obstructive pulmonary disease. Intern Emerg Med 1: 279–286.
22. Baydin A, Aygun D, Yazici M, Karatas A, Deniz T, et al. (2007) Is there a relationship between the blood cholinesterase and QTc interval in the patients with acute organophosphate poisoning? Int J Clin Pract 61: 927–930.
23. Anand S, Singh S, Nahar Saikia U, Bhalla A, Paul Sharma Y, et al. (2009) Cardiac abnormalities in acute organophosphate poisoning. Clin Toxicol 47: 230–235.
24. Yurumez Y, Yavuz Y, Saglam H, Durukan P, Ozkan S, et al. (2009) Electrocardiographic findings of acute organophosphate poisoning. J Emerg Med 36: 39–42.
25. Shadnia S, Okazi A, Akhlaghi N, Sasanian G, Abdollahi M (2009) Prognostic value of long QT interval in acute and severe organophosphate poisoning. J Med Toxicol 5: 196–199.
26. Akdur O, Durukan P, Ozkan S, Avsarogullari L, Vardar A, et al. (2010) Poisoning severity score, Glasgow coma scale, corrected QT interval in acute organophosphate poisoning. Hum Exp Toxicol 29: 419–425.
27. Vijayakumar S, Fareedullah M, Ashok Kumar E, Mohan Rao K (2011) A prospective study on electrocardiographic findings of patients with organophosphorus poisoning. Cardiovasc Toxicol 11: 113–117.
28. Su HM, Chiu HC, Lin TH, Voon WC, Liu HW, et al. (2006) Longitudinal study of the ageing trends in QT interval and dispersion in healthy elderly subjects. Age Ageing 35: 636–638.
29. Burns TR, Klima M, Teasdale TA, Kasper K (1990) Morphometry of the aging heart. Mod Pathol 3: 336–342.
30. Capasso JM, Malhotra A, Remily RM, Scheuer J, Sonnenblick EH (1983) Effects of age on mechanical and electrical performance of rat myocardium. Am J Physiol 245: H72–81.
31. Pfeifer MA, Weinberg CR, Cook D, Best JD, Reenan A, et al. (1983) Differential changes of autonomic nervous system function with age in man. Am J Med 75: 249–258.
32. Hasler RM, Nuesch E, Juni P, Bouamra O, Exadaktylos AK, et al. (2012) Systolic blood pressure below 110 mmHg is associated with increased mortality in penetrating major trauma patients: Multicentre cohort study. Resuscitation 83: 476–481.
33. Gaspari RJ, Paydarfar D (2009) Respiratory failure induced by acute organophosphate poisoning in rats: effects of vagotomy. Neurotoxicology 30: 298–304.

8

Analysis of the Transcriptome in Hyperoxic Lung Injury and Sex-Specific Alterations in Gene Expression

Krithika Lingappan[1]*, Chandra Srinivasan[2], Weiwu Jiang[1], Lihua Wang[1], Xanthi I. Couroucli[1], Bhagavatula Moorthy[1]

1 Department of Pediatrics, Section of Neonatology, Texas Children's Hospital, Baylor College of Medicine, Houston, Texas, United States of America, **2** Division of Pediatric Cardiology, Department of Pediatrics, University of Texas Medical School at Houston, Houston, Texas, United States of America

Abstract

Exposure to high concentration of oxygen (hyperoxia) leads to lung injury in experimental animal models and plays a role in the pathogenesis of diseases such as Acute Respiratory Distress Syndrome (ARDS) and Bronchopulmonary dysplasia (BPD) in humans. The mechanisms responsible for sex differences in the susceptibility towards hyperoxic lung injury remain largely unknown. The major goal of this study was to characterize the changes in the pulmonary transcriptome following hyperoxia exposure and further elucidate the sex-specific changes. Male and female (8–10 wk) wild type (WT) (C57BL/6J) mice were exposed to hyperoxia (FiO_2>0.95) and gene expression in lung tissues was studied at 48 h. A combination of fold change ≥ 1.4 and false discovery rate (FDR)<5% was used to define differentially expressed genes (DEGs). Overrepresentation of gene ontology terms representing biological processes and signaling pathway impact analysis (SPIA) was performed. Comparison of DEG profiles identified 327 genes unique to females, 585 unique to males and 1882 common genes. The major new findings of this study are the identification of new candidate genes of interest and the sex-specific transcriptomic changes in hyperoxic lung injury. We also identified DEGs involved in signaling pathways like MAP kinase and NF-kappa B which may explain the differences in sex-specific susceptibility to hyperoxic lung injury. These findings highlight changes in the pulmonary transcriptome and sex-specific differences in hyperoxic lung injury, and suggest new pathways, whose components could serve as sex-specific biomarkers and possible therapeutic targets for acute lung injury (ALI)/acute respiratory distress (ARDS) in humans.

Editor: M. Firoze Khan, University of Texas Medical Branch, United States of America

Funding: This work was supported in part by the National Institutes of Health (NIH) ES-019689, ES-001932, HL-087174, and HL-112516 to B.M. and HL-088343 to X.C. (www.nih.gov). The funders had no role in study design, data collection and analysis, decision to publish, or preparation of the manuscript.

Competing Interests: The authors have declared that no competing interests exist.

* Email: lingappa@bcm.edu

Introduction

Exposure to high concentration of oxygen (hyperoxia) leads to lung injury in experimental animal models and plays a major role in the pathogenesis of diseases such as Acute Respiratory Distress Syndrome (ARDS) and Bronchopulmonary dysplasia (BPD) in humans [1–3]. Reactive oxygen species (ROS) generated during hyperoxia exposure result in damage of many cellular components including DNA, proteins and lipids and ultimately leading to epithelial and endothelial cell death in the lung. Hyperoxia is also associated with increased expression of cytokines that sequester and activate inflammatory cells, most notably, neutrophils [4,5]. Together these events lead to pulmonary edema and atelectasis, which are the key histopathological findings in acute lung injury [6]. Hyperoxia exposure leads to pathological changes similar to ARDS in other mammalian species [1–5,7,8].

Sex-specific differences in lung injury have been established both in animal models of acute lung injury (ALI) and observed in epidemiological studies in human patients. Males with ARDS have a higher mortality rate compared to females [9–11]. Sex-based differences have also been observed in diseases such as idiopathic pulmonary fibrosis and asthma [12–15]. In premature neonates, male sex is considered to be an independent risk factor for the development of BPD [12,16–18]. The reasons behind these sex-biased differences in lung injury are not well elucidated yet. Differences in lung development among male and female fetuses may contribute to these differences. Hormonal differences between males and females are also thought to play a role [19,20]. Estrogen is known to have a stimulatory and androgens an inhibitory effect on lung development [19]. Expression of enzymes involved in antioxidant defense pathways have also been shown to be different between male and female premature neonates [21,22]. In acute lung injury models, testosterone was found to increase [23] and estrogen to ameliorate inflammation and injury [24]. Studies on sex hormones have identified some potential mechanisms behind the sexually dimorphic differences but more work is needed.

Like many other diseases genetic and non-genetic factors play a role in hyperoxic lung injury. Genetic susceptibility is thought to contribute to the development of BPD in human neonates [25]. Some mouse strains are resistant (C3, 129X1/SvJ), while others are susceptible (B6, A/J and D2) to hyperoxic lung injury [26]. *Nrf2*-ARE (antioxidant response element) signaling pathway has

Table 1. List of genes selected for validation by qPCR analysis.

Gene symbol	Assay ID
Slc7a11	Mm00442530_m1
Ankrd1	Mm00496512_m1
Slc7a5	Mm00441516_m1
Nqo1	Mm01253561_m1
Egr1	Mm00656724_m1
BDNF	Mm04230607_s1
Pdk4	Mm01166879_m1
Agr2	Mm01291804_m1
IL1b	Mm00434228_m1
18s	Mm03928990_g1

been identified as significant in many acute lung injury models [27]. QTL (quantitative trait loci) analyses has revealed other candidate genes; angiopoietin-1 (*Angpt1*) and oxidation resistance-1 (*Oxr1*) which may determine susceptibility to hyperoxic lung injury [28].

We have recently shown that after hyperoxia exposure, adult male mice show greater pulmonary edema, lung injury, inflammation and cell death compared to female mice [29]. However, the molecular mechanisms of sex differences are not completely understood. Sex-specific global gene expression in an animal model of hyperoxic lung injury has not been reported. In this study, we employed a non-biased approach to measure global changes in gene expression following hyperoxia exposure in the lung at 48 h and further studied the sex-specific changes in male and female mice.

Materials and Methods

Animals

This study was conducted in strict accordance with the recommendations in the Guide for the Care and use of Laboratory Animals of the National Institutes of Heath. The Institutional Animal Care and Use Committee (IACUC) of Baylor College of Medicine approved the protocol (Protocol number AN-907). All efforts were made to minimize suffering. Breeding pairs of mice were obtained from the Jackson Laboratory (Bar Harbor, ME). 8–10 week old male (C57BL/6J) or female mice were maintained at Texas Children's Hospital animal facility and used for the study. They were fed standard mice food and water *ad libitum*. Animals were maintained in a 12 h day/night cycle.

Oxygen exposure

Mice were maintained in either room air (21% oxygen) or exposed to hyperoxia (95–100% oxygen) environment using pure O_2 at 5 l/min for 24–72 h in a sealed Plexiglass chamber, as reported previously [30]. After sealing the chamber, the oxygen concentration in the plexiglass chamber was measured frequently by an analyzer (Getronics, Kenilworth, New Jersey). Purified tap water and food (Purina Rodent Lab Chow 5001 from Purina Mills, Inc., Richmond, IN) were available *ad libitum*. After hyperoxia exposure, the animals were anesthetized with 200 mg/kg of sodium pentobarbital (i.p.) and euthanized by exsanguination while under deep pentobarbital anesthesia. The lung tissues were harvested for further analysis.

RNA isolation

We used a total of 12 animals per sex per treatment group. Total RNA from lung samples in mice exposed to room air or hyperoxia for 48 h was isolated using the miRNeasy kit as per the manufacturer's standard protocols (Qiagen, Valencia, CA, USA). Following total RNA isolation, sample concentration was assayed using a Nanodrop-8000 (Thermo Scientific, Wilmington, DE, USA). Sample Quality checks were done using the NanoDrop spectrophotometer and Agilent Bioanalyzer.

Affymetrix Gene Chip Array Analysis

We used the Ambion (Life Technologies, Grand Island, NY, USA) WT Expression Kit protocol and reagents to convert total RNA into sense-strand cDNA. The cDNA was then fragmented and labeled using the Affymetrix GeneChip (Affymetrix, Santa Clara,CA,USA) WT Terminal Labeling Kit.

Data analysis

We used 3 biological replicates in each group. The groups were: 1) Room air-male, 2) Room air-female, 3) Hyperoxia-male and 4) Hyperoxia-female (NCBI GEO accession number: GSE51039). To minimize the impact of individual mouse to mouse variability on the microarray data, each biological replicate was comprised of a randomized pool of lung RNA prepared from n = 4 mice. Gene expression in lung tissue was studied using the Mouse Gene 1.0 ST Array (Affymetrix). Raw gene expression data was preprocessed using 'Robust Multichip Average' methodology. A combination of fold-change (FC)≥1.4 and false discovery rate (FDR)<5% was used to define differentially expressed genes (DEGs). Overrepresentation of gene ontology terms representing biological processes among the DEGs was tested using a conditional hypergeometric test (p-value <0.01). Signaling pathway impact analysis (SPIA), was also performed, as this approach combines two types of evidence: (i) the over- representation of DEGs in a given pathway and (ii) the abnormal perturbation of that pathway, as measured by propagating measured expression changes across the pathway topology [31]. A significance threshold of 5% was used on the FDR corrected p-values in order to detect pathway significance.

Real time qPCR validation

To validate microarray results, a subset of genes was validated by quantitative real-time PCR (qRT-PCR). Non-random sampling strategies have limited utility as gene selection procedures because the validation results may not generalize to the entire set of DEGs

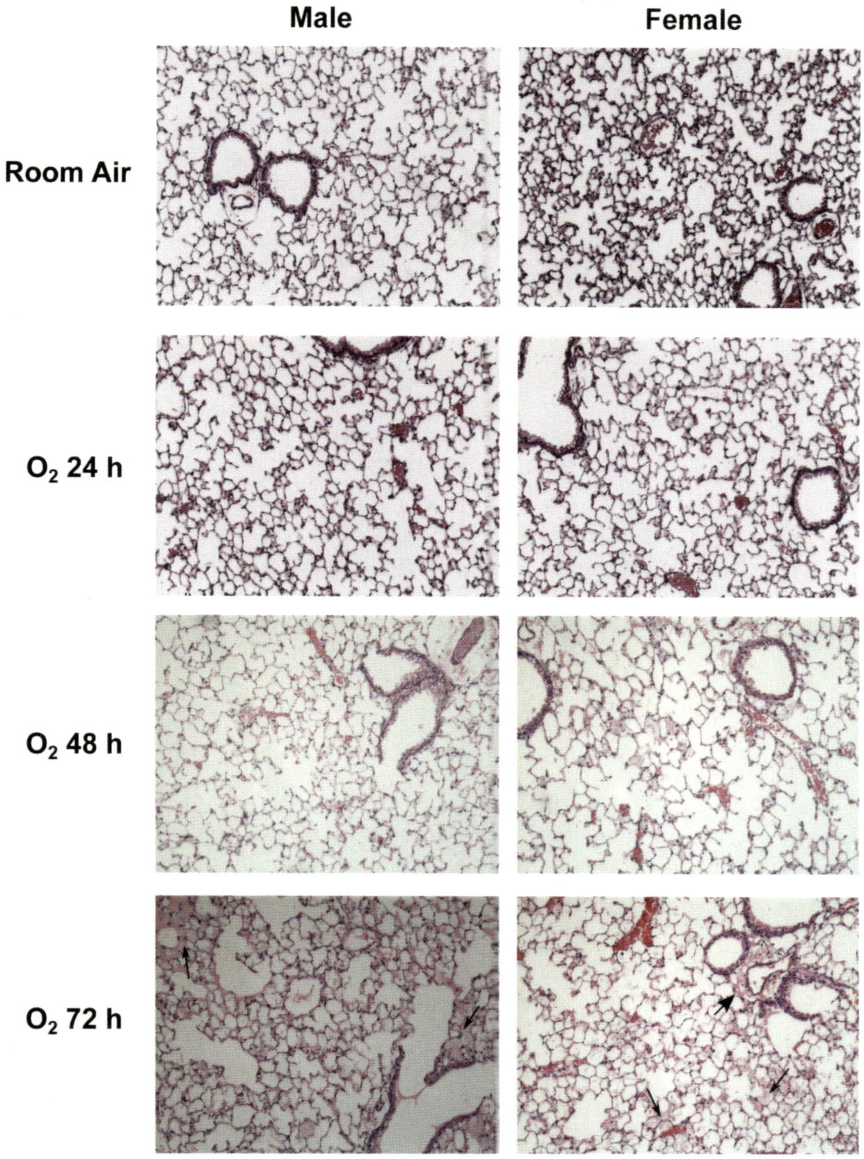

Figure 1. Representative hematoxylin eosin stained images from the lungs of male and female mice (n = 5 mice per group) exposed to room air or 24–72 h of hyperoxia. WT males show more alveolar edema and hemorrhage when compared to female mice. Thin arrows point to areas of alveolar edema. Thick arrow points to area of perivascular edema.

[32]. Therefore, we selected 5 genes (*Ankrd1*, *Slc7a5*, *Slc7a11*, *Egr1* and *Nqo1*) from the pool of DEGs in a random-stratified manner. For random- stratified sampling, the entire list of upregulated genes was rank ordered according to fold change; the data were then divided into 5 equal-sized bins and one gene per bin was selected randomly. In addition, we also selected five additional genes from the pool of genes showing sex-specific differential expression in the microarray experiment. RNA (50 ng), isolated as above, was subjected to one step real time quantitative TaqMan RT-PCR using 7900HT Fast Real-Time PCR System (Applied Biosystems, Foster City, CA). Gene-specific primers purchased from life science technologies (Table 1) in the presence of TaqMan reverse transcription reagents and RT reaction mix (Applied Biosystems, Foster City, CA) were used to reverse transcribe RNA, and TaqMan Gene Expression probes and TaqMan Universal PCR Master Mix (Applied Biosystems, Foster City, CA), were used for PCR amplification. 18S was used as the reference gene. Concordance correlation coefficient (CCC) was used to measure the agreement between the $\log_2$ FC results from microarray and FC from qRT-PCR in both males and females. Data was processed and analyzed using Bioconductor software packages (*'oligo'*, *'limma'*, *'GOstats'*, *'SPIA'*, *'HTqPCR'*) in R programming language [33,34].

Histopathology, immunohistochemistry and western blot

The mice were maintained in either room air (21% oxygen) or exposed to hyperoxia (95–100% oxygen) environment using pure O_2 at 5 l/min for 24 h, 48 h or 72 h in a sealed Plexiglass chamber, as described previously. Tracheotomy was performed on the anesthetized mice (n = 5/group) and the lung tissue was fixed by intratracheal instillation of 10% zinc formalin at constant pressure of 25 cm of H_2O. Samples were left in solution for 24 h in formaldehyde, and then transferred to 70% ethanol for long-term storage. Routine histology was performed on lung tissues

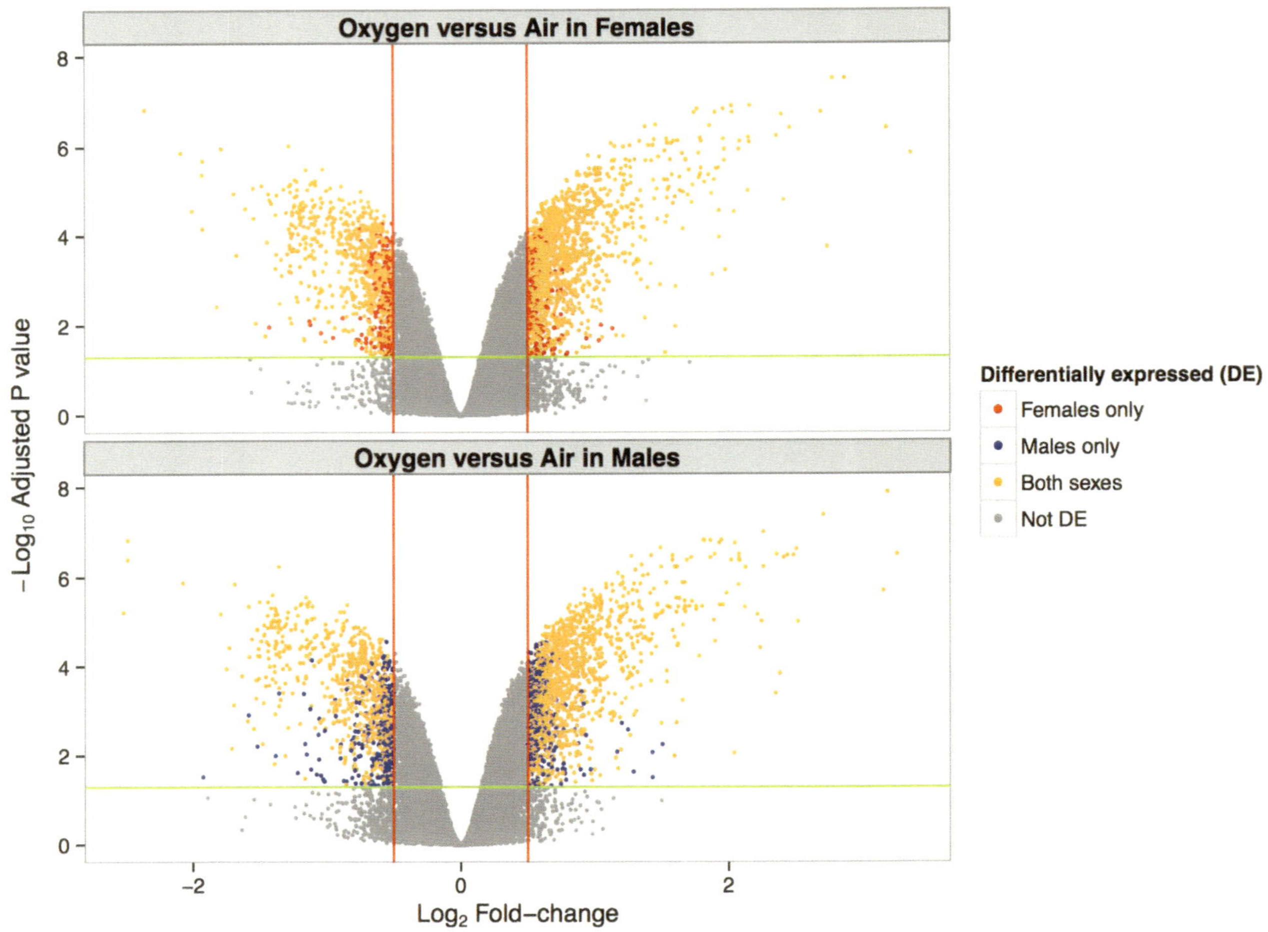

Figure 2. Volcano plot for differentially expressed genes in male and female mice after hyperoxia (FiO_2>95%) exposure for 48 h compared to room air controls. The x-axis is log_2fold change. Each point represents an individual transcript. The vertical lines represents 1.4 fold change with upregulated genes on the right and downregulated genes on the left. The horizontal lines represent an adjusted p value of 0.05.

from individual animals following staining of the paraffin sections with hematoxylin and eosin. Five microns deparaffinized lung sections were immunostained with Anti xCT antibody (ab37186; dilution 1:1000) followed by staining with biotinylated secondary antibodies (Vector Laboratories Burlingame, CA). For western blotting, lung whole protein (20 µg of protein) from individual male animals (n = 5/group) exposed to room air or to hyperoxia for 48 h, was prepared in Milliplex MAP lysis buffer (EMD

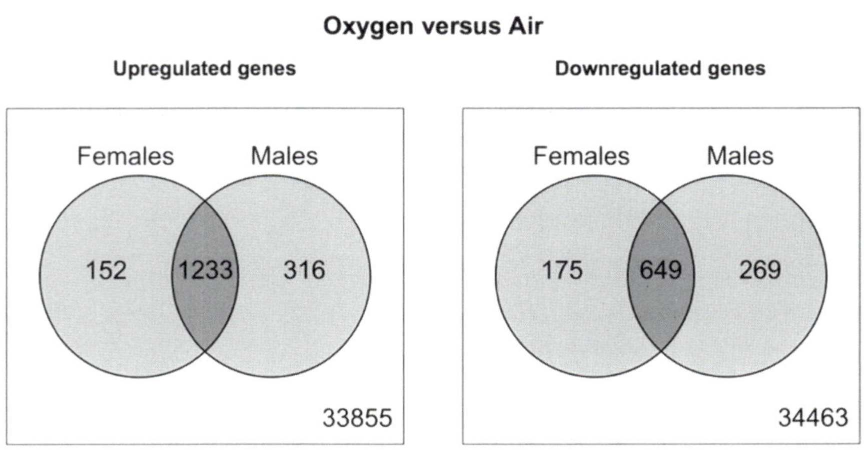

Figure 3. Venn diagram showing the comparison of upregulated and downregulated DEGs in the lung between male and female mice after hyperoxia exposure (FiO_2>95%) for 48 hours.

Table 2. List of pulmonary DEGs after hyperoxia exposure.

Affymetrix ID	Symbol	Chromosome	log_2FC
Common in both males and females (≥4 fold change)			
10579331	Gdf15	chr8	3.36
10498024	Slc7a11	chr3	3.18
10534667	Serpine1	chr5	2.87
10545672	Mthfd2	chr6	2.78
10467191	Ankrd1	chr19	2.74
10361091	Atf3	chr1	2.69
10495675	F3	chr3	2.46
10598976	Timp1	chrX	2.42
10523182	Areg	chr5	2.40
10424400	Myc	chr15	2.36
10543067	Asns	chr6	2.16
10556297	Adm	chr7	2.16
10537146	Akr1b8	chr6	2.15
10513739	Tnc	chr4	2.15
10350516	Ptgs2	chr1	2.09
10448307	Tnfrsf12a	chr17	2.08
10467136	Ch25h	chr19	2.05
10582275	Slc7a5	chr8	2.03
10545130	Gadd45a	chr6	2.03
Males only (≥2 fold change)			
10543017	Pdk4	chr6	1.50
10507908	Fhl3	chr4	1.29
10587323	Gsta1	chr9	1.25
10517067	Sfn	chr4	1.17
Females only (≥2 fold change)			
10574427	Impdh2	chr8	1.03

Millipore) and used for apoprotein estimation. The primary antibody was the same as used in immunohistochemistry at a dilution of 1:3000. For loading controls, the membranes were stripped and incubated with antibodies against β-actin, followed by electrochemical detection of bands. The statistical analysis of densitometric values was done using Students t-test and p value< 0.05 was considered significant.

Results

Lung histopathology after hyperoxia exposure and sex-specific differences

Figure 1 shows representative lung fields at 10× magnification from male and female mice exposed to room air or 24 h, 48 h or 72 h of hyperoxia. Qualitative assessment of lung injury showed that at 24 h there were no appreciable signs of lung injury due to hyperoxia exposure on histopathology. After 48 h of hyperoxia exposure, there are signs of lung injury in the form of alveolar edema. After 72 h, extensive lung injury in the form of alveolar, perivascular and peribronchial edema and alveolar hemorrhage was seen. Male mice showed more injury compared to female mice.

Hyperoxia and sex-biased gene expression

After 48 h of hyperoxia exposure, a total of 2209 (upregulated (UR): 1385, downregulated (DR): 824) and 2467 (UR: 1549, DR: 918) genes were differentially expressed compared to room-air in females and males, respectively. Comparison of DEG profiles identified 327 genes unique to females, 585 unique to males, and 1882 common genes. Figure 2 shows the volcano plot of the DEGs (upregulated and downregulated) in males and females only and those that were differentially regulated irrespective of sex. Figure 3 shows the number of genes up and downregulated after hyperoxia exposure and the distribution in males and females, and those that were common to both male and female mice. Interestingly, 152 genes were upregulated in females only and 316 in males only. Among the downregulated genes, 175 were in females and 269 in males only as shown in Figure 3. Table 2 shows the genes with the highest fold change (≥4) in both males and females and (≥2) in males and females separately.

Pathway analysis of DEGs

To identify the biological processes that were enriched in the subsets of DEGs that were common to males and females, males only, and females only, we performed both over-representation and pathway topology analyses in these subsets of genes to

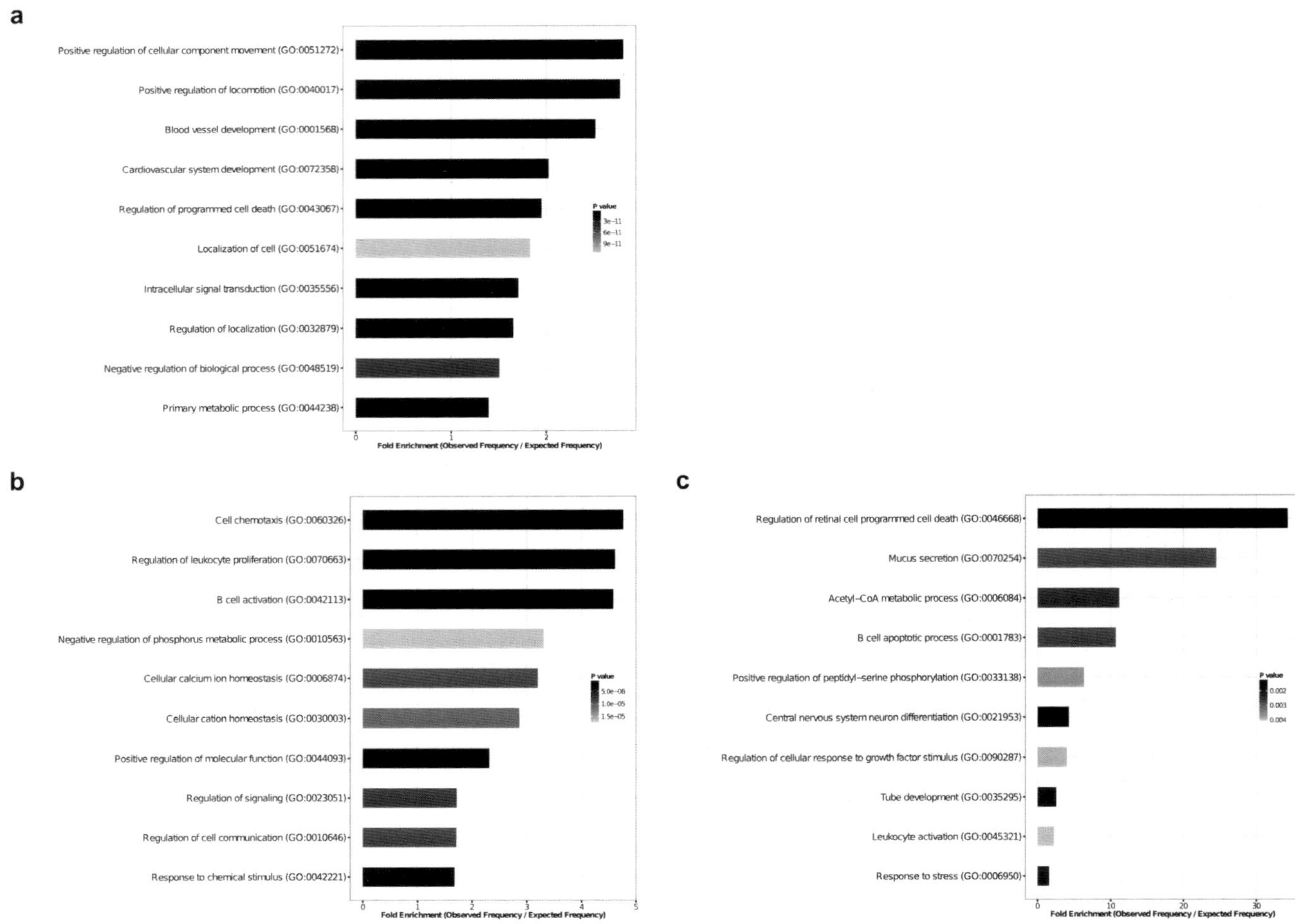

Figure 4. Pathway analysis by ORA (over representation analysis). Analysis of enrichment of biological processes in the three groups; 4a: analysis of DEGs common in both male and female animals after hyperoxia exposure 4b: analysis of DEGs in male animals 4c: analysis of DEGs in female animals. Overrepresentation of gene ontology terms representing biological processes among the DEGs was tested using a conditional hypergeometric test (p-value <0.01).

highlight the differences in the results obtained by these two methods. There are many drawbacks to the over-representation analysis method (ORA) for pathway analysis. ORA typically only considers the number of genes and ignores any values associated with them such as probe intensities; it typically uses only the most significant genes and discards the others. By treating each gene equally, ORA assumes that each gene is independent of the other genes and that each pathway is independent of other pathways [35]. To overcome these drawbacks, we also performed pathway topology analysis. This type of analysis considers the structure and dynamics of an entire pathway by incorporating a number of important biological factors, including changes in gene expression, types of interactions, and the positions of genes in a pathway [31].

Figure 4a shows the major biological processes for the group of genes that were differentially regulated both in males and females. Among these were regulation of programmed cell death and angiogenesis. We then identified the enriched biological processes in DEGs, which showed sex-specific expression upon exposure to hyperoxia. Figure 4b shows the biological processes that were found to be significant among the DEGs in males only, and figure 4c shows the biological pathways that were found to be significant in females only. In males, the molecular pathways regulating leukocyte proliferation, adhesion, and chemotaxis were significant. In females, acetyl-CoA metabolic process and mucus secretion were among the most significantly enriched biological processes.

Table 3 shows the results of pathway topology analysis by Signaling Pathway Impact Analysis (SPIA). SPIA uses the information from a set of differentially expressed genes and their fold changes, as well as pathways topology in order to assess the significance of the pathways in the condition under the study [31]. These two aspects are captured by the probability values: P_{NDE} (probability of obtaining a number of differentially expressed genes on the given pathway at least as large as the observed one), where NDE stands for the number of differentially expressed genes and P_{PERT} which is calculated based on the amount of perturbation measured in each pathway. The two types of evidence, P_{NDE} and P_{PERT}, are finally combined into one global probability value, P_G, which is used to rank the pathways and test the research hypothesis that the pathway is significantly perturbed in the condition under the study. A significance threshold of 5% was used on the FDR corrected p-values (pGFDR) in order to detect pathway significance. The Kyoto Encyclopedia of Genes and Genomes (KEGG) pathway ID enriched in each group are shown in Table 3. Based on this analysis, we found the KEGG pathways common to both males and females (Table 3) were; p53 signaling, cytokine-cytokine receptor interaction, transcriptional misregulation in cancer, mitogen-activated protein kinase (MAPK) signal-

Table 3. Signaling Pathway Impact Analysis of DEGs.

Table 3a: DEGs exclusive to females in response to oxygen					
Pathway name (KEGG)	**Pathway ID**	**Size**	**NDE**	**pGFDR**	**Status**
Systemic lupus erythematosus	05322	124	23	8.46e-18	Activated
Alcoholism	05034	175	22	2.15e-13	Activated
Transcriptional misregulation in cancer	05202	171	12	0.0004	Inhibited
Table 3b: DEGs exclusive to males in response to oxygen					
Pathway name (KEGG)	**Pathway ID**	**Size**	**NDE**	**pGFDR**	**Status**
Dilated cardiomyopathy	05414	88	5	0.0460	Activated
NF-kappa B signaling pathway	04064	89	6	0.0460	Inhibited
Table 3c: DEGs common to both sexes in response to oxygen					
Pathway name (KEGG)	**Pathway ID**	**Size**	**NDE**	**pGFDR**	**Status**
Rheumatoid arthritis	05323	80	19	0.0006	Activated
HTLV-I infection	05166	275	40	0.0020	Inhibited
Cytokine-cytokine receptor interaction	04060	239	34	0.0020	Activated
p53 signaling pathway	04115	67	14	0.0020	Inhibited
Transcriptional misregulation in cancer	05202	171	30	0.0020	Inhibited
RNA transport	03013	156	27	0.0038	Activated
Focal adhesion	04510	199	30	0.0161	Activated
Osteoclast differentiation	04380	117	20	0.0177	Inhibited
MAPK signaling pathway	04010	260	36	0.0177	Activated
Epstein-Barr virus infection	05169	204	26	0.0218	Inhibited
Small cell lung cancer	05222	83	12	0.0218	Activated
Chemokine signaling pathway	04062	177	25	0.0218	Activated
Axon guidance	04360	129	20	0.0302	Inhibited
Toll-like receptor signaling pathway	04620	100	17	0.0474	Activated

Notes. The KEGG IDs of the pathways are specified. NDE: Number of differentially expressed genes in the pathway; pGFDR: False discovery rate corrected p value.

ing, chemokine signaling and toll-like receptor signaling. In male mice, the pathways of dilated cardiomyopathy and NF kappa B signaling were significant based on the DEGs. In female mice, alcoholism, systemic lupus erythematosus (SLE) and transcriptional misregulation in cancer were the significant pathways.

Real time qPCR validation

Microarray results were verified by qPCR. Usually, validation of differential expression of genes is performed on a gene to gene basis. The disadvantage of following this approach is that it is not possible to generalize validation results to the remaining majority of non-validated genes or to evaluate the overall quality of these studies. Miron *et al.* [32] showed that the common method of selecting only the most differentially expressed genes for validation generally fails as a global validation strategy and proposed random-stratified sampling as a better gene selection method. Therefore, we selected 5 genes (*Ankrd1*, *Slc7a5*, *Slc7a11*, *Egr1* and *Nqo1*) from the pool of DEGs in a random-stratified manner based on their fold change as described in materials and methods. In addition, we also selected five additional genes from the pool of genes showing sex-specific differential expression in the microarray experiment. Figure 5 shows the PCR results for DEGs common to both males and females (5a) and the changes in transcript levels of genes showing sex-specific differences (5b) in expression after hyperoxia exposure. Table 4 shows the comparison of results between microarray and PCR for the selected genes. To better estimate the global validation of the microarray experiment with the PCR, we calculated the concordance correlation coefficient (CCC), which combines the accuracy and precision coefficients in one index. This is depicted in Figure 6. All the genes tested in males and females by microarray and PCR are represented as dots in this graph. It is used to determine how far the observed data deviate from the line of perfect concordance. CCC increases in value as a function of the nearness of the data's reduced major axis to the line or perfect concordance (the accuracy of the data) and of the tightness of the data about its reduced major axis (the precision of the data). We achieved a CCC of 0.71 for males and 0.69 for females, which shows good validity of our microarray experiment findings [32].

Immunohistochemistry and western blot

For validation at the protein level we performed immunohistochemistry for one of the DEGs (*Slc7a11*) in the hyperoxia group, which was common to both males and females. Compared to the room air controls, after 48 h of hyperoxia exposure, intense positive staining is seen in the lung sections in the peribronchiolar epithelial and type II alveolar epithelial cells (Figure 7) similar to the results seen in the microarray and the PCR results. Figure 8A shows Slc7a11 protein expression assessed by western blot assay in whole lung protein from male mice, at room air and after 48 h

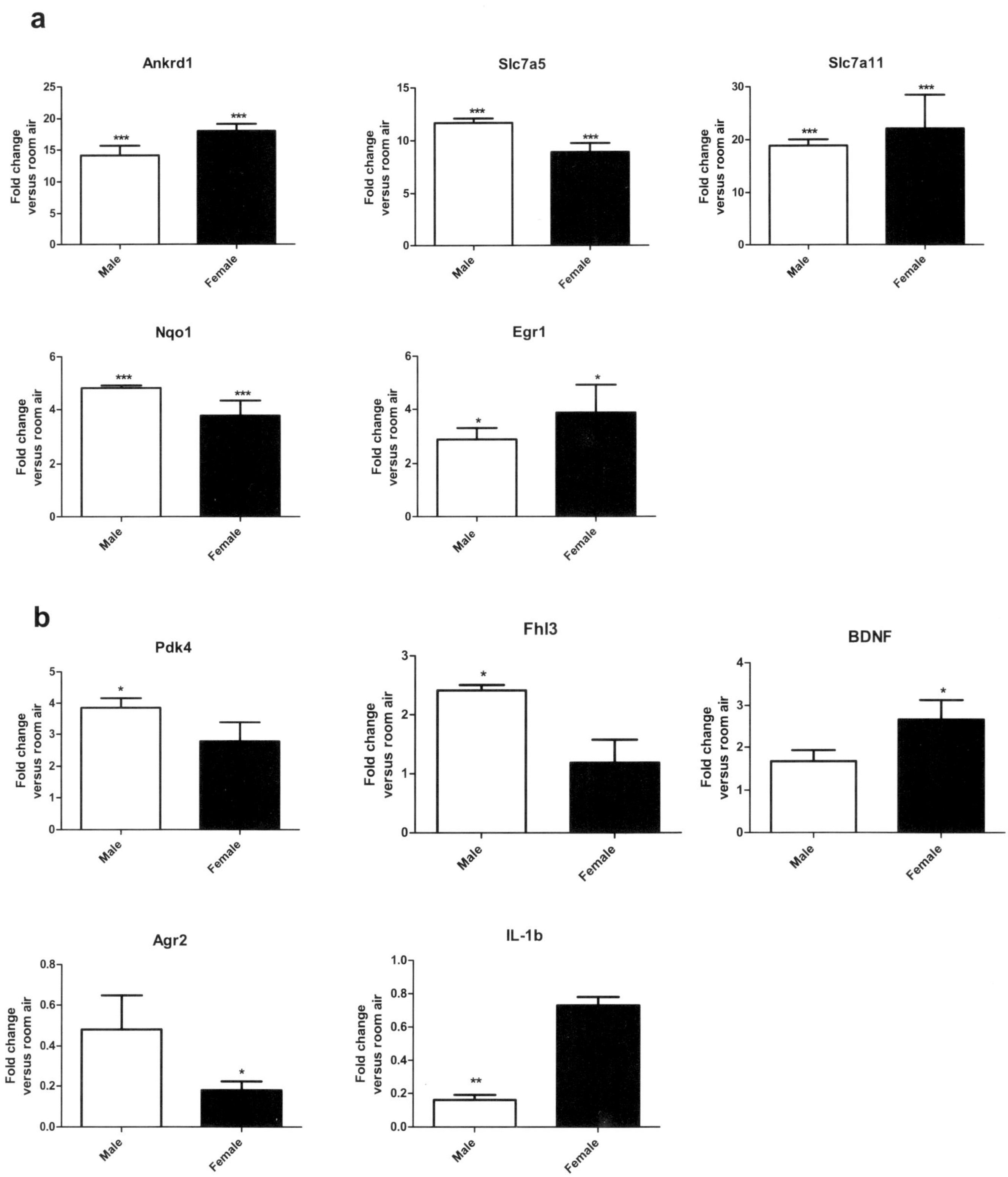

Figure 5. Real time RT-PCR analysis of mRNA from the lungs of male and female mice exposed to room air or hyperoxia for 48 h. Values are means ± SEM from n = 3 groups. Each group consisted of pooled RNA from four animals. Figure 5a: Real time RT-PCR analysis of differentially expressed genes common to both male and female mice. Significant upregulation over room air levels are indicated by * $p<0.05$ and *** $p<0.001$(one-way ANOVA). Figure 5b: Real time RT-PCR analysis of genes showing sex-specific changes. Fold change over room air levels are represented on the y-axis. Significant up or downregulation over room air levels are indicated by *$p<0.05$ and **$p<0.01$ (one-way ANOVA).

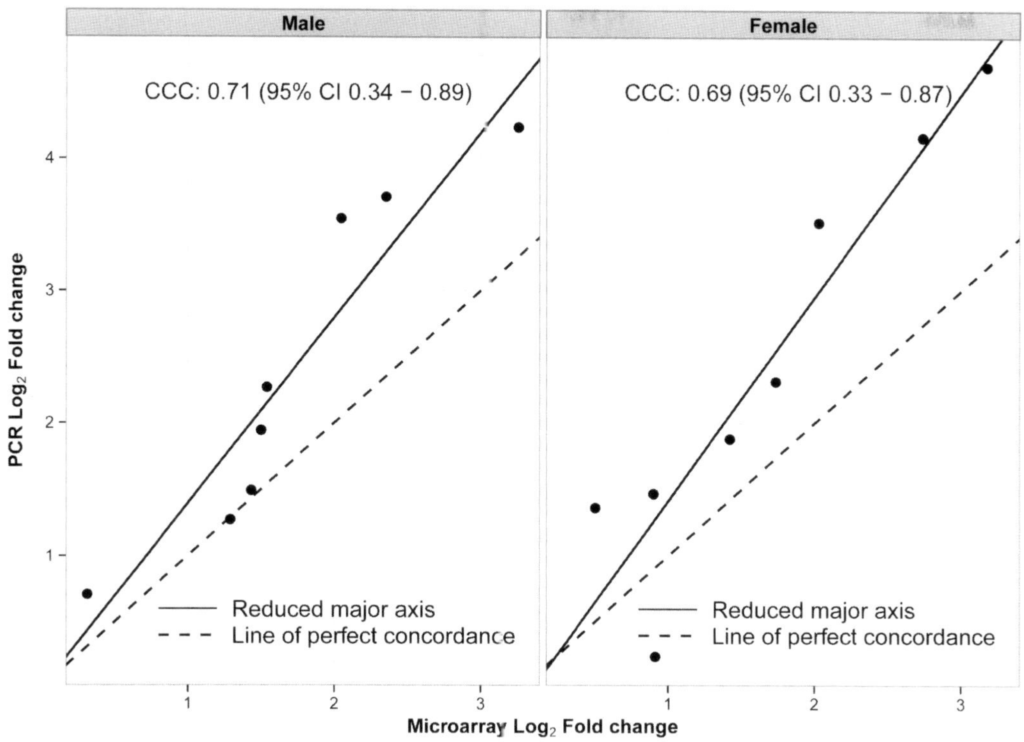

Figure 6. Concordance correlation coefficient (CCC) between qPCR and microarray results. Used to measure the agreement between the log_2 FC results from qRT-PCR and microarray in both males and females. The dashed line represents the line of perfect concordance. The solid line represents the reduced major axis.

hyperoxia exposure. There is increased expression (8B; $p<0.01$) of Slc7a11 after hyperoxia exposure compared to room air controls. The expression pattern was similar in females (results not shown).

Discussion

The major new findings of this study are the identification of new candidate genes of interest and the sex-specific transcriptomic changes in hyperoxic lung injury. We also identified pathways that are differentially regulated in a sex-specific manner. These findings could in part explain the differences in susceptibility between males and females in diseases such as ARDS and BPD. The hyperoxic lung injury model is a type of oxidant stress to the lung and the findings from this study could explain the sex-specific differences in the pathophysiology of many other diseases, in which increased oxidative stress plays a role such as pulmonary fibrosis, asthma and COPD [36]. While transcriptomic differences

Table 4. Fold change for the selected genes in the microarray and qPCR experiment.

Affymetrix ID	Gene Symbol	Gene Name	Group	Microarray		PCR	
				M	F	M	F
10498024	Slc7a11	Solute carrier family 7 (cationic amino acid transporter, y+ system), member 11	C	9.513	9.063	18.83	25.83
10467191	Ankrd1	Ankyrin repeat domain 1	C	5.098	6.68	13.08	17.91
10582275	Slc7a5	Solute carrier family 7 (cationic amino acid transporter, y+ system), member 5	C	4.141	4.084	11.67	11.42
10454782	Egr1	Early growth response 1	C	2.694	3.340	2.82	4.97
10581538	Nqo1	NAD(P)H dehydrogenase, quinone 1	C	2.908	2.676	4.82	3.68
10474399	BDNF	Brain derived neurotrophic factor	F		1.424	1.63	2.57
10543017	Pdk4	Pyruvate dehydrogenase kinase, isozyme 4	M	2.83		3.85	2.77
10487597	IL1b	Interleukin 1 beta	M	−2.55		0.16	0.73
10395365	Agr2	Anterior gradient 2	F		−2.64	0.48	0.18

Notes: C: Common to both male and female animals; F: In females only; M: In males only.

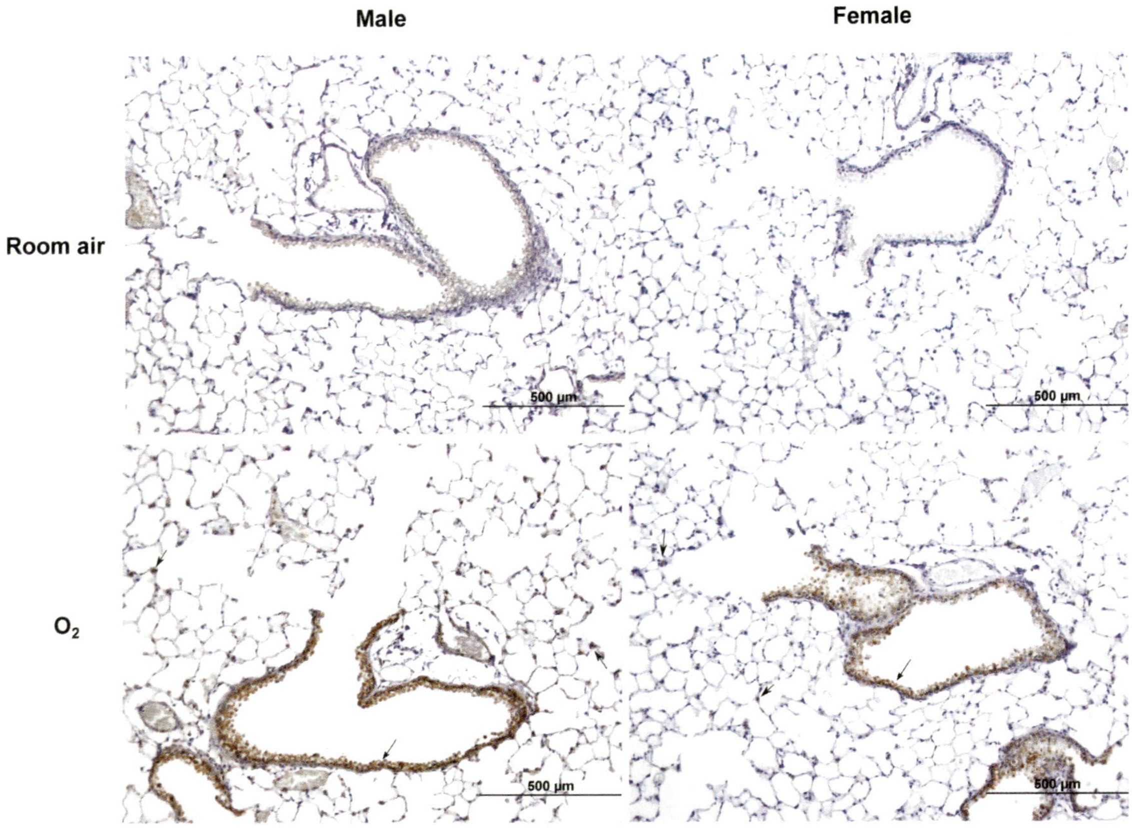

Figure 7. Increased Slc7a11 expression in the lungs (male or female) following hyperoxia exposure. Representative sample of immunohistochemical staining for *Slc7a11* in the lungs of male or female mice at room air and after exposure to hyperoxia for 48 h (n = 5 animals/ group).

have been described in hyperoxic lung injury [37] sex-specific changes in the transcriptome following hyperoxic lung injury have not been not been well described in the past studies.

Using microarrays to examine differential gene expression in the lungs after hyperoxia exposure for 48 hours, we identified genes that are differentially expressed unique to each of the sexes as well as those that are common to both the sexes. Of those genes that were differentially expressed following hyperoxia exposure, 1882 were common to both males and females; there were 585 genes unique to males and 327 unique to females. We selected the 48 h time point, as major differences in lung injury by histopathological analysis and markers of inflammation were found at 72 h with most animals dying between 60–90 h of exposure [6]. This study, therefore, focuses on the initiation phase of hyperoxic lung injury when cellular activation instead of cellular injury is taking place [5].

The study reveals potential candidate genes that could explain the sex-specific differences in the pathophysiology of hyperoxic lung injury. Of particular note are the genes *Pdk4, Fhl3, BDNF, Agr2 and CCl17*. *Pdk4* (pyruvate dehydrogenase lipoamide kinase 4), was upregulated in males after hyperoxia exposure. *Pdk4* is an inhibitory kinase, which phosphorylates and inhibits the activity of pyruvate dehydrogenase. The role of this gene in hyperoxic lung injury has not been tested. Grassian *et al* (2011) reported that *Pdk4* overexpression decreased de novo lipogenesis and cell proliferation. Hyperoxia exposure is known to decrease cell proliferation in pulmonary epithelial cell lines when exposed to hyperoxia [38], and *Pdk4* could have a potential role in this effect. Another candidate gene, *Agr2* was downregulated in female mice after hyperoxia exposure. *Agr2* inhibits p53 [39] and hyperoxia is known to induce p53 expression [40]. The downregulation of *Agr2* in female could in part explain this phenomenon in female mice. *Fhl3* (The four-and-a-half LIM domain 3) gene was upregulated in males after hyperoxia exposure. The four-and-a-half LIM domain (FHL) proteins have a highly conserved double zinc finger motif and have been implicated in transcriptional regulation [41] and suppression of tumor growth [42]. *Fhl3* has been shown to inhibit the transactivation of hypoxia-inducible factor 1 (*HIF-1*) [43]. *HIF-1* in turn has been shown to be downregulated in neonatal mice exposed to hyperoxia [44,45]. *Fhl3* could also have effects on cell cycle progression and apoptosis. It has been shown to cause cell-cycle arrest through upregulation of p21 and induce caspase-3 mediated apoptosis in glioma cells [46]. *BDNF* (Brain derived neurotrophic factor) was upregulated in females following hyperoxia exposure. Neurotrophins like BDNF have been implicated in many lung diseases [47]. *BDNF* was upregulated in the lung specifically in the peribronchial smooth muscles in 5- day old rat pups exposed to >95% oxygen for 7 days [48]. *Ccl17* was upregulated in females after hyperoxia exposure. This gene is one of several Cys-Cys (CC) cytokine genes. The cytokine encoded by this gene displays chemotactic activity for T lymphocytes, but not monocytes or granulocytes. In a study by Bhattacharya *et al* [49] in human lung samples in patients with BPD, *CCl17* was downregulated.

Pathway analysis based on sex-specific gene expression patterns showed sex-specific differences in enrichment of biological processes (Figure 4 and Table 3). The MAP kinase pathway is activated under hyperoxic conditions [50–52]. At the 48 h time

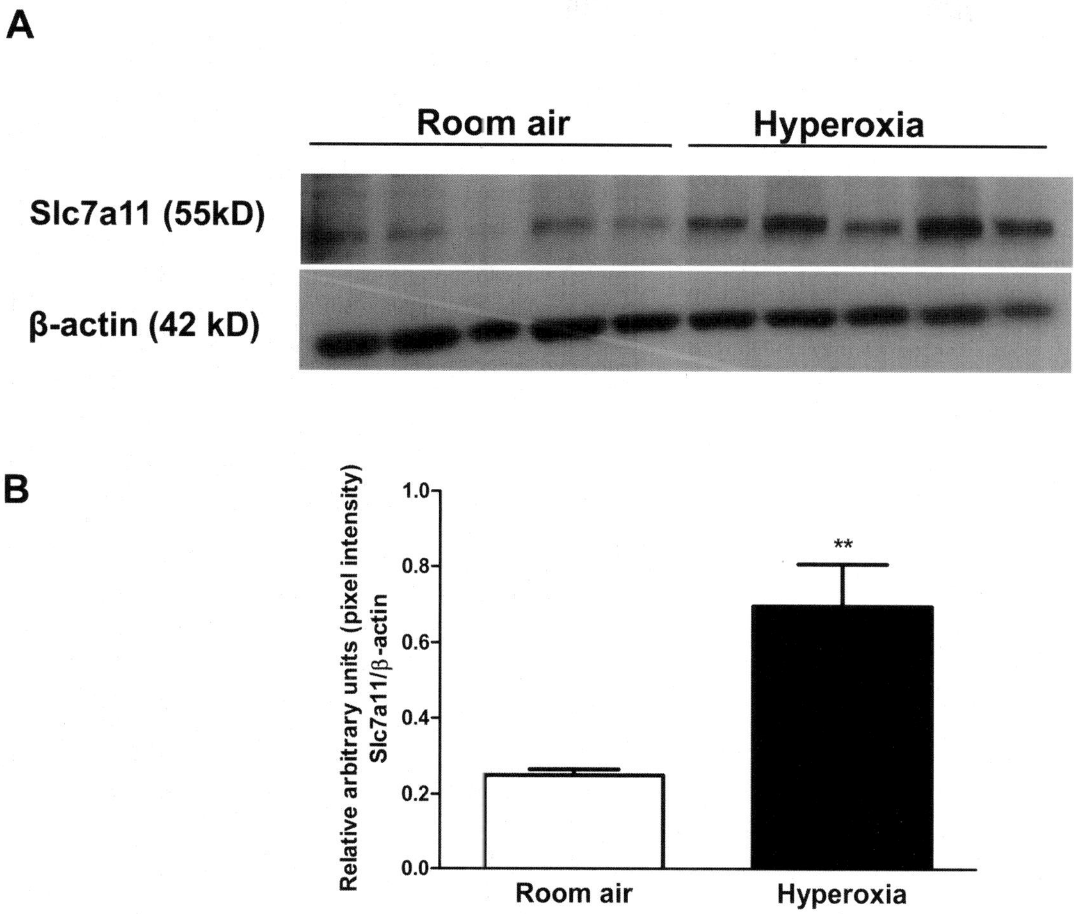

Figure 8. Increased Slc7a11 expression in the lungs (male) following hyperoxia exposure. 8A: Western blot assay for Slc7a11 expression in lungs following hyperoxia exposure. Twenty μg of whole lung protein from male animals at room air and exposed to 48 h of hyperoxia was subjected to western blotting using antibodies against Slc7a11. Under each sample lane is the corresponding β-actin blot to assess for protein loading. **8B:** Densitometry analysis of pulmonary Slc7a11 immunoblots at room air and after 48 h of hyperoxia exposure. Significant differences from room air controls are indicated by **, $p<0.01$.

point, in our study, the MAP kinase pathway was inhibited in males but activated in females. Interestingly, *IL-1β* was found to be downregulated in males at the 48 h time point and not in females and this could explain the differential regulation of this pathway in males. Similarly, the NFκ-B pathway was inhibited in males by pathway topology analysis. NFκ-B also plays an important role in hyperoxic lung injury [53–55]. The pathway is activated in hyperoxic conditions but this may be a part of a survival mechanism to escape cell death [56–58]. Enhanced NF-κB protected the lung from acute hyperoxic injury in neonatal mice via inhibition of apoptosis (Yang *et al.*, 2004). Specifically, *IL-1β* was downregulated and *Iκbα* was upregulated (data not shown) both of which could play a role in the inhibition of this pathway. Also, higher levels of oxidative stress can lead to inhibition of NFκ-B rather than its activation through other mechanisms [55].

In addition to the genes, which showed sex-specific changes in their response to hyperoxia exposure, we identified important differentially expressed genes common to both sexes. Gene expression pattern in the lung after exposure to hyperoxia has been reported previously in adult and neonatal mice. In the study by Perkowski *et al* in 2003 [59] using a total of five mice, *p21, metallothionein and cysteine-rich protein 61* were the top three upregulated genes in 8–10 week old female mice after hyperoxia exposure for 48 h. We also found these genes to be upregulated both in male and female mice in our study at this time point. We also found similar upregulation in *elastin, galectin 3, glutathione reductase, heme oxygenase-1, p53 and connective tissue growth factor. connective tissue growth factor.*

Slc7a11 (solute carrier family (anionic amino acid transporter light chain Xc-system), Member 11) was upregulated in both male and female mice in our study and we validated this at the protein level using immunohistochemistry and western blot (Figure 7 and 8). To our knowledge, this is the first documentation of induction of this gene and protein in a hyperoxic lung injury model in adult mice. This gene codes the protein, xCT, which is upregulated after exposure to hyperoxia [60]. xCT is regulated in part by *Nrf2*, which has an important protective role in hyperoxia induced ALI [61]. Howden *et al* [62] exposed adult mice to 100% oxygen for 96 hours in different mouse strains to study the cardiopulmonary response and identify candidate susceptibility genes in hyperoxic lung injury. *Slc7a11* emerged as one of the candidate genes by linkage analysis. *Slc7a11* was also upregulated in neonatal mice following hyperoxia exposure [37]. The protective role of xCT against oxidative stress in the lung was also shown in a model of paraquat induced oxidative stress. xCT deficient mice had decreased survival, increased injury and inflammation. It was upregulated in lungs exposed to oxidative stress and contributed to the maintenance of glutathione levels under these conditions [63].

Nqo1 (NAD(P)H:quinone oxidoreductase 1) is a phase II antioxidant enzyme that has been shown to be induced in murine lung in response to hyperoxia by *Nrf2* to protect against lung injury [37] was upregulated following 48 h of hyperoxia exposure in our study. Single nucleotide polymorphisms in this gene have been linked to susceptibility to ALI [64]. *Serpine-1 or plasminogen activator inhibitor (PAI)-1* was also upregulated in our study. This gene has been shown to play a major deleterious role in hyperoxic lung injury [65]. *PAI-1* upregulation impairs fibrinolytic activity in the alveoli and leads to fibrin accumulation.

We have reported previously on sex-specific differences in hyperoxic lung injury and the possible protective role of cytochrome P450 (CYP)1A1. We did not find this gene to be significantly differentially regulated at the 48 h time point in this study. In our experiments *Cyp1a1* shows the most upregulation at the 24 h time point (data not shown), which could explain its absence in the list of DEGs at the 48 h time point.

Although the array data provides a comprehensive overview of gene expression in the lung after hyperoxia, our study has its limitations. First, array data provides information on gene expression levels. Changes in gene expression levels may not necessarily reflect actual protein levels. Also, important functional changes induced by post-translational modifications cannot be identified. In this study, we examined whole lung tissue gene expression that includes endothelial cells, epithelial cells, interstitial cells, as well as circulating or adherent hematopoietic cells. Hence, most of the genes on the array are likely to be expressed by many cell types. In this investigation, we did not time our experiments with the estrous cycle in female mice, which could have led to some of the variability in our findings. The data is from 12 female adult mice whose lung RNA was pooled in this study. However, there is emerging data that mammalian cells differ intrinsically based on the sex and also respond differently to stressors irrespective of the past or current concentrations of sex hormones [66].

In conclusion, we present the changes in the mouse pulmonary transcriptome after hyperoxia exposure at the 48 h time point and identified new potential candidate genes of interest. Furthermore, our results support the hypothesis that there is sex-specific modulation of gene expression and biological processes in the lung under hyperoxic conditions, which may contribute to sex-based differences in hyperoxic lung injury. It is increasingly appreciated that gender differences impact disease presentation and clinical trajectory of patients with ALI. While hormonal factors and differences in lung development are described as contributing factors, comprehensive evaluation of the transcriptomic profile as in this study provides a substantial opportunity to advance the understanding of sex-specific differences in the pathophysiology of hyperoxic lung injury, and could lead to insights about sex-related individualized therapy.

Author Contributions

Conceived and designed the experiments: KL BM. Performed the experiments: KL LW WJ. Analyzed the data: KL CS. Contributed reagents/materials/analysis tools: BM KL WJ LW. Contributed to the writing of the manuscript: BM CS XC KL.

References

1. Kallet RH, Matthay MA (2013) Hyperoxic acute lung injury. respir care 58: 123–141. doi:10.4187/respcare.01963.
2. Hilgendorff A, Reiss I, Ehrhardt H, Eickelberg O, Alvira CM (2013) Chronic Lung Disease in the Preterm Infant: Lessons Learned From Animal Models. American Journal of Respiratory Cell and Molecular Biology. doi:10.1165/rcmb.2013-0014TR.
3. Buczynski BW, Maduekwe ET, O'Reilly MA (2013) The role of hyperoxia in the pathogenesis of experimental BPD. Semin Perinatol 37: 69–78. doi:10.1053/j.semperi.2013.01.002.
4. Freeman BA, Crapo JD (1981) Hyperoxia increases oxygen radical production in rat lungs and lung mitochondria. J Biol Chem 256: 10986–10992.
5. Clark JM, Lambertsen CJ (1971) Pulmonary oxygen toxicity: a review. Pharmacol Rev 23: 37–133.
6. Matute-Bello G, Frevert CW, Martin TR (2008) Animal models of acute lung injury. Am J Physiol Lung Cell Mol Physiol 295: L379–L399. doi:10.1152/ajplung.00010.2008.
7. Bryan CL, Jenkinson SG (1988) Oxygen toxicity. Clin Chest Med 9: 141–152.
8. Budinger GRS, Mutlu GM, Urich D, Soberanes S, Buccellato LJ, et al. (2011) Epithelial cell death is an important contributor to oxidant-mediated acute lung injury. Am J Respir Crit Care Med 183: 1043–1054. doi:10.1164/rccm.201002-0181OC.
9. Ware LB, Matthay MA (2000) The acute respiratory distress syndrome. N Engl J Med 342: 1334–1349. doi:10.1056/NEJM200005043421806.
10. Moss M, Mannino DM (2002) Race and gender differences in acute respiratory distress syndrome deaths in the United States: an analysis of multiple-cause mortality data (1979–1996). Crit Care Med 30: 1679–1685.
11. Agarwal R, Aggarwal AN, Gupta D, Behera D, Jindal SK (2006) Etiology and outcomes of pulmonary and extrapulmonary acute lung injury/ARDS in a respiratory ICU in North India. Chest 130: 724–729. doi:10.1378/chest.130.3.724.
12. Natarajan G, Pappas A, Shankaran S, Kendrick DE, Das A, et al. (2012) Outcomes of extremely low birth weight infants with bronchopulmonary dysplasia: impact of the physiologic definition. Early Hum Dev 88: 509–515. doi:10.1016/j.earlhumdev.2011.12.013.
13. Olson AL, Swigris JJ, Lezotte DC, Norris JM, Wilson CG, et al. (2007) Mortality from pulmonary fibrosis increased in the United States from 1992 to 2003. Am J Respir Crit Care Med 176: 277–284. doi:10.1164/rccm.200701-044OC.
14. Gribbin J, Hubbard RB, Le Jeune I, Smith CJP, West J, et al. (2006) Incidence and mortality of idiopathic pulmonary fibrosis and sarcoidosis in the UK. Thorax 61: 980–985. doi:10.1136/thx.2006.062836.
15. Rhodes L, Moorman JE, Redd SC (2005) Sex differences in asthma prevalence and other disease characteristics in eight states. J Asthma 42: 777–782. doi:10.1080/02770900500308387.
16. Kraybill EN, Runyan DK, Bose CL, Khan JH (1989) Risk factors for chronic lung disease in infants with birth weights of 751 to 1000 grams. J Pediatr 115: 115–120.
17. Ambalavanan N, Carlo WA, McDonald SA, Yao Q, Das A, et al. (2011) Identification of extremely premature infants at high risk of rehospitalization. Pediatrics 128: e1216–e1225. doi:10.1542/peds.2011-1142.
18. Slaughter JL, Pakrashi T, Jones DE, South AP, Shah TA (2011) Echocardiographic detection of pulmonary hypertension in extremely low birth weight infants with bronchopulmonary dysplasia requiring prolonged positive pressure ventilation. J Perinatol 31: 635–640. doi:10.1038/jp.2010.213.
19. Carey MA, Card JW, Voltz JW, Germolec DR, Korach KS, et al. (2007) The impact of sex and sex hormones on lung physiology and disease: lessons from animal studies. Am J Physiol Lung Cell Mol Physiol 293: L272–L278. doi:10.1152/ajplung.00174.2007.
20. Carey MA, Card JW, Voltz JW, Arbes SJ, Germolec DR, et al. (2007) It's all about sex: gender, lung development and lung disease. Trends Endocrinol Metab 18: 308–313. doi:10.1016/j.tem.2007.08.003.
21. Hamon I, Valdes V, Franck P, Buchweiller M-C, Fresson J, et al. (2011) [Gender-dependent differences in glutathione (GSH) metabolism in very preterm infants]. Arch Pediatr 18: 247–252. doi:10.1016/j.arcped.2010.12.004.
22. Vento M, Aguar M, Escobar J, Arduini A, Escrig R, et al. (2009) Antenatal steroids and antioxidant enzyme activity in preterm infants: influence of gender and timing. Antioxid Redox Signal 11: 2945–2955. doi:10.1089/ars.2009.2671.
23. Card JW, Carey MA, Bradbury JA, DeGraff LM, Morgan DL, et al. (2006) Gender differences in murine airway responsiveness and lipopolysaccharide-induced inflammation. J Immunol 177: 621–630.
24. Speyer CL, Rancilio NJ, McClintock SD, Crawford JD, Gao H, et al. (2005) Regulatory effects of estrogen on acute lung inflammation in mice. Am J Physiol, Cell Physiol 288: C881–C890. doi:10.1152/ajpcell.00467.2004.
25. Shaw GM, O'Brodovich HM (2013) Progress in understanding the genetics of bronchopulmonary dysplasia. Semin Perinatol 37: 85–93. doi:10.1053/j.semperi.2013.01.004.
26. Hudak BB, Zhang LY, Kleeberger SR (1993) Inter-strain variation in susceptibility to hyperoxic injury of murine airways. Pharmacogenetics 3: 135–143.
27. CHO H, KLEEBERGER S (2007) Genetic mechanisms of susceptibility to oxidative lung injury in mice☆. Free Radic Biol Med 42: 433–445. doi:10.1016/j.freeradbiomed.2006.11.021.

28. Prows DR, Hafertepen AP, Winterberg AV, Gibbons W, Liu C, et al. (2007) Genetic analysis of hyperoxic acute lung injury survival in reciprocal intercross mice. Physiol Genomics 30: 271–281. doi:10.1152/physiolgenomics.00038.2007.
29. Lingappan K, Jiang W, Wang L, Couroucli XI, Barrios R, et al. (2013) Sex-specific differences in hyperoxic lung injury in mice: Implications for acute and chronic lung disease in humans. Toxicol Appl Pharmacol. doi:10.1016/j.taap.2013.06.007.
30. Gonder JC, Proctor RA, Will JA (1985) Genetic differences in oxygen toxicity are correlated with cytochrome P-450 inducibility. Proc Natl Acad Sci USA 82: 6315–6319.
31. Tarca AL, Draghici S, Khatri P, Hassan SS, Mittal P, et al. (2009) A novel signaling pathway impact analysis. Bioinformatics 25: 75–82. doi:10.1093/bioinformatics/btn577.
32. Miron M, Woody OZ, Marcil A, Murie C, Sladek R, et al. (2006) A methodology for global validation of microarray experiments. BMC Bioinformatics 7: 333. doi:10.1186/1471-2105-7-333.
33. R Core Team (2013) R: A Language and Environment for Statistical Computing. Vienna, Austria.
34. Gentleman RC, Carey VJ, Bates DM, others (2004) Bioconductor: Open software development for computational biology and bioinformatics. Genome Biology 5: R80.
35. Khatri P, Sirota M, Butte AJ (2012) Ten years of pathway analysis: current approaches and outstanding challenges. PLoS Comput Biol 8: e1002375. doi:10.1371/journal.pcbi.1002375.
36. Park HS, Kim SR, Lee YC (2009) Impact of oxidative stress on lung diseases. Respirology 14: 27–38. doi:10.1111/j.1440-1843.2008.01447.x.
37. Cho H-Y, van Houten B, Wang X, Miller-DeGraff L, Fostel J, et al. (2012) Targeted deletion of nrf2 impairs lung development and oxidant injury in neonatal mice. Antioxid Redox Signal 17: 1066–1082. doi:10.1089/ars.2011.4288.
38. O'Reilly MA (2001) DNA damage and cell cycle checkpoints in hyperoxic lung injury: braking to facilitate repair. Am J Physiol Lung Cell Mol Physiol 281: L291–L305.
39. Chevet E, Fessart D, Delom F, Mulot A, Vojtesek B, et al. (2012) Emerging roles for the pro-oncogenic anterior gradient-2 in cancer development. Oncogene. doi:10.1038/onc.2012.346.
40. O'Reilly MA, Staversky RJ, Stripp BR, Finkelstein JN (1998) Exposure to hyperoxia induces p53 expression in mouse lung epithelium. American Journal of Respiratory Cell and Molecular Biology 18: 43–50. doi:10.1165/ajrcmb.18.1.2950m.
41. Johannessen M, Møller S, Hansen T, Moens U, Van Ghelue M (2006) The multifunctional roles of the four-and-a-half-LIM only protein FHL2. Cell Mol Life Sci 63: 268–284. doi:10.1007/s00018-005-5438-z.
42. Ding L, Wang Z, Yan J, Yang X, Liu A, et al. (2009) Human four-and-a-half LIM family members suppress tumor cell growth through a TGF-beta-like signaling pathway. J Clin Invest 119: 349–361. doi:10.1172/JCI35930.
43. Hubbi ME, Gilkes DM, Baek JH, Semenza GL (2012) Four-and-a-half LIM domain proteins inhibit transactivation by hypoxia-inducible factor 1. J Biol Chem 287: 6139–6149. doi:10.1074/jbc.M111.278630.
44. Popescu CR, Sutherland MR, Cloutier A, Benoît G, Bertagnolli M, et al. (2013) Hyperoxia exposure impairs nephrogenesis in the neonatal rat: role of HIF-1α. PLoS ONE 8: e82421. doi:10.1371/journal.pone.0082421.
45. Park H-S, Park J-W, Kim J-H, Choi C-W, Lee H-J, et al. (2012) Sildenafil Alleviates Bronchopulmonary Dysplasia in Neonatal Rats by Activating the Hypoxia-Inducible Factor Signaling Pathway. American Journal of Respiratory Cell and Molecular Biology. doi:10.1165/rcmb.2012-0043OC.
46. Han W, Xin Z, Zhao Z, Bao W, Lin X, et al. (2013) RNA-binding protein PCBP2 modulates glioma growth by regulating FHL3. J Clin Invest 123: 2103–2118. doi:10.1172/JCI61820DS1.
47. Prakash YS, Thompson MA, Meuchel L, Pabelick CM, Mantilla CB, et al. (2010) Neurotrophins in lung health and disease. Expert Review of Respiratory Medicine 4: 395–411. doi:10.1586/ers.10.29.
48. Yao Q, Haxhiu MA, Zaidi SI, Liu S, Jafri A, et al. (2005) Hyperoxia enhances brain-derived neurotrophic factor and tyrosine kinase B receptor expression in peribronchial smooth muscle of neonatal rats. Am J Physiol Lung Cell Mol Physiol 289: L307–L314. doi:10.1152/ajplung.00030.2005.
49. Bhattacharya SS, Go DD, Krenitsky DLD, Huyck HLH, Solleti SKS, et al. (2012) Genome-wide transcriptional profiling reveals connective tissue mast cell accumulation in bronchopulmonary dysplasia. Am J Respir Crit Care Med 186: 349–358. doi:10.1164/rccm.201203-0406OC.
50. Li L-F, Liao S-K, Ko Y-S, Lee C-H, Quinn DA (2007) Hyperoxia increases ventilator-induced lung injury via mitogen-activated protein kinases: a prospective, controlled animal experiment. Crit Care 11: R25. doi:10.1186/cc5704.
51. Barazzone C, Horowitz S, Donati YR, Rodriguez I, Piguet PF (1998) Oxygen toxicity in mouse lung: pathways to cell death. American Journal of Respiratory Cell and Molecular Biology 19: 573–581. doi:10.1165/ajrcmb.19.4.3173.
52. Romashko J, Horowitz S, Franek WR, Palaia T, Miller EJ, et al. (2003) MAPK pathways mediate hyperoxia-induced oncotic cell death in lung epithelial cells. Free Radic Biol Med 35: 978–993.
53. Jacobson JR, Birukov KG (2009) Activation of NFkB and coagulation in lung injury by hyperoxia and excessive mechanical ventilation: one more reason "low and slow" is the way to go? Transl Res 154: 219–221. doi:10.1016/j.trsl.2009.07.012.
54. Liu Y-Y, Liao S-K, Huang C-C, Tsai Y-H, Quinn DA, et al. (2009) Role for nuclear factor-kappaB in augmented lung injury because of interaction between hyperoxia and high stretch ventilation. Transl Res 154: 228–240. doi:10.1016/j.trsl.2009.06.006.
55. Michiels C, Minet E, Mottet D, Raes M (2002) Regulation of gene expression by oxygen: NF-kappaB and HIF-1, two extremes. Free Radic Biol Med 33: 1231–1242.
56. Beg AA, Baltimore D (1996) An essential role for NF-kappaB in preventing TNF-alpha-induced cell death. Science 274: 782–784.
57. Barinaga M (1996) Life-death balance within the cell. Science 274: 724.
58. Horowitz S (1999) Pathways to cell death in hyperoxia. Chest 116: 64S–67S.
59. Perkowski S (2003) Gene Expression Profiling of the Early Pulmonary Response to Hyperoxia in Mice. American Journal of Respiratory Cell and Molecular Biology 28: 682–696. doi:10.1165/rcmb.4692.
60. Bannai S, Sato H, Ishii T, Sugita Y (1989) Induction of cystine transport activity in human fibroblasts by oxygen. J Biol Chem 264: 18480–18484.
61. Cho H-Y, Jedlicka AE, Reddy SPM, Kensler TW, Yamamoto M, et al. (2002) Role of NRF2 in protection against hyperoxic lung injury in mice. American Journal of Respiratory Cell and Molecular Biology 26: 175–182. doi:10.1165/ajrcmb.26.2.4501.
62. Howden R, Cho HY, Miller-DeGraff L, Walker C, Clark JA, et al. (2012) Cardiac Physiologic and Genetic Predictors of Hyperoxia-Induced Acute Lung Injury in Mice. American Journal of Respiratory Cell and Molecular Biology 46: 470–478. doi:10.1165/rcmb.2011-0204OC.
63. Kobayashi S, Kuwata K, Sugimoto T, Igarashi K, Osaki M, et al. (2012) Enhanced expression of cystine/glutamate transporter in the lung caused by the oxidative-stress-inducing agent paraquat. Free Radic Biol Med 53: 2197–2203. doi:10.1016/j.freeradbiomed.2012.09.040.
64. Reddy AJ, Christie JD, Aplenc R, Fuchs B, Lanken PN, et al. (2009) Association of human NAD(P)H:quinone oxidoreductase 1 (NQO1) polymorphism with development of acute lung injury. Journal of Cellular and Molecular Medicine 13: 1784–1791. doi:10.1111/j.1582-4934.2008.00581.x.
65. Barazzone C, Belin D, Piguet PF, Vassalli JD, Sappino AP (1996) Plasminogen activator inhibitor-1 in acute hyperoxic mouse lung injury. J Clin Invest 98: 2666–2673. doi:10.1172/JCI119089.
66. Penaloza C, Estevez B, Orlanski S, Sikorska M, Walker R, et al. (2009) Sex of the cell dictates its response: differential gene expression and sensitivity to cell death inducing stress in male and female cells. FASEB J 23: 1869–1879. doi:10.1096/fj.08-119388.

Wnt5a through Noncanonical Wnt/JNK or Wnt/PKC Signaling Contributes to the Differentiation of Mesenchymal Stem Cells into Type II Alveolar Epithelial Cells *In Vitro*

Airan Liu[1]ᶿ, Song Chen[2]ᶿ, Shixia Cai[1], Liang Dong[1], Le Liu[1], Yi Yang[1], Fengmei Guo[1], Xiaomin Lu[1], Hongli He[1], Qihong Chen[1], Shuling Hu[1], Haibo Qiu[1]*

1 Department of Critical Care Medicine, Zhongda Hospital, School of Medicine, Southeast University, Nanjing, P. R. China, **2** State Key Laboratory of Natural Medicines, School of Life Science and Technology, China Pharmaceutical University, Nanjing, P. R. China

Abstract

The differentiation of mesenchymal stem cells (MSCs) into type II alveolar epithelial (AT II) cells is critical for reepithelization and recovery in acute respiratory distress syndrome (ARDS), and Wnt signaling was considered to be the underlying mechanisms. In our previous study, we found that canonical Wnt pathway promoted the differentiation of MSCs into AT II cells, however the role of the noncanonical Wnt pathway in this process is unclear. It was disclosed in this study that noncanonical Wnt signaling in mouse bone marrow–derived MSCs (mMSCs) was activated during the differentiation of mMSCs into AT II cells in a modified co-culture system with murine lung epithelial-12 cells and small airway growth media. The levels of surfactant protein (SP) C, SPB and SPD, the specific markers of AT II cells, increased in mMSCs when Wnt5a was added to activate noncanonical Wnt signaling, while pretreatment with JNK or PKC inhibitors reversed the promotion of Wnt5a. The differentiation rate of mMSCs also depends on their abilities to accumulate and survive in inflammatory tissue. We found that the Wnt5a supplement promoted the vertical and horizontal migration of mMSCs, ameliorated the cell death and the reduction of Bcl-2/Bax induced by H_2O_2. The effect of Wnt5a on the migration of mMSCs and their survival after H_2O_2 exposure were partially inhibited with PKC or JNK blockers. In conclusion, Wnt5a through Wnt/JNK signaling alone or both Wnt/JNK and Wnt/PKC signaling promoted the differentiation of mMSCs into AT II cells and the migration of mMSCs; through Wnt/PKC signaling, Wnt5a increased the survival of mMSCs after H_2O_2 exposure *in vitro*.

Editor: Pranela Rameshwar, Rutgers - New Jersey Medical School, United States of America

Funding: This work was co-financed by three national natural science foundations of China (No. 81070049, 81300060, 81170057 URL:http://isisn.nsfc.gov.cn/egrantweb/), two natural science foundations of the Jiangsu province (No. Bk2010399, BK2011600 URL: http://210.73.128.90/XMSB/Eve_Login.jsp) and the new teacher fund for doctor station sponsored by the Ministry of Education China (No. 2010009212006). The funders had no role in study design, data collection and analysis, decision to publish, or preparation of the manuscript.

Competing Interests: The authors have declared that no competing interests exist.

* E-mail: haiboq2000@gmail.com

ᶿ These authors contributed equally to this work

Introduction

Despite extensive studies on the pathophysiology and treatment of acute respiratory distress syndrome (ARDS), the mortality remains at 34–44 percent [1]. The damage of the alveolar epithelial barrier, which mainly consists of type I and type II alveolar epithelial cells, is the main pathological characteristic and the therapeutic target of ARDS. AT II cells play an important role in pulmonary physiology and pathology because they are capable of synthesizing and secreting alveolar surfactant to reduce surface tension and prevent the collapse of the alveoli and because they may differentiate into the type I alveolar epithelial cells (AT I cells) to serve as progenitor cells for the reepithelization of impaired alveoli [2]. Thus, promoting the regeneration and repair of injured AT II cells is critical for patient recovery from ARDS.

Recently, the potential of multipotent mesenchymal stem cells (MSCs) in the treatment of ARDS has been revealed in several investigations [3–6]. It was found that MSCs, which can differentiate into AT II cells *in vitro* and *in vivo*, were involved in the repair of the alveolar epithelium in ARDS [7–10]. However, their engraftment and differentiation rates in injured lungs were limited [5], and further exploration is needed to improve these rates. Thus, it is necessary to explore the mechanisms underlying the differentiation of MSCs into AT II cells and their migration to injured lung tissue.

Wnt pathway is considered to be important in regulating mechanisms for the proliferation, development, differentiation of cells and organisms and can be divided into canonical and noncanonical Wnt pathway. In our previous study, we found that the activation of the canonical Wnt pathway promoted the differentiation of mice bone marrow-derived MSCs (mMSCs) into AT II cells based on a model for the differentiation of mice bone marrow derived MSCs (mMSCs) into AT II cells with indirectly co-cultured with murine lung epithelial (MLE)-12 cells plus small airway growth media (SAGM) [10]. However, the role of noncanonical Wnt pathway which functions independent of the accumulation of β-catenin and is as critical as canonical wnt signaling in modulating differentiation, proliferation, migration of cells, in the differentiation of MSC into AT II cells have not been well explored.. In the noncanonical Wnt pathway, Wnt ligand such as Wnt5a induces calcium influx through Dvl, followed by the phosphorylation of the downstream Calmodulin-dependent protein kinase (CaMK) or Protein kinase C (PKC), which regulates target gene expression through the activation of the nuclear factor of activated T cells (NFAT). JNK is another downstream effector of Wnt5a that activates activator protein 1 (AP-1), thereby regulating PCP (planar cell polarity) signaling [11,12].

Several recent studies have shown that noncanonical Wnt signaling has critical effects on the differentiation of MSCs, which express a number of ligands, receptors and pathway inhibitors [13]. Boland, et al. [14] found that Wnt5a could promote MSC differentiation into osteoblasts. Topol, et al. [15] also found that Wnt5a hinders the chondrogenic lineage commitment of MSCs, promotes chondrocyte differentiation, and delays chondrocyte maturation into hypertrophic stages. Additionally, the overexpression or shortage of noncanonical Wnt signaling could induce dysplasia of the alveolar epithelium [16], therefore we believe that noncanonical Wnt signaling may have a critical effect on the differentiation of MSCs into AT II cells, although this has not yet been investigated.

The aims of our study were to explore the role and underlying mechanisms of noncanonical Wnt signaling in the differentiation of mice bone marrow derived (mMSCs) into AT II cells according to the detection of the some AT II cells related markers as well as the ability of mMSCs to survive under oxidative stress conditions and migrate to injured lung tissue *in vitro*. The latter two properties can promote the localization and survival of MSCs in impaired lung tissue, thus indirectly influencing the differentiation of MSCs into AT II cells.

Materials and Methods

Ethics statement

All experimental procedures with animals used in the present study were complied with the National Research Council's guidelines and had been given prior approval by Care of Experimental Animals Committee of the Southeast University (approval ID: 2011-0122).

Cell culture

mMSCs and MLE-12 cells were used in the present study. mMSCs, obtained from Cyagen Biosciences Inc. (Guangzhou, China), were isolated from the bone marrow of C57BL/6 mice. The cells were verified as mesenchymal stem cells according to the identification of cell surface phenotypes (CD34+, CD44+, CD29+, SCA-1+ and CD117−) and the multipotent differentiation potential along the adipogenic, osteogenic, and chondrogenic lineages offered by the supplier [10]. MLE-12 cells, purchased from American Type Culture Collection (ATCC, Manassas, VA, USA), and mMSCs were cultured in Dulbecco's modified Eagle media/nutrient F-12 (DMEM/F12) 1:1 mixture (Thermo Scientific Hyclone, Beijing, China) supplemented with 2% (for MLE-12 cells) or 10% (for mMSCs) fetal bovine serum (FBS; Wisent Inc., St-Bruno, Quebec, Canada), 100 U/ml penicillin and 100 μg/ml streptomycin (Thermo Scientific Hyclone) in a humidified 5% CO_2 incubator at 37°C. The culture media was changed every 3 days, and the cells were passaged when they reached 90% confluency.

The differentiation of mMSCs into AT II cells

According to our previous study [10], a co-culture system with MLE-12 cells and SAGM (Lonza Group Ltd., Basel, Swizerland) was adopted for driving the differentiation of mMSCs into AT II cells. Briefly, 1×10^4 mMSCs and MLE-12 cells in 1.5 ml or 1 ml DMEM/F12 media supplemented with 10% FBS were, respectively, seeded in the lower or upper chambers of Transwell inserts (0.4-μm pore size, 4.5 cm^2, Corning, Inc., Corning, NY, USA) to establish the co-culture system. After mMSCs reached 80% confluency three days later, the culture media was replaced with SAGM, which consisted of small airway epithelial basal media and supplements, including 0.5 mg/ml bovine serum albumin, 30 μg/ml bovine pituitary extract, 0.5 μg/ml hydrocortisone, 0.5 ng/ml epithelial growth factor, 0.5 μg/ml epinephrine, 5 μg/ml insulin, 6.5 ng/ml triiodothyronine, 10 μg/ml transferring and 0.1 ng/ml retinoic acid, for another 7 days. To investigate the role of noncanonical Wnt signaling in mMSC differentiation, 500 ng/ml Wnt5a (R&D Systems, Minneapolis, MN, USA), in the presence or absence of 5 μmol/L SP600125 (Merck Biosciences, Darmstadt, Germany), a blocker of JNK, or 2.5 μmol/L GF109203X (Enzo Life Science, Farmingdale, NY, USA), a blocker of PKC were added to the co-cultured conditions. After differentiation, the inserts were removed, and mMSCs were harvested for western blotting and quantitative real-time PCR (qRT-PCR) analysis.

Cell proliferation and viability assay

To evaluate the effect of the noncanonical Wnt pathway on the proliferation and tolerance to H_2O_2-induced oxidative stress in mMSCs, 1×10^3 cells in 100 μl DMEM/F12 supplemented with 2% FBS were seeded into flat-bottomed 96-well culture plates. When the cell confluency reached 30–40% (for the proliferation test) or 75–85% (for the tolerance to H_2O_2 test), the growth media were supplemented with certain concentrations of Wnt5a, SP600125 or GF109203X for the indicated time in the absence or presence of H_2O_2. Then, the cell number was evaluated using a modified 3-(4, 5-dimethylthiazol-2-yl)-2, 5-diphenyltetrazolium (MTT) assay (Sigma, St. Louis, MO, USA), and the absorbance of resulting formazan was measured at 570 nm (630 nm as a reference).

Cell migration assay

The vertical and horizontal migrations of mMSCs were determined through a Transwell migration assay or wound healing assay, respectively. In the vertical migration test, 1×10^4 mMSCs in 200 μl serum-free DMEM/F12 containing 500 ng/ml Wnt5a or 500 ng/ml Wnt5a plus 5 μmol/L SP600125 or 2.5 μmol/L GF109203X were loaded into the Transwell inserts (6.5 mm diameter and 8 μm pore size, Corning, Inc.). Then, either 600 μl DMEM/F12 supplemented with 10% FBS or conditioned media of lung tissue obtained from normal or ARDS mice was added in the 96-well culture plates below the inserts. The conditioned media of mice lung tissue were obtained in accordance with our previous study [10]. Briefly, male C57BL/6 mice between 8 to 10 weeks of age were randomly intratracheally administrated with lipopolysaccharide (LPS, Escherichia coli strain 0111:B4, Sigma-Aldrich) dissolved in sterile phosphate-buffered saline (PBS) (2 mg/kg) or the same amount of PBS after anaesthesia with butaylone (Sigma-Aldrich) intraperitoneal administration. After being sacrificed 24 hours later, their right lung lobes were harvested then cut into small pieces, which were incubated with 2% FBS-DMEM/F12 media for another 6 hours to acquire the conditioned media, and the left lung lobes were used to detect the expression of Wnt5a using western blotting. After 10 hours of migration in a humidified CO_2 incubator at 37°C, the average number of migratory cells were detected by counting the cells stained with crystal violet (Beyotime Institute of Biotechnology, Haimen, China) in five fields under a microscope (×200).

In the wound healing assay, after the mMSCs reached 90% confluency in 96-well culture plates, the cell monolayer was scraped in a straight line to create a "scratch" with a 10 μl pipet tip. The original culture media and the debris were replaced with 2% FBS-DMEM/F12 media supplemented with 500 ng/ml Wnt5a or 500 ng/ml Wnt5a plus 5 μmol/L SP600125 or 2.5 μmol/L GF109203X. The cells were incubated in a humidified 5% CO_2 incubator at 37°C for 12 hours, and images under a phase-contrast microscope were acquired for further measurement of the intervals.

Western blotting analysis

Total protein and nucleoprotein from cells and lung tissue were extracted using RIPA lysis buffer (Beyotime Institute of Biotechnology) or a nuclear protein extraction kit (Beyotime Institute of Biotechnology) supplemented with 1 mmol/L PMSF, 1 mmol/L NaF and 1 mmol/L Na_3VO_4, respectively, according to the manufacturer's instructions. Following separation by 10 or 12% sodium dodecyl sulfate-polyacrylamide gel electrophoresis (SDS-PAGE), the proteins were electro-transferred to PVDF membranes (Millipore, Bedford, MA, USA), which were then blocked for 1 hour at room temperature and incubated at 4°C overnight with primary antibodies against β-catenin, p-CamK II, p-SAPK/JNK (Thr183/Tyr185), SAPK/JNK, p-PKCα/β II (Thr638/641), p-PKC (pan) (β II Ser660), Wnt5a/b (Cell Signaling Technology, Beverly, MA, USA), CamK II β/γ/δ, PKC pan (Bioworld Technology inc., MN, USA), pro-surfactant protein C (pro-SPC) (Millipore), Bax, Bcl-2 and β-actin (Santa Cruz Biotechnology, Inc., Santa Cruz, CA, USA). On the following day, the immunoreactive bands were detected with a chemiluminescence imaging system (ChemiQ 4800mini, Ouxiang, Shanghai, China) after incubation with a horseradish peroxidase-conjugated secondary antibody (Zhongshan Golden Bridge Biotechnology Co., Ltd., Beijing, China) for 1 hour at room temperature.

Quantitative real-time polymerase chain reaction

The levels of surfactant protein (SP) B, SPC, SPD and aquaporin (AQP) 5 mRNA in mMSCs after differentiation into AT II cells were analyzed via qRT-PCR. Total RNA was extracted using TRIzol reagent (Takara Bio, Inc., Kyoto, Japan), according to the manufacturer's instructions. Then, an equal volume of isopropanol was added to the collected aqueous phase to precipitate the RNA, which was subsequently reverse transcribed to yield single-stranded cDNAs using the qPCR RT Kit (Toyobo Co., Ltd., Osaka, Japan), based on the manufacturer's instructions. The qRT-PCR reaction was performed using THUNDERBIRD qPCR Mix (Toyobo Co., Ltd.) and the ABI Prism 7300 Sequence Detection System (Applied Biosystems, Foster City, CA, USA). Each sample was analyzed in triplicate with 40 PCR cycles, each of which consisted of a denaturation step at 95°C for 15 seconds, an annealing step at 56°C for 20 seconds, and an extension step at 72°C for 40 seconds. The primer sequences used for PCR amplification in our study were designed based on the sequences of the genomic clones as follows:

SPB (175 bp: NM_147779) 5′-CTGCTTCCTACCCTCTGCTG-3′ (forward)

5′-CTTGGCACAGGTCATTAGCTC-3′ (reverse)

SPC (137 bp: NM_011359) 5′-CATCGTTGTGTATGACTACCA-3′ (forward)

5′-CCTGGAAGTTCTGGAGTTTTCT-3′ (reverse)

SPD (75 bp: NM_009160) 5′-CCTGACAAACAGAGGTGCATT-3′ (forward)

5′-GAGAAAGGGCAGCATGTCAG-3′ (reverse)

AQP5 (220 bp: NM_009701) 5′-AGAAGGAGGTGTGTTCAGTTGC-3′ (forward)

5′-GCCAGAGTAATGGCCGGAT-3′ (reverse)

GAPDH (149 bp: NM_008084) 5′-TATGTCGTGGAGTCTACTGGT-3′ (forward)

5′-GAGTTGTCATATTTCTCGTGG-3′ (reverse)

Statistical analysis

Data were presented as the means ± standard deviation (SD). Comparison among groups was performed by the analysis of variance (ANOVA), followed by Tukey's test. *P* values less than 0.05 were considered statistically significant.

Results

Regulation of noncanonical Wnt signaling in mMSCs by Wnt5a, SP600125 and GF109203X

Under normal cultural conditions, phosphorylated PKC, JNK and CaMK II expression were up-regulated in a dose-dependent manner by 2-hour incubations with increasing concentrations of Wnt5a (50, 100, 200 or 500 ng/ml) and reached maximum levels after 500 ng/ml Wnt5a treatment. The PKC inhibitor, GF109203X, at 2.5 μmol/L or the JNK blocker, SP600125, at 5 μmol/L inhibited the up-regulation of phosphorylation of PKC and/or JNK caused by the 500 ng/ml Wnt5a incubation. (**Figs. 1A, 1B**) The regulatory effects of Wnt5a, SP600125 and GF109203X on the noncanonical Wnt pathway were similarly observed in mMSCs differentiated into AT II cells. (**Fig. 2**) Additionally, we investigated the effect of Wnt5a on canonical Wnt signaling through the detection of nuclear β-catenin in mMSCs by western blotting, and β-catenin was found to be elevated with the incubation of Wnt5a in mMSCs in differentiation conditions but was unchanged in mMSCs in general culture media. (**Figs. 1A, 1B, Fig. 2**)

The noncanonical Wnt pathway was activated during the differentiation of mMSCs into AT II cells

According to our previous study, we drove the differentiation of mMSCs into AT II cells in an indirect co-culture system with murine lung epithelial (MLE)-12 cells plus small airway growth media (SAGM) [10]. As we confirmed before, after 10 days of differentiation, some mMSCs changed from a typical fibroblast-like spindle appearance to an epithelia-like cobblestone cell morphology. Also, lamellar body-like structures, a typical organelles of AT II cells, and numerous vacuoles were found within the cytoplasm and near the cell surface in some mMSCs after differentiation. The expression of specific markers of AT II cells, pro-SPC protein and the level of SPB, SPC and SPD mRNA in mMSCs elevated after differentiation [10]. We then examined the activation of noncanonical Wnt pathway in mMSCs during the differentiation and found that the phosphorylated and total PKC levels were significantly increased on the first, third or tenth day of differentiation of mMSCs into AT II cells, and reached their highest levels on the tenth day; the phosphorylated and total CaMK II levels were also found to be up-regulated from the seventh day, and their maximum values were observed on the seventh or tenth day. Also, the phosphorylated and total JNK levels were elevated on the third or seventh day and reached their highest levels on the tenth or seventh day, respectively. (**Fig. 3**)

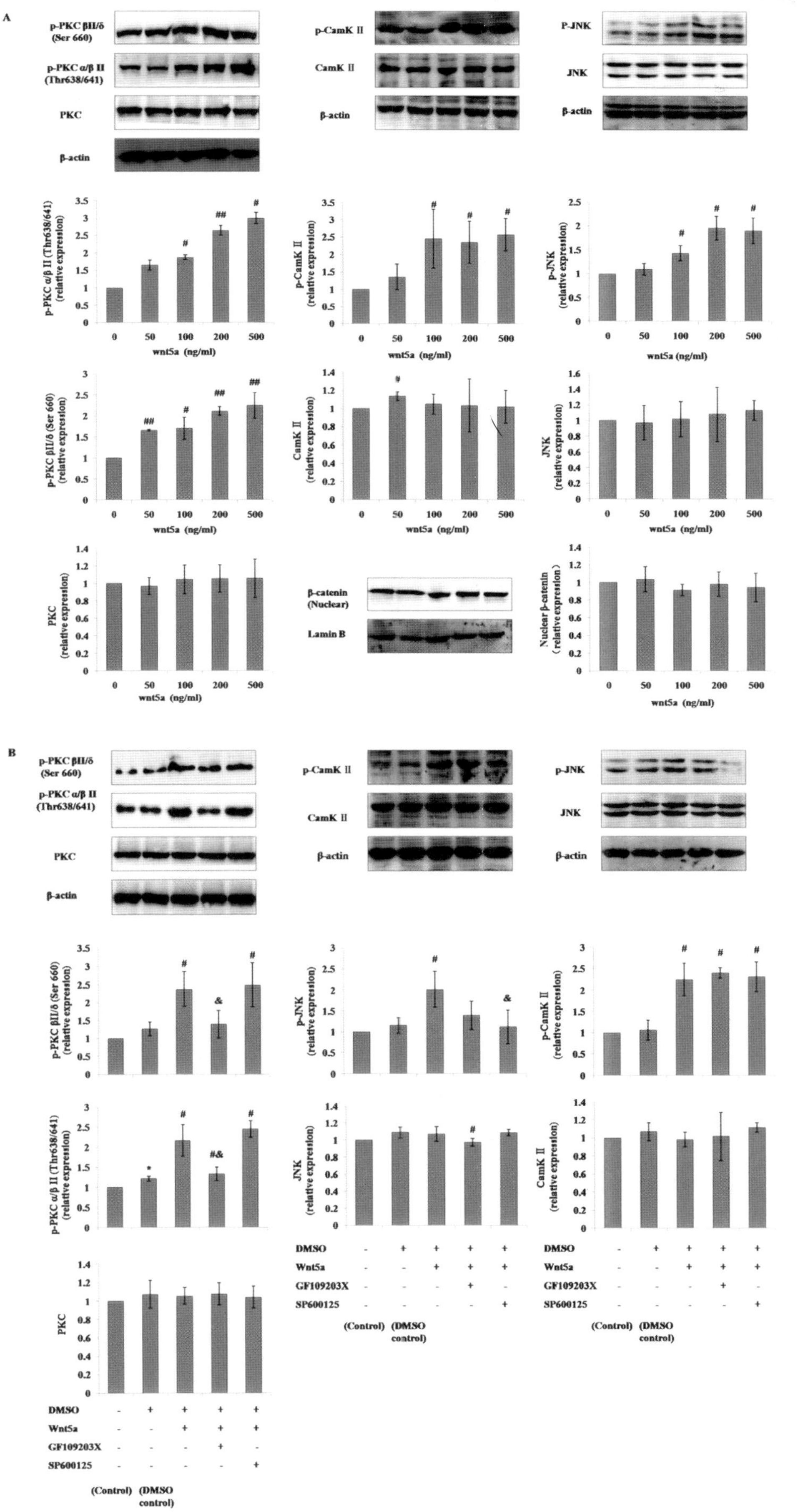
A
p-PKC βII/δ (Ser 660)
p-PKC α/β II (Thr638/641)
PKC
β-actin
p-CamK II
CamK II
β-actin
P-JNK
JNK
β-actin
p-PKC α/β II (Thr638/641) (relative expression)
p-CamK II (relative expression)
p-JNK (relative expression)
wnt5a (ng/ml)
0 50 100 200 500
p-PKC βII/δ (Ser 660) (relative expression)
CamK II (relative expression)
JNK (relative expression)
PKC (relative expression)
β-catenin (Nuclear)
Lamin B
Nuclear β-catenin (relative expression)
B
p-PKC βII/δ (Ser 660)
p-PKC α/β II (Thr638/641)
PKC
β-actin
p-CamK II
CamK II
β-actin
p-JNK
JNK
β-actin
p-PKC βII/δ (Ser 660) (relative expression)
p-JNK (relative expression)
p-CamK II (relative expression)
p-PKC α/β II (Thr638/641) (relative expression)
JNK (relative expression)
CamK II (relative expression)
PKC
DMSO
Wnt5a
GF109203X
SP600125
(Control) (DMSO control)

Figure 1. Modulation of noncanonical Wnt signaling in mMSCs with the supplementation of Wnt5a, SP600125 or GF109203X in general culture conditions. The p-PKC (pan) (β II Ser660), p-PKCα/β II (Thr638/641), PKC pan, p-SAPK/JNK (Thr183/Tyr185), SAPK/JNK, p-CamK II, CamK II β/γ/δ, and nuclear β-catenin levels in mMSCs cultured in 10% FBS-DMEM/F12 media added with different concentrations of Wnt5a (**A**) or 500 ng/ml Wnt5a plus 5 μmol/L SP600125 or 2.5 μmol/L GF109203X for 2 hours were evaluated through western blotting (**B**). (n = 3; $^*P<0.05$ *vs* Control; $\#P<0.05$, $\#\#P<0.01$ *vs* Wnt5a 0 ng/ml or DMSO Control; $\&P<0.05$ *vs* DMSO + Wnt5a + GF109203X- SP600125-).

Activation of the noncanonical Wnt pathway promoted mMSCs differentiation into AT II cells

After 10 days of differentiation, the pro-SPC protein and the SPB, SPC and SPD mRNA in the mMSCs were significantly elevated after incubation with 500 ng/ml Wnt5a. Additionally, pre-incubation with either 5 μmol/L SP600125 or 2.5 μmol/L GF109203X before the 500 ng/ml Wnt5a treatment reversed the promotion of Wnt5a on pro-SPC protein and SPB and SPC mRNA, and SP600125 seemed to have a greater inhibitory effect than GF109203X treatment. However, Wnt5a, SP600125 and GF109203X had no effect on the expression of AQP5 mRNA. (**Fig. 4**)

Activation of the noncanonical Wnt pathway had no significant effect on the proliferation of mMSCs

The effect of activation of the noncanonical Wnt pathway on mMSC proliferation was evaluated using MTT assays after incubation for 3 days with increasing concentrations of Wnt5a (100, 200, or 500 ng/ml), and no significant differences were observed after 100–500 ng/ml Wnt5a intervention. Interestingly, the supplementation of GF109203X plus Wnt5a reduced the number of mMSCs. (**Figs. 5A, 5B**)

Effect of cellular toxicity from oxidative stress on viability and noncanonical Wnt signaling in mMSCs

In the present study, oxidative stress in mMSCs was induced with H_2O_2. Increasing H_2O_2 concentrations (0.05, 0.1, 0.2, 0.3, 0.4, 0.5 and 0.6 mmol/L) reduced the viability of mMSCs in a concentration-dependent manner after 12 hours of incubation, as evaluated using the MTT assay (**Fig. 6A**). The minimum concentration of H_2O_2 that significantly inhibited viability, 0.2 mmol/L, was chosen for subsequent experiments. We then evaluated the expression of the apoptosis-related proteins Bax and Bcl-2 in mMSCs incubated with 0.2 mmol/L H_2O_2. We found that the Bcl-2/Bax ratio in mMSCs exposed to 0.2 mmol/L H_2O_2 assessed by western blotting analysis was significantly reduced compared to control (**Fig. 6D**). Additionally, noncanonical Wnt pathway-related proteins, including p-JNK, p-PKC and p-CaMK II, were all up-regulated in mMSCs after H_2O_2 treatment (**Fig. 6B**).

Activation of noncanonical Wnt pathway-protected mMSCs from oxidative stress-induced injury

mMSCs pre-incubated with 500 ng/ml Wnt5a for one hour offered significant protection against cell death induced by 12 hours of 0.2 mmol/L H_2O_2 incubation (**Fig. 6C**). Correspondingly, the decreased Bcl-2/Bax ratio in the H_2O_2-treated mMSCs was reversed by the activation of the noncanonical Wnt pathway by Wnt5a. Supplementation with GF109203X significantly reversed the effect of Wnt5a, but supplementation with SP600125 showed no significant difference from the H_2O_2 vehicle (**Fig. 6D**).

Activation of the noncanonical Wnt pathway-promoted migration of mMSCs

Compared to control, supplementation with 500 ng/ml Wnt5a significantly reduced the gap of the wound in the wound healing assay and enhanced the vertical migration of mMSCs towards the higher concentration of FBS in the lower chambers in the Transwell inserts assay. However, the Wnt5a effect was significantly blocked by GF109203X and partly inhibited by SP600125 (**Figs. 7A, 7B**). We subsequently examined mMSCs migration to conditioned media from normal or ARDS mice-derived lung tissue in the lower chambers of the Transwell inserts and the influence of noncanonical Wnt pathway activation on this process. We found that ARDS lung tissue attracted more mMSCs than normal lung tissue and the migration of mMSCs towards the conditioned medium of ARDS mice-derived lung tissue was further enhanced with Wnt5a, whose effect was reversed with the incubation of SP600125 or GF109203X (**Fig. 7C**).

Higher levels of noncanonical Wnt ligands in lung tissue of ARDS mice

To explore the levels of noncanonical Wnt ligands in normal or inflammatory lung tissue, Wnt5a in lung tissue was analyzed via western blotting. We found a significantly higher expression of Wnt5a in ARDS mouse-derived lung tissues than in normal ones. (**Fig. 8**)

Discussion

AT II cells are considered critical for the repair of injured lung tissue in ARDS patients [2,17]. Many investigations, including our previous study, have disclosed that multipotent MSCs could differentiate into AT II cells in ARDS animals and in some *in vitro* conditions [6–10,18]. These findings partly contribute to the efficacy of MSCs in ARDS treatment. Elucidation of the mechanisms underlying the differentiation of mMSCs into AT II cells, which has not yet been fully explored, may promote the development of ARDS therapy. The role of the canonical Wnt pathway in the differentiation of mMSCs into AT II cells has been elucidated in our previous study [10]; however, the effect of the noncanonical Wnt pathway, which transduces a signal independent of the accumulation of β-catenin, in this process has little been discussed. In the present study, we found that the noncanonical Wnt signaling pathway was involved in the differentiation of mMSCs into AT II cells in vitro and that the activation of the Wnt/PCP (Wnt/JNK) or Wnt/Ca^{2+}/PKC pathway with Wnt5a favored the differentiation of MSCs into AT II cells in a co-culture system.

As we know, about nine pathways in the transduction of noncanonical Wnt signaling have been disclosed, although they have not yet been well described. Wnt/PCP (or Wnt/JNK) and Wnt/Ca^{2+} signaling are the two most studied molecular signaling pathways. The Wnt/JNK pathway is initiated by the activation of FZD and Ror2 with Wnts [11,12]. This signal is transduced through Dvl and Ras homologue GTPases (RhoGTPases) to activate the nuclear transcription factor activator protein 1 (AP-1), which is composed of proteins of the Jun family (e.g., c-Jun, Jun-B, Jun-D), Fos family (e.g., c-Fos, foxB, Fra-1, Fra-2), ATF family

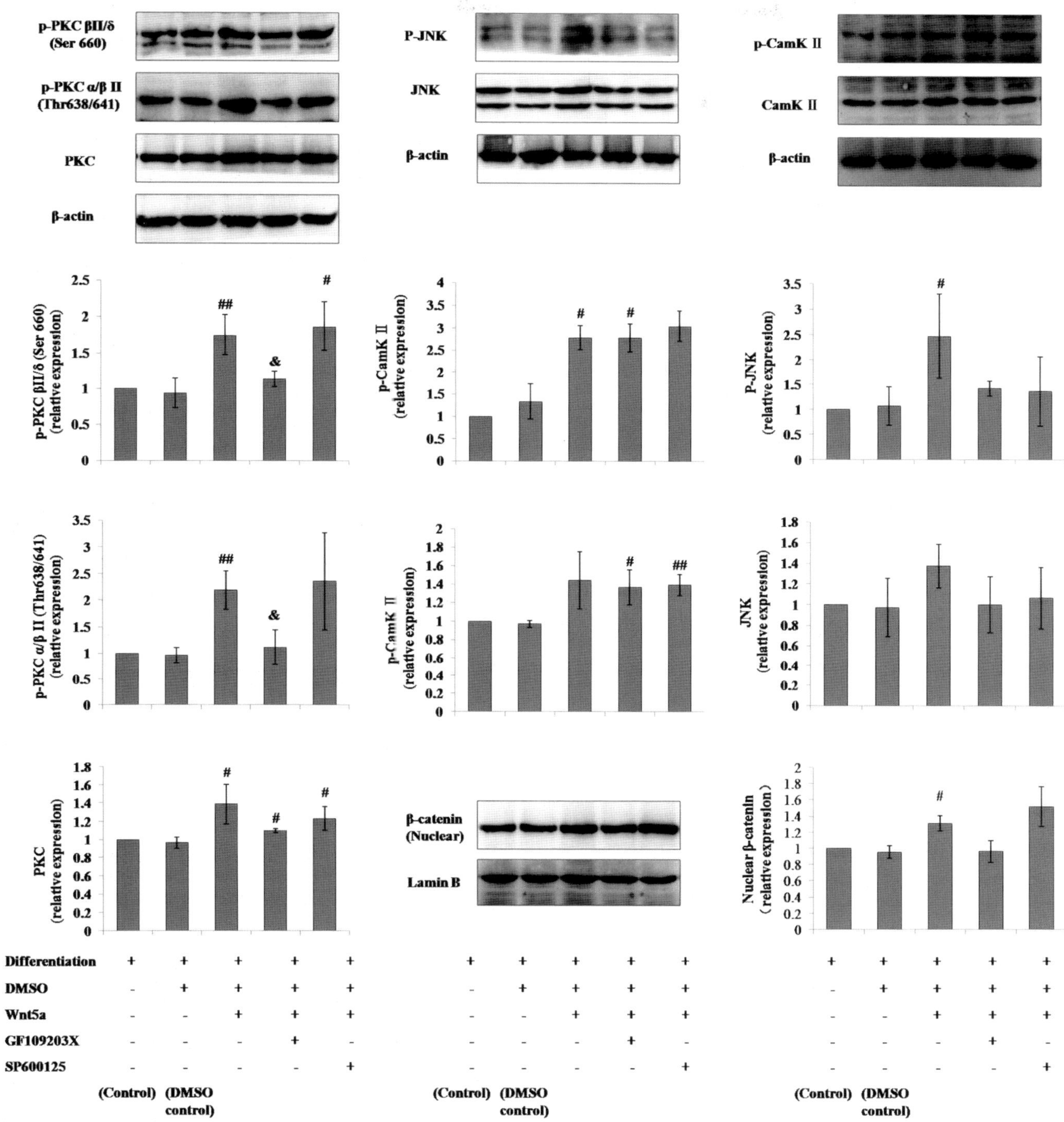

Figure 2. Regulation of noncanonical Wnt signaling in mMSCs with the supplementation of Wnt5a, SP600125 or GF109203X in differentiation conditions into AT II cells. The p-PKC (pan) (β II Ser660), p-PKCα/β II (Thr638/641), PKC pan, p-SAPK/JNK (Thr183/Tyr185), SAPK/JNK, p-CamK II, CamK II β/γ/δ, and nuclear β-catenin levels in mMSCs co-cultured with MLE-12 cells and SAGM with the supplementation of 500 ng/ml Wnt5a or 500 ng/ml Wnt5a plus 5 μmol/L SP600125 or 2.5 μmol/L GF109203X for 10 days were evaluated through western blotting. (n = 3; #*P*<0.05, ##*P*<0.01 *vs* DMSO control; &*P*<0.05 *vs* differentiation + DMSO + Wnt5a + GF109203X- SP600125-).

(e.g., ATF-α, ATF-2, ATF-3) and JDP family (e.g., JDP-1, JDP-2). The activation of AP-1 is critical for many biological behaviors, including cell differentiation, proliferation, and apoptosis [19–21]. In the Wnt/Ca^{2+} pathway, the binding of the Wnts to their receptors, including Frz2, 3, 4 and 5, increases the intracellular release of Ca^{2+} or the extracellular Ca^{2+} influx, which then activates PKC and CaMK II. It was found that PKC could regulate cell adhesion and tissue development during the development of vertebrates [22,23].

Through the activation of PKC, CaMK II and JNK, the noncanonical Wnt pathway plays important roles in diverse biological behaviors of cells and organisms that are different from the roles of the canonical Wnt pathway. Many ligands and receptors belonging to this pathway are expressed in MSCs and can influence the biological functions of MSCs, including

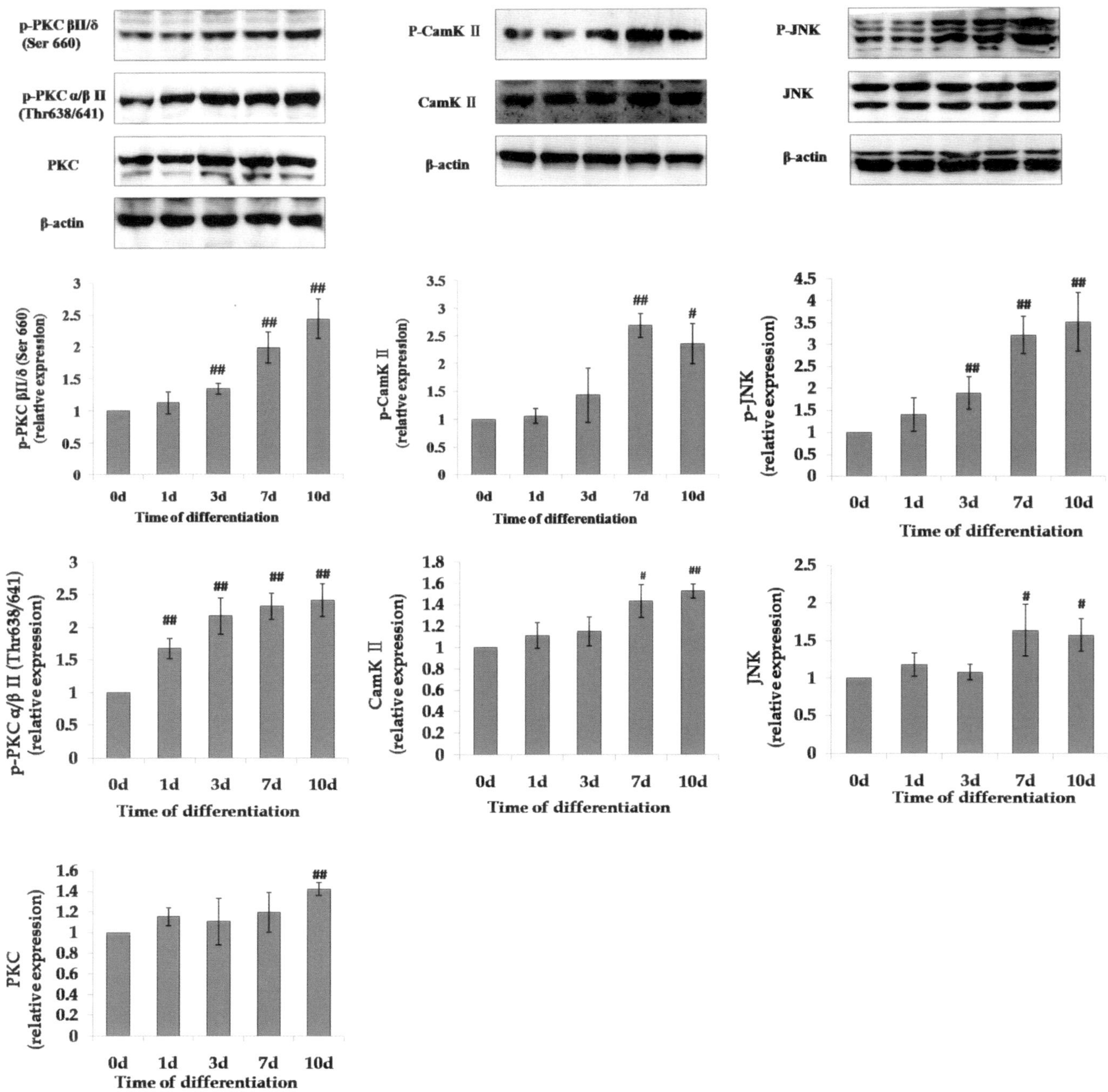

Figure 3. The activity of noncanonical Wnt signaling during the differentiation of mMSCs into AT II cells. The levels of the noncanonical Wnt pathway-related proteins, p-PKC (pan) (β II Ser660), p-PKCα/β II (Thr638/641), PKC pan, p-SAPK/JNK (Thr183/Tyr185), SAPK/JNK, p-CamK II, and CamK II β/γ/δ, in mMSCs on the first, third, seventh and tenth days of differentiation into AT II cells were detected through western blot. (n = 3, #$P<0.05$, ##$P<0.01$ *vs* 0 d).

migration, differentiation, and development. He et al. [24] found that Wnt11 could promote MSC differentiation into myocardial cells via the noncanonical Wnt pathway. A similar effect of Wnt4 on the differentiation of MSCs into osteoblasts in vitro and in vivo was observed in the study by Chang et al. [25]. Diverse effects of noncanonical Wnt signaling on the differentiation of MSCs, according to the target cell of differentiation, were observed in other studies. Some studies showed that the up-regulation of Wnt/JNK signaling inhibited adipogenesis while stimulating osteoblastogenesis in MSCs. Furthermore, even for the same type of target cells, the developmental stage of the target cells can also influence the effect of the noncanonical Wnt pathway. A study by Bergwitz, et al. [26] suggested that Wnt4 could inhibit chondrocyte differentiation while favoring late maturation. Topol, et al. [15] also found that the opposing noncanonical signals of Wnt5a hinder the chondrogenic lineage commitment of MSCs, promote chondrocyte differentiation, and delay chondrocyte maturation into hypertrophic stages, but their effects on the differentiation of MSCs into AT II cells have not been explored.

In our study, we firstly examined the regulation of noncanonical Wnt signaling in mMSCs with Wnt5a, a specific ligand that activates the noncanonical Wnt pathway and GF109203X, an

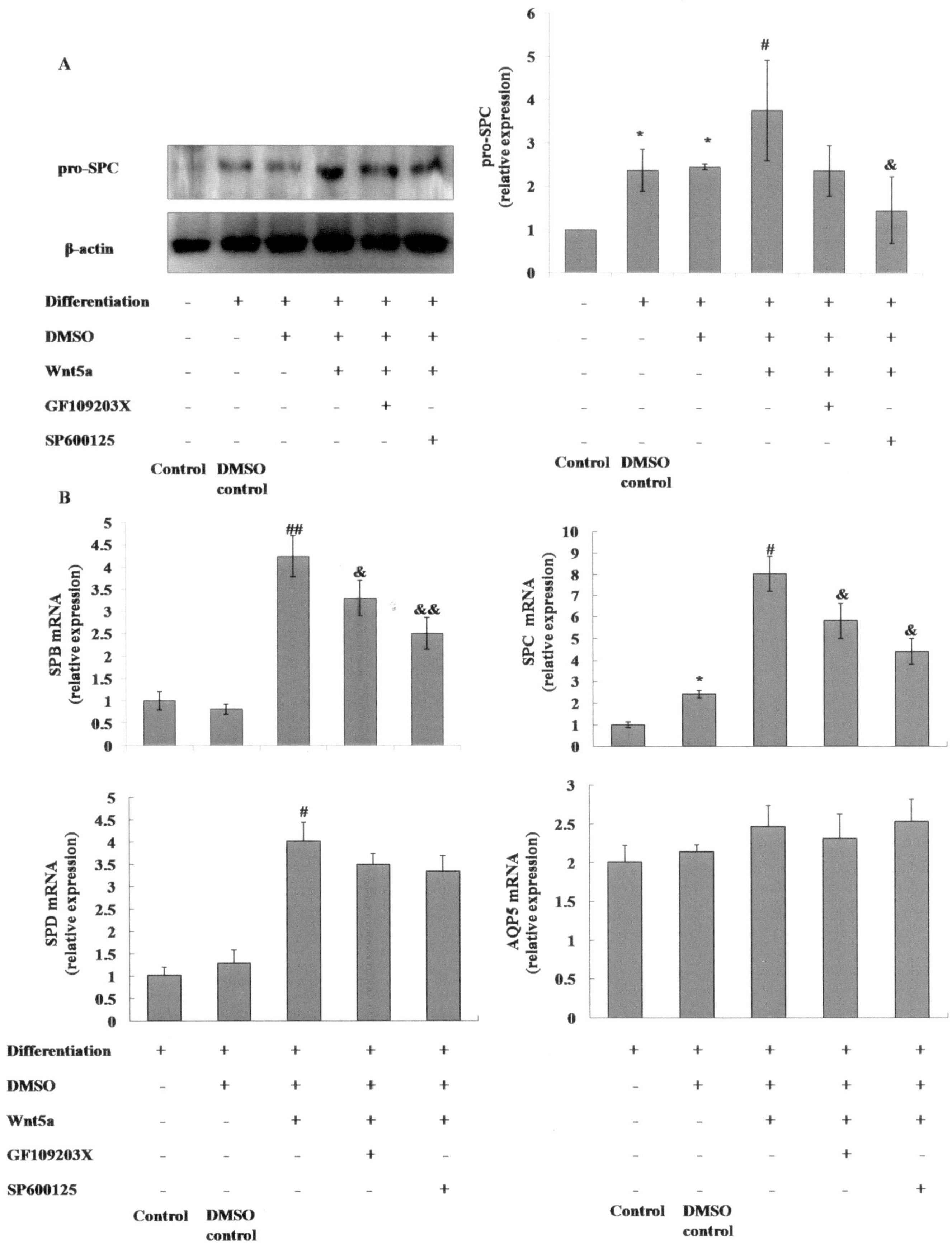
A
pro-SPC
β-actin
pro-SPC (relative expression)
Differentiation
DMSO
Wnt5a
GF109203X
SP600125
Control
DMSO control
B
SPB mRNA (relative expression)
SPC mRNA (relative expression)
SPD mRNA (relative expression)
AQP5 mRNA (relative expression)
Differentiation
DMSO
Wnt5a
GF109203X
SP600125
Control
DMSO control

Figure 4. The effect of noncanonical Wnt pathway on the expression of specific markers of alveolar epithelial cells in mMSCs differentiating into AT II cells. The expression of pro-SPC protein (**A**) and SPB, SPC, SPD and AQP5 mRNA (**B**) in mMSCs after 10 days of differentiation driven by co-culture with MLE-12 cells and SAGM with supplementation of 500 ng/ml Wnt5a plus 5 μmol/L SP600125 or 2.5 μmol/L GF109203X were evaluated with western blotting and qRT-PCR. ($n=3$; *$P<0.05$ *vs* Control; #$P<0.05$, ##$P<0.01$ *vs* DMSO control; &$P<0.05$, &&$P<0.01$ *vs* differentiation + DMSO + Wnt5a + GF109203X- SP600125-).

inhibitor of PKC, or SP600125, an inhibitor of JNK. Interestingly, GF109203X was found to inactivate JNK in MSCs while SP600125 did not influence the activation of PKC, suggesting that phophorylated PKC might be the upstream effector of JNK; this finding was in accordance with other studies [27,28]. Additionally, crosstalk between canonical and noncanonical Wnt signaling has been shown previously. It was found that Wnt/Ca^{2+} signaling could activate the TAK1-NLK MAPK pathway, which might reduce the transcription of TCF/LEF 1 without influencing the accumulation of β-catenin, thus, inhibiting canonical Wnt signaling [29,30]. However, some recent studies suggested that noncanonical Wnt signaling also could stimulate the canonical Wnt pathway and the effect of noncanonical Wnt ligands on the activation of canonical Wnt signaling might be related to the kind of FZD receptors on the target cells [31,32]. In the present study, no significant difference in the nuclear accumulation of β-catenin was observed after 2 hours of incubation with Wnt5a, whereas a rised accumulation of β-catenin was found after 10 days of treatment with Wnt5a in the differentiation conditions to some extent. There might be some unclear signaling mechanisms in the differentiation, which may need more investigations.

Like the canonical Wnt pathway, the noncanonical Wnt pathway-related proteins are expressed in embryonic and adult lung tissues and are involved in physiological and pathological processes of the lung [33]. The overexpression of Wnt5a in transgenic mice and in chicks has been reported to result in severe pulmonary hypoplasia. [34]. Increasing the downregulated non-canonical Wnt receptor Fzd2 with GATA 6 mutants was found to be able to partly reduce the lung epithelial defects induced by GATA6 mutants [35]. In addition to their physiological effects, the noncanonical Wnt pathway also participates in the carcinogenesis and invasion of lung cancer [36,37]. In the present study, the upregulation of Wnt5a was also observed in lung tissue of ARDS mice induced with LPS through intratracheal administration. Therefore, the noncanonical Wnt pathway is hypothesized to be involved and potentially effective in the differentiation of MSCs into pulmonary cells.

To examine the role of the noncanonical Wnt pathway in the differentiation of MSCs into AT II cells, a co-culture condition with MLE-12 cells plus SAGM, verified to be effective at driving the differentiation of MSCs into AT II cells in our previous study, was used in the present study [10]. As the phosphorylation levels of JNK, PKC, and CaMK II were increased in the third to tenth days of co-culture, the noncanonical Wnt pathway was considered to be involved in the differentiation process. Further supplementation of Wnt5a increased the expression of the pro-SPC protein and the SPB, SPC and SPD mRNA, and this effect could be inhibited with the addition of either the PKC or JNK inhibitors. As phophorylated PKC might be an upstream effector of JNK, we were not able to elucidate whether Wnt/JNK alone or both Wnt/JNK and Wnt/PKC are the signaling pathways that regulate the differentiation. Either PKC or JNK was reported to be involved in regulating the differentiation of the noncanonical Wnt pathway. Yu, et al. found that the inactivation of PKC could reverse the promotion of differentiation into neural progenitor cells by Wnt5a [38]. A similar suppression effect of Wnt/PKC signaling was also observed in the investigation of the pro-differentiation of circulating progenitor cells into cardiomyogenic cells [39]. In another study, Wnt2 activating the noncanonical Wnt pathway through JNK/AP1 signaling induced the differentiation of embryonic stem cells into cardiac myocytes [40]. In the investigation by Qiu, et al, the activation of Wnt/JNK signaling by anisomycin enhanced osteoblast differentiation, whereas its inhibition by SP600125 enhanced adipocyte differentiation of human MSCs [41]. Some studies have reviewed the importance of both JNK and PKC in the pro-differentiation effect of the noncanonical Wnt pathway [42].

The migration and concentration of MSCs into injured or inflammatory sites after administration *in vivo* occurs prior to the exertion of their biological functions, including an anti-inflammation function, specialized cell-type differentiation and repair of injured tissues. Several studies have observed an enhanced

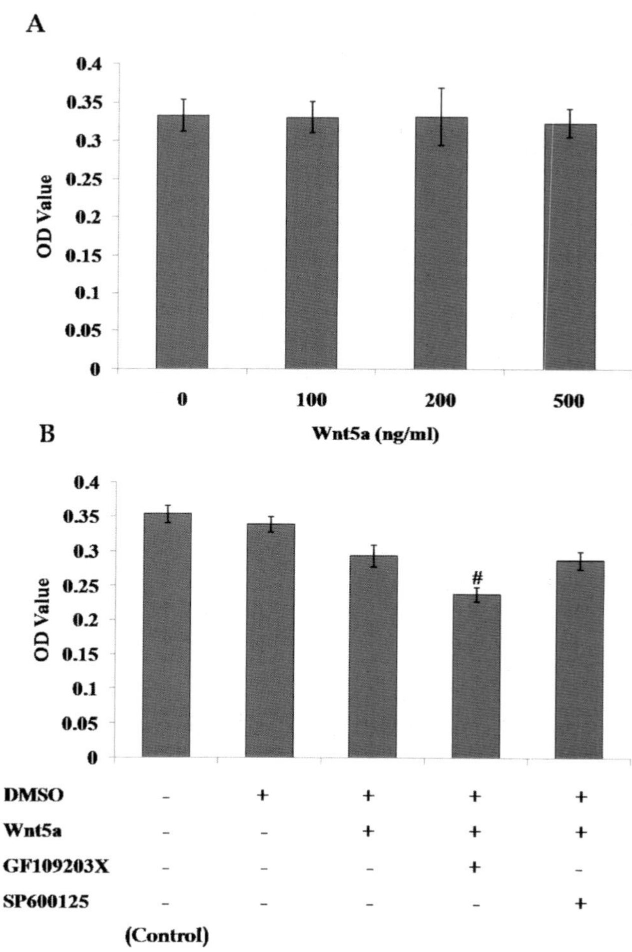

Figure 5. Role of noncanonical Wnt signaling in the proliferation of mMSCs. The proliferation of mMSCs was evaluated using MTT assay after incubation in 2% FBS-DMEM/F12 media supplemented with increasing concentrations of Wnt5a (**A**) or 500 ng/ml Wnt5a plus 5 μmol/L SP600125 or 2.5 μmol/L GF109203X (**B**) for 72 h. ($n=4$; #$P<0.05$ *vs* Control).

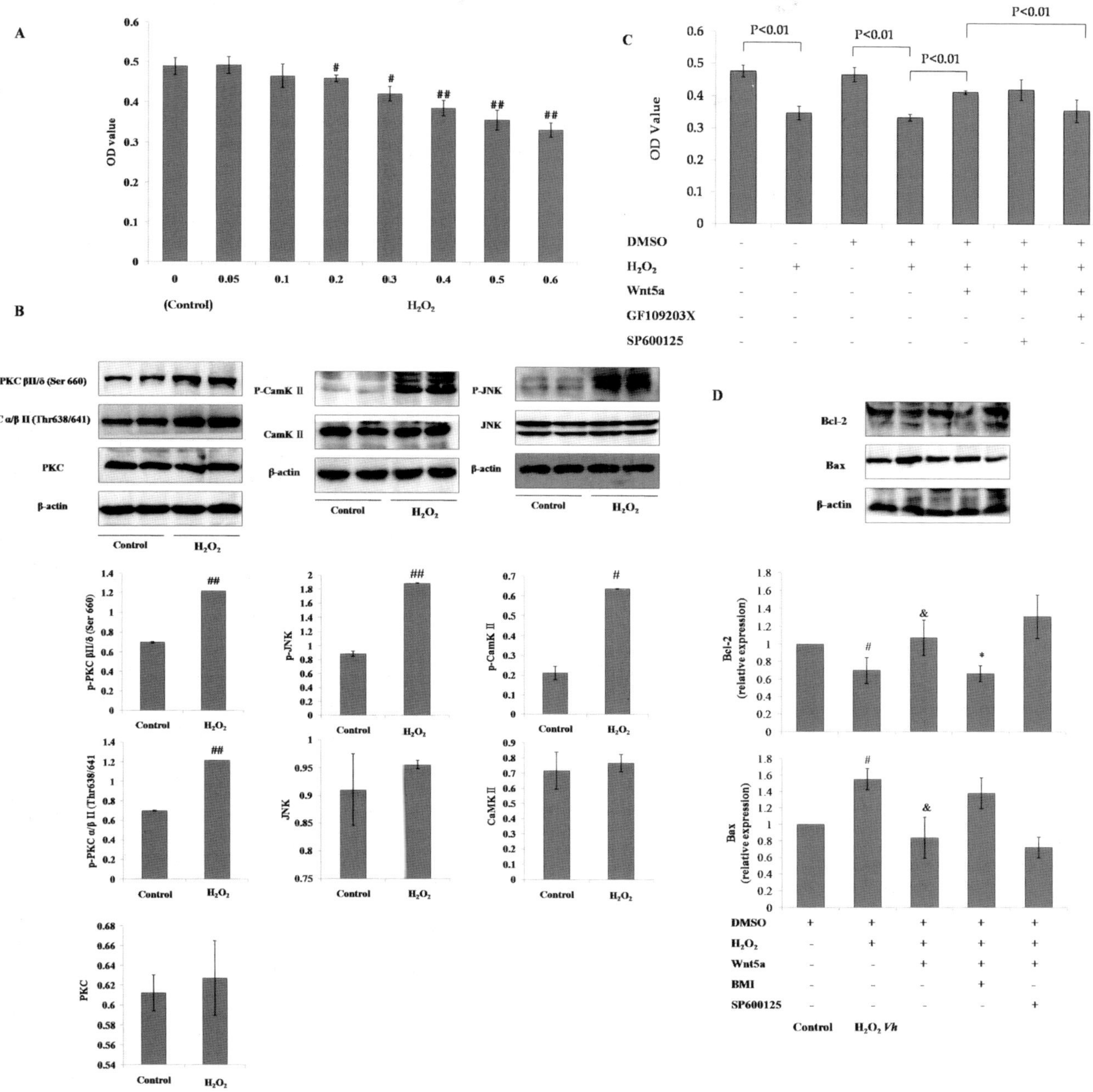

Figure 6. Role of noncanonical Wnt pathway in the H_2O_2-induced cellular toxicity of mMSCs. The viability of mMSCs after treatment with increasing concentrations of H_2O_2 supplemented in 2% FBS-DMEM/F12 growth media for 12 hours was determined using an MTT assay (**A**, $n = 4$). The expressions of p-PKCα/β II (Thr638/641), p-PKC (pan) (β II Ser660), p-SAPK/JNK (Thr183/Tyr185), p- CamK II, PKC pan, SAPK/JNK, CamK II β/γ/δ in mMSCs with 0.2 mmol/L H_2O_2 treatment for 12 hours were analyzed using western blotting (**B**, $n = 3$). The effect of pretreatment mMSCs with 500 ng/ml Wnt5a plus 5 μmol/L SP600125 or 2.5 μmol/L GF109203X for 1 hour on mMSC survival (**C**, $n = 4$) and the expression of Bcl-2 and Bax (**D**, $n = 3$) influenced by 0.2 mmol/L H_2O_2 for 12 hours were analyzed using MTT assay and western blotting. (#$P<0.05$, ##$P<0.01$ *vs* control, &$P<0.05$ *vs* H_2O_2 *Vh*, *$P<0.05$ *vs* DMSO+ H_2O_2+ Wnt5a- SP600125- GF109203X-).

recruitment of transplanted MSCs to the injured lung tissue in ARDS mice compared to the recruitment in control mice [43]. Some potential molecular mechanisms, including the cell derived factor-1α (SDF-1α) and its cellular receptor CXCR4, canonical Wnt signaling and so on, that drive the migration of MSCs have been presented in several previous studies [10,44–47]. A role for noncanonical Wnt signaling in the migration of endothelial cells, gastric cancer cells, pancreatic cancer cells, and breast cancer cells, among others, has been shown by recent studies [48–51]; however, its effect on the migration of mMSCs has not been thoroughly explored. Our results showed that the activation of the noncanonical Wnt pathway through the incubation of mMSCs with Wnt5a significantly increased the migration of the mMSCs and blockers of either PKC or JNK could decrease or block the enhancement of migration caused by Wnt5a. The promotion of Wnt/PCP signaling in the migration of MSCs might be mediated through the up-regulation of some receptor of chemokines. Jin, et al. found that the inactivation of JNK led to the reduced expression of CXCR4 in Ewing sarcoma cells upregulated by Wnt5a [52]. In other investigations, JNK, through its downstream

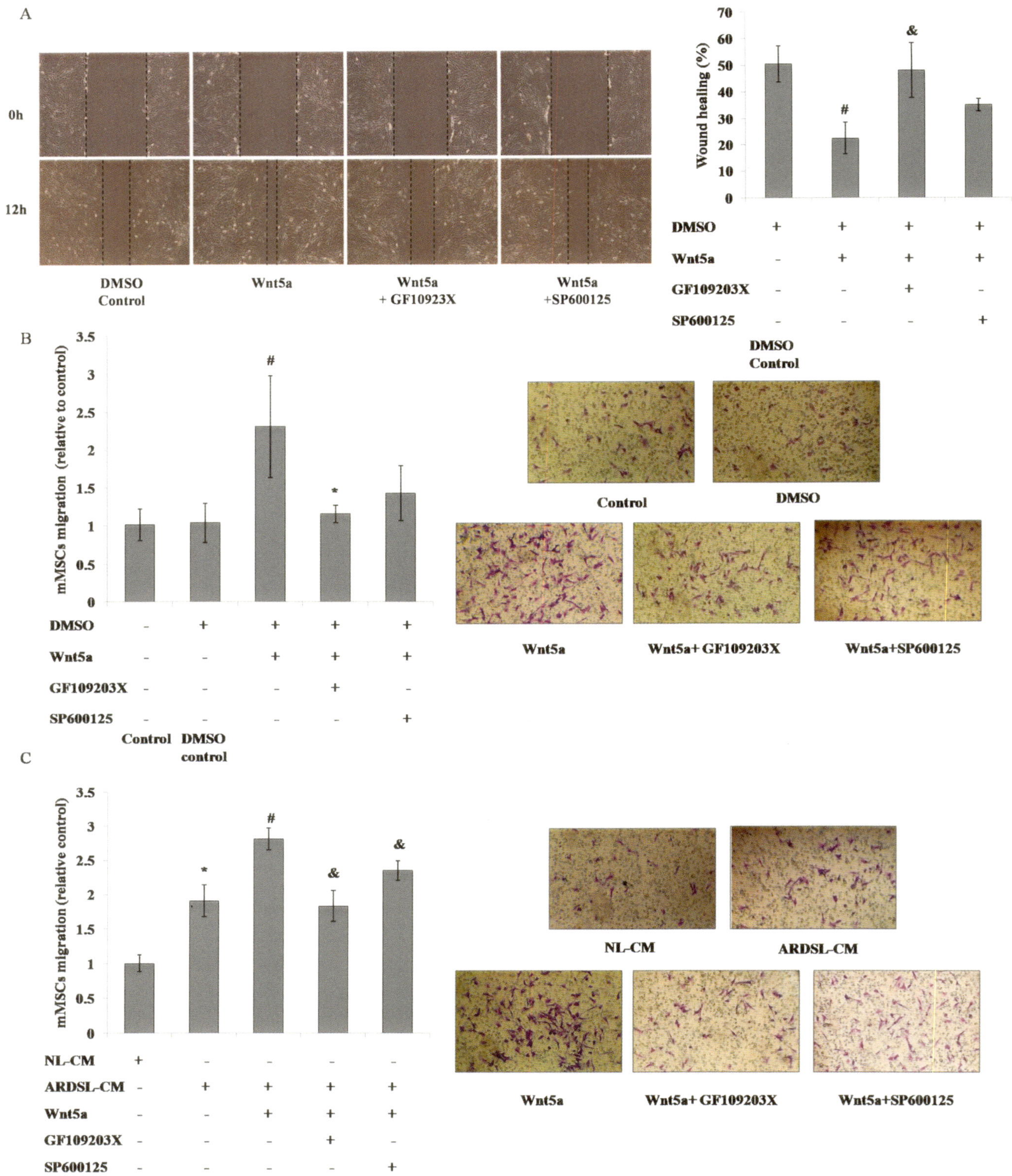

Figure 7. Role of noncanonical Wnt pathway in the migration of mMSCs. The horizontal migration of mMSCs incubated in 2% DMEM/F12 media supplemented with 500 ng/ml Wnt5a or 500 ng/ml Wnt5a plus 2.5 μmol/L GF109203X or 5 μmol/L SP600125 was examined by wound healing assay (**A** ×200; $n=3$; #$P<0.05$ *vs* DMSO control; &$P<0.05$ *vs* DMSO+ Wnt5a+ GF109203X- SP600125-). The vertical migration of mMSCs incubated in 2% DMEM/F12 media supplemented with 500 ng/ml Wnt5a or 500 ng/ml Wnt5a plus 2.5 μmol/L GF109203X or 5 μmol/L SP600125 towards 10% FBS-DMEM/F12 media (10% FBS-GM) (**B** ×200; $n=3$; #$P<0.05$ *vs* DMSO control; *$P<0.05$ *vs* DMSO+ Wnt5a+ GF109203X- SP600125-) or conditioned media from normal (NL-CM) or ARDS mouse-derived lung tissue (ARDSL-CM) (**C** ×200; $n=3$; *$P<0.05$ *vs* NL-CM; #$P<0.05$ *vs* ARDSL-CM; &$P<0.05$ *vs* ARDSL-CM+ Wnt5a+) was examined through Transwell inserts migration assay.

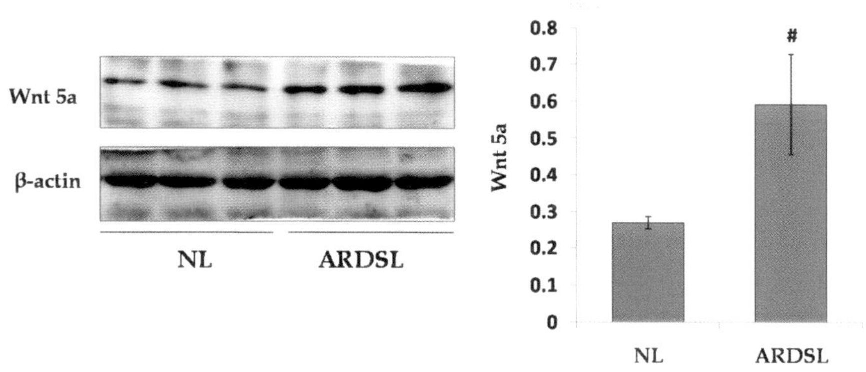

Figure 8. Wnt5a ligand in lung tissue of normal or ARDS mice. The expression of Wnt5a in normal or ARDS mouse-derived lung tissue was evaluated through western blotting analysis. ($n = 3$; #$P<0.05$ *vs* NL).

transcriptional factor AP-1, upregulated metalloproteinase (MMP)-9 or the phosphorylation of paxillin to regulate the migration of cells [53,54]. The activation of MMP-9 and the regulation of the cytoskeleton might also be the underlying mechanisms for the enhanced migration induced by Wnt/PKC signaling [55]. In our present study, it was hard to tell whether the Wnt/PKC and Wnt/JNK pathways or the Wnt/JNK pathway alone mediated the enhancement of migration by Wnt5a in mMSCs.

The proliferation and survival of MSCs in the injured tissues after transplantation also played an important role in their differentiation to the target cells. Cell numbers in the target tissue decreased rapidly after the administration of MSCs [56]. Mei et al. [57] found that approximately 47% of MSCs injected into the lung tissue of ARDS mice 15 minutes after induction of ARDS decreased to less than 8% 3 days later. The low survival of grafted MSCs limits their transdifferentiation and effects on target tissue repair [58]. Both the excitatory and inhibitory effects of the noncanonical Wnt pathway on cell proliferation have been previously reported. Some studies found that Wnt5a could increase the proliferation of fibroblasts or endothelial cells [59], while some investigators insisted that Wnt5a had a negative effect on human endothelial cell proliferation [60]. In our present study, no significant difference in the proliferation of mMSCs was observed after Wnt5a treatment compared to the control. The effect of Wnt5a on the mMSC proliferation might need further exploration.

There are several factors in complex *in vivo* situations that negatively influence the survival of transplanted MSCs. Oxidants, which are produced from inflammatory lung tissue and are a causative factor of lung injury [61], are detrimental to MSCs transplanted *in vivo* and trigger their apoptosis [62]. Hydrogen peroxide (H_2O_2), a typical oxidant, was adopted in our study to induce oxidative damage to mMSCs. We found a H_2O_2 dose-dependent decrease in the survival of mMSCs and the down-regulation of Bcl-2/Bax, the balance of which determines whether a cell undergoes apoptosis [63]. The activation of the noncanonical Wnt pathway in mMSCs by H_2O_2 *in vitro* was observed in our study. Vuga, et al. found that Wnt5a intervention could enhance resistance to apoptosis caused by H_2O_2 [64], but the role of the noncanonical Wnt pathway in the injury of mMSCs induced by H_2O_2 has not yet been explored. In our study, the supplement of Wnt5a prior to H_2O_2 treatment reversed the decline of survival and the Bcl-2/Bax ratio in mMSCs induced by H_2O_2 treatment. Interestingly, no significant difference was found after SP600125 intervention, and a reverse in the deterioration induced by H_2O_2 was detected with GF109203X treatment. It appeared that Wnt5a, through Wnt/PKC signaling, mediated the protection against the damage of mMSCs induced by H_2O_2. This finding was in accordance with the results of the investigation of Bluwstein et al [65]. JNK was found in some other studies to participate in cell death, and the inhibition of JNK activation ameliorated the H_2O_2 induced apoptosis [66–68].

Conclusions

Our results demonstrated the importance of the noncanonical Wnt pathway in the differentiation of mMSCs into AT II cells in a co-cultured system with MLE-12 cells and SAGM. Wnt5a, either through Wnt/JNK signaling alone or through the combination of Wnt/JNK and Wnt/PKC signaling, promoted the differentiation of mMSCs into AT II cells and their migration towards ARDS lung tissue. Furthermore, Wnt5a supplementation, through Wnt/PKC signaling, increased the survival of mMSCs after being treated with H_2O_2 *in vitro* but had no significant influence on the proliferation of mMSCs. From these results, we speculate that noncanonical Wnt signaling plays a critical role in the differentiation of mMSCs into pneumonocytes and in the repair of injured lung tissue *in vivo*, and this needs to be confirmed by future studies.

Author Contributions

Conceived and designed the experiments: ARL SC HBQ. Performed the experiments: ARL SXC LD LL HLH SLH QHC. Analyzed the data: ARL SC XML. Contributed reagents/materials/analysis tools: YY FMG HBQ. Wrote the paper: ARL SC.

References

1. Phua J, Badia JR, Adhikari NK, Friedrich JO, Fowler RA, et al. (2009) Has mortality from acute respiratory distress syndrome decreased over time?: A systematic review. Am J Respir Crit Care Med 179: 220–227.
2. Matthay MA, Robriquet L, Fang X (2005) Alveolar epithelium: role in lung fluid balance and acute lung injury. Proc Am Thorac Soc 2: 206–213.
3. Lee JW, Fang X, Gupta N, Serikov V, Matthay MA (2009) Allogeneic human mesenchymal stem cells for treatment of E. coli endotoxin-induced acute lung injury in the ex vivo perfused human lung. Proc Natl Acad Sci USA 106: 16357–16362.
4. Gupta N, Su X, Popov B, Lee JW, Serikov V, et al. (2007) Intrapulmonary delivery of bone marrow-derived mesenchymal stem cells improves survival and attenuates endotoxin-induced acute lung injury in mice. J Immunol 179: 1855–1863.
5. Ortiz LA, Gambelli F, McBride C, Gaupp D, Baddoo M, et al. (2003) Mesenchymal stem cell engraftment in lung is enhanced in response to

bleomycin exposure and ameliorates its fibrotic effects. Proc Natl Acad Sci USA 100: 8407–8411.
6. Zhao F, Zhang YF, Liu YG, Zhou JJ, Li ZK, et al. (2008) Therapeutic effects of bone marrow-derived mesenchymal stem cells engraftment on bleomycin-induced lung injury in rats. Transplant Proc 40: 1700–1705.
7. Rojas M, Xu J, Woods CR, Mora AL, Spears W, et al. (2005) Bone marrow-derived mesenchymal stem cells in repair of the injured lung. Am J Respir Cell Mol Biol 33: 145–152.
8. Serikov VB, Popov B, Mikhailov VM, Gupta N, Matthay MA (2007) Evidence of temporary airway epithelial repopulation and rare clonal formation by BM-derived cells following naphthalene injury in mice. Anat Rec (Hoboken) 290: 1033–1045.
9. Berger MJ, Adams SD, Tigges BM, Sprague SL, Wang XJ, et al. (2006) Differentiation of umbilical cord blood-derived multilineage progenitor cells into respiratory epithelial cells. Cytotherapy 8: 480–487.
10. Liu AR, Liu L, Chen S, Yang Y, Zhao HJ, et al. (2013) Activation of canonical wnt pathway promotes differentiation of mouse bone marrow-derived MSCs into type II alveolar epithelial cells, confers resistance to oxidative stress, and promotes their migration to injured lung tissue in vitro. J Cell Physiol 228: 1270–1283.
11. Ling L, Nurcombe V, Cool SM (2009) Wnt signaling controls the fate of mesenchymal stem cells. Gene 433: 1–7.
12. Rao TP, Kühl M (2010) An updated overview on Wnt signaling pathways: a prelude for more. Circ Res 106: 1798–1806.
13. Etheridge SL, Spencer GJ, Heath DJ, Genever PG (2004) Expression profiling and functional analysis of wnt signaling mechanisms in mesenchymal stem cells. Stem Cells 22: 849–860.
14. Boland GM, Perkins G, Hall DJ, Tuan RS (2004) Wnt 3a promotes proliferation and suppresses osteogenic differentiation of adult human mesenchymal stem cells. Cell Biochem 93: 1210–1230.
15. Topol L, Jiang X, Choi H, Garrett-Beal L, Garolan PJ, et al. (2003) Wnt-5a inhibits the canonical Wnt pathway by promoting GSK-3-independent beta-catenin degradation. J Cell Biol 162: 899–908.
16. Loscertales M, Mikels AJ, Hu JK, Donahoe PK, Roberts DJ (2008) Chick pulmonary Wnt5a directs airway and vascular tubulogenesis. Development 135: 1365–1376.
17. Rackley CR, Stripp BR (2012) Building and maintaining the epithelium of the lung. J Clin Invest 122: 2724–2730.
18. Ma N, Gai H, Mei J, Ding FB, Bao CR, et al. (2011) Bone marrow mesenchymal stem cells can differentiate into type II alveolar epithelial cells in vitro. Cell Biol Int 35: 1261–1266.
19. Liebermann DA, GregoryB HoffnlanB (1998) AP-1 (Fos/Jun) transcription factors in hematopoietic differentiation and apoptosis. Int J Oncol 12: 685–700.
20. Caelles C, González-Sancho JM, Muñoz A (1997) Nuclear hormone receptor antagonism with AP-1 by inhibition of the JNK pathway. Genes Dev 11: 3351–3364.
21. Leppä S, Eriksson M, Saffrich R, Ansorge W, Bohmann D (2001) Complex functions of AP-1 transcription factors in differentiation and survival of PC12 cells. Mol Cell Biol 21: 4369–4378.
22. De A (2011) Wnt/Ca^{2+} signaling pathway: a brief overview. Acta Biochim Biophys Sin (Shanghai) 43: 745–756.
23. Kühl M, Sheldahl LC, Park M, Miller JR, Moon RT (2000) The Wnt/Ca^{2+} pathway: a new vertebrate Wnt signaling pathway takes shape. Trends Genet 16: 279–283.
24. He Z, Li H, Zuo S, Pasha Z, Wang Y, et al. (2011) Transduction of Wnt11 promotes mesenchymal stem cell transdifferentiation into cardiac phenotypes. Stem Cells Dev 20: 1771–1778.
25. Chang J, Sonoyama W, Wang Z, Jin Q, Zhang C, et al. (2007) Noncanonical Wnt-4 signaling enhances bone regeneration of mesenchymal stem cells in craniofacial defects through activation of p38 MAPK. J Biol Chem 282: 30938–30948.
26. Bergwitz C, Wendlandt T, Kispert A, Brabant G (2001) Wnts differentially regulate colony growth and differentiation of chondrogenic rat calvaria cells. Biochim Biophys Acta 1538: 129–140.
27. Lang W, Wang H, Ding L, Xiao L (2004) Cooperation between PKC-alpha and PKC-epsilon in the regulation of JNK activation in human lung cancer cells. Cell Signal 16: 457–467.
28. Hara T, Namba H, Yang TT, Nagayama Y, Fukata S, et al. (1998) Ionizing radiation activates c-Jun NH2-terminal kinase (JNK/SAPK) via a PKC-dependent pathway in human thyroid cells. Biochem Biophys Res Commun 244: 41–44.
29. Yuzugullu H, Benhaj K, Ozturk N, Senturk S, Celik E, et al. (2009) Canonical Wnt signaling is antagonized by noncanonical Wnt5a in hepatocellular carcinoma cells. Mol Cancer 8:90.
30. Ishitani T, Kishida S, Hyodo-Miura J, Ueno N, Yasuda J, et al. (2003) The TAK1-NLK mitogen-activated protein kinase cascade functions in the Wnt5a/Ca^{2+} pathway to antagonize Wnt/β-catenin signaling. Mol Cell Biol 23: 131–139.
31. Ring L, Neth P, Weber C, Steffens S, Faussner A (2014) β-Catenin-dependent pathway activation by both promiscuous "canonical" WNT3a-, and specific "noncanonical" WNT4- and WNT5a-FZD receptor combinations with strong differences in LRP5 and LRP6 dependency. Cell Signal 26:260–267.
32. van Amerongen R, Fuerer C, Mizutani M, Nusse R (2012) Wnt5a can both activate and repress Wnt/β-catenin signaling during mouse embryonic development. Dev Biol 369:101–114.
33. Pongracz JE, Stockley RA (2006) Wnt signalling in lung development and diseases. Respir Res 7: 15.
34. Li C, Xiao J, Hormi K, Borok Z, Minoo P (2002) Wnt5a participates in distal lung morphogenesis. Dev Biol 248: 68–81.
35. Zhang Y, Goss AM, Cohen ED, Kadzik R, Lepore JJ, et al. (2008) A Gata6-Wnt pathway required for epithelial stem cell development and airway regeneration. Nat Genet 40: 862–870.
36. Zhao Y, Yang ZQ, Wang Y, Miao Y, Liu Y, et al. (2010) Dishevelled-1 and dishevelled-3 affect cell invasion mainly through canonical and noncanonical Wnt pathway, respectively, and associate with poor prognosis in nonsmall cell lung cancer. Mol Carcinog 49: 760–770.
37. Bartis D, Csongei V, Weich A, Kiss E, Barko S, et al. (2013) Down-regulation of canonical and up-regulation of non-canonical Wnt signaling in the carcinogenic process of squamous cell lung carcinoma. PLoS One 8, e57393.
38. Yu JM, Kim JH, Song GS, Jung JS (2006) Increase in proliferation and differentiation of neural progenitor cells isolated from postnatal and adult mice brain by Wnt-3a and Wnt-5a. Mol Cell Biochem 288: 17–28.
39. Koyanagi M, Haendeler J, Badorff C, Brandes RP, Hoffmann J, et al. (2005) Non-canonical Wnt signaling enhances differentiation of human circulating progenitor cells to cardiomyogenic cells. J Biol Chem 280: 16838–16842.
40. Onizuka T, Yuasa S, Kusumoto D, Shimoji K, Egashira T, et al. (2012) Wnt2 accelerates cardiac myocyte differentiation from ES-cell derived mesodermalcells via non-canonical pathway. J Mol Cell Cardiol 52: 650–659.
41. Qiu W, Chen L, Kassem M (2011) Activation of non-canonical Wnt/JNK pathway by Wnt3a is associated with differentiation fate determination of human bone marrow stromal (mesenchymal) stem cells. Biochem Biophys Res Commun 413: 98–104.
42. Flaherty MP, Abdel-Latif A, Li Q, Hunt G, Ranjan S, et al. (2008) Noncanonical Wnt11 signaling is sufficient to induce cardiomyogenic differentiation in unfractionated bone marrow mononuclear cells. Circulation 117: 2241–2252.
43. Yamada M, Kubo H, Kobayashi S, Ishizawa K, Numasaki M, et al. (2004) Bone marrow-derived progenitor cells are important for lung repair after lipopolysaccharide-induced lung injury. J Immunol 172: 1266–1272.
44. Zhuang Y, Chen X, Xu M, Zhang LY, Xiang F (2009) Chemokine stromal cell-derived factor 1/CXCL12 increases homing of mesenchymal stem cells to injured myocardium and neovascularization following myocardial infarction. Chin Med J (Engl) 122: 183–187.
45. Wang Y, Deng Y, Zhou GQ (2008) SDF-1alpha/CXCR4-mediated migration of systemically transplanted bone marrow stromal cells towards ischemic brain lesion in a rat model. Brain Res 1195: 104–112.
46. Karow M, Popp T, Egea V, Ries C, Jochum M, et al. (2009) Wnt signalling in mouse mesenchymal stem cells: impact on proliferation, invasion and MMP expression. J Cell Mol Med 13: 2506–2520.
47. Shang YC, Wang SH, Xiong F, Zhao CP, Peng FN, et al. (2007) Wnt3a signaling promotes proliferation, myogenic differentiation, and migration of rat bone marrow mesenchymal stem cells. Acta Pharmacol Sin 28: 1761–1774.
48. Cheng CW, Yeh JC, Fan TP, Smith SK, Charnock-Jones DS (2008) Wnt5a-mediated non-canonical Wnt signalling regulates human endothelial cell proliferation and migration. Biochem Biophys Res Commun 365: 285–290.
49. Kurayoshi M, Oue N, Yamamoto H, Kishida M, Inoue A, et al. (2006) Expression of Wnt-5a is correlated with aggressiveness of gastric cancer by stimulating cell migration and invasion. Cancer Res 66: 10439–10448.
50. Ripka S, König A, Buchholz M, Wagner M, Sipos B, et al. (2007) WNT5A–target of CUTL1 and potent modulator of tumor cell migrationand invasion in pancreatic cancer. Carcinogeniesis 28: 1178–1187.
51. Zhu Y, Tian Y, Du J, Hu Z, Yang L, et al. (2012) Dvl2-dependent activation of Daam1 and RhoA regulates Wnt5a-induced breast cancer cell migration. PLoS One 7: e37823.
52. Jin Z, zhao C, Han X, Han Y (2012) Wnt5a promotes ewing sarcoma cell migration through upregulating CXCR4 expression. BMC Cancer 12: 480.
53. Huang C, Rajfur Z, Borchers C, Schaller MD, Jacobson K (2003) JNK phosphorylates paxillin and regulates cell migration. Nature 424: 219–223.
54. Yamamoto H, Oue N, Sato A, Hasegawa Y, Yamamoto H, et al. (2010) Wnt5a signaling is involved in the aggressiveness of prostate cancer and expression of metalloproteinase. Oncogene 29: 2036–2046.
55. Shi MD, Shih YW, Lee YS, Cheng YF, Tsai LY (2013) Suppression of 12-O-tetradecanoylphorbol-13-acetate-induced MCF-7 breast adenocarcinoma cells invasion/migration by α-tomatine through activating PKCα/ERK/NF-κB-dependent MMP-2/MMP-9 expressions. Cell Biochem Biophys 66: 161–174.
56. Muller-Ehmsen J, Krausgrill B, Burst V, Schenk K, Neisen UC, et al. (2006) Effective engraftment but poor mid-term persistence of mononuclear and mesenchymal bone marrow cells in acute and chronic rat myocardial infarction. J Mol Cell Cardiol 41: 876–884.
57. Mei SH, McCarter SD, Deng Y, Parker CH, Liles WC, et al. (2007) Prevention of LPS-induced acute lung injury in mice by mesenchymal stem cells overexpressing angiopoietin 1. PLoS Med 4: e269.
58. Copland IB, Lord-Dufour S, Cuerquis J, Coutu DL, Annabi B, et al. (2009) Improved autograft survival of mesenchymal stromal cells by plasminogen activator inhibitor 1 inhibition. Stem Cells 27: 467–477.

59. Masckauchán TN, Agalliu D, Vorontchikhina M, Ahn A, Parmalee NL, et al. (2006) wnt5a signaling induces proliferation and survival of endothelial cells in vitro and expression of MMP-1 and Tie-2. Mol Biol Cell 17: 5163–5172.
60. Cheng CW, Yeh JC, Fan TP, Smith SK, Charnock-Jones DS (2008) Wnt5a-mediated non-canonical Wnt signalling regulates human endothelial cell proliferation and migration. Biochem Biophys Res Commun 365: 285–290.
61. Ward PA (2010) Oxidative stress: acute and progressive lung injury. Ann N Y Acad Sci 1203: 53–59.
62. Yang YJ, Qian HY, Huang J, Geng YJ, Gao RL, et al. (2008) Atorvastatin treatment improves survival and effects of implanted mesenchymal stem cells in post-infarct swine hearts. Eur Heart J 29: 1578–1590.
63. Hotchkiss RS, Strasser A, McDunn JE, Swanson PE (2009) Cell death. N Engl J Med 361: 1570–1583.
64. Vuga LJ, Ben-Yehudah A, Kovkarova-Naumovski E, Oriss T, Gibson KF, et al. (2009) WNT5A is a regulator of fibroblast proliferation and resistance to apoptosis. Am J Respir Cell Mol Biol 41: 583–589.
65. Bluwstein A, Kumar N, Léger K, Traenkle J, Oostrum Jv, et al. (2013) PKC signaling prevents irradiation-induced apoptosis of primary human fibroblasts. Cell Death Dis 14: 4:e498.
66. Zhang JY, Jiang H, Gao W, Wu J, Peng K, et al. (2008) The JNK/AP1/ATF2 pathway is involved in H_2O_2-induced acetylcholinesterase expression during apoptosis. Cell Mol Life Sci 65: 1435–1445.
67. Yoon SO, Kim MM, Park SJ, Kim D, Chung J, et al. (2002) Selenite suppresses hydrogen peroxide-induced cell apoptosis through inhibition of ASK1/JNK and activation of PI3-K/Akt pathways. FASEB 16: 111–113.
68. Wang L, Matsushita K, Araki I, Takeda M (2002) Inhibition of c-Jun N-terminal kinase ameliorates apoptosis induced by hydrogen peroxide in the kidney tubule epithelial cells (NRK-52E). Nephron 91: 142–147.

10

Concomitant Pulmonary Tuberculosis in Hospitalized Healthcare-Associated Pneumonia in a Tuberculosis Endemic Area

Jia-Yih Feng[1,2], Wen-Feng Fang[3,4], Chieh-Liang Wu[5,6], Chong-Jen Yu[7,8], Meng-Chih Lin[3,4], Shih-Chi Ku[9], Yu-Chun Chen[10,11], Chang-Wen Chen[12], Chih-Yen Tu[13,14,15], Wei-Juin Su[1,11]❡, Kuang-Yao Yang[1,11]*❡

1 Department of Chest Medicine, Taipei Veterans General Hospital, Taipei, Taiwan, **2** Institute of Clinical Medicine; School of Medicine, National Yang-Ming University, Taipei, Taiwan, **3** Division of Pulmonary and Critical Care Medicine and Department of Respiratory Therapy, Kaohsiung Chang Gung Memorial Hospital and Chang Gung University College of Medicine, Kaohsiung, Taiwan, **4** Department of Respiratory Care, Chang Gung University of Science and Technology, Chiayi, Taiwan, **5** Department of Internal Medicine, Chiayi Branch, Taichung Veterans General Hospital, Taichung, Taiwan, **6** Department of Respiratory Therapy, College of Health Care, China Medical University, Taichung, Taiwan, **7** Department of Internal Medicine, National Taiwan University Hospital, Taipei, Taiwan, **8** School of Medicine, National Taiwan University, Taipei, Taiwan, **9** Division of Pulmonary and Critical Care Medicine, Department of Internal Medicine, National Taiwan University Hospital, Taipei, Taiwan, **10** Department of Medical Research and Education, National Yang-Ming University Hospital, Yilan, Taiwan, **11** School of Medicine, National Yang-Ming University, Taipei, Taiwan, **12** Medical Intensive Care Unit, Department of Internal Medicine, National Cheng-Kung University Hospital, Tainan, Taiwan, **13** Division of Pulmonary and Critical Care Medicine, Department of Internal Medicine, China Medical University Hospital, Taichung, Taiwan, **14** School of Medicine, China Medical University, Taichung, Taiwan, **15** Department of Life Science, National Chung Hsing University, Taichung, Taiwan

Abstract

Background: In tuberculosis (TB) endemic areas, *Mycobacterium tuberculosis* is an important but easily misdiagnosed pathogen in community-acquired pneumonia (CAP). However, the occurrence of concomitant pulmonary tuberculosis (PTB) in hospitalized healthcare-associated pneumonia (HCAP) has never been investigated.

Methods and Findings: Seven hundred and one hospitalized HCAP and 934 hospitalized CAP patients from six medical centers in Taiwan were included in this nationwide retrospective study. Concomitant PTB was defined as active PTB diagnosed within 60 days of admission due to HCAP or CAP. The predictors for concomitant PTB and the impact of PTB on the outcomes of pneumonia were investigated. Among the enrolled subjects, 21/701 (3%) of the HCAP patients and 25/934 (2.7%) of the CAP patients were documented to have concomitant PTB. In multivariate analysis, a history of previous anti-TB treatment (OR = 5.84, 95% CI: 2.29–20.37 in HCAP; OR = 3.33, 95% CI: 1.09–10.22 in CAP) and escalated pneumonia severity index (PSI) scores (OR = 1.014, 95% CI: 1.002–1.026, in HCAP; OR = 1.013, 95% CI: 1.001–1.026, in CAP) were independent predictors for concomitant PTB in both CAP and HCAP patients. Regarding treatment outcomes, HCAP patients with concomitant PTB were associated with more acute respiratory failure within 48 hours of admission (47.6% vs. 22.6%, $p = 0.008$), higher intensive care unit admission rate (61.9% vs. 35.7%, $p = 0.014$), longer hospitalization (39.6±34.1 vs. 23.7±27 days, $p = 0.009$), and higher in-hospital mortality (47.6% vs. 26.3%, $p = 0.03$) than those without concomitant PTB. Exposure to certain groups of antibiotics for the treatment of pneumonia was not associated with the occurrence of concomitant PTB.

Conclusions: In HCAP patients, the occurrence of concomitant PTB is comparable with that in CAP patients and associated with higher PSI scores, more acute respiratory failure, and higher in-hospital mortality.

Editor: Olivier Neyrolles, Institut de Pharmacologie et de Biologie Structurale, France

Funding: This work was supported, in part, by research grants from Taiwan National Science Council Research Grant (NSC 97-2314-B-075-046, NSC 100-2314-B-075-047-MY3), and Taipei Veterans General Hospital (V97C1-143, V98C1-072, V99C1-167, V100C-159, V99C1-181, V99A-023 and V100A-002). The funders had no role in study design, data collection and analysis, decision to publish, or preparation of the manuscript.

Competing Interests: The authors have declared that no competing interests exist.

* E-mail: kyyang@vghtpe.gov.tw

❡ These authors contributed equally to this work.

Introduction

Tuberculosis (TB) is an important infectious disease associated with high mortality and morbidity. According to estimates of the World Health Organization (WHO), there were 9.4 million incident cases of TB, and 1.7 million people who died from TB worldwide in 2009 [1]. In Taiwan, the incidence and mortality of TB were 62 and 3.3 cases per 100,000 population, respectively, in 2008 [2]. Due to the non-specific symptoms and diverse radiographic presentations, it is not always easy to differentiate pulmonary tuberculosis (PTB) from bacterial pneumonia in a clinical setting [3]. In TB endemic areas, TB studies are frequently ordered in patients treated for community-acquired pneumonia (CAP). Empirical antibiotics, especially newer fluoroquinolones

(FQNs), are used with caution as they may delay the diagnosis of PTB and are associated with worse outcomes [4,5].

Healthcare-associated pneumonia (HCAP) is a relatively new category of pneumonia that was first defined in 2005 with unique microbiological characteristics and treatment outcomes [6,7]. It represents a pulmonary infection that occurs before hospitalization in patients who had contact with or an exposure history to a healthcare environment [8]. HCAP patients are generally older with multiple comorbidities, which are also risk factors for the development of PTB. However, the occurrence of concomitant PTB in HCAP patients has never been evaluated. Unawareness of concomitant PTB in hospitalized HCAP patients may lead to a delayed diagnosis and transmission of *Mycobacterium tuberculosis* (MTB) in healthcare facilities. The main purpose of the present study was to investigate the occurrence and clinical predictors of concomitant PTB in hospitalized HCAP patients, and compare them to those of CAP patients. The relationship of exposure to antibiotics for the treatment of pneumonia to PTB occurrence, and the impact of concomitant PTB in the outcomes of pneumonia in these patients were also evaluated.

Materials and Methods

Ethics

This study was approved by the Institutional Review Boards of Taipei Veterans General Hospital; Kaohsiung Chang Gung Memorial Hospital; Taichung Veterans General Hospital; National Taiwan University Hospital; National Cheng-Kung University Hospital; and China Medical University Hospital. Being a retrospective study, informed consent was waived according to the regulations of the Department of Health, Taiwan.

Patients

This was a nationwide retrospective cohort study conducted at six tertiary medical centers in Taiwan. Patients admitted to these hospitals with a final diagnosis of HCAP from 1 January 2007 to 31 December 2007 were eligible for inclusion. We also included hospitalized CAP patients from these hospitals during the same study period for comparison. HCAP and CAP were defined as in previous reports [9,10]. Patients presenting with pneumonia diagnosed within 48 hours after hospitalization were included as HCAP if at least one of the following criteria was satisfied: (1) receiving regular dialysis at an outpatient clinic; (2) receiving radiation therapy or chemotherapy at an outpatient clinic; (3) undergoing repeated hospitalization within 90 days prior to the episode of current pneumonia; or (4) residing in a nursing home. Pneumonia patients diagnosed within 48 hours after hospitalization were included as CAP if none of the HCAP criteria were met. The diagnosis of pneumonia was confirmed by chest radiographic manifestations with the growth of microorganisms from cultures of respiratory specimens or clinical improvement after antibiotic therapy. Patients who had lung cancer with obstructive pneumonitis, inadequate data for review, or were younger than 18 years old were excluded from analysis.

Clinical evaluation

Demographic profiles (age, sex), clinical characteristics (smoking habits and comorbidities), and usage of antibiotics were obtained

Table 1. Demographic profiles between hospitalized HCAP and CAP patients[a].

	Overall, =1635	Type of pneumonia		P value
		CAP, n=934	HCAP, n=701	
Mean age (SD)	72.8 (15.7)	72.5(16.6)	73.1 (14.5)	0.47
Male gender	1172 (71.7%)	674 (72.2%)	498 (71%)	0.62
Smoking habit	603 (36.9%)	329 (35.2%)	274 (39.1%)	0.11
Previous anti-TB treatment	82 (5%)	49 (5.2%)	33 (4.7%)	0.62
Comorbidities				
Malignancy	322 (19.7%)	79 (8.5%)	243 (34.7%)	<0.001
Renal insufficiency	199 (12.2%)	69 (7.4%)	130 (18.5%)	<0.001
Chronic liver disease	86 (5.3%)	41 (4.4%)	45 (6.4%)	0.07
Diabetes	443 (27.1%)	235 (25.2%)	208 (29.7%)	0.042
COPD	250 (15.3%)	154 (16.5%)	96 (13.7%)	0.12
Pneumonia severity				
PSI score	133.3 (34.5)	126.5 (31.7)	142.3 (36.0)	<0.001
CURB65 score	1.81 (1.07)	1.77 (1.05)	1.87 (1.10)	0.08
Chest film presentation				
Upper lung involvement	661 (40.4%)	339 (36.3%)	322 (45.9%)	<0.001
Bilateral lung involvement	703 (43%)	378 (40.5%)	325 (46.4%)	0.017
TB testing when admission	562 (34.4%)	375 (40.1%)	187 (26.7%)	<0.001
Pathogen in sputum culture (n=744)				
Gram-positive bacteria	209 (28.1%)	131 (31.3%)	78 (24%)	0.08
Gram-negative bacteria	535 (71.9%)	288 (68.7%)	247 (76%)	0.06

[a]The data are presented as n (%) unless otherwise stated.

HCAP, healthcare-associated pneumonia; CAP, community acquired pneumonia; TB, tuberculosis; SD, standard deviation; COPD, chronic obstructive pulmonary disease; PSI, pneumonia severity index; CURB65, confusion, urea, respiratory rate, blood pressure, age 65.

from medical records. A history of previous anti-TB treatment was determined according to the registration database of the Centers for Disease Control (CDC), Taiwan, and the medical records in each study hospital. The chest radiographs on the day of admission were reviewed by the responsible pulmonologist at each hospital. The pneumonia scoring indices, including CURB65 (confusion, urea, respiratory rate, blood pressure, age 65) score and pneumonia severity index (PSI) were calculated as described in previous studies [11,12]. The antibiotics used during hospitalization were classified as cephalosporin, penicillin, macrolide, and newer quinolone (including moxifloxacin and levofloxacin) groups. Exposure to these groups of antibiotics was defined if the antibiotics had been used within the last 7 days. The outcomes of pneumonia were evaluated by organ dysfunction within 48 hours, intensive care unit (ICU) admission rate, length of hospital stay, number of antibiotics used, long-term ventilator dependence rate, and mortality rate. Organ dysfunction was defined as per a previous study [13]. The severity of pneumonia was stratified according to the PSI scores ($\leq$130, 131~149, and $\geq$150) and the number of organ dysfunctions to compare with the occurrence of concomitant PTB. All the patients were followed until mortality or discharge after an improvement in pneumonia.

Identification of concomitant PTB

As conventional TB culture methods generally require six to eight weeks to obtain the final results, pneumonia patients with active PTB diagnosed within 60 days of admission were defined as cases with concomitant PTB. The occurrence of PTB was determined according to the records in the CDC registration database, Taiwan. Only PTB that was proven by TB cultures or typical pathological findings from respiratory specimens were included for analysis.

Statistical analysis

Statistical analysis was performed using SPSS version 17.0 software (SPSS, Chicago, IL, USA). Continuous variables between subgroups were compared with Mann-Whitney U or independent t tests, and categorical variables were compared using Pearson's chi-square or Fisher's exact tests. Binary logistic regression analysis with stepwise selection was performed to determine the independent variables for the occurrence of concomitant PTB, and odds ratios with their 95% confidence intervals were presented. A p value less than 0.1 in the univariate analysis was required for a variable to be entered into the multivariate model. Survival time was estimated by the Kaplan-Meier method, and the log-rank test was used to compare mortality in HCAP and CAP patients with or without concomitant PTB. Censored analysis was used because the observation time was limited by discharge from the hospitals. All tests were two-tailed, and a p value less than 0.05 was considered to be statistically significant.

Results

Patients characteristics

During the study period, a total of 718 HCAP patients were identified from the six study hospitals. Of these patients, seven

Table 2. Demographic profiles and clinical characteristics of CAP and HCAP patients with and without concomitant pulmonary tuberculosis[a].

	Overall patient, n = 1635		P value	CAP patients, n = 934		P value	HCAP patients, n = 701		P value
	With TB, n = 46	Without TB, n = 1589		With TB, n = 25	Without TB, n = 909		With TB, n = 21	Without TB, n = 680	
Mean age (SD)	76.2 (15.3)	72.7 (15.7)	0.14	74.1 (16.8)	72.5 (16.6)	0.65	79.6 (13.4)	72.9 (14.5)	0.034
Male gender	38 (82.6%)	1134 (71.4%)	0.10	22 (88%)	652 (71.7%)	0.07	16 (76.2%)	482 (70.9%)	0.60
Smoking habit	20 (43.5%)	583 (36.7%)	0.35	12 (48%)	317 (34.9%)	0.18	8 (38.1%)	266 (39.1%)	0.93
Previous anti-TB treatment	9 (19.6%)	73 (4.6%)	<0.001	4 (16%)	45 (5%)	0.015	5 (23.8%)	28 (4.1%)	<0.001
Comorbidities									
Malignancy	14 (30.4%)	308 (19.4%)	0.06	5 (20%)	74 (8.1%)	0.036	9 (42.9%)	234 (34.4%)	0.42
Renal insufficiency	6 (13%)	193 (12.1%)	0.85	3 (12%)	66 (7.3%)	0.37	3 (14.3%)	127 (18.7%)	0.61
Chronic liver disease	1 (2.2%)	85 (5.3%)	0.34	1 (4%)	40 (4.4%)	0.92	0	45 (6.6%)	0.39
Diabetes	14 (30.4%)	429 (27%)	0.61	8 (32%)	227 (25%)	0.42	6 (28.6%)	202 (29.7%)	0.91
COPD	11 (23.9%)	239 (15%)	0.10	7 (28%)	147 (16.2%)	0.12	4 (19%)	92 (13.5%)	0.47
Pneumonia severity									
PSI score (SD)	149.9 (35.7)	132.8 (34.4)	0.001	140.3 (36.1)	126.1 (31.5)	0.033	161.3 (32.5)	141.7 (36.0)	0.017
CURB65 score (SD)	1.91 (1.05)	1.81 (1.08)	0.60	1.80 (1.00)	1.77 (1.05)	1.00	2.05 (1.12)	1.87 (1.10)	0.46
Chest film presentation									
Upper lung involvement	19 (41.3%)	642 (40.4%)	0.90	8 (32%)	331 (36.4%)	0.65	11 (52.4%)	311 (45.7%)	0.55
Bilateral lung involvement	24 (52.2%)	679 (42.7%)	0.20	12 (48%)	366 (40.3%)	0.44	12 (57.1%)	313 (46%)	0.31
Type of pneumonia			0.73			-			-
CAP	25 (54.3%)	905 (57%)		-	-		-	-	
HCAP	21 (45.7%)	684 (43%)		-	-		-	-	
TB testing on admission	25 (54.3%)	537 (33.8%)	0.004	16 (64%)	359 (39.5%)	0.014	9 (42.9%)	178 (26.2%)	0.089

[a]The data are presented as n (%) unless otherwise stated.
HCAP, healthcare-associated pneumonia; CAP, community acquired pneumonia; TB, tuberculosis; SD, standard deviation; COPD, chronic obstructive pulmonary disease; PSI, pneumonia severity index; CURB65, confusion, urea, respiratory rate, blood pressure, age 65.

Table 3. Relationships between antibiotics exposure and the occurrence of concomitant pulmonary tuberculosis in HCAP and CAP patients[a].

Antibiotics exposure	CAP patients, n = 934		P value	HCAP patients, n = 701		P value
	With TB, n = 25	Without TB, n = 909		With TB, n = 21	Without TB, n = 680	
Penicillin						
Yes	15 (2.4%)	602 (97.6%)	0.52	16 (3.9%)	395 (96.1%)	0.10
No	10 (3.2%)	307 (96.8%)		5 (1.7%)	285 (98.3%)	
Cephalosporin						
Yes	6 (3.4%)	171 (96.6%)	0.51	3 (1.7%)	169 (98.3%)	0.27
No	19 (2.5%)	738 (97.5%)		18 (3.4%)	511 (96.6%)	
Macrolide						
Yes	5 (2.3%)	210 (97.7%)	0.72	1 (2.6%)	38 (97.4%)	1.00
No	20 (2.8%)	699 (97.2%)		20 (3%)	642 (97%)	
Carbapenem						
Yes	0	17 (100%)	1.00	0	27 (100%)	1.00
No	25 (2.7%)	892 (97.3%)		21 (3.1%)	653 (96.9%)	
Newer fluoroquinolones[b]						
Yes	4 (2%)	192 (98%)	0.47	4 (2.5%)	155 (97.5%)	0.69
No	21 (2.9%)	717 (97.1%)		17 (3.1%)	525 (96.1%)	

[a]The data are presented as n (%) unless otherwise stated.
[b]Included levofloxacin and moxifloxacin.
HCAP, healthcare-associated pneumonia; CAP, community acquired pneumonia; TB, tuberculosis.

were excluded due to lung cancer with obstructive pneumonitis, and 10 were excluded due to incomplete data for review. In total, 701 hospitalized HCAP patients were included for analysis. Among these patients, 323 (46.1%) were hospitalized in an acute care hospital for two or more days within 90 days before the current admission; 164 (23.4%) resided in a nursing home or long-term care facility; 136 (19.4%) had received intravenous antibiotic therapy, chemotherapy, or wound care within the past 30 days of the current infection; and 77 (11%) attended a hospital or hemodialysis clinic. We also included 934 CAP patients from the study hospitals for comparison. The flow diagram showing the number of cases and reasons for exclusion is shown in Figure S1. The demographic characteristics of the HCAP and CAP patients are shown in Table 1. Compared with the CAP patients, the HCAP patients were more likely to have a malignancy, renal insufficiency, diabetes, higher PSI score, and present with upper lung and/or bilateral lung involvement.

The pathogens isolated from respiratory specimens of the included patients are shown in Table S1.

Occurrence of concomitant PTB and clinical predictors

Seven HCAP patients had active PTB on admission, and a further 14 were diagnosed with PTB within 60 days after admission. Six CAP patients had active PTB on admission, and a further 19 were diagnosed with PTB within 60 days. The occurrence of concomitant PTB was comparable between the HCAP and CAP patients (3% vs. 2.7%, p = 0.73).

Table 4. Univariate and multivariate logistic regression analysis of predictors associated with concomitant pulmonary tuberculosis in hospitalized HCAP and CAP patients[a].

	CAP patients				HCAP patients			
	Univariate		Multivariate		Univariate		Multivariate	
	OR (95% CI)	P value	OR (95% CI)	P value	OR (95% CI)	P value	OR (95% CI)	P value
Age	1.01 (0.98–1.03)	0.65			1.04 (1.003–1.086)	0.034		
Male gender	2.89 (0.86–9.74)	0.07			1.32 (0.48–3.64)	0.60		
Previous anti-TB treatment	3.66 (1.21–11.1)	0.015	3.33 (1.09–10.22)	0.035	7.28 (2.49–21.3)	<0.001	5.84 (2.29–20.37)	0.001
Malignancy	2.82 (1.03–7.72)	0.036			1.43 (0.59–3.44)	0.42		
Upper lobe involvement	0.82 (0.35–1.93)	0.65			1.31 (0.55–3.11)	0.55		
PSI score	1.01 (1.002–1.027)	0.033	1.013 (1.001–1.026)	0.038	1.015 (1.003–1.026)	0.015	1.014 (1.002–1.026)	0.023

[a]Univariate and multivariate OR are derived from logistic regression analysis with stepwise selection procedure.
HCAP, healthcare-associated pneumonia; CAP, community acquired pneumonia; TB, tuberculosis; OR, odds ratio; CI, confidence interval.

The demographic and clinical characteristics of the HCAP and CAP patients with or without concomitant PTB are shown in Table 2. In the HCAP group, patients with concomitant PTB were more likely to be older in age (79.6±13.4 vs. 72.9±14.5 years, $p = 0.034$), have a history of previous anti-TB treatment (23.8% vs. 4.1%, $p < 0.001$), and have higher PSI scores (161.3±32.5 vs. 141.7±36, $p = 0.017$), as compared with those without concomitant PTB. In the CAP group, patients with concomitant PTB were more likely to have a previous history of anti-TB treatment (16% vs. 5%, $p = 0.015$), malignancy (20% vs. 8.1%, $p = 0.036$), and higher PSI scores (140.3±36.1 vs. 126.1±31.5, $p = 0.033$).

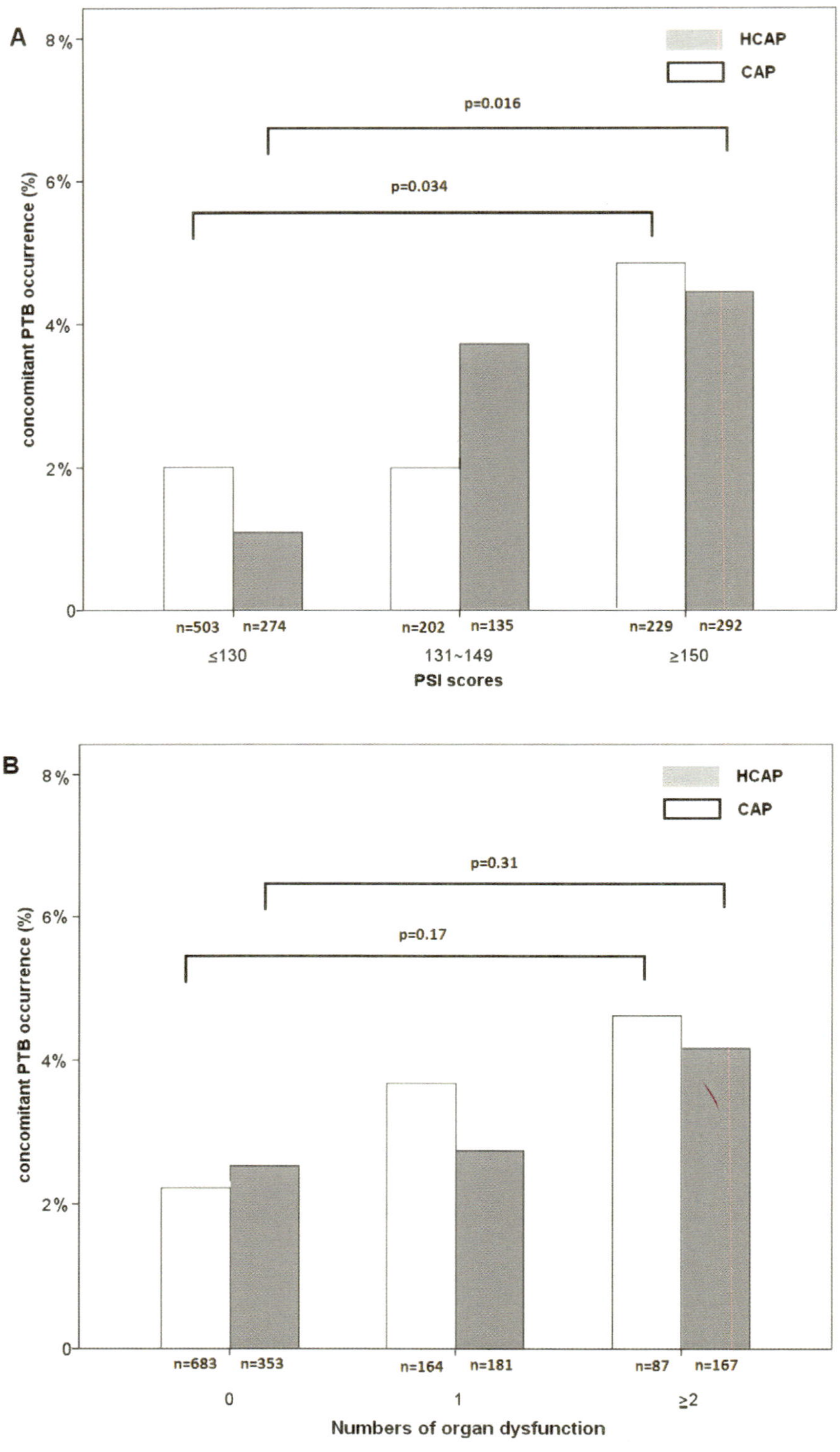

Figure 1. Occurrence of concomitant PTB among hospitalized HCAP and CAP patients with various severity. Patients are divided according to (A) PSI scores and (B) number of organ dysfunctions. HCAP, healthcare-associated pneumonia; CAP, community acquired pneumonia; PSI, pneumonia severity index; PTB, pulmonary tuberculosis.

The association between exposure to antibiotics and the occurrence of concomitant PTB is shown in Table 3. In both HCAP and CAP patients, the exposure to certain groups of antibiotics were comparable between patients with or without concomitant PTB.

In multivariate analysis, higher PSI scores (OR = 1.014, 95% CI: 1.002–1.026 in HCAP; OR: 1.013, 95% CI: 1.001–1.026 in CAP) and a previous history of anti-TB treatment (OR = 5.84, 95% CI: 2.29–20.37 in HCAP; OR: 3.33, 95% CI: 1.09–10.22 in CAP) were independent predictors of concomitant PTB in both HCAP and CAP patients (Table 4).

The occurrence of concomitant PTB in HCAP and CAP patients stratified by the severity of PSI scores and the number of organ dysfunctions is shown in Figure 1. The occurrence of concomitant PTB increased as the PSI scores increased. Patients with PSI scores ≥150 had significantly more concomitant PTB than those with PSI scores ≤130, in both the HCAP (p = 0.016) and CAP (p = 0.034) groups. The occurrence of concomitant PTB also increased as the number of organ dysfunctions increased, although without statistical significance.

The demographic characteristics of the HCAP and CAP patients with or without concomitant PTB within 90 days and their clinical predictors are shown in Table S2 and Table S3.

Impact of concomitant PTB in outcomes of the pneumonia patients

The treatment outcomes of the HCAP and CAP patients with or without concomitant PTB are shown in Table 5. In the HCAP group, patients with concomitant PTB had more acute respiratory failure within 48 hours of admission (47.6% vs. 22.6%, p = 0.008), higher ICU admission rate (61.9% vs. 35.7%, p = 0.014), and longer hospital stay (39.6±34.1 days vs. 23.7±27 days, p = 0.009) compared to those without concomitant PTB. In the CAP group, patients with concomitant PTB had a higher probability of ICU admission (44% vs. 19.7%, p = 0.003) and longer hospital stay (32±27.4 days vs. 19±20.3 days, p = 0.002).

Regarding mortality, the in-hospital mortality rate was higher in the HCAP patients with concomitant PTB (47.6% vs. 26.3%, p = 0.03) compared to those without PTB, although the 30-day and 60-day mortality rates were similar. The mortality rates were comparable in the CAP patients with or without concomitant PTB. Kaplan-Meier analysis of survival according to the presence or absence of concomitant PTB in the HCAP and CAP patients is shown in Figure 2. HCAP patients with concomitant PTB had significantly higher mortality (p = 0.041) compared to those without PTB. The survival curves overlapped between CAP patients with or without concomitant PTB.

Univariate and multivariate analysis of clinical predictors for in-hospital mortality in CAP and HCAP patients are shown in Table S4.

Discussion

To the best of our knowledge, this is the first study to evaluate the predictors and outcomes of concomitant PTB in HCAP patients in a TB endemic area. We found that the occurrence of concomitant PTB in hospitalized HCAP patients was not rare and was comparable to those with CAP. A history of previous anti-TB

Table 5. Impact of concomitant tuberculosis in treatment outcome of HCAP and CAP patients[a].

	CAP patients, n = 934		P value	HCAP patients, n = 701		P value
	With TB, n = 25	Without TB, n = 909		With TB, n = 21	Without TB, n = 680	
Organs dysfunction within 48 hours						
Respiratory failure	3 (12%)	115 (12.7%)	0.92	10 (47.6%)	154 (22.6%)	0.008
Septic shock	4 (16%)	91 (10%)	0.33	5 (23.8%)	135 (19.9%)	0.66
Altered mental status	4 (16%)	66 (7.3%)	0.10	6 (28.6%)	145 (21.3%)	0.43
Renal dysfunction	2 (8%)	67 (7.4%)	0.91	1 (4.8%)	104 (15.3%)	0.18
Liver dysfunction	0	1 (0.1%)	1.00	0	3 (0.4%)	0.76
Coagulopathy	0	6 (0.7%)	1.00	1 (4.8%)	13 (1.9%)	0.36
Thrombocytopenia	2 (8%)	26 (2.9%)	0.14	1 (4.8%)	50 (7.4%)	0.65
ICU admission	11 (44%)	179 (19.7%)	0.003	13 (61.9%)	243 (35.7%)	0.014
Length of hospital stay (SD)						
All patients	32.0 (27.4)	19.0 (20.3)	0.002	39.6 (34.1)	23.7 (27.0)	0.009
Survivors	24.5 (17.9)	18.4 (19.7)	0.19	46.2 (42.6)	23.1 (23.9)	0.002
Non-survivors	56.1 (39.3)	23.4 (24.4)	0.003	32.4 (21.4)	25.7 (34.6)	0.54
28 days hospital free day (SD)	7.2 (8.9)	11.9 (8.8)	0.008	4.2 (7.5)	7.8 (8.5)	0.039
Mean Numbers of antibiotics used (SD)	1.74 (0.69)	1.61 (0.75)	0.41	1.29 (0.46)	1.37 (0.62)	0.52
Long-term ventilator dependent	1 (4%)	18 (2%)	0.48	1 (4.8%)	32 (4.7%)	0.99
Mortality						
30-day mortality	2 (8%)	73 (8%)	1.00	4 (19%)	133 (19.6%)	0.95
60-day mortality	3 (12%)	99 (10.9%)	0.86	7 (33.3%)	166 (24.4%)	0.35
In-hospital mortality	6 (24%)	106 (11.7%)	0.06	10 (47.6%)	179 (26.3%)	0.030

[a]The data are presented as n (%)unless otherwise stated.
HCAP, healthcare-associated pneumonia; CAP, community acquired pneumonia; TB, tuberculosis; SD, standard deviation; ICU, intensive care unit.

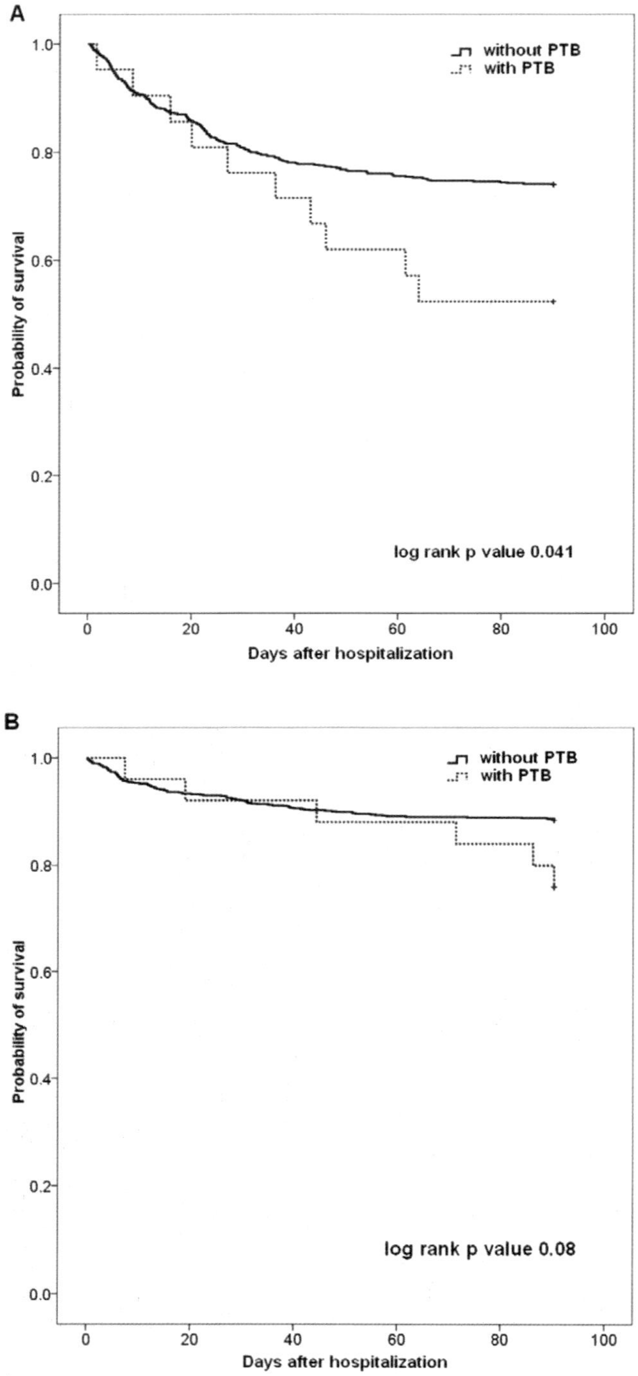

Figure 2. Kaplan-Meier survival curves of hospitalized pneumonia patients with or without concomitant PTB. Patients with (A) HCAP and (B) CAP were stratified by the presence or absence of concomitant PTB within 60 days. HCAP, healthcare-associated pneumonia; CAP, community acquired pneumonia; PTB, pulmonary tuberculosis.

treatment and higher PSI scores were independent predictors for the occurrence of PTB in both HCAP and CAP patients. We also found that HCAP patients with concomitant PTB were associated with worse outcomes of pneumonia, including more acute respiratory failure, higher ICU admission rate, longer hospital stay, and higher in-hospital mortality.

HCAP is a relatively new category of pneumonia that refers to pneumonias that occur prior to hospital admission in patients with specific risk factors [9]. In contrast to CAP, which is typically attributable to antibiotic-susceptible bacteria [14], patients with HCAP have a higher probability of being infected with antibiotic-resistant bacteria, and HCAP is usually associated with multiple comorbidities, higher disease severity and higher mortality [15–17]. There is a lack of an ideal scoring index for HCAP, however the applicability of PSI scores and CURB65 was reported in one recent study [18]. Compared with the CAP patients, the HCAP patients in our study had higher PSI scores and more advanced pulmonary involvement on chest radiographs. These patients also had a higher proportion of malignancies, renal insufficiency, and diabetes, which are well documented risk factors for PTB [19,20]. Considering the multiple comorbidities and higher severity in HCAP patients, identifying the occurrence of concomitant PTB is an important issue, especially in TB endemic areas.

The association between CAP and PTB in TB endemic areas has been reported in previous studies [21,22]. The latest guidelines for CAP also recommend TB studies as initial survey in TB endemic areas [10]. However, studies evaluating the association between HCAP and PTB are surprisingly rare. According to the latest HCAP guidelines, PTB should be considered only in non-responders to antibiotics treatment [9]. In our study, 3% of the hospitalized HCAP patients were documented to have concomitant PTB, which is comparable to the CAP patients. This indicates that PTB is not rare in HCAP patients in TB endemic areas, and that clinicians should keep PTB in mind when evaluating HCAP patients. Early diagnosis of concomitant PTB in HCAP is also important to prevent TB transmission in medical facilities.

The identification of clinical predictors associated with PTB in pneumonia patients helps in the early recognition of PTB. A prospective study performed in the Unites States indicated that typical CXR presentations, a history of previous TB, immigration status, weight loss and homelessness are independent predictors for PTB in patients presenting to the emergency department with a diagnosis of pneumonia [23]. In line with that report, a history of previous anti-TB treatment was an independent clinical predictor of PTB in the present study. We also found that higher PSI scores were independently associated with the presence of concomitant PTB in both HCAP and CAP patients. By comparison, age was not an independent predictor for concomitant PTB in multivariate analysis. One possible explanation is that the calculation of PSI scores already takes the factor of age into consideration. Another possible reason is that the correlation between age and higher disease severity may lessen the statistical significance of age in multivariate analysis. Furthermore, we clearly demonstrated that patients with PSI scores >130, which have been reported to have the highest risk of mortality [12], had a higher occurrence of PTB compared to those with PSI scores ≤ 130. Patients with higher disease severity may be associated with more comorbidities that increase the risk of PTB occurrence. Meanwhile, the presence of concomitant PTB may also complicate the disease course of pneumonia and increase disease severity. The higher disease severity and possible complications associated with anti-TB treatment may further worsen the treatment outcomes of these patients with pneumonia.

The impact of PTB on the outcomes of hospitalized pneumonia patients has been evaluated before with controversial results. Penner et al. reported higher mortality in patients with pneumonia and PTB requiring mechanical ventilation compared to those without PTB [24]. Another case control study reported comparable mortality rates between ICU admitted pneumonia patients with or without active PTB [25]. In our study, we found that HCAP patients with concomitant PTB were associated with higher in-hospital mortality. In multivariate analysis, the independent predictors for mortality of the HCAP patients were the presence of malignancy, higher PSI scores, higher CURB65 scores, and bilateral involvement in chest radiograms, but did not include the occurrence of concomitant PTB (data not shown). Our findings imply that the worse treatment outcomes of HCAP patients with PTB are more likely to result from the underlying comorbidities and higher disease severity, but not TB disease per se. Nevertheless, our findings still have important clinical implications. Given the fact that concomitant PTB is not rare in hospitalized HCAP patients, and that the higher disease severity in these patients lead to higher mortality, it is important that clinicians should consider PTB in HCAP patients with more comorbidities and higher severity. In addition, we also found that HCAP patients with concomitant PTB had more acute respiratory failure within 48 hours of admission, higher ICU admission rate, and longer hospital stay. Therefore, early diagnosis and early treatment of PTB may not only potentially reduce mortality, but also avoid TB transmission within healthcare facilities.

Our study has several limitations. This is a retrospective study and some clinical information may be incomplete. All of the participating hospitals are tertiary medical centers, and the enrolled patients were of older age with more comorbidities. Therefore, the incidence of concomitant PTB in these patients may be higher than that of the general population. Nevertheless, our findings can be applied to patients with more comorbidities. TB testing on admission was not routinely done in each patient. The occurrences of concomitant PTB may be underdiagnosed in HCAP group because of the lower TB testing rate on admission. However, our findings also clearly indicate the lack of awareness of PTB by clinicians, especially in HCAP patients. We did not stratify deaths as being due to either TB or HCAP in the study design because it is not always easy to clarify the causes of death in a retrospective study. All-cause mortality is more objective and applicable in clinical practice. Being a retrospective study, the MTB specimens from our patients could not be completely obtained, so drug susceptibility profiles were not demonstrated. Finally, this study was conducted in a TB endemic area with a low HIV prevalence rate, which may limit the application of our findings to non-HIV endemic areas.

In conclusion, our findings suggest that the occurrence of concomitant PTB in hospitalized HCAP patients in a TB endemic area is not rare and frequently overlooked by clinicians. Higher PSI scores and a history of previous anti-TB treatment were independent predictors for concomitant PTB in both hospitalized HCAP and CAP patients. Regarding treatment outcomes, hospitalized HCAP patients with concomitant PTB were associated with higher in-hospital mortality and more acute respiratory failure within 48 hours. These patients also had a higher ICU admission rate and longer hospital stay, which may lead to TB transmission if the diagnosis of PTB is delayed. Our results provide important evidence to remind clinicians to keep a high suspicion of and identify concomitant PTB early in hospitalized HCAP patients by examining the risk factors and pneumonia severity. Further prospective studies are warranted to elucidate this issue, especially in TB endemic areas.

Supporting Information

Figure S1 Study profile demonstrating the number of cases and reasons for exclusion.

Table S1 Pathogens isolated in respiratory specimens of CAP and HCAP patients[a].

Table S2 Demographic profiles and clinical characteristics of CAP and HCAP patients with and without concomitant pulmonary tuberculosis within 90 days of admission[a].

Table S3 Univariate and multivariate logistic regression analysis of predictors associated with concomitant pulmonary tuberculosis within 90 days of admission in hospitalized HCAP and CAP patients[a].

Table S4 Univariate and multivariate logistic regression analysis of predictors associated with in-hospital mortality in hospitalized CAP and HCAP patients[a].

Acknowledgments

The authors would like to thank all those who contributed to the study: Kuo-Hsuan Hsu at VGHTC, Wei Chen at CMUH, Wen-Chien Fan and Shiang-Fen Huang at VGHTPE, Chih-Ying Ou at CKUH.

Author Contributions

Conceived and designed the experiments: JYF WFF CLW CJY MCL CWC SCK CYT WJS KYY. Analyzed the data: JYF YCC WJS KYY. Contributed reagents/materials/analysis tools: JYF WFF CLW CJY MCL CWC SCK CYT WJS KYY. Wrote the paper: JYF KYY.

References

1. Global tuberculosis control 2010 (2011) Geneva: World Health Organization.
2. Taiwan tuberculosis control report 2008 (2009) Taipei: Centers of Disease Control, Department of Health, R.O.C (Taiwan).
3. Miller LG, Asch SM, Yu EI, Knowles L, Gelberg L, et al. (2000) A population-based survey of tuberculosis symptoms: how atypical are atypical presentations? Clin Infect Dis 30: 293–299.
4. Chang KC, Leung CC, Yew WW, Lau TY, Leung WM, et al. (2010) Newer fluoroquinolones for treating respiratory infection: do they mask tuberculosis? Eur Respir J 35: 606–613.
5. Wang JY, Hsueh PR, Jan IS, Lee LN, Liaw YS, et al. (2006) Empirical treatment with a fluoroquinolone delays the treatment for tuberculosis and is associated with a poor prognosis in endemic areas. Thorax 61: 903–908.
6. Kollef MH, Shorr A, Tabak YP, Gupta V, Liu LZ, et al. (2005) Epidemiology and outcomes of health-care-associated pneumonia: results from a large US database of culture-positive pneumonia. Chest 128: 3854–3862.
7. Carratala J, Mykietiuk A, Fernandez-Sabe N, Suárez C, Dorca J, et al. (2007) Health care-associated pneumonia requiring hospital admission: epidemiology, antibiotic therapy, and clinical outcomes. Arch Intern Med 167: 1393–1399.
8. Micek ST, Kollef KE, Reichley RM, Roubinian N, Kollef MH (2007) Healthcare-associated pneumonia and community-acquired pneumonia: a single-center experience. Antimicrob Agents Chemother 51: 3568–3573.
9. American Thoracic Society, Infectious Diseases Society of America (2005) Guidelines for the management of adults with hospital-acquired, ventilator-associated, and healthcare-associated pneumonia. Am J Respir Crit Care Med 171: 388–416.
10. Mandell LA, Wunderink RG, Anzueto A, Bartlett JG, Campbell GD, et al. (2007) Infectious Diseases Society of America/American Thoracic Society consensus guidelines on the management of community-acquired pneumonia in adults. Clin Infect Dis 44: S27–S72.
11. Lim WS, van der Eerden MM, Laing R, Boersma WG, Karalus N, et al. (2003) Defining community acquired pneumonia severity on presentation to hospital: an international derivation and validation study. Thorax 58: 377–382.
12. Fine MJ, Auble TE, Yealy DM, Hanusa BH, Weissfeld LA, et al. (1997) A prediction rule to identify low-risk patients with community-acquired pneumonia. N Engl J Med 336: 243–250.

13. Bernard GR, Vincent JL, Laterre PF, LaRosa SP, Dhainaut JF, et al. (2001) Efficacy and safety of recombinant human activated protein C for severe sepsis. N Engl J Med 344: 699–709.
14. Mandell LA, Bartlett JG, Dowell SF, Dowell SF, File TM, Jr., et al. (2003) Update of practice guidelines for the management of community-acquired pneumonia in immunocompetent adults. Clin Infect Dis 37: 1405–1433.
15. Shindo Y, Sato S, Maruyama E, Ohashi T, Ogawa M, et al. (2009) Health-care-associated pneumonia among hospitalized patients in a Japanese community hospital. Chest 135: 633–640.
16. Carratalà J, Garcia-Vidal C (2008) What is healthcare-associated pneumonia and how is it managed? Curr Opin Infect Dis 21: 168–167.
17. Venditti M, Falcone M, Corrao S, Licata G, Serra P, et al. (2009) Outcomes of patients hospitalized with community-acquired, health care-associated, and hospital-acquired pneumonia. Ann Intern Med 150: 19–26.
18. Fang WF, Yang KY, Wu CL, Yu CJ, Chen CW, et al. (2011) Application and comparison of scoring indices to predict outcomes in patients with healthcare-associated pneumonia. Crit Care 15: R32.
19. Walker C, Unwin N (2010) Estimates of the impact of diabetes on the incidence of pulmonary tuberculosis in different ethnic groups in England. Thorax 65: 578–581.
20. Kim HR, Hwang SS, Ro YK, Jeon CH, Ha DY, et al. (2008) Solid-organ malignancy as a risk factor for tuberculosis. Respirology 13: 413–419.
21. Liam CK, Pang YK, Poosparajah S (2006) Pulmonary tuberculosis presenting as community-acquired pneumonia. Respirology 11: 786–792.
22. Nyamande K, Lalloo UG, John M (2007) TB presenting as community-acquired pneumonia in a setting of high TB incidence and high HIV prevalence. Int J Tuberc Lung Dis 11: 1308–1313.
23. Moran GJ, Barrett TW, Mower WR, Krishnadasan A, Abrahamian FM, et al. (2009) Decision instrument for the isolation of pneumonia patients with suspected pulmonary tuberculosis admitted through US emergency departments. Ann Emerg Med 53: 625–632.
24. Penner C, Roberts D, Kunimoto D, Manfreda J, Long R (1995) Tuberculosis as a primary cause of respiratory failure requiring mechanical ventilation. Am J Respir Crit Care Med 151: 867–872.
25. Hui C, Wu CL, Chan MC, Kuo IT, Chiang CD (2003) Features of severe pneumonia in patients with undiagnosed pulmonary tuberculosis in an intensive care unit. J Formos Med Assoc 102: 563–569.

Inhaled NO Contributes to Lung Repair in Piglets with Acute Respiratory Distress Syndrome via Increasing Circulating Endothelial Progenitor Cells

Yuanyuan Qi[1], Liling Qian[1,2]*, Bo Sun[1,2,3], Lijuan Liu[1], Panpan Wu[1], Libo Sun[1]

1 Departments of Pediatrics, Children's Hospital of Fudan University, Shanghai, China, **2** The Key Laboratory of Neonatal Disease, Ministry of Health, Shanghai, China, **3** The Institutes of Biomedical Sciences of Fudan University, Shanghai, China

Abstract

Background: Nitric oxide (NO) plays an important role in mobilization of endothelial progenitor cells (EPCs). We hypothesized that inhaled NO (iNO) would induce EPC mobilization and therefore promote lung repair in acute respiratory distress syndrome (ARDS).

Methodology/Principal Findings: Healthy piglets were randomized into four groups (n = 6): Control (Con; mechanical ventilation only); ARDS (established by oleic acid infusion and mechanical ventilation); ARDS plus granulocyte-colony stimulating factor (G-CSF; 10 μg/kg/d subcutaneously); ARDS plus NO inhalation (iNO; 10 ppm). EPCs and mobilizing cytokines were assayed at different time points (baseline, 0, 24, 72 and 168 h) and injury reparation was assessed at 168 h. Compared to the Con group, the levels of EPCs were increased in bone marrow but not in blood in the ARDS group at 24 h. Compared to the ARDS group, inhaled NO induced a rapid elevation in the number of $CD34^+KDR^+$, KDR^+CD133^+ and $CD34^+KDR^+CD133^+$ EPCs in blood (2163 ± 454 vs. 1094 ± 416, 1302 ± 413 vs. 429 ± 244, 1140 ± 494 vs. 453 ± 273 cells/ml, respectively, $P<0.05$), and a reduction in the percentage of KDR^+CD133^+ cells in bone marrow. Lung CD34, CD133, VEGF, VEGF receptor 2, endothelial NO synthase mRNA, and VEGF and VEGF receptor 2 protein expression levels were augmented in the iNO group, but not in the G-CSF group, compared to ARDS. Furthermore, iNO treatment reduced vascular permeability, increased pulmonary vessel density, and alleviated pulmonary edema and inflammation compared to ARDS treatment. Plasma VEGF, stromal cell-derived factor-1 (SDF-1) and bone marrow NO_2^-/NO_3^- were significantly higher in the iNO group compared to the ARDS group at 72 h.

Conclusions: These results suggest that iNO induces mobilization of EPCs from bone marrow into circulation, contributes to vascular repair, and thereby alleviates lung damage.

Editor: Rory Edward Morty, University of Giessen Lung Center, Germany

Funding: This work was supported by the National Natural Science Foundation of China (No. 30600687), Shanghai Rising-Star Program (No. 09QA1400700) and the Project 211 (phase III), Ministry of Education. The funders had no role in study design, data collection and analysis, decision to publish, or preparation of the manuscript.

Competing Interests: The authors have declared that no competing interests exist.

* E-mail: llqian@126.com

Introduction

Acute lung injury (ALI) and acute respiratory distress syndrome (ARDS) remain important challenges for pediatric intensive care units [1]. Mortality from ARDS approximates 40% despite the advances in supportive and pharmacologic treatment [2–4]. Diffuse endothelial damage plays a critical role in the pathogenesis of ALI/ARDS. Data from animal models of ALI demonstrate that up to 50% of lung capillaries are lost and large and small vessels within the lung are damaged during ALI/ARDS [5]. Regeneration of pulmonary endothelium has been suggested as one of the potential therapeutic targets for ARDS [6].

Accumulating evidence suggests that EPCs are mobilized from bone marrow and recruited into tissue to contribute to lung repair after injury. The number of EPCs has been shown to be acutely elevated in circulation, and this increase was associated with the repair of damaged pulmonary endothelium in mice with lung injury [7]. Moreover, patients with low EPC counts reportedly have persistent fibrotic changes in lung tissue after recovery from pneumonia [8], the numbers of EPCs were increased in ALI patients and an adverse outcome was associated with a lower EPC number [9]. Our previous study showed that the level of EPCs was increased in blood and unaltered in bone marrow in animals with moderate lung injury (200 mmHg$\leq PaO_2/FiO_2 \leq$300 mmHg). In contrast, the level of EPCs was unaltered in blood but elevated in bone marrow in animals with severe lung injury ($PaO_2/FiO_2\leq$200 mmHg; unpublished observations). These studies suggest that increased circulating EPCs contribute to lung repair in ALI, however the mobilization of EPCs from bone marrow is inhibited in severe lung injury, and thus a lack of sufficient EPCs in circulation might result in an impaired repair process. Therefore, we hypothesize that mobilization of EPCs might provide an effective strategy for restoring pulmonary endothelial function and reducing severity of ARDS.

Table 1. General conditions and oxygenation values at 0 h.

Group (n = 6)	Weight (kg)	Sex (M/F)	PaO_2/FiO_2 (mmHg)	Cdyn (ml/cmH_2O/kg)
Con	7.8±0.8	3/3	357±39.0	1.2±0.3
ARDS	8.3±1.4	3/3	133±15.0	0.5±0.2
G-CSF	8.3±0.7	4/2	140±22.1	0.6±0.1
iNO	8.8±0.9	2/4	135±25.3	0.6±0.1

Values are means ± SD. Cdyn, dynamic compliance.

Several cytokines have been used to mobilize EPCs from bone marrow in cardiovascular diseases [10]. However, currently the use of mobilizing cytokines in ALI is hampered by the fact that most powerful mobilizers, such as granulocyte colony-stimulating factor (G-CSF), also exert a pro-inflammatory effect and may have the potential to promote tumor growth [11]. There is a critical need to search for more safe and effective mobilizers for EPC therapy in ARDS.

Recent studies have demonstrated that endothelial nitric oxide synthase (eNOS) and nitric oxide (NO) play an important role in EPC mobilization [12–14]. eNOS transcription enhancer and NO donor supplementation could increase EPC number and improve EPC function in ischemic diseases [15–18]. Inhaled NO (iNO) was first used as a vasodilator to selectively dilate pulmonary vessels, and was then shown to have anti-inflammatory effects on the lung [19]. More recent studies have shown that iNO therapy could improve pulmonary angiogenesis. Experimental studies showed that iNO preserved vascular growth and enhanced alveolarisation in newborn rat models of vascular endothelial growth factor receptor (VEGFR2) inhibition, eNOS-deficient and hyperoxia [20–22]. Recently, it has been reported that iNO restored vessel density and improved lung structure in neonatal rat model of bronchopulmonary dysplasia (BPD) [23]. Our previous animal studies also indicated that inhaled NO can attenuate the lung

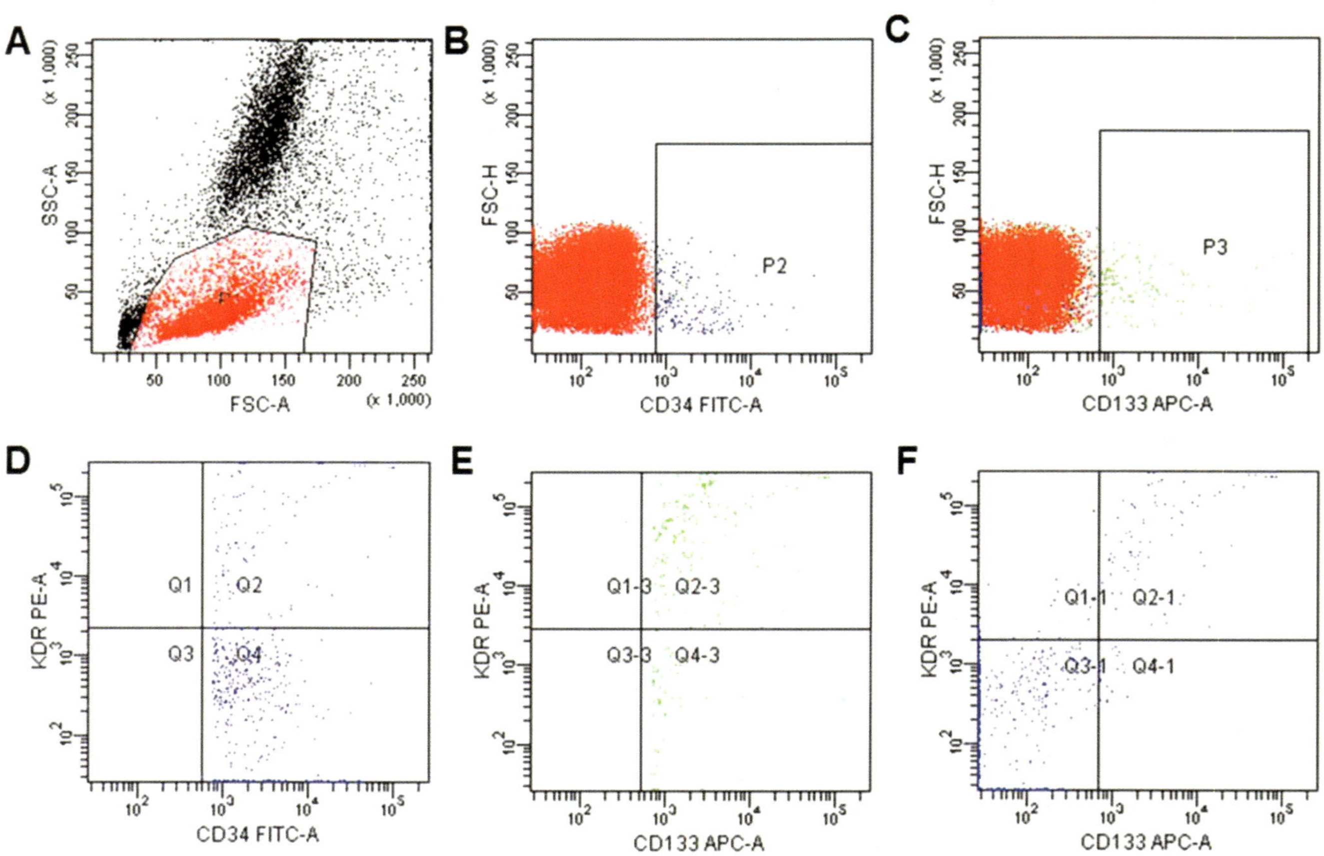

Figure 1. Representative cytograms for the determination of CD34$^+$, CD133$^+$, CD34$^+$KDR$^+$, KDR$^+$CD133$^+$ and CD34$^+$KDR$^+$CD133$^+$ cells from animals. (A) A gate P1 enclosing the mononuclear cells for further selection. P1 selected mononuclear cells are examined for the expression of CD34$^+$ cells (B) or CD133$^+$ cells(C). (D) CD34$^+$ events from P2 are examined further for the expression of VEGFR2 (KDR). (E) CD133$^+$ events from P3 are examined for the expression of KDR. (F) CD34$^+$ events from P2 are examined for expression of KDR and CD133. The upper right represents events that are CD34$^+$KDR$^+$CD133$^+$.

injury score in hyperoxic lung injury and ALI animals [24,25]. However, it is unknown whether iNO can mobilize bone marrow EPCs and consequently promote lung vascular repair.

The aim of this study was to observe the dynamic changes of circulating EPCs, and to further investigate the effect of iNO on EPC mobilization and lung vascular reparation in both acute and recovery phases, using an oleic acid induced ARDS model in young piglets.

Methods

Ethics statement

Animal study protocols were approved by the Scientific and Ethics Committees at Children's Hospital of Fudan University (Approval Number: 2007001), and were in compliance with the Chinese national regulations on the use of experimental animals.

Study animals and protocols

Twenty-four healthy piglets were used in this study. Each animal was anesthetized intramuscularly with 50 mg/kg ketamine and orally intubated with a cuffed endotracheal tube. Mechanical ventilation was initiated in pressure-control ventilation (PCV) mode (Servo 300, Siemens-Elema, Sweden), with a frequency of 15 breaths/min, a positive end-expiratory pressure (PEEP) of 2 cmH_2O, an inspiration time of 0.33 s, and an inspired oxygen fraction (FiO_2) of 0.21. The PEEP was adjusted to 6 cmH_2O after the induction of ARDS, and the ventilator settings were adjusted to provide a tidal volume of 6–8 ml/kg and to maintain target PaO_2 (>60 mmHg) and $PaCO_2$ (30–50 mmHg). The anesthesia was maintained by continuous infusion of ketamine (10 mg/kg/h) and fentanyl (5 µg/kg/h). A central venous catheter was placed into the right external jugular vein for drug administration. A thermodilution catheter (4 Fr, PiCCO plus system, Pulsion Medical Systems) was placed into the right internal carotid artery and connected to a PiCCOplus monitor (Pulsion Medical Systems). The baseline (B) was defined upon stabilization of animals after the operation.

The animals were randomly assigned into each of the following 4 groups (n = 6 each): Con group, where normal animals were ventilated; ARDS group, which was established and treated with mechanical ventilation; G-CSF group, where a subcutaneous injection of G-CSF (a commonly used agent for EPCs mobilizing) was administered to ARDS animals at a dose of 10 µg/kg daily for 7 days; and iNO group, where inhaled NO (10 ppm) was administered to ARDS animals during ventilation and NO gas at 1000 ppm (Noventek) was supplied to the inspiratory line of the ventilator circuit [25–27].

ARDS was established by a slow, 30-min intravenous infusion of 0.13–0.15 ml/kg oleic acid (01008; Sigma) suspended in 15 ml of saline via a central venous catheter. ARDS was defined as $PaO_2/FiO_2 \leq 200$ mmHg, with dynamic lung compliance (Cdyn) decreased by more than 50% from its baseline level, and histological evidence of bilateral infiltration of inflammatory cells in the lung (verified by our pilot study in 2 additional piglets) according to previous reports [25,26]. The moment lung injury was established was defined as treatment time 0 h. There were no differences in the body weight among the four groups, and no difference in PaO_2/FiO_2 and Cdyn was found among ARDS, iNO and G-CSF group at time 0 (Table 1, Table S1). Animals were ventilated for 48–72 h and then weaned and fed for recovery until day 7. At different time points (B, 0, 24, 72 and 168 h), blood or bone marrow samples were collected for further analysis.

Lung hemodynamics

Extravascular lung water (EVLW), EVLW index (ELWI) and pulmonary vascular permeability index (PVPI) were determined using the PiCCOplus monitor to evaluate the pulmonary vascular permeability and pulmonary edema at B, 0, 2, 6, 12 and 24 h.

Flow cytometric analysis

Blood was collected from the arterial catheter in each animal. Bone marrow was obtained by aspiration of the posterior iliac crest. The EPC levels were assessed by flow cytometry using cell surface antigens in different combinations ($CD34^+KDR^+$, KDR^+CD133^+, and $CD34^+KDR^+CD133^+$ cells) as previously reported [8,28,29]. Briefly, before staining with specific monoclonal antibodies, cells were treated with fetal calf serum for 10 minutes, and then the samples were washed with PBS. Then, 100 µl of peripheral blood or bone marrow sample was incubated with 10 µl FITC-conjugated CD34 monoclonal antibodies (mAbs) (348053, BD Biosciences, San Jose, CA, USA), 5 µl of APC-conjugated CD133 mAb (130-090-826, Miltenyi Biotec, Bergisch Gladbach, Germany), and 10 µl of PE-conjugated KDR mAb (FAB357P, R&D Systems, Minneapolis, MN), followed by incubation at 4°C for 30 min. Red cells were lysed and the frequency of EPCs was determined by a two-dimensional forward scatter/fluorescence dot plot analysis of the samples (FACSAria; BD Biosciences, Franklin Lakes, NJ). Isotype controls were used for setting gates and determining the positive/negative boundaries, and the analysis was confirmed by running the FMO (fluorescence-minus-one) controls. After morphological gating to exclude granulocyte and cell debris, we gated $CD34^+$ or $CD133^+$ cells and then examined the resulting population for dual expression of KDR, and triple positive cells were identified by the dual expression of KDR and CD133 in the CD34 gate (Figure 1A–F). About 500,000 cells were acquired. The levels of EPC were expressed as number of cells per milliliter of blood, and as percentage of total mononuclear cells (MNC) in bone marrow. We did not test the absolute number of EPCs in bone marrow due to the inability to obtain the bone marrow cell counts by the hematology analyzer. The same trained operator, who was blind to the experiment, performed all the tests throughout the study.

ELISA

The plasma concentrations of VEGF and stromal cell-derived factor-1 (SDF-1) were quantified by commercial ELISA kits. The ELISA was performed according to the manufacturer's instructions.

Lung processing

At the end of the experiment, the animals were sacrificed with intravenous injection of 10% potassium chloride. After the thorax was opened, lungs and heart were removed en bloc. Lung tissue from the tip of the right mid-lobe was used for wet-to-dry weight (W/D) ratio analysis. The rest of the mid-lobe was immediately frozen in liquid

Table 2. Primers used in quantitative PCR.

Gene	Forward-sense primer	Reverse-antisense primer
VEGFR2	5'CGGAAATGACACTGGAGC3'	5'TTCTGGATACCTCGCACA3'
CD34	5'ACTGCCTGCTGCTGGTCT3'	5'GCTCTGGTGGCTCCTAACAT3'
CD133	5'TCTTTTGTTCCTGCCGTTG3'	5'ACCATAGATGATACCGATGCTTA3'
VEGF	5'CCTTGCTGCTCTACCTCC3'	5'CTCCAGTCCTTCGTCGTT3'
eNOS	5'GTGGTAACCAGCACCTTTGG3'	5'GCAGGAAACACTATTGAAGC3'
GAPDH	5'GGTCGGAGTGAACGGATTTG3'	5'TTCTCAGCCTTGACTGTGCC3'

Table 3. Total numbers of WBCs ($\times 10^9$/L) in different groups at different time points.

Group	Baseline (n=6)	0 h (n=6)	24 h (n=6)	72 h (n=5–6)	168 h (n=5–6)
Con	19.1±3.5	18.4±3.3	19.2±4.1*	18.3±3.3	17.1±1.7*
ARDS	20.9±6.4	17.6±3.1	12.2±1.8†	15.9±1.5†	13.7±1.4†
G-CSF	18.1±3.6	16.8±2.8	30.5±9.1**†	38.3±21.5**†	42.6±29.8**†
iNO	21.3±5.9	18.6±4.4	19.5±8.1*	19.9±5.6	16.8±3.6

Values are means ± SD.
*$P<0.05$ vs. ARDS;
**$P<0.01$ vs. ARDS;
†$P<0.05$ vs. Baseline.

nitrogen for further measurement of RNA and protein. Bronchoalveolar lavage of the right lung was performed with sterile saline via an intracheal tube [30]. The left lung was fixed by perfusion for 30 min via the pulmonary artery with 4% paraformaldehyde in PBS. Lung permeability index (LPI) was measured by determining the ratio of bronchoalveolar lavage fluid protein to plasma protein.

Morphometric analysis

Sections stained with hematoxylin and eosin were examined by light microscopy for injury patterns and severity as assessed by lung injury scores for edema, neutrophil infiltration, hemorrhage and bronchiole epithelial desquamation [25,26,30].

Immunohistochemistry and vessel density

Fixed lungs were paraffin-embedded and sections were prepared by subsequent deparaffinization and rehydration [27]. The sections were incubated with rabbit polyclonal antibodies against factor VIII (CP039A, 1:200, Biocare Medical, Walnut Creek, USA), VEGFR2 (KDR) (ab45010, 1:100; Abcam, Cambridge, UK) and eNOS (ab5589, 1:100; Abcam, Cambridge, UK) at room temperature for 2 h and then overnight at 4°C. Sections were then incubated with corresponding biotinylated secondary antibodies for 45 min at 37°C followed by avidin-biotin-peroxidase for 45 min at 37°C (Vectastain Elite ABC kit; 1:200, Vector Laboratories). The sections were then developed with diaminobenzidine (DAB) and H_2O_2 and lightly counterstained with hematoxylin. To analyze the vessel density, 5 fields in each slice were randomly selected. The number of vessels was counted using a light microscope at 200× magnification. Results were expressed as number of vessels per field.

Apoptosis

Lung tissue was analyzed for terminal deoxynucleotidyl transferase dUTP-mediated nick-end labeling (TUNEL) using the DeadEnd Colorimetric TUNEL System (Promega, Madison, WI) according to the manufacturer' protocol. As a negative control, the TdT enzyme was omitted in parallel reactions. All sections were counterstained with hematoxylin after TUNEL staining. The ratio of TUNEL-positive cells to total cells (apoptotic index) was calculated from three random, non-overlapping fields at 400× magnification for each section.

Quantitative real-time PCR

Total lung RNA was extracted from frozen lung tissue using Trizol Reagent and was reverse-transcribed into cDNA. The primer sequences of target genes VEGF, VEGFR2, eNOS, CD34 and CD133 are described in Table 2. GAPDH was used as a loading control. Real-time PCR was conducted for quantitative analysis using SYBR Green PCR Master Mix as per manufacturer's instructions (TOYOBO, Japan). The endpoint used in the real-time PCR quantification was defined as the PCR cycle number that crossed the signal threshold (Ct). After validation of amplification efficiencies of two genes, quantification of target gene expression was calculated by the comparative Ct method.

Western blot analysis

Lung tissue samples were analyzed for VEGF and VEGFR2 protein expression with western blot analysis. Briefly, forty micrograms of total protein were separated by SDS-PAGE and then transferred to a nitrocellulose membrane by electroblotting. Blots were blocked for 2 h in 10% nonfat dry milk in TBST with 0.1% Tween 20 at room temperature. Immunodetection was performed

Table 4. EPC number in peripheral blood from animals of different groups.

	Group	Baseline (n=6)	0 h (n=6)	24 h (n=6)	72 h (n=5–6)	168 h (n=5–6)
$CD34^+KDR^+$ cells(cells/ml)	Con	1164±799	955±536	1238±643	1166±685	1032±634
	ARDS	1145±703	975±637	1094±416	1176±603	1024±330
	G-CSF	1160±440	966±539	1430±1011	4097±1468*	5715±3505*
	iNO	1151±277	955±375	2163±454*	2198±671*	2100±794*†
$CD34^+KDR^+CD133^+$ cells (cells/ml)	Con	424±314	478±381	497±268	400±216	455±287
	ARDS	404±275	423±278	453±273	366±191	313±198
	G-CSF	416±225	377±127	451±230	797±323	901±506*
	iNO	435±125	382±74	1140±494*†	822±321	739±303
KDR^+CD133^+ cells(cells/ml)	Con	486±364	509±375	544±303	498±276	507±227
	ARDS	459±300	356±202	429±244	468±249	406±281
	G-CSF	446±264	360±182	553±375	867±488	1420±572*
	iNO	514±175	442±113	1302±413*†	1056±347*	952±272*

Values are means ± SD.
*$P<0.05$ vs. ARDS;
†$P<0.05$ vs. G-CSF.

Table 5. EPC level in bone marrow from animals of different groups.

	Group	Baseline (n = 6)	24 h (n = 6)	72 h (n = 5–6)
$CD34^+KDR^+$ cells/MNC, %	Con	0.014±0.005	0.017±0.005	0.014±0.004
	ARDS	0.014±0.009	0.050±0.020†	0.018±0.005
	G-CSF	0.013±0.009	0.021±0.014	0.017±0.013
	iNO	0.012±0.006	0.026±0.014	0.015±0.008
$CD34^+KDR^+CD133^+$ cells/MNC, %	Con	0.008±0.003	0.011±0.003	0.007±0.003
	ARDS	0.007±0.004	0.022±0.007†	0.016±0.006
	G-CSF	0.008±0.005	0.009±0.004*	0.004±0.003
	iNO	0.008±0.004	0.012±0.005	0.007±0.004
KDR^+CD133^+ cells/MNC, %	Con	0.008±0.003	0.011±0.005	0.011±0.006
	ARDS	0.007±0.004	0.028±0.012†	0.014±0.005
	G-CSF	0.009±0.004	0.011±0.006*	0.005±0.003
	iNO	0.009±0.004	0.013±0.007*	0.008±0.003

Values are means ± SD. MNC, mononuclear cells.
*$P<0.05$ vs. ARDS;
†$P<0.05$ vs. Con.

with rabbit polyclonal VEGF antibody (bs-0279R, 1:500, Biosynthesis Biotechnology) and rabbit polyclonal VEGFR2 antibody (ab45010, 1:250, Abcam, Cambridge, UK) at room temperature for 1 h and overnight at 4°C. After the blots were washed to remove unbound antibody, a horseradish peroxidase-conjugated secondary antibody (Jackson Immunoresearch, West Grove, PA) was applied for 1 h at room temperature. After washing, bands were visualized with SuperSignal West Pico chemiluminescent substrate (Thermo Fisher Scientific, Rockford, IL). β-actin (bs-0061R, 1:500, Biosynthesis Biotechnology) was used as a loading control. Image J software was used to perform densitometry measurements.

NO assay

NO production in bone marrow plasma was evaluated by measuring the total NO_2^-/NO_3^- by Griess reaction (Nanjing Jiancheng Bioengineering Institute).

Gelatin zymography

Gelatin zymography was performed as described elsewhere [31]. Bone marrow samples were diluted in non-reducing sample buffer and 4 il of sample was added to each lane. The samples were electrophoresed in 10% polyacrylamide gels containing 2 mg/ml gelatin. After electrophoresis, gels were washed in 2.5% Triton X-100 for 1 h, incubated for 18 h at 37°C in development buffer, and stained for 3 h with 0.1% Coomassie Brilliant Blue. Gelatinolytic activity of matrix metallopeptidase 9 (MMP-9) was detected as transparent bands on the Coomassie Brilliant Blue-stained gels.

Statistical analysis

All the continuous data are presented as means and SD. Continuous parametric variables were subjected to ANOVA, followed by post-hoc test of Bonferroni for between-group differences, and by paired samples t test for within-group differences. Nonparametric variables were subjected to Kruskal-Wallis test for differences among groups, followed by Wilcoxon-Mann-Whitney test for between-group differences. A P value<0.05 was regarded as statistically significant.

Results

Inhaled NO induces rapid mobilization of bone marrow EPCs into circulation

In the G-CSF group, the WBC counts gradually increased compared to the ARDS group (Table 3). Moreover, the total

Table 6. Cytokine concentrations in plasma evaluated by ELISA.

Group	VEGF (ng/l)					SDF-1 (ìg/l)				
	Baseline (n = 6)	0 h (n = 6)	24 h (n = 6)	72 h (n = 5–6)	168 h (n = 5–6)	Baseline (n = 6)	0 h (n = 6)	24 h (n = 6)	72 h (n = 5–6)	168 h (n = 5–6)
Con	264±47.3	288±60.9	316±98.5	292±27.7	248±110	4.7±0.9	4.4±0.9	3.9±0.8	4.4±1.0	4.2±1.2
ARDS	299±33.7	294±54.8	314±116	256±81.1	257±83.9	4.4±0.5	5.4±0.8	4.1±1.2	4.3±1.3	4.0±1.2
G-CSF	279±29.0	316±33.3	309±63.3	387±45.1‡	293±76.5	5.1±1.3	3.9±1.3	4.1±1.2	4.3±0.8	4.4±1.4
iNO	308±27.8	331±40.1	357±44.9	478±63.3*§‡	352±31.9	5.1±1.2	5.0±1.2	5.1±0.9	6.0±1.2*†	5.8±0.6

Values are means ± SD.
*$P<0.05$ vs. ARDS;
§$P<0.05$ vs. Con;
†$P<0.05$ vs. Baseline,
‡$P<0.01$ vs. Baseline.

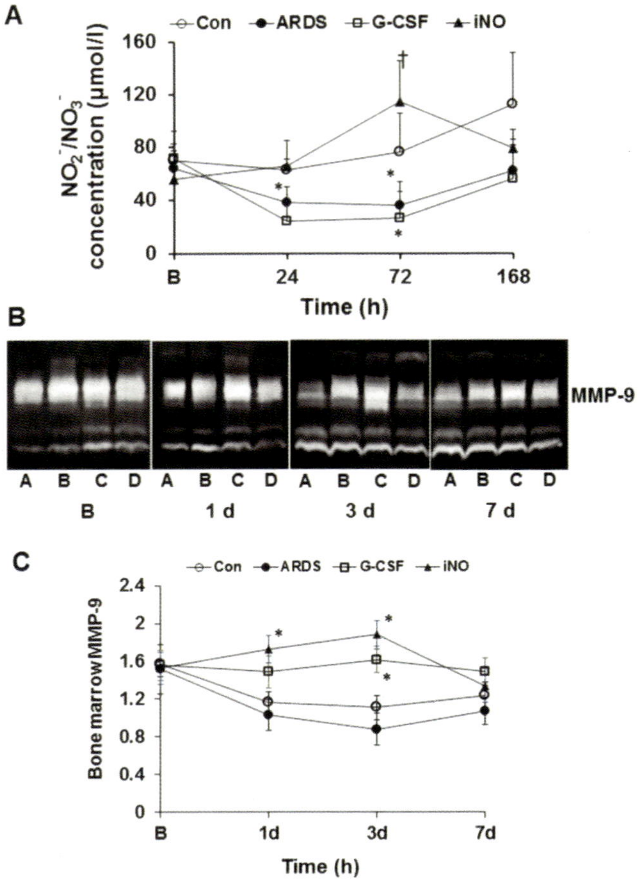

Figure 2. Effects of iNO on NO_2^-/NO_3^- and MMP-9 in bone marrow. (A) In the iNO group, the NO_2^-/NO_3^- concentration was increased at 72 h compared to the ARDS group. In the ARDS group, the NO_2^-/NO_3^- level decreased at 24 and 72 h compared to baseline. (B) MMP-9 expression measured by Zymography in bone marrow, A–D represent ARDS, G-CSF, iNO and Con, respectively. (C) Inhaled NO enhanced the MMP-9 expression at day 1 and 3. (* $P<0.05$ vs. B; † $P<0.05$ vs. ARDS group. n = 5–6 in each group).

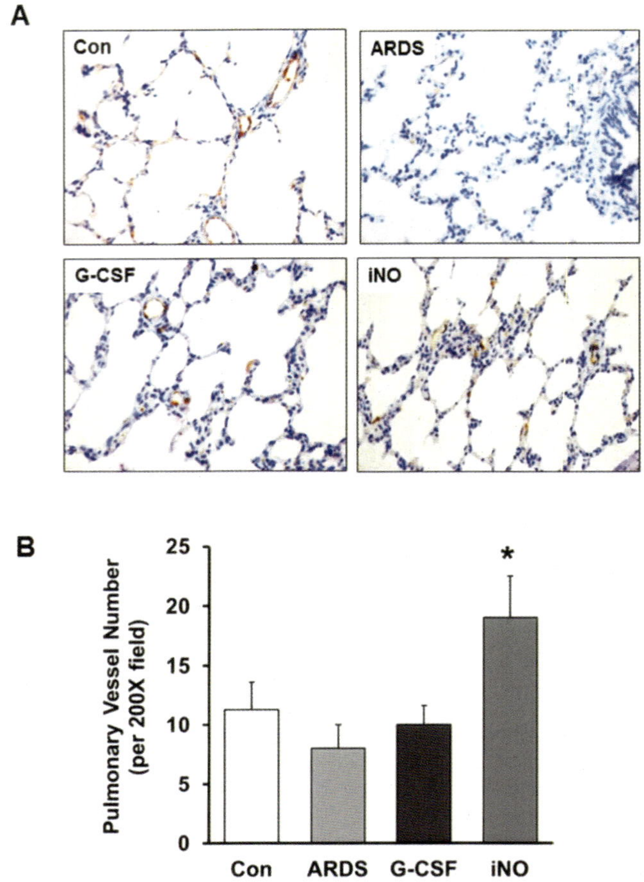

Figure 3. Vessel density of animals in different groups at day 7. (A) Representative photomicrographs (×400) illustrating Factor VIII staining to identify blood vessels in the lung. (B) The number of vessels per high-powered field is significantly higher in the iNO group relative to the ARDS group. (* $P<0.05$ vs. ARDS group, n = 5–6 in each group).

WBC counts fell dramatically at 24 h in ARDS group, G-CSF and iNO increased the WBC counts compared with ARDS (Table 3). There was no difference in the level of EPCs ($CD34^+KDR^+$, KDR^+CD133^+, and $CD34^+KDR^+CD133^+$ cells) among the four groups either in peripheral blood or in bone marrow at baseline (Table 4). In the blood, the numbers of various EPC types in the ARDS group did not differ from those in the Con group at any time point (Table 4). These results suggest impairment in EPC mobilization from bone marrow into circulation in ARDS. Inhaled NO significantly increased circulating EPC numbers (in all three EPC typs) compared to ARDS at 24 h, and this increase was sustained up to 168 h for $CD34^+KDR^+$ and KDR^+CD133^+ EPCs. The percentage of $CD34^+KDR^+$/MNC was also higher in iNO than ARDS at 24 and 72 h (Table S2). No differences were detected in the EPC numbers between G-CSF and ARDS at 24 h. However, we observed an elevation in the number of $CD34^+KDR^+$ cells at 72 h and in the number of all types of EPCs at 168 h in G-CSF compared to ARDS, along with

Table 7. Lung injury score, LPI and W/D ratio in different groups.

Group	Edema	Neutrophil infiltration	Hemorrhage	Bronchiole epithelial desquamation	W/D	LPI
Con (n = 6)	0.2±0.4	0.3±0.5	0.2±0.4	0.4±0.5	4.8±0.4	2.5±0.9
ARDS (n = 5)	1.3±0.9	2.0±1.2	1.5±1.2	1.4±0.6	5.9±0.3	11.4±5.0
G-CSF (n = 5)	0.4±0.5	2.3±0.9	0.3±0.5	0.6±0.4*	5.3±0.2	4.3±2.4*
iNO (n = 6)	0.3±0.5*	1.0±0*†	0.2±0.4	0.5±0.5*	5.2±0.3*	3.7±1.5*

Values are means ± SD. W/D, wet-to-dry lung weight ratio; LPI, lung permeability index.
*$P<0.05$ vs. ARDS,
†$P<0.05$ vs. G-CSF.

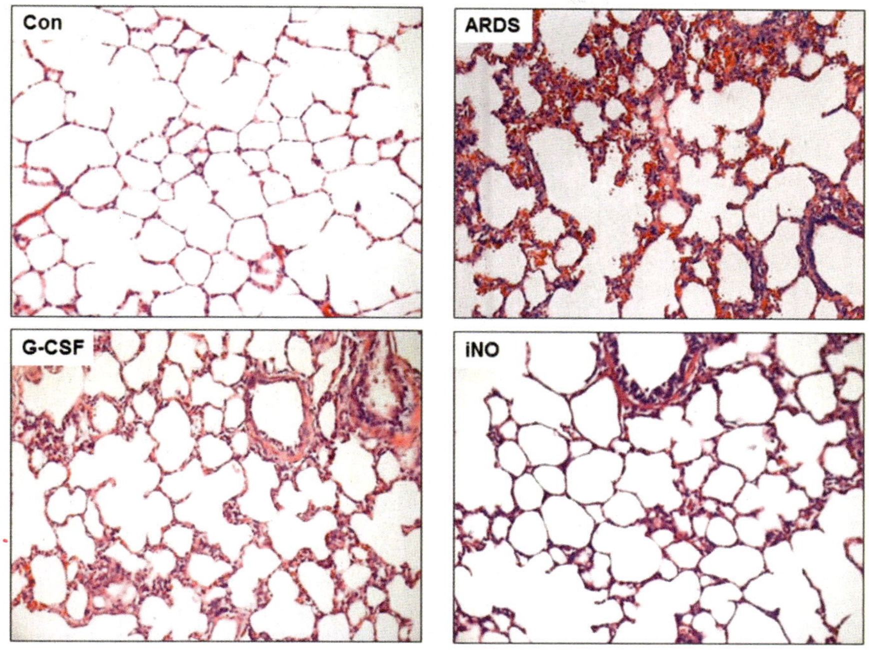

Figure 4. Lung histology from animals of different groups at day 7. Lung sections were stained with hematoxylin and eosin (HE) and inflammation cell infiltration, edema and hemorrhage were visualized at 200× magnification. Oleic acid and mechanical ventilation resulted in atelectatic, congested and edematous lung, with hemorrhagic spots in the lung. There was significantly alleviated edema, neutrophil infiltration and alveolar epithelial desquamation in the iNO group compared to the ARDS group.

elevation in the percentage of $CD34^+KDR^+$ at 72 h and $CD34^+KDR^+$ and KDR^+CD133^+ at day 7 (Table S2). The increase of $CD34^+KDR^+$ cells in the G-CSF group compared to ARDS group was more pronounced than that of the iNO group compared to ARDS group at 168 h.

In bone marrow, the percentages of all three types of EPCs were higher in ARDS versus Con at 24 h. Interestingly, iNO and G-CSF reduced the percentage of KDR^+CD133^+ cells in bone marrow at 24 h compared to the ARDS. The percentage of $CD34^+KDR^+CD133^+$ EPCs was also lower in the G-CSF group relative to ARDS group. There was a trend towards a reduction in the percentage of bone marrow $CD34^+KDR^+$ cells in both iNO and G-CSF groups compared to ARDS at 24 h (Table 5).

Effects of iNO on plasma and bone marrow EPC mobilizing cytokines during lung injury

There was no significant difference in plasma SDF-1 and VEGF concentrations between groups at baseline (Table 6). The plasma VEGF and SDF-1 levels were not change significantly different between ARDS and Con at any time point. In comparison with the ARDS group, the iNO group showed an elevation in the plasma VEGF (256±81.1 vs. 478±63.3 ng/l, $p<0.05$, respectively) and SDF-1 (4.3±1.3 vs. 6.0±1.2 μg/l, $p<0.05$, respectively) at 72 h. G-CSF treatment increased the VEGF concentration but did not affect the level of SDF-1 at any time point.

No significant difference was observed in bone marrow plasma NO_2^-/NO_3^- concentrations between groups at baseline. ARDS animals demonstrated a marked decline in the concentrations of NO_2^-/NO_3^- at 24 and 72 h (Figure 2A). The NO_2^-/NO_3^- level in bone marrow was higher in iNO animals versus ARDS at 72 h (Figure 2A). However, NO_2^-/NO_3^- was not increased in bone marrow in the G-CSF group.

Gelatin zymography analysis demonstrated that, compared to ARDS, iNO augmented the expression of MMP-9 in bone marrow at 24 and 72 h, while bone marrow MMP-9 expression was increased in the G-CSF group at 72 h (Figure 2B and C).

Inhaled NO restores lung vascular growth and improves lung histology via EPC mobilization

There was a trend towards improvement in ELWI and PVPI in the iNO and G-CSF groups, whereas the ARDS group showed deterioration, during the first 12 h. The values of ELWI and PVPI were dramatically decreased in iNO compared to ARDS (13.2±1.6 vs. 24.7±9.2 and 4.6±0.6 vs. 6.1±1.1, respectively) at 24 h. The LPI was lower in iNO than in ARDS. The Lung W/D ratio was also decreased in the iNO group compared to the ARDS group at day 7 (Table 7).

The iNO animals exhibited higher factor VIII-positive vessel density than the ARDS group (Figure 3A and B). G-CSF treatment did not significantly change the vessel density compared to the ARDS group.

Lung histology from the ARDS group was characterized by atelectatic, congested and edematous with hemorrhagic spots (Figure 4). As indicated by the lung injury score, there was mildly less severe hemorrhage, but dramatically alleviated edema, neutrophil infiltration and alveolar epithelial desquamation in the iNO group compared to the ARDS group (Table 7). There was also attenuated alveolar epithelial desquamation in the G-CSF group. However, lung inflammation was more prominent in the G-CSF than the iNO group.

TUNEL staining exhibited little or no labeling in Con animals, while more cells with intense labeling were present in lungs of ARDS group animals. The apoptotic index was markedly reduced in the iNO group compared to the ARDS group (Figure 5).

CD34 mRNA level did not change greatly in the ARDS group, as compared to Con. CD34 mRNA expression was 4-fold greater in the iNO group than in the ARDS group. CD133 mRNA expression was also elevated in the iNO group compared to the

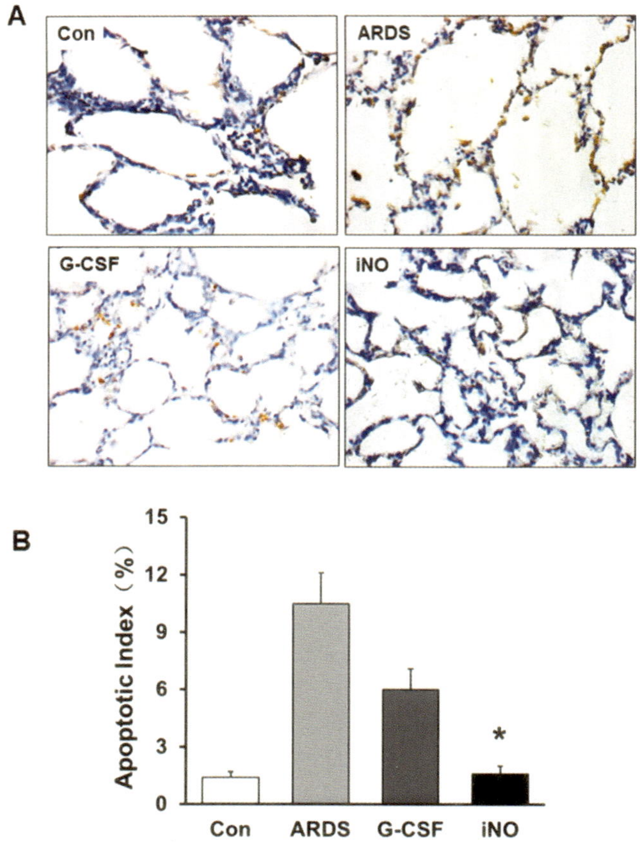

Figure 5. Effects of iNO on apoptosis of lung tissue cells at day 7. (A) Representative images of lung sections showing the TUNEL staining. (B) Bar graph showed the ratio of TUNEL-positive cells was decreased in the iNO group compared to the ARDS group. (* $P<0.05$ vs. ARDS group, n = 5–6 in each group).

ARDS group (Figure 6). No difference was found in CD34 and CD133 mRNA expression between G-CSF and ARDS groups.

Inhaled NO increases VEGF, VEGFR2, and eNOS expression

There was no difference in VEGF and VEGFR2 mRNA expression between ARDS and Con groups. Lung VEGF and VEGFR2 mRNA expression was significantly higher in iNO animals, but not G-CSF animals, compared to ARDS (Figure 7A). As determined by western blot analysis, lung VEGF and VEGFR2 protein was elevated in iNO relative to ARDS (Figure 7B). Moreover, immunochemistry of lung sections also showed stronger VEGFR2 staining in the iNO group than in the ARDS group (Figure 7C). Increased eNOS mRNA expression was also noted in the iNO group, as reflected by the immunohistochemical staining (Figure 8A and B).

Discussion

Diffuse endothelial damage is a hallmark of ARDS. Potential therapies targeted at repair of endothelial damage have not been thoroughly explored. It is believed that EPCs could be a prognostic biological marker and that EPC mobilization could ameliorate lung injury. However, little is known about the dynamics of EPC mobilization and homing during the course of ARDS or the long term therapeutic efficacy of EPC mobilization on lung vascular and tissue repair.

To date, no consensus has yet been reached on the definition of EPCs or methods for their identification. The $CD34^+$ KDR^+CD133^+ cells are widely accepted as circulating EPC. Flow cytometric analyses of three surface antigens and corresponding subpopulations of EPCs ($CD34^+KDR^+$, KDR^+CD133^+ and $CD34^+KDR^+CD133^+$ cells) have been used for EPCs enumeration, and have been shown to correlate with severity of disease state in many studies [8,28,32]. Subsequently, some studies indicated different phenotype of EPC, for example, Case et al [33] reported that $CD34^+CD133^+VEGFR2^+$ cells do not spontaneously form capillary-like structures with lumens. Further studies are required regarding the specific phenotypic of EPC to develop the consensus definition on EPC and to understand its role in vascular repair. Despite the controversy, the triple-positive cell population was still used for the enumeration of EPC in recent published articles [34,35]. Therefore, we still chose the combinations of antigens to detect different EPC populations.

Previous studies have shown that bone marrow EPCs are released into peripheral blood during ALI/ARDS [7,8], and notably, an insufficient number of circulating EPCs has been correlated with adverse outcomes in ARDS [8,9]. Recent evidence suggests that intravenous EPC transplantation promotes the integrity of lung vessels after lung injury [36–38]. However, the clinical application of cell-therapy is limited by several factors, such as the scarcity of circulating EPCs and the technical difficulty

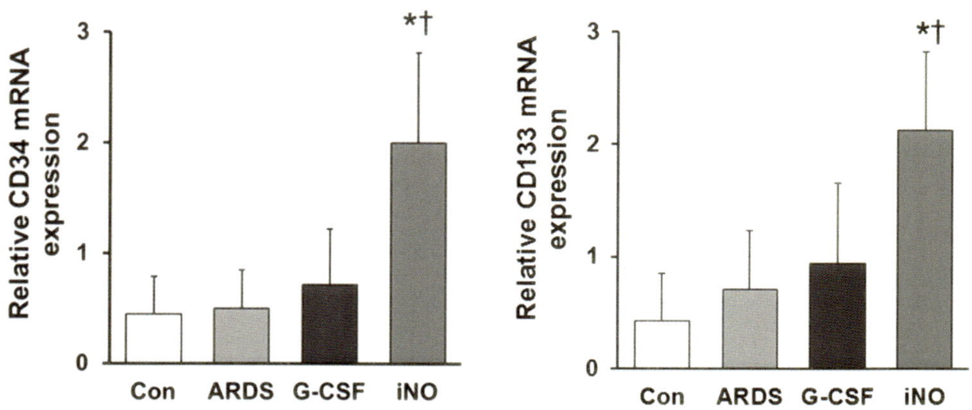

Figure 6. Lung CD34 and CD133 mRNA expression at day 7. In the iNO group, lung CD34 (A) and CD133 (B) mRNA levels were increased compared to the Con and ARDS groups. (* $P<0.05$ vs. ARDS group; † $P<0.05$ vs. Con group; n = 5–6 in each group).

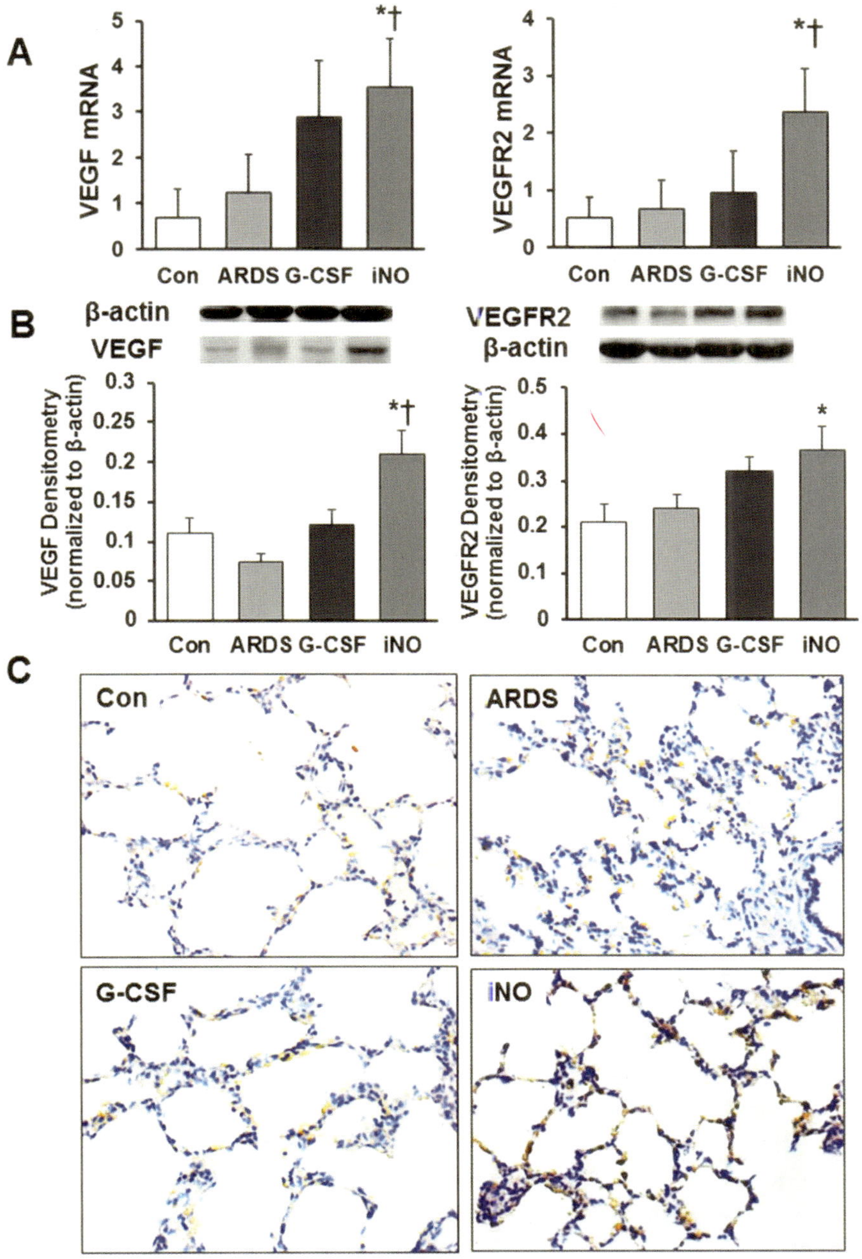

Figure 7. Effects of iNO on lung VEGF and VEGFR2 expression at day 7. (A) VEGF and VEGFR2 mRNA expression levels (normalized to GAPDH) were increased in the iNO group compared to the ARDS and Con groups. (B) Representative blots for VEGF and VEGFR2 (top) and bar graph for band densitometry (bottom). (C) Representative immunohistochemical images showed enhanced VEGFR2 expression in the iNO group compared to the ARDS group. (* $P<0.05$ vs. ARDS group; † $P<0.05$ vs. Con group. n = 5–6 in each group).

of purifying EPCs. Exogenous mobilization of EPCs from bone marrow may provide a less cumbersome and potentially more effective strategy to achieve therapeutic angiogenesis. G-CSF is one of the prototypical mobilizing cytokines that has been used for stem cell and EPC mobilization in cardiovascular diseases. NO-mediated EPC release into circulation and subsequent angiogenesis has been described previously. Inhaled NO has been demonstrated to improve oxygenation and preserve vascular growth of lung in a BPD model [21–23]. In the present study, we used iNO treatment as a strategy to stimulate the mobilization of EPCs and compared its effects with G-CSF. Our results showed that G-CSF mobilized EPCs from the bone marrow after 3 days' administration, which was consistent with previous reports [39], but iNO treatment increased the number of EPCs more rapidly than G-CSF. Higher levels of EPCs in the blood were observed on day 7 in the G-CSF group, possibly due to the 7 day administration of G-CSF, while NO inhalation was only administered for 48–72 h along with mechanical ventilation. These findings suggest that iNO has a profound effect on EPC mobilization.

It is well established that endothelial-active cytokines, such as VEGF and SDF-1 induce EPC mobilization [10]. Previous studies have demonstrated that activation of VEGF/eNOS signaling induces bone marrow NO production and subsequent up-regulation of MMP-9 expression [40]. Of interest here, plasma concentrations of SDF-1 and VEGF were elevated in the iNO

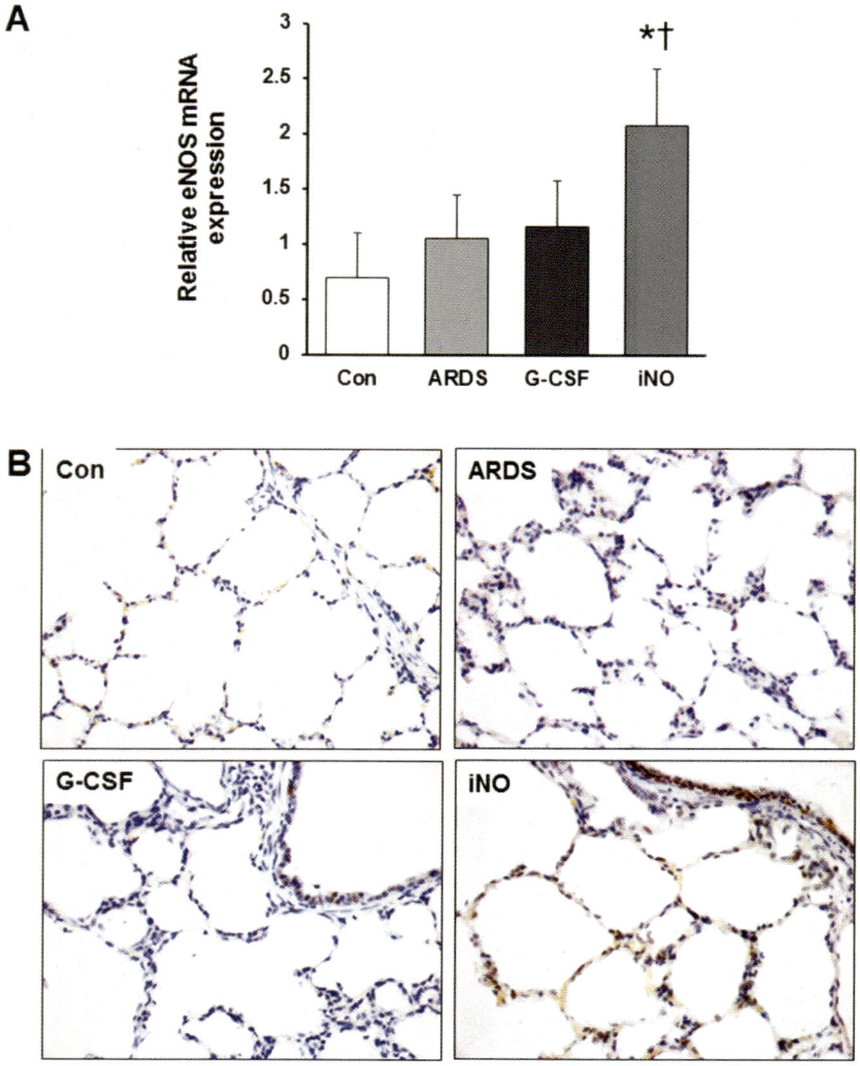

Figure 8. Effects of iNO on lung eNOS expression at day 7. (A) eNOS mRNA expression (normalized to GAPDH) increased in the iNO group compared to the Con group. (B) Representative immunohistochemical images show enhanced eNOS expression in iNO relative to ARDS. (* $P<0.05$ vs. Con group. n = 5–6 in each group).

group. Moreover, we also found that iNO increased MMP-9 expression in bone marrow. These data suggest a possible mechanism whereby iNO acts to increase the mobilization factors, SDF-1 and VEGF, and therefore promote EPC mobilization. However, the precise mechanism by which inhaled NO enhances EPC mobilization and improves the lung repair remains to be defined.

Mobilization of EPCs might result in accelerated regeneration and a promotion in the repair process of injured vessels [41]. We found that iNO promoted the integrity of pulmonary endothelium, increased the vascular density and alleviated the lung histological injury compared to ARDS. Multiple lines of evidence suggest that EPCs are recruited to sites of injury and participate in the tissue repair [42]. Here, we showed that iNO treatment augmented the mRNA expression of EPC surface markers CD34 and CD133 in lung tissue. VEGF is an important growth factor in vasculogenesis and angiogenesis during lung development. Moreover, accumulating evidence suggests that VEGF and eNOS play critical roles in EPC mobilization, adhesion and incorporation into damaged vessels [12,43,44]. VEGF exerts its biological effect on vascular endothelium through specific receptors, especially VEGFR2. In accordance with previous studies [20,23,45], we found that iNO up-regulated VEGF and VEGFR2 expression in the lung on day 7, compared to the ARDS group. Our data also showed that iNO enhanced the lung tissue eNOS expression. Collectively, our data suggests that inhaled NO promotes angiogenesis and reendothelization of pulmonary vascular endothelium, thereby improving lung repair. The beneficial effects of iNO are likely due to the promotion of mobilization and homing of EPCs.

One of the major limitations of this study is that we did not measure the EPC number in lung tissue and therefore were unable to evaluate the incorporation of circulating EPCs into the lung. However, we determined the CD34 and CD133 mRNA expression levels, which partially reflects the EPC levels in lung. The effects of iNO on the VEGF/eNOS or SDF/CXCR4 signal pathways of EPCs homing and recruitment have not been demonstrated. Some studies showed that multiple pathways affect trafficking of EPCs to sites of injury. More studies are needed to determine the role of iNO on homing and recruitment of EPCs to lung tissue. In addition, studies have shown that the role of EPCs is not only to repair or regenerate damaged vasculature, but also to produce several cytokines, such as IL-10. Cytokine levels were not examined in this study.

In conclusion, we have provided substantial evidence demonstrating that inhaled NO mobilizes bone marrow EPCs into circulation and attenuates damage of lung alveolar-capillary barrier in ARDS. These findings suggest a feasible therapy for ARDS. The mechanism of EPC mobilization, homing to injured lungs and subsequent involvement in lung repair is a more complicated process, requiring further investigation.

Supporting Information

Table S1 Blood gas values and PaO_2/FiO_2 during ventilation time.

Table S2 The number of EPCs/MNC in peripheral blood at different time points.

Author Contributions

Conceived and designed the experiments: YQ LQ BS. Performed the experiments: YQ LL PW LS. Analyzed the data: YQ LL. Contributed reagents/materials/analysis tools: YQ LQ BS. Wrote the paper: YQ LQ BS.

References

1. Ware LB, Matthay MA (2000) The acute respiratory distress syndrome. N Engl J Med 342: 1334–1349.
2. The Acute Respiratory Distress Syndrome Network (2003) Effects of recruitment maneuvers in patients with acute lung injury and acute respiratory distress syndrome ventilated with high positive end-expiratory pressure. Crit Care Med 31: 2592–2597.
3. The National Heart, Lung, and Blood Institute Acute Respiratory Distress Syndrome (ARDS) Clinical Trials Network (2006) Efficacy and safety of corticosteroids for persistent acute respiratory distress syndrome. N Engl J Med 354: 1671–1684.
4. The National Heart, Lung, and Blood Institute Acute Respiratory Distress Syndrome (ARDS) Clinical Trials Network (2006) Comparison of two fluid management strategies in acute lung injury. N Engl J Med 354: 2564–2575.
5. Tomashefski JF, Jr., Davies P, Boggis C, Greene R, Zapol WM, et al. (1983) The pulmonary vascular lesions of the adult respiratory distress syndrome. Am J Pathol 112: 112–126.
6. Orfanos SE, Mavrommati I, Korovesi I, Roussos C (2004) Pulmonary endothelium in acute lung injury: From basic science to the critically ill. Intensive Care Med 30: 1702–1714.
7. Yamada M, Kubo H, Kobayashi S, Ishizawa K, Numasaki M, et al. (2004) Bone marrow-derived progenitor cells are important for lung repair after lipopolysaccharide-induced lung injury. J Immunol 172: 1266–1272.
8. Yamada M, Kubo H, Ishizawa K, Kobayashi S, Shinkawa M, et al. (2005) Increased circulating endothelial progenitor cells in patients with bacterial pneumonia: evidence that bone marrow derived cells contribute to lung repair. Thorax 60: 410–413.
9. Burnham EL, Taylor WR, Quyyumi AA, Rojas M, Brigham KL, et al. (2005) Increased circulating endothelial progenitor cells are associated with survival in acute lung injury. Am J Respir Crit Care Med 172: 854–860.
10. Aicher A, Zeiher AM, Dimmeler S (2005) Mobilizing endothelial progenitor cells. Hypertension 45: 321–325.
11. Natori T, Sata M, Washida M, Hirata Y, Nagai R, et al. (2002) G-CSF stimulates angiogenesis and promotes tumor growth: potential contribution of bone marrow-derived endothelial progenitor cells. Biochem Biophys Res Commun 297: 1058–1061.
12. Aicher A, Heeschen C, Mildner-Rihm C, Urbich C, Ihling C, et al. (2003) Essential role of endothelial nitric oxide synthase for mobilization of stem and progenitor cells. Nat Med 9: 1370–1376.
13. Duda DG, Fukumura D, Jain RK (2004) Role of eNOS in neovascularization: NO for endothelial progenitor cells. Trends Mol Med 10: 143–145.
14. Leone AM, Valgimigli M, Giannico MB, Zaccone V, Perfetti M, et al. (2009) From bone marrow to the arterial wall: the ongoing tale of endothelial progenitor cells. Eur Heart J 30: 890–899.
15. Sasaki K, Heeschen C, Aicher A, Ziebart T, Honold J, et al. (2006) Ex vivo pretreatment of bone marrow mononuclear cells with endothelial NO synthase enhancer AVE9488 enhances their functional activity for cell therapy. Proc Natl Acad Sci USA 103: 14537–14541.
16. Segal MS, Shah R, Afzal A, Perrault CM, Chang K, et al. (2006) Nitric oxide cytoskeletal-induced alterations reverse the endothelial progenitor cell migratory defect associated with diabetes. Diabetes 55: 102–109.
17. Chen YH, Lin SJ, Lin FY, Wu TC, Tsao CR, et al. (2007) High glucose impairs early and late endothelial progenitor cells by modifying nitric oxide-related but not oxidative stress mediated mechanisms. Diabetes 56: 1559–1568.
18. Javanmard SH, Gheisari Y, Soleimani M, Nematbakhsh M, Monajemi A (2010) Effect of L-arginine on circulating endothelial progenitor cells in hypercholesterolemic rabbits. Int J Cardiol 143: 213–216.
19. Thomassen MJ, Buhrow LT, Connors MJ, Kaneko FT, Erzurum SC, et al. (1997) Nitric oxide inhibits inflammatory cytokine production by human alveolar macrophages. Am J Respir Cell Mol Biol 17: 279–283.
20. Tang JR, Markham NE, Lin YJ, McMurtry IF, Maxey A, et al. (2004) Inhaled nitric oxide attenuates pulmonary hypertension and improves lung growth in infant rats after neonatal treatment with a VEGF receptor inhibitor. Am J Physiol Lung Cell Mol Physiol 287: L344–L351.
21. Balasubramaniam V, Maxey AM, Morgan DB, Markham NE, Abman SH (2006) Inhaled NO restores lung structure in eNOS-deficient mice recovering from neonatal hypoxia. Am J Physiol Lung Cell Mol Physiol 291: L119–L127.
22. Lin YJ, Markham NE, Balasubramaniam V, Tang JR, Maxey A, et al. (2005) Inhaled nitric oxide enhances distal lung growth after exposure to hyperoxia in neonatal rats. Pediatr Res 58: 22–29.
23. Tourneux P, Markham N, Seedorf G, Balasubramaniam V, Abman SH (2009) Inhaled nitric oxide improves lung structure and pulmonary hypertension in a model of bleomycin-induced bronchopulmonary dysplasia in neonatal rats. Am J Physiol Lung Cell Mol Physiol 297: L1103–L1111.
24. Hu XW, Guo CB, BoSun (2007) Inhaled nitric oxide attenuates hyperoxic and inflammatory injury without alteration of phosphatidylcholine synthesis in rat lungs. Pulm Pharmacol Ther 20: 75–84.
25. Song J, Palmer K, Sun B (2010) Effects of inhaled nitric oxide and surfactant with extracorporeal life support in recovery phase of septic acute lung injury in piglets. Pulm Pharmacol Ther 23: 78–87.
26. Zhu YR, Guo CB, Cao L, Gong XH, Wang CQ, et al. (2005) Different effects of surfactant and inhaled nitric oxide in modulation of inflammatory injury in ventilated piglet lungs. Pulm Pharmacol Ther 18: 303–313.
27. Qian L, Liu H, Yu W, Wang X, Sun Z, et al. (2008) Effects of positive end-expiratory pressure, inhaled nitric oxide and surfactant on expression of proinflammatory cytokines and growth factors in preterm piglet lungs. Pediatr Res 64: 17–23.
28. Fadini GP, Sartore S, Albiero M, Baesso I, Murphy E, et al. (2006) Number and function of endothelial progenitor cells as a marker of severity for diabetic vasculopathy. Arterioscler Thromb Vasc Biol 26: 2140–2146.
29. Kondo T, Hayashi M, Takeshita K, Numaguchi Y, Kobayashi K, et al. (2004) Smoking cessation rapidly increases circulating progenitor cells in peripheral blood in chronic smokers. Arterioscler Thromb Vasc Biol 24: 1442–1447.
30. Zhou ZH, Sun B, Lin K, Zhu LW (2000) Prevention of rabbit acute lung injury by surfactant, inhaled nitric oxide, and pressure support ventilation. Am J Respir Crit Care Med 161: 581–588.
31. Hawkes SP, Li H, Taniguchi GT (2001) Zymography and reverse zymography for detecting MMPs, and TIMPs. Clark II (Ed.), Matrix Metalloproteinases Protocols. Humana Press. pp 399–410.
32. Timmermans F, Plum J, Yoder MC, Ingram DA, Vandekerckhove B, et al. (2009) Endothelial progenitor cells: identity defined? J Cell Mol Med 13: 87–102.
33. Case J, Mead LE, Bessler WK, Prater D, White HA, et al. (2007) Human CD341AC1331VEGFR-2 cells are not endothelial progenitor cells but distinct, primitive hematopoietic progenitors. Exp Hematol 35: 1109–1118.
34. Kheirandish-Gozal L, Bhattacharjee R, Kim J, Clair HB, Gozal D (2010) Endothelial progenitor cells and vascular dysfunction in children with obstructive sleep apnea. Am J Respir Crit Care Med 182: 92–97.
35. Padfield GJ, Tura O, Haeck ML, Short A, Freyer E, et al. (2010) Circulating endothelial progenitor cells are not affected by acute systemic inflammation. Am J Physiol Heart Circ Physiol 298: H2054–2061.
36. Lam CF, Liu YC, Hsu JK, Yeh PA, Su TY, et al. (2008) Autologous Transplantation of Endothelial Progenitor Cells Attenuates Acute Lung Injury in Rabbits. Anesthesiology 108: 392–401.
37. Kähler CM, Wechselberger J, Hilbe W, Gschwendtner A, Colleselli D, et al. (2007) Peripheral infusion of rat bone marrow derived endothelial progenitor cells leads to homing in acute lung injury. Respir Res 8: 50.
38. Balasubramaniam V, Ryan SL, Seedorf GJ, Roth EV, Heumann TR, et al. (2010) Bone marrow-derived angiogenic cells restore lung alveolar and vascular structure after neonatal hyperoxia in infant mice. Am J Physiol Lung Cell Mol Physiol 298: L315–L323.
39. Pitchford SC, Furze RC, Jones CP, Wengner AM, Rankin SM (2009) Differential Mobilization of Subsets of Progenitor Cells from the Bone Marrow. Cell Stem Cell 4: 62–72.

40. Fukumura D, Gohongi T, Kadambi A, Izumi Y, Ang J, et al. (2001) Predominant role of endothelial nitric oxide synthase in vascular endothelial growth factor-induced angiogenesis and vascular permeability. Proc Natl Acad Sci USA 98: 2604–2609.
41. Kong D, Melo LG, Gnecchi M, Zhang L, Mostoslavsky G, et al. (2004) Cytokine-induced mobilization of circulating endothelial progenitor cells enhances repair of injured arteries. Circulation 110: 2039–2046.
42. Dzau VJ, Gnecchi M, Pachori AS, Morello F, Melo LG (2005) Therapeutic potential of endothelial progenitor cells in cardiovascular diseases. Hypertension 46: 7–18.
43. Balasubramaniam V, Mervis CF, Maxey AM, Markham NE, Abman SH (2007) Hyperoxia reduces bone marrow, circulating, and lung endothelial progenitor cells in the developing lung: implications for the pathogenesis of bronchopulmonary dysplasia. Am J Physiol Lung Cell Mol Physiol 292: L1073–L1084.
44. Voelkel NF, Vandivier RW, Tuder RM (2006) Vascular endothelial growth factor in the lung. Am J Physiol Lung Cell Mol Physiol 290: L209–L221.
45. Lopez E, Boucherat O, Franco-Montoya ML, Bourbon JR, Delacourt C, et al. (2006) Nitric oxide donor restores lung growth factor and receptor expression in hyperoxia-exposed rat pups. Am J Respir Cell Mol Biol 34: 738–745.

12

Curcumin Modulates the Inflammatory Response and Inhibits Subsequent Fibrosis in a Mouse Model of Viral-induced Acute Respiratory Distress Syndrome

Sreedevi Avasarala[❡¤], **Fangfang Zhang**[❡], **Guangliang Liu, Ruixue Wang, Steven D. London, Lucille London***

Department of Oral Biology and Pathology, School of Dental Medicine, Stony Brook University, Stony Brook, New York, United States of America

Abstract

Acute Respiratory Distress Syndrome (ARDS) is a clinical syndrome characterized by diffuse alveolar damage usually secondary to an intense host inflammatory response of the lung to a pulmonary or extrapulmonary infectious or non-infectious insult often leading to the development of intra-alveolar and interstitial fibrosis. Curcumin, the principal curcumoid of the popular Indian spice turmeric, has been demonstrated as an anti-oxidant and anti-inflammatory agent in a broad spectrum of diseases. Using our well-established model of reovirus 1/L-induced acute viral pneumonia, which displays many of the characteristics of the human ALI/ARDS, we evaluated the anti-inflammatory and anti-fibrotic effects of curcumin. Female CBA/J mice were treated with curcumin (50 mg/kg) 5 days prior to intranasal inoculation with 10^7 PFU reovirus 1/L and daily, thereafter. Mice were evaluated for key features associated with ALI/ARDS. Administration of curcumin significantly modulated inflammation and fibrosis, as revealed by histological and biochemical analysis. The expression of IL-6, IL-10, IFNγ, and MCP-1, key chemokines/cytokines implicated in the development of ALI/ARDS, from both the inflammatory infiltrate and whole lung tissue were modulated by curcumin potentially through a reduction in the phosphorylated form of NFκB p65. While the expression of TGFß1 was not modulated by curcumin, TGFß Receptor II, which is required for TGFß signaling, was significantly reduced. In addition, curcumin also significantly inhibited the expression of α-smooth muscle actin and Tenascin-C, key markers of myofibroblast activation. This data strongly supports a role for curcumin in modulating the pathogenesis of viral-induced ALI/ARDS in a pre-clinical model potentially manifested through the alteration of inflammation and myofibroblast differentiation.

Editor: Raju Reddy, University of Pittsburgh, United States of America

Funding: This work was supported by a U.S. Public Health Service grant NCCAM 5R21AT003824 (LL)(http://nccam.nih.gov/). The funders had no role in study design, data collection and analysis, decision to publish, or preparation of the manuscript.

Competing Interests: The authors have declared that no competing interests exist.

* E-mail: lucille.london@stonybrook.edu

❡ These authors contributed equally to this work.

¤ Current address: Department of Medicine, University of Colorado, Aurora, Colorado, United States of America

Introduction

Acute Respiratory Distress Syndrome (ARDS), the most severe form of acute lung injury (ALI), is a clinical manifestation of the response of the lung to pulmonary insults brought on by infectious, non-infectious and other damaging events and affects up to 200,000 patients annually in the US with a mortality rate approaching 50% with inflammation and tissue fibrosis being the leading cause of morbidity and mortality [1,2]. Pulmonary fibrosis, itself, is a devastating disease with an almost universally terminal outcome affecting five million people worldwide, including some 200,000 cases culminating in 40,000 deaths/year in the US [3]. Factors that predispose to ARDS are diverse and include sepsis, aspiration, and pneumonias [1,2]. Although supportive therapy has improved survival somewhat, there are no effective therapeutic agents for improving clinical outcomes in ARDS patients [1,2]. Therefore, there is an urgent need for the development of treatments to halt the progression of this devastating syndrome.

There are limited models to study ALI/ARDS and no good model systems currently available to study ALI/ARDS and/or pulmonary fibrosis initiated by an infectious (viral) insult [4]. Pulmonary infection of CBA/J mice with 10^7 PFU reovirus serotype 1, strain Lang (reovirus 1/L) induces ALI/ARDS, providing a model that recapitulates both its acute exudative phase, including the formation of hyaline membranes, as well as its regenerative phase with healing by repair, leading to intra-alveolar and interstitial fibrosis [5,6]. As with ARDS in human patients, corticosteroids were ineffective in attenuating the infiltration of inflammatory leukocytes, suppressing key cytokine/chemokine expression, and inhibiting the development of fibrotic lesions in reovirus 1/L-ALI/ARDS [7,8]. Finally, aberrant apoptosis has been proposed as one mechanism leading to fibrotic lesion development in ALI/ARDS, and we have demonstrated an indirect role for the Fas/FasL pathway in reovirus 1/L-ALI/ARDS [9]. Therefore, our model provides a very clinically relevant model for infection-induced acute viral pneumonia leading to ALI/ARDS.

Curcumin, a natural phytochemical present in turmeric, the ground powder of the rhizomes of *Curcuma longa*, has been described as having anti-oxidant, anti-inflammatory, and anti-carcinogenic properties and has been used to treat cancer, arthritis, digestive and liver abnormalities, and respiratory infections [10–16]. Toxicity studies conducted on animals have indicated no adverse effects with prolonged use [14,17–19]. While curcumin's effects have been studied in many diseases, the full potential benefits of curcumin and its mechanisms of action have just begun to be elucidated for the treatment of pulmonary diseases including fibrosis and ALI/ARDS [20–28]. Pretreatment with curcumin showed beneficial effects on ALI induced by oleic acid [29], by paraquat toxicity [26], by sepsis-induced ALI [30–34] and by aspiration-induced ALI [35]. Although the precise mechanism by which curcumin mediated it's beneficial effects in these model systems is not clear, it has been suggested that the modulation of both pro-inflammatory and anti-inflammatory factors may be involved in curcumin's effects [14,17–19]. In this study, curcumin treatment *in vivo* effected both inflammatory (diffuse alveolar damage, DAD) and fibrotic lesion development leading to a significant reduction in the development of ALI/ARDS in reovirus 1/L-infected mice in this pre-clinical model, which may be manifested, at least in part, through the modulation of cytokine/chemokine expression through NFκB and through modulation of myofibroblast differentiation and fibrosis through the regulation of TGFß receptor II (RII).

Materials and Methods

Animals

Four to five week-old female CBA/J mice were obtained from Jackson Laboratory (Bar Harbor, ME, USA) and maintained in micro-isolator cages under specific pathogen free conditions in a BL-2 facility. Cages were housed in a HEPA-filtered animal isolator clean room (Nuaire Inc., Plymouth, MN, USA) and all animal manipulations were performed in class II biological safety cabinets. Virally primed mice were kept physically isolated from all other experimental and stock mice.

Ethics Statement

This study was carried out in strict accordance with the recommendations in the Guide for the Care and Use of Laboratory Animals of the National Institutes of Health. The protocol was approved by the Stony Brook University Institutional Animal Care and Use Committee (IACUC) (Protocol # 235392-5).

Virus

Reovirus 1/L was originally obtained from Dr. W. Joklik (Duke University School of Medicine, Durham, NC, USA). Third-passage gradient-purified stocks were obtained by re-cloning and amplifying parental stocks on L-929 fibroblast cells (American Type Culture Collection, Rockville, MD, USA) [5,6]. Following the purification of new stocks, infectious viral titers were obtained by limiting dilution on L-929 monolayers [5,6].

Inoculation Protocol

Animals were lightly anesthetized with an i.p. injection of 100 µl of 18% Ketamine (Vetalar 100 mg/ml; Fort Dodge Laboratories, Inc., Fort Dodge, IA, USA) and 10% Xylazine (Xylazine HCl 20 mg/ml; Phoenix Scientific, Inc., St. Joseph, MO, USA) in sterile injectable grade 0.9% NaCl (Baxter Healthcare Corp., Deerfield, IL, USA) prior to immunization. Animals were inoculated by the intranasal (i.n.) application of 10^7 PFU of reovirus 1/L in 30 µl (15 µl in each nostril) in 0.9% NaCl. Control animals were inoculated with 30 µl (15 µl in each nostril) 0.9% NaCl. Mice were treated with curcumin (≥94% curcuminoid content) (Sigma-Aldrich, St. Louis, MO, USA) at a concentration of 50 mg/kg in 2% carboxymethylcellulose (CMC) in a total volume of 100 µl delivered by an i.p. injection 5 days prior to infection and daily, thereafter. A curcumin dosage of 50 mg/kg was chosen after a series of initial experiments analyzing histologically the inflammatory infiltrate and fibrotic lesions using curcumin concentrations ranging from 50 mg/kg to 200 mg/kg (data not shown). As controls, either saline or reovirus 1/L-infected mice received a daily i.p. injection of 2% CMC (vehicle). Saline mice treated with 2% CMC (vehicle) did not develop any significant pathology (not shown). Likewises, reovirus 1/L-infected mice treated with 2% CMC (vehicle) did not show any significant improvement in lung pathology (not shown). Since our initial finding indicated that vehicle treatment alone does not modulate key features of reovirus 1/L-ALI/ARDS (inflammation and fibrosis), we compared untreated reovirus 1/L-ALI/ARDS to curcumin-treated reovirus 1/L-ALI/ARDS to minimize stressing the animals unnecessarily. After the indicated time points, animals were sacrificed via carbon dioxide inhalation (Euthanex™ CO_2 system).

Titration of infectious virions

Freshly harvested lungs (without the associated lymph nodes) were flash frozen in liquid nitrogen and stored at −80°C until use. Frozen lungs were freeze-thawed three times in 1 ml MEM containing 10% FBS followed by homogenization for 1.5 minutes with a Mini-Beadbeater (Biospec Products, Bartlesville, OK). Lung supernatants were then subjected to centrifugation at 2000 g for 10 minutes at 4°C. Serial dilutions of tissue homogenates (100 µl) in gel-saline were used in a standard plaque assay to determine reovirus 1/L PFU/ml on L-929 cell monolayers as previously described [36].

Histology

Lungs were inflated *in situ* with 2% paraformaldehyde (Sigma-Aldrich) by intra-tracheal intubation, removed, and suspended in an additional 2% paraformaldehyde for 2 hours at 4°C before being embedded in paraffin. Histological staining was performed on 4-micron sections by McClain Laboratories (Smithtown, NY, USA). Mason's Trichrome and Sirius red staining were used to visualize collagen deposition. With Mason's Trichrome, the nuclei stain a dark red/purple, muscle stains red, and connective tissue including collagen stains blue. With Sirius red, in bright-field microscopy, collagen is red on a yellowish background. Nuclei, if stained, are black but may often be grey or brown. To score lung inflammation and fibrosis, lung samples were screened for the following three histopathological parameters: (a) deposition of extracellular matrix; (b) leukocyte infiltration (interstitial inflammation); and (c) airway obliteration due to granulation tissue formation and/or fibrosis. Each slide was blindly evaluated using low (4X and 10X) and high (20X and 40X) magnification and scored on a scale of 0–3 with 0 as absent (normal); 1 as mild; 2 as moderate; and 3 as severe [5,6]. The final histology score was based on evaluation of whole lung sections (one section per mouse) and values reported are an average of 18 (reovirus 1/L–ALI/ARDS d9 and d14), 12 (curcumin-treated reovirus 1/L-ALI/ARDS d9) and 28 (reovirus 1/L-ALI/ARDS d14) individual assessments. Images from low (20X) and high (40X) magnification on an Olympus BX40 microscope (Olympus, Melville, NY, USA) were captured with a Polaroid digital microscope camera and edited using Adobe Photoshop 5.0 software.

Sircol Assay for Collagen Content

Soluble lung collagen was measured in lung homogenates using the Sircol Assay (Biocolor Ltd, UK), following manufacturer's instructions. Briefly, the right lobe of the lung was suspended at 30 mg/tissue/ml in 0.5 M acetic acid and homogenized for 3 min with a Mini-Beadbeater (Biospec Products, Bartlesville, OK, USA). Cellular debris was pelleted by centrifugation and 100 μl of the supernatant was mixed with the Sircol dye and centrifuged. The pellets were dissolved with alkaline reagent, as directed. Absorbance was read at 540 nm. Total soluble collagen was determined using a standard curve. The Sircol Assay is suitable for monitoring collagen produced *in situ* where collagen that is soluble in cold acid/pepsin can be recovered and measured from mammalian soft tissues, cartilages and fluids.

Flow Cytometric Analysis

Lungs were harvested and digested with 5 ml 1 mg/ml collagenase H (Roche, Nutley, NJ, USA) at 37°C for single cell isolation. Cells were washed three times with PBS containing 5% FCS and 0.05% azide, and resuspended at 10^6 cells/ml. Cells were stained for surface markers as described previously [5,6]. The following antibodies (Abs) were purchased from BD Biosciences (San Jose, CA, USA) and used in this analysis: CD4 (GK1.5, L3T4; R-PE-labeled); CD8a (53–6.7, PerCP-labeled); CD11b/Mac-1 (M1/70, integrinα_m chain, Mac-1 α chain, APC-labeled); CD19 (1D3, FITC-labeled); Ly6G (RB6-8C5, Gr-1, PerCP-Cy5.5-labeled); and R-PE-conjugated rat anti-mouse Pan-NK cells (DX5). Isotype matched controls were run for each sample (not shown). Flow cytometric analysis was performed using a dual-laser Accuri C6 flow cytometer (BD Accuri, Ann Arbor, MI, USA) and data was analyzed using FlowJo Analysis Software (Tree Star Inc., Ashland, OR, USA).

Immunofluorescence (IF)

Immunostaining of paraformaldehyde-fixed and paraffin embedded lung sections was performed by IF procedures. Five to eight-micron sequential sections were collected on poly-L-lysine treated slides (Sigma-Aldrich), deparaffinized in xylene and dehydrated in graded alcohol. Tissue sections were then heat treated for 10 minutes with a Target Retrieval Solution (Dako Corp. S1700; Carpinteria, CA, USA) following manufacture's instructions. Tissue sections were permeabilized in 0.2% Triton X-100 in PBS for 45 minutes at room temperature, followed by incubation in 10% BSA for 1 hr. The sections were then incubated overnight at 4°C with a rat anti-tenascin-C (TN-C) Ab (1:200, Sigma-Aldrich), a mouse anti-α-smooth muscle actin (α-SMA) Ab (1:400, Sigma-Aldrich), or a goat anti-E-cadherin Ab (1:200, R & D Systems, Minneapolis, MN, USA). After three washes in PBS, slides were incubated with the corresponding secondary Abs conjugated with photostable Alexa Fluor® dye (1:1000, Life Technologies Corporation, Grand Island, NY, USA) for 1 hr at room temperature. Slides were treated with Vectashield anti-fade mounting medium with DAPI to stain nuclei (Vector Laboratories), and viewed with a Nikon Eclipse TE2000-S microscopy system. For control incubations, primary Abs was replaced by normal mouse, goat, or rat serum (Vector Laboratories).

Serum aspartate aminotransferase (AST), alanine aminotransferase (ALT) and alkaline phosphatase (AP) activities

Serum was collected by cardiac puncture at the time of euthanasia and was stored at −80°C until use. Serum AST, ALT and AP activities were measured enzymatically using standardized enzyme assays kits obtained from Stanbio Laboratory (Boerne, TX, USA).

RNA Preparation and Quantitative RT-PCR (qRT-PCR)

Lung tissue was homogenized in the presence of TRI Reagent® Solution and total RNA was isolated according to the manufacturer's instructions (Applied Biosystems, Life Technologies, Carlsbad, CA, USA). qRT-PCR was carried out in 20 μl total volume containing 100 ng of RNA and 200 nM of each primer using a Power SYBR® Green RNA-to-C_T™ 1-Step Kit (Applied Biosystems). After reverse transcription for 30 min at 48°C and a starting denaturation for 10 minutes at 95°C, 40 PCR cycles (15 s 95°C and 1 min 60°C) were performed using the ABI StepOne Plus™ Real-Time PCR System® (Applied Biosystems). Oligonucleotide primers used in qRT-PCR are listed in Table 1. Each sample was evaluated in triplicate. Specificity of PCR products was evaluated at the end of each run by melt curve analysis. A non-template control and an endogenous control (GAPDH) were used for relative quantification. All quantitations (threshold cycle [CT] values) were normalized to that of GAPDH to generate ΔCT, and the difference between the ΔCT value of the sample and that of the reference (saline (control)) was calculated as ΔΔCT. The relative level of gene expression was expressed as $2^{-\Delta\Delta CT}$ [R].

Western Blot Analysis

For western blotting, lungs were removed and homogenized in 1.5 ml Tissue PE LB™ tissue protein extraction lysis buffer containing a cocktail of protease inhibitors (N-Ethylmaleimide [10 mM], benzamidine [5 mM], leupeptin [50 μg/ml], pepstatin A [5 μg/ml], PMSF [2 mM]) using a Mini-Beadbeater (Geno Technology, St. Louis, MO, USA). Total protein was determined using a modified Bradford protein assay (Sigma-Aldrich). Twenty micrograms of total protein were mixed with 4X sample buffer containing 5% 2-mercaptoethanol, resolved by SDS-PAGE (Ready Gels Tris HCl 10%; Bio-Rad, Hercules, CA, USA), and transferred to PVDF membranes. Membranes were then blocked for 2 hours in 5% non-fat milk in TBST, and incubated overnight at 4°C with either a rat anti-TN-C (Sigma-Aldrich), a mouse monoclonal anti-α-SMA (Sigma-Aldrich), a polyclonal goat anti-E-cadherin (R&D Systems), a rabbit anti-phosph-p65-NFκB, a rabbit anti-phosph-p38 or a rabbit anti-ß actin (Cell Signaling Technology, Danvers, MA, USA) Ab. The membranes were then washed 3X and incubated with the appropriate secondary Abs conjugated to horseradish peroxidase (Thermo-Scientific) for one and a half hours at room temperature. Western analysis using an anti-ß actin Ab (Santa Cruz Biotechnology, Inc.) was performed to demonstrate equal loading. Immunostained bands were visualized with SuperSignal® West Pico Chemiluminescent Substrate kit (Thermo-Scientific) followed by exposure to HyBlot CL™ Autoradiography Film (Denville Scientific Inc, Metuchen, NJ, USA). Band intensities on scanned gels were analyzed using the public domain National Institutes of Health ImageJ program.

Statistical analysis

Statistical analyses were performed by using an ANOVA with treatment and time of study included as factors. When appropriate, comparisons between two variables were performed using a Student's t test. A p value less than 0.05 was considered significant.

Table 1. Primers used for qRT-PCR and RT-PCR.

Gene	Forward (5′–3′)	Reverse (5′–3′)
Pro-collagen 1	TTCACCTACAGCACGCTTGTG	GATGACTGTCTTGCCCCAAGTT
IL-6	GAGGATACCACTCCCAACAGACC	AAGTGCATCATCGTTGTTCATACA
IL-10	CCCTTTGCTATGGTGTCCTT	TGGTTTCTCTTCCCAAGACC
IFNγ	AGCGGCTGACTGAACTCAGATTGTAG	GTCACAGTTTTCAGCTGTATAGGG
GM-CSF	CACCCGCTCACCCATCAC	TTCTTTGATGGCCTCTACATGCT
MCP-1	GTCTGTGCTGACCCCAAGAAG	TGGTTCGATCCAGGTTTTTA
TGFß1	GACTCTCCACCTGCAAGACCA	GGGACTGGCGAGCCTTAGTT
TGFß-RII	CACGACCCCAAGCTCACCTA	TTGGGAGAAGCGGCATCTT
TN-C	ACGGCTACCACAGAAGCTG	CGCGGCTTATTCCATAGAGTTC
α-SMA	GTCCCAGACATCAGGGAGTAA	TCGGATACTTCAGCGTCAGGA
E-cadherin	CAGGTCTCCTCATGGCTTTGC	CTTCCGAAAAGAAGGCTGTCC
Reovirus M3	TCACAACCCTTCACTCCGTCTG	AAATAATCCGCAGTCTCCAACG
GAPDH	CATGGCCTTCCGTGTTCCTA	GCGGCACGTCAGATCCA

Results

Administration of Curcumin protects CBA/J mice from the Development of ALI/ARDS in Response to reovirus 1/L

In order to determine the efficacy of treatment with curcumin on the development of either ARDS associated DAD or fibrosis, CBA/J mice were inoculated i.n. with 10^7 PFU reovirus 1/L and were either untreated or treated with 50 mg/kg curcumin by i.p. injection 5 days prior to infection and daily, thereafter. We first evaluated whether daily curcumin treatment of mice *in vivo* affected the ability of reovirus 1/L to infect or replicate in reovirus 1/L-inoculated mice (Fig. 1). We demonstrate on day 9 post-reovirus 1/L-inoculation that both the number of reovirus 1/L infectious virions (Fig. 1A) as well as the ability of reovirus 1/L to replicate *in vivo* (Fig. 1B) are not affected by curcumin treatment. Thus, we demonstrate that the mechanism of action of curcumin in this model is not due to affects on replication or clearance of reovirus 1/L from infected lungs. To determine the extent of inflammation and fibrosis, paraffin-embedded lung sections were stained with H&E, Sirius Red, or Masson's Trichrome (Fig. 2). Inflammation (as evidenced by DAD) was evaluated on day 9 and fibrosis was evaluated on day 14. All untreated, reovirus 1/L-ALI/ARDS mice developed a viral pneumonia including symptoms and histological features of ARDS, as previously described [5,6]. Specifically, reovirus 1/L-ALI/ARDS mice developed a significant diffuse cellular infiltrate leading to DAD and severe pneumonia (Fig. 2A; day 9, grade: 2.3 +/−0.46). Accompanying this DAD are edema, capillary dilation and hemorrhage, and the formation of hyaline membranes (not shown). Those mice that survive the acute phase of the disease develop interstitial fibrosis and intra-alveolar fibrosis (Fig. 2A; day 14, grade: 2.1 +/−0.50). In contrast, curcumin-treated reovirus 1/L-ALI/ARDS mice developed significantly less of a cellular infiltrate with a patchy distribution and formation of condensed focal lymphocytic accumulations (Fig. 2A; day 9, grade: 1.31 +/−0.44; $p<0.05$ versus reovirus 1/L-ALI/ARDS). In addition, the intra-alveolar and interstitial fibrosis associated with the late phase of reovirus 1/L-ALI/ARDS was also significantly inhibited by treatment with curcumin (Fig. 2A; day 14, grade: 1.31 +/−0.49; $p<0.05$ versus reovirus 1/L-ALI/ARDS). To more clearly demonstrate the presence of fibrotic lesions histologically, tissue sections were stained with Mason's Trichrome or Sirius red on day 14 post-infection (Fig. 2B). In normal or saline (control) lung sections, Sirius red or Mason's Trichrome staining for collagen is evident only within the walls of the bronchioles and arterioles, which contain connective tissue including collagen, while the lung alveolar airspaces are not stained (Fig. 2B). As can be observed, significant staining for collagen via either Mason's Trichrome (blue) or Sirius red (bright red) is evident in reovirus 1/L-ALI/ARDS mice, which is dramatically reduced in curcumin-treated reovirus 1/L-ALI/ARDS mice (Fig. 2B).

To support the histological evaluation of fibrosis, the Sircol™ Collagen Assay demonstrated significant collagen accumulation in the lungs at day 14-post infection in untreated, reovirus 1/L-ALI/ARDS mice as compared to saline (control) lungs (approximately a 2-fold increase) (Fig. 3A). In contrast, the amount of collagen accumulation in the lungs of curcumin-treated reovirus 1/L-ALI/ARDS mice is significantly reduced versus the reovirus 1/L-ALI/ARDS mice, even though they still accumulate more collagen than saline (control) mice (Fig. 3A). As an additional measure of collagen accumulation, mRNA for pro-collagen I was measured on day 14 post-infection (Fig. 3B). Reovirus 1/L-ALI/ARDS mice expressed a significantly higher level of pro-collagen I mRNA as compared to saline (control) mice, which was significantly reduced in curcumin-treated, reovirus 1/L-ALI/ARDS mice (Fig. 3B).

To provide further evidence for the anti-fibrogenic action of curcumin in reovirus 1/L-ALI/ARDS, we analyzed pulmonary expression of TN-C, an extracellular matrix glycoprotein that is highly expressed in adult lung parenchyma following acute lung injury [37–40] and pulmonary levels of α-SMA and E-cadherin, two well-established markers of epithelial to mesenchymal transition (Fig. 4). As evaluated by western, TN-C is minimally expressed in adult saline (control) lung tissue (Fig. 4A). In untreated, reovirus 1/L-ALI/ARDS lung tissue, the 190-kDa isoform of TN-C is highly expressed on day 14 post-infection. However, in the presence of curcumin, induction of TN-C is significantly reduced on day 14 post-reovirus 1/L inoculation (Fig. 4A). Western analysis data for TN-C expression was confirmed by mRNA expression via qRT-PCR (Fig. 4B). By IF, TN-C expression is minimal in saline (control) lung (Fig. 4C). However, TN-C is highly induced in untreated, reovirus 1/L-

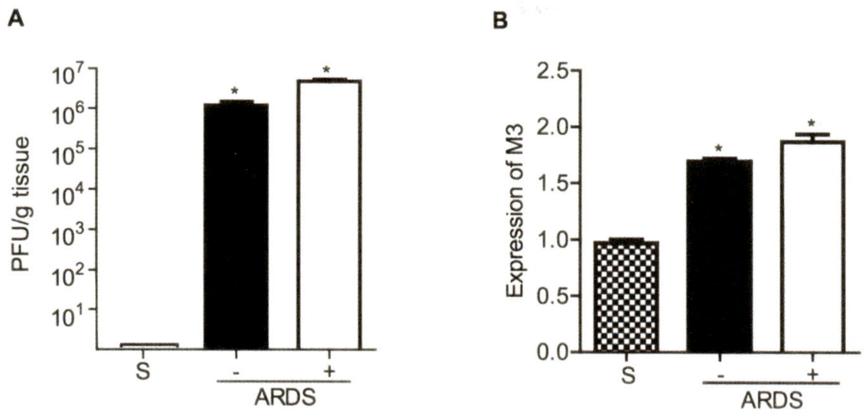

Figure 1. Administration of curcumin does not effect reovirus 1/L clearance or replication in vivo. CBA/J mice were inoculated i.n. with 10^7 PFU reovirus 1/L and were either untreated (−) or treated (+) with 50 mg/kg curcumin by i.p. injection beginning 5 days prior to infection and daily, thereafter. Whole lungs were removed or day 9 post-infection. (A) Lungs were individually homogenized and PFU were determined by a standard plaque assay. Results are expressed as the average number of PFU per g lung tissue. No plaques were detected in saline inoculated mice. Histograms are the mean +/− S.D. of one experiment with three mice per time point. *p<0.05 versus saline (control). (B) RNA was prepared from whole lung tissue from saline (S) or from untreated (−, solid bars) or curcumin-treated (+, open bars) reovirus 1/L-ALI/ARDS and relative expression of reovirus 1 L M3 gene was assessed by qRT-PCR. Histograms are the mean +/− S.D. of one experiment with three mice per time point. *p<0.05 versus saline (control).

ALI/ARDS lungs on day 14 especially visible in areas of lung injury (Fig. 4C, red). In curcumin-treated reovirus 1/L-ALI/ARDS mice, the presence of TN-C was significantly reduced (Fig. 4C). Similarly by IF, expression of α-SMA was negligible in saline (control) mice being observed only within the walls of the bronchioles and vasculature (Fig. 4C, red). However, a marked induction of α-SMA expression was observed in reovirus 1/L-ALI/ARDS, in agreement with the increased deposition of fibrotic tissue (Fig. 4C, red). In contrast, curcumin-treated reovirus 1/L-ALI/ARDS mice demonstrated a marked reduction in α-SMA expression (Fig. 4C). The expression of α-SMA was confirmed by protein expression via western analysis and by mRNA expression via qRT-PCR (Fig. 4A and B). In saline (control) lungs, E-cadherin is clearly expressed by the alveolar epithelial cells (Fig. 4C, green). However, during post injury, lung remodeling is associated with increased E-cadherin expression, which occurs simultaneously with the peak of cellular proliferation and repair and E-cadherin expression is reduced in curcumin-treated reovirus 1/L-ALI/ARDS (Fig. 4C, green). The expression of E-cadherin was confirmed by protein expression via western analysis and by mRNA expression via qRT-PCR (Fig. 4A and B).

Administration of Curcumin suppresses serum liver enzyme levels in reovirus 1/L-ALI/ARDS

We also analyzed changes in liver enzymes to detect hepatic dysfunction as evidence of a systemic response after reovirus 1/L-ALI/ARDS and whether treatment with curcumin affected

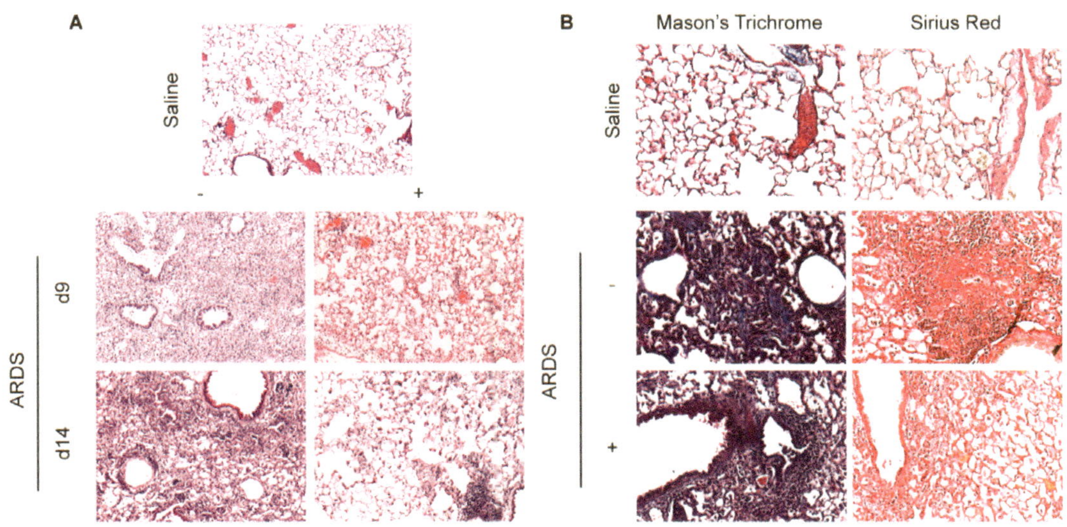

Figure 2. Administration of curcumin protects CBA/J mice from the development of ALI/ARDS in response to reovirus 1/L. CBA/J mice were inoculated i.n. with 10^7 PFU reovirus 1/L and were either untreated (−) or treated (+) with 50 mg/kg curcumin by i.p. injection beginning 5 days prior to infection and daily, thereafter. Whole lungs were removed at the indicated time points, fixed in 2% paraformaldehyde and embedded in paraffin. Staining was performed on 4-micron sections. (A) H&E Staining on days 9 and 14; (B) Mason's Trichrome and Sirius Red Staining on day 14. Objective magnification: 10X (A) and 20X (B). Representative of at least four independent experiments evaluating 3 mice per time point.

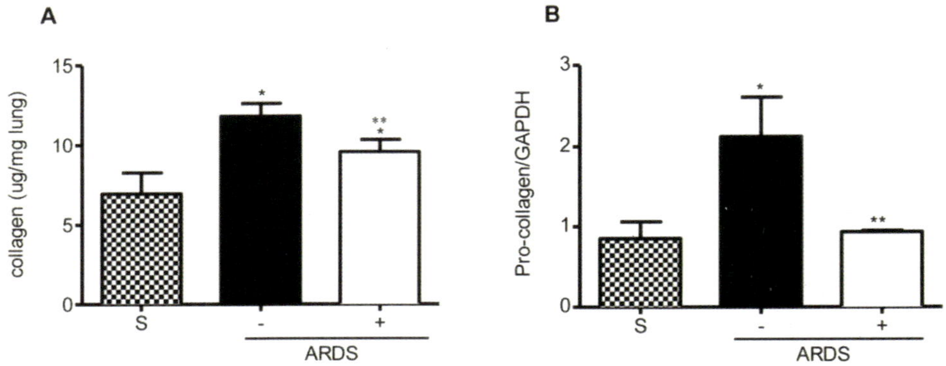

Figure 3. Administration of curcumin reduces collagen deposition in reovirus 1/L-ALI/ARDS. CBA/J mice were inoculated i.n. with 10^7 PFU reovirus 1/L and were either untreated (−) or treated (+) with 50 mg/kg curcumin by i.p. injection beginning 5 days prior to infection and daily, thereafter. (A) Whole lungs were removed from saline (S), untreated (−, solid bars) or curcumin-treated (+, open bars) reovirus 1/L-ALI/ARDS on day 14 post-infection and soluble lung collagen was measured using the Sircol Assay as per manufacturer's instructions; (B) RNA was prepared from whole lung tissue from saline (S) or from untreated (-, solid bars) or curcumin-treated (+, open bars) reovirus 1/L-ALI/ARDS on day 14 post-infection and relative expression of pro-collagen 1 was assessed by qRT-PCR. Histograms are the mean +/− S.D. of two experiments with three mice per time point. *p<0.05 versus saline (control), **p<0.05 versus reovirus 1/L-ALI/ARDS.

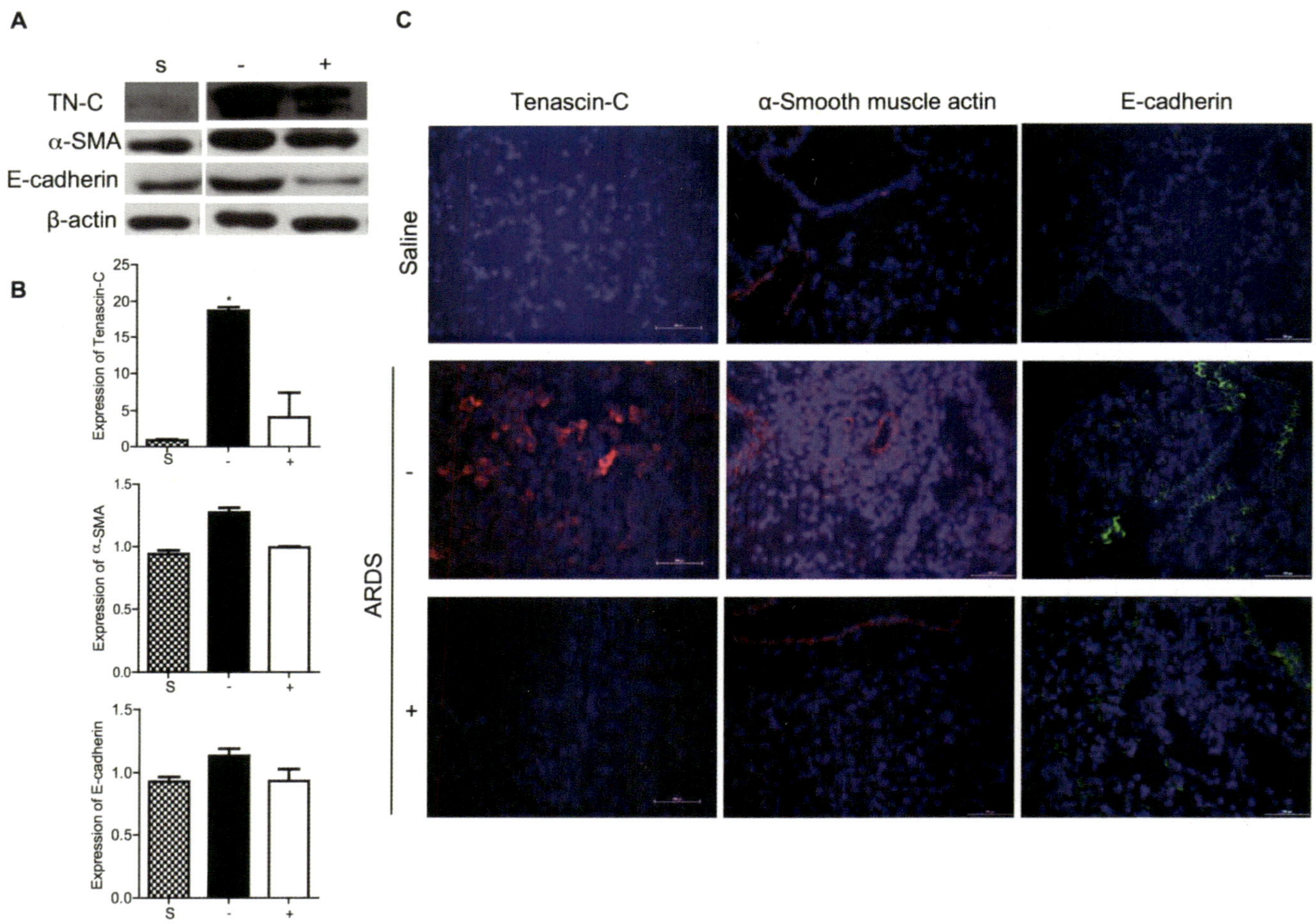

Figure 4. Administration of curcumin reduces expression of the myofibroblast cell phenotype in reovirus 1/L-ALI/ARDS. CBA/J mice were inoculated i.n. with 10^7 PFU reovirus 1/L and were either untreated (−) or treated (+) with 50 mg/kg curcumin by i.p. injection beginning 5 days prior to infection and daily, thereafter. (A) Western analysis from whole lung lysates for protein expression of TN-C, α-SMA, and E-cadherin from either saline (S), untreated (−), or curcumin-treated (+) reovirus 1/L-ALI/ARDS mice on day 14 post-inoculation. ß-actin expression demonstrated equal loading. Representative of three mice per time point; (B) RNA was prepared from whole lung tissue on day 14 post-inoculation and the relative expression of TN-C, α-SMA, and E-cadherin was assessed by qRT-PCR from untreated (−, solid bars) or treated (+, open bars) reovirus 1/L-ALI/ARDS mice. Saline inoculated mice were used as controls (S, stippled bars). Histograms are the mean +/− S.D. of three mice per time point. *p<0.05 versus saline (control). (C) Lungs of saline, untreated (−) or curcumin-treated (+) reovirus 1/L-ALI/ARDS mice on day 14 post-inoculation were paraffin embedded and stained with an Abs to TN-C (red), α-SMA (red), or E-cadherin (green). Representative of two independent experiments.

potential hepatic dysfunction (Fig. 5). Serum enzyme analysis indicated an early significant increase in serum AST activity over saline (control) mice on day 5 post-inoculation in either untreated or curcumin-treated reovirus 1/L-ALI/ARDS mice which was reduced to control levels on day 9 post-inoculation (Fig. 5A). However, on day 14 a significant increase in serum AST activity was observed in untreated, reovirus 1/L-ALI/ARDS which was reduced to control levels in curcumin-treated, reovirus 1/L-ALI/ARDS mice (Fig. 5A). Both serum ALT activity (Fig. 5B) on day 14 and AP activity (Fig. 5C) on both days 9 and 14 post-inoculation were significantly increased over saline (control) levels in reovirus 1/L-ALI/ARDS mice that was reduced to control levels in curcumin-treated, reovirus 1/L-ALI/ARDS mice.

Curcumin modulates the Phenotype of the Inflammatory Cellular Infiltrate in Reovirus 1/L-ALI/ARDS Mice

To determine the percentage over time of different leukocyte subsets present in the inflammatory infiltrate, infiltrating cells from whole lung preparations were obtained on days 5, 9, and 14 post reovirus 1/L inoculation and analyzed by flow cytometry using monoclonal Abs specific for T cell subsets (CD4, CD8), B cells (CD19), Macrophages (CD11b), neutrophils (GR-1), and NK cells (CD49B (pan-NK)) (Fig. 6). In saline or saline + curcumin-treated (control) mice, approximately $0.77+/-0.20\times10^6$ cells were recovered from the interstitial spaces with macrophages and PMNs being the predominate cells present (Table 2; not shown). A significant increase in the total number of inflammatory cells was recovered from either untreated reovirus 1/L-ALI/ARDS or curcumin-treated reovirus 1/L-ALI/ARDS mice on days 5, 9, or 14 as compared to saline or saline + curcumin-treated (control) mice (Table 2). Further, the number of recovered cells on days 5 and 14 from curcumin-treated reovirus 1/L-ALI/ARDS mice was significantly less than the number recovered from untreated reovirus 1/L-ALI/ARDS (Table 2). In regards to phenotype, a significant decrease in the number of PMNs ($GR1^+$) and $CD4^+$ cells on day 5 and $CD19^+$ B cells on day 9 was observed in curcumin-treated reovirus 1/L-ALI/ARDS mice versus untreated reovirus 1/L-ALI/ARDS mice (Fig. 6A and B). On day 14, as compared to reovirus 1/L-ALI/ARDS, a significant decrease in PMNs, NK cells, CD8+ T cells and CD19+ B cells was observed in curcumin-treated reovirus 1/L-ALI/ARDS mice (Fig. 6C).

To determine whether the cytokine/chemokine expression profile of the infiltrating cells from reovirus 1/L-ALI/ARDS mice was modulated during curcumin treatment, RNA from infiltrating cells on days 5, 9, and 14 was evaluated for expression of key cytokines/chemokines including IL-6, IL-10, IFNγ, G/M-CSF, and MCP-1 via qRT-PCR (Fig. 7). Interestingly, an early significant increase in the expression of IL-6, G/M-CSF and MCP-1 was observed on day 5 in curcumin-treated reovirus 1/L-ALI/ARDS as compared to untreated reovirus 1/L-ALI/ARDS mice or saline (control) mice (Fig. 7A). However, by day 9 post-inoculation, the expression of IL-6, G/M-CSF and MCP-1 was significantly higher in both untreated versus curcumin treated reovirus 1/l-ALI/ARDS mice as compared to saline (control) mice (Fig. 7A). In addition, on day 9 the expression of IFNγ, was significantly increased in curcumin-treated reovirus 1/L-ALI/ARDS mice as compared to untreated reovirus 1/L-ALI/ARDS mice and saline (control) mice (Fig. 7A). By day 14 in either untreated or curcumin-treated reovirus 1/L-ALI/ARDS, the expression of IL-6, IL-10, IFNγ, GM-CSF and MCP-1 were similar to that of saline (control) mice (Fig. 7A). In addition, cytokine/chemokine mRNA expression from whole lung tissue (including the infiltrating cells) was also evaluated on days 9 and 14 post-inoculation by qRT-PCR. Expression of IL-6, IL-10, IFNγ, and MCP-1 was significantly increased over saline (control) in both untreated and curcumin-treated reovirus 1/L-ALI/ARDS on day 9 post-inoculation (Fig. 7B). However, at day 14 post-inoculation, the expression of IL-6, IL-10, IFNγ, and MCP-1 in reovirus 1/L-ALI/ARDS mice was still significantly increased over saline (control) mice, which was significantly inhibited in curcumin-treated reovirus 1/L-ALI/ARDS mice (Fig. 7B).

Curcumin differentially modulates the TGFß1 NFκB, and the p38 signaling pathways

Three key pathways involved in the pathogenesis of ALI/ARDS, TGFß1, NFκB, and p38 were investigated in reovirus 1/L-ALI/ARDS. RNA from whole lung tissue on days 9 and 14 post inoculation was evaluated for expression of TGFß1 and TGFß RII by RT-PCR or qRT-PCR (Fig. 8) and protein extracts from whole lung tissue were evaluated for expression of the phosphorylated form of the p65 subunit of NFκB or the phosphorylated form of p38, an additional key molecule in the TGFß signaling pathway (Fig. 9). While the expression of TGFß1 was not modulated by curcumin on either day 9 or day 14 in reovirus 1/L-ALI/ARDS (Fig. 8A and B), TGFß RII, which is required for TGFß signaling, was significantly reduced on day 9 in the presence of curcumin (Fig. 8B). Curcumin also demonstrated differential effects on expression of the phosphorylated (P) forms of p38 and the p65

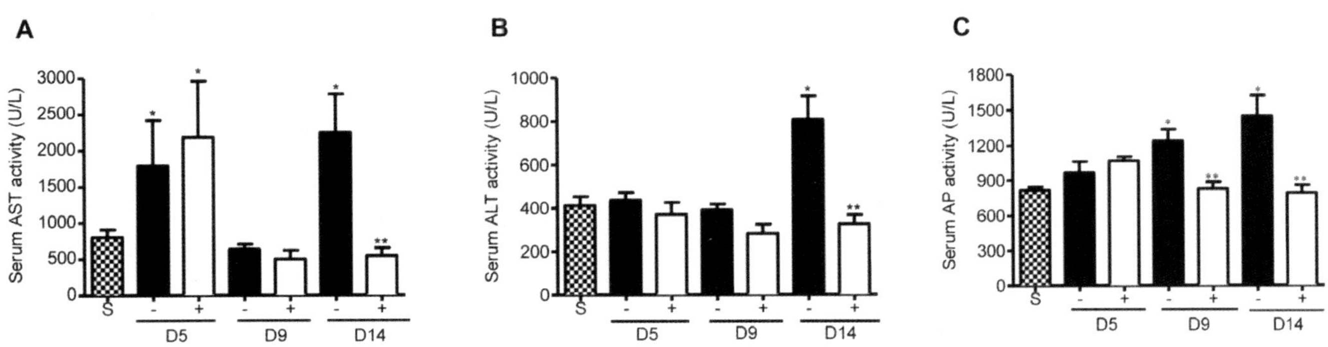

Figure 5. Administration of curcumin reduces expression of the key liver enzymes in the serum during reovirus 1/L-ALI/ARDS. CBA/J mice were inoculated i.n. with 10^7 PFU reovirus 1/L and were either untreated (−, solid bars) or treated (+, open bars) with 50 mg/kg curcumin by i.p. injection beginning 5 days prior to infection and daily, thereafter. Saline inoculated mice were used as controls (S, stippled bars). Serum was collected at the indicated time points. (A) Serum AST activity; (B) Serum ALT activity; (C) Serum AP activity. Histograms are the mean +/− S.D. of two experiments with three mice per time point. *p<0.05 versus saline (control), **p<0.05 versus reovirus 1/L-ALI/ARDS.

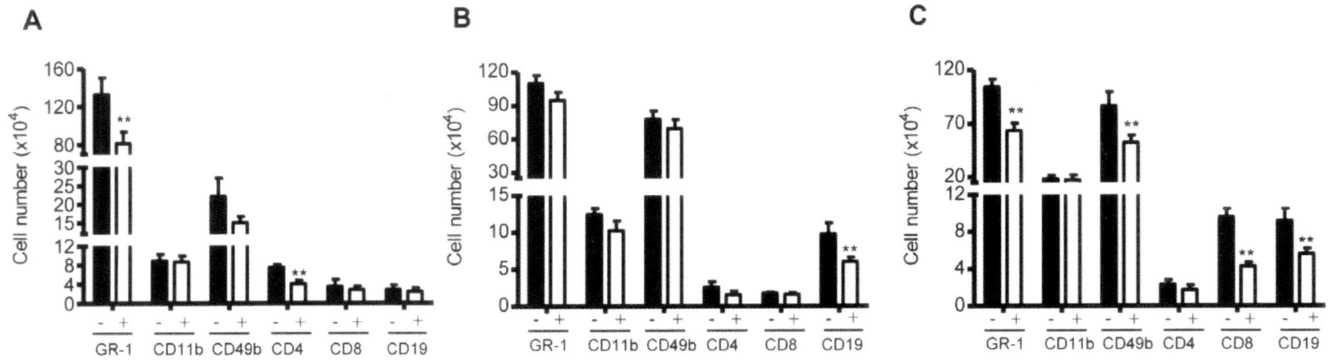

Figure 6. Administration of curcumin modulates the inflammatory cell infiltrate during reovirus 1/L-ALI/ARDS. CBA/J mice were inoculated i.n. with 10^7 PFU reovirus 1/L and were either untreated (−, solid bars) or treated (+, open bars) with 50 mg/kg curcumin by i.p. injection beginning 5 days prior to infection and daily, thereafter. Infiltrating cells were recovered from the lungs and analyzed for the expression of the indicated cell surface phenotype markers, as described. (A) Day 5; (B) Day 9; (C) Day 14. Histograms are the mean +/− S.D. of two experiments with three mice per time point. **$p<0.05$ versus reovirus 1/L-ALI/ARDS.

subunit of NFκB (Fig. 9). Treatment of reovirus 1/L-ALI/ARDS with curcumin resulted in a significant increase in P-p38 evident on day 9 post-inoculation as compared to untreated reovirus1/L-ALI/ARDS (Fig. 9A and B). However, treatment of reovirus 1/L-ALI/ARDS with curcumin resulted in a significant reduction of P-p65 NFκB as compared to untreated reovirus1/L-ALI/ARDS (Fig. 9A and B).

Discussion

This study was conducted in a mouse model of infection (reovirus 1/L)-induced *acute viral pneumonia*, which leads to ARDS, the most severe form of ALI. Reovirus 1/L-ALI/ARDS mice demonstrated severely damaged lungs as evidenced by DAD followed by infiltration of the interstitium and alveolar spaces with fibroblasts with excessive collagen deposition [5–8]. However, in reovirus 1/L-ALI/ARDS undergoing treatment with curcumin in a pre-clinical model, these inflammatory and fibrotic changes were significantly reduced. Key markers of fibrosis including expression of α-SMA, TN-C and E-cadherin were modified by curcumin. Curcumin also modulated the expression of key chemokines/cytokines implicated in the development of ALI/ARDS including IL-6, IL-10, IFNγ, and MCP-1 from both the inflammatory infiltrate and from whole lung tissue potentially through the modulation of NFκB. While the expression of TGFß1 was not modulated by curcumin, TGFß RII, which is required for TGFß signaling, was significantly reduced. In reovirus 1//L-ALI/ARDS, we also observed dramatic increases in systemic levels of liver enzymes including AST, ALT, and AP especially on day 14 when significant fibrotic lesions are observed. This is similar to many patients with ARDS who die not from hypoxemia but from multiple organ failure [41,42]. However, curcumin-treated reovirus 1/L-ALI/ARDS mice demonstrated a significant decrease is all three systemic indicators suggesting that curcumin prevents not only the inflammatory reaction but also the later systemic reactions due to continued lung fibrosis and hypoxemia. We also demonstrate in reovirus 1/L-ALI/ARDS an increase in expression of ãSMA and TN-C especially visible in areas of lung injury in agreement with the increased deposition of fibrotic tissue. In contrast, reovirus 1/L-ALI/ARDS mice treated with curcumin demonstrated a marked reduction in α-SMA and TN-C. These data confirm that curcumin induces anti-fibrogenic actions, related at least in part to a lower accumulation of myofibroblasts during the course of the fibrogenic process. Our results also suggest that the curcumin further manifests its effects through the induction of the p38 MAPK, a subfamily of serine-threonine protein kinases, having pro-apoptotic effects in response to extracellular stimuli [43]. Since the effects of curcumin are likely pleotropic and complex, determining the downstream effectors of curcumin will be crucial in analyzing the full potential value of curcumin as a potential therapeutic.

In this report, we demonstrate a differential effect of curcumin on the inflammatory infiltrate versus whole lung tissue, which would include an inflammatory response associated with resident epithelial, endothelial and/or fibroblast cells. We demonstrate from the inflammatory infiltrate an early (day 5) and significant rise in IL-6, G/M-CSF, and MCP-1 in curcumin-treated reovirus 1/L-ALI/ARDS which is not mirrored by untreated reovirus 1/L-ALI/ARDS until day 9. In addition, on day 9, IFNγ expression

Table 2. Number of cells recovered from untreated and curcumin-treated reovirus 1/L-ALI/ARDS[a]

Group	Day 5[b]	Day 9	Day 14
Reovirus 1/L-ALI/ARDS	1.76+/−0.61*	2.14+/−0.42*	2.30+/−0.65*
Curcumin-treated Reovirus 1/L-ALI/ARDS	1.15+/−0.34*, **	1.84+/−0.40*	1.45+/−0.46*, **

[a]CBA/J mice were inoculated i.n. with 10^7 PFU reovirus 1/L and were either untreated or treated with 50 mg/kg curcumin by i.p. injection at 5 days prior to infection and daily, thereafter. At the indicated time points, infiltrating cells were recovered from the lungs. In saline or saline + curcumin-treated mice (controls), approximately $0.77+/-0.20\times10^6$ cells were recovered from the interstitial spaces.

[b]Mean number of cells $\times10^6$ +/−S.D. of two experiments with four mice per time point.

*$p<0.05$ versus saline

**$p<0.05$ versus reovirus 1/L-ALI/ARDS

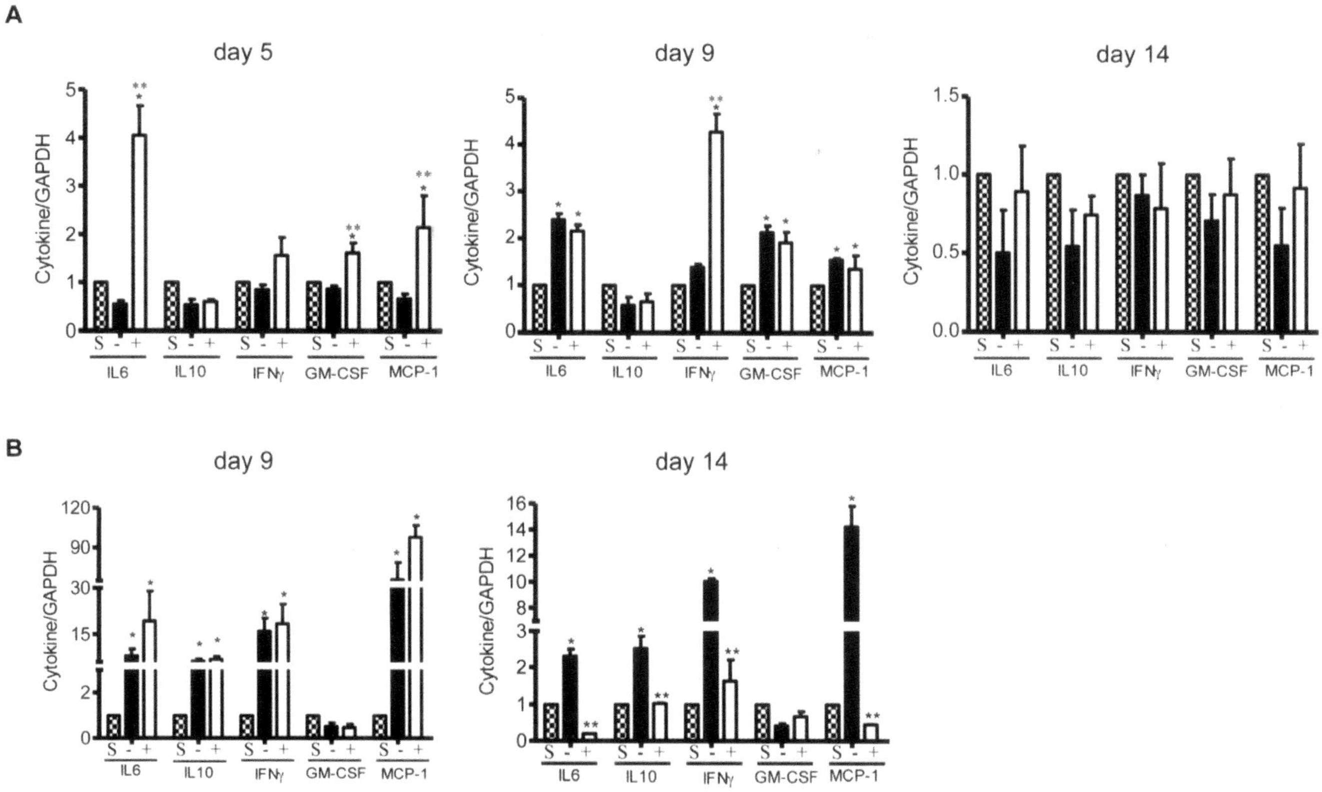

Figure 7. Administration of curcumin modulates key cytokine/chemokine expression during reovirus 1/L-ALI/ARDS. CBA/J mice were inoculated i.n. with 10^7 PFU reovirus 1/L and were either untreated (−, solid bars) or treated (+, open bars) with 50 mg/kg curcumin by i.p. injection beginning 5 days prior to infection and daily, thereafter. At the indicated time points, RNA was prepared from (A) the infiltrating cells; or (B) whole lung tissue and relative expression of key cytokines/chemokines was assessed by qRT-PCR. Saline inoculated mice were used as controls (S, stippled bars). Histograms are the mean +/− S.D. of two experiments with three mice per time point. *p<0.05 versus saline (control), **p<0.05 versus reovirus 1/L-ALI/ARDS.

from the inflammatory infiltrate in curcumin-treated reovirus 1/L-ALI/ARDS is significantly higher than in untreated reovirus 1/L-ALI/ARDS. However, by day 14, the inflammatory infiltrate from either reovirus 1/L-ALI/ARDS or curcumin-treated reovirus 1/L-ALI/ARDS no longer significantly expresses any of these key cytokines/chemokines. However, when evaluating whole lung mRNA for cytokine/chemokine expression, it is evident that resident pulmonary alveolar epithelial, endothelial, and fibroblast cells contribute to the overall cytokine/chemokine storm especially as evident on day 14. While curcumin down regulates the

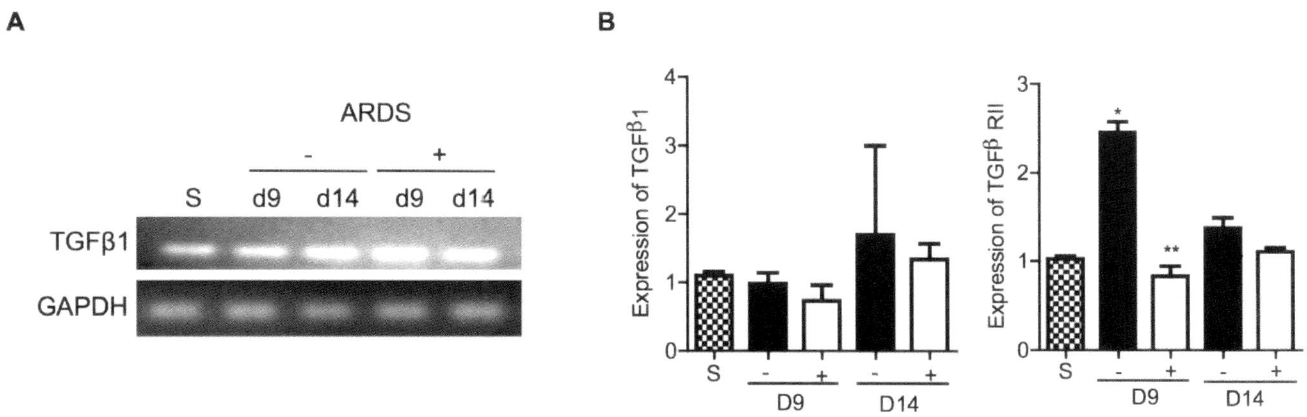

Figure 8. Administration of curcumin modulates TGFß RII expression during reovirus 1/L-ALI/ARDS. CBA/J mice were inoculated i.n. with 10^7 PFU reovirus 1/L and were either untreated (−, solid bars) or treated (+, open bars) with 50 mg/kg curcumin by i.p. injection beginning 5 days prior to infection and daily, thereafter. At the indicated time points, RNA was prepared from whole lung tissue and the relative expression of (A) TGFß1 was assessed by RT-PCR; (B) TGFß1 and TGFß RII mRNA expression was also assessed by qRT-PCR. Saline inoculated mice were used as controls (S, stippled bars). Histograms are the mean +/−S.D. of two experiments with three mice per time point. *p<0.05 versus saline (control), **p<0.05 versus reovirus 1/L-ALI/ARDS.

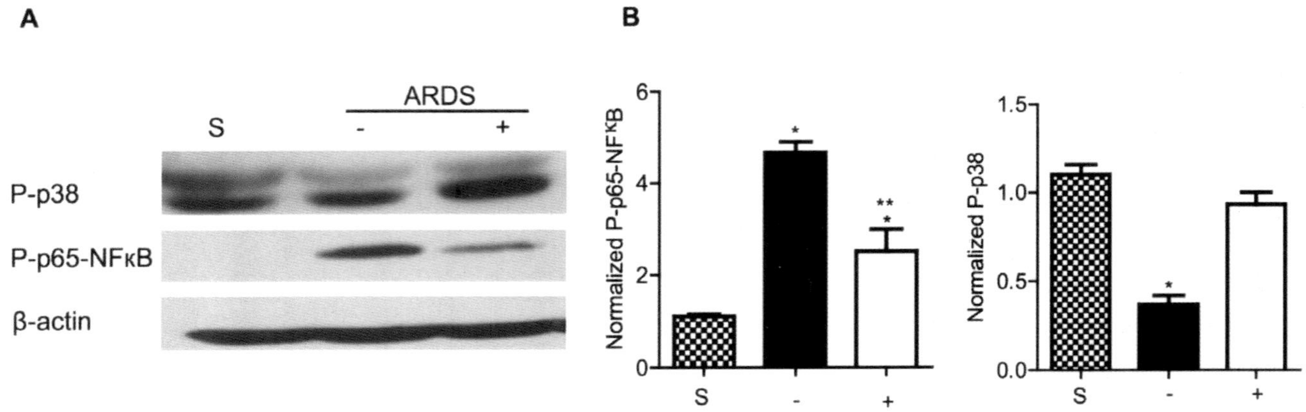

Figure 9. Administration of curcumin modulates the phosphorylation status of the p65 subunit of NFkB and p38 MAPK. CBA/J mice were inoculated i.n. with 10^7 PFU reovirus 1/L and were either untreated (−) or treated (+) with 50 mg/kg curcumin by i.p. injection beginning 5 days prior to infection and daily, thereafter. (A) On day 9 post-inoculation, protein was extracted from whole lung tissue from untreated (−) or curcumin-treated (+) reovirus 1/L-ALI/ARDS mice and analyzed for the expression of phosphorylated p38 (P-p38) and phosphorylated p65-NFκB (P-p65-NFκB) by western analysis. Saline inoculated mice were used as controls (S). Analysis of ß actin was performed to demonstrate equal loading. Representative of two experiments with three mice per time point. (B) Relative expression of P-p38 and P-p65-NFκB was determined by comparing their expression to that of ß-actin. Histograms represent densitometric data from the mean +/− SD autoradiogram signals from three mice for the saline, untreated (−, solid) or curcumin-treated (+, open) reovirus 1/L-ALI/ARDS*$p<0.05$ versus saline (control), **$p<.0.05$ versus reovirus 1/L-ALI/ARDS.

expression IL-6, IL-10, IFNγ and MCP-1 in curcumin-treated reovirus 1/L-ALI/ARDS on day 14, untreated reovirus 1/L-ALI/ARDS express high levels of these cytokines/chemokines especially, IFNγ and MCP-1. These results suggest a consistent and prolonged inflammatory response most likely initiating from resident pulmonary alveolar epithelial cells and fibroblasts in untreated reovirus 1/L-ALI/ARDS, contributed to the pathology associated with ALI/ARDS. We have previously demonstrated a role for IFNγ in the pathophysiology of reovirus 1/L pulmonary pathologies and suggest that prolonged and high levels of IFNγ are associated with more severe pulmonary pathologies [7,8]. The reduced pathology associated with curcumin treatment and the reduced expression of IFNγ by curcumin would support this hypothesis. We have also demonstrated the potential effect of curcumin on NFκB activation by a decrease in the levels of the P-p65. This result is clearly consistent with the decreased expression of IFNγ and MCP-1, which is observed in curcumin-treated reovirus 1/L-ALI/ARDS. The literature clearly links canonical activation of NFκB in cells to the pathogenesis of inflammatory diseases [44–48]. NFκB is activated in the lungs of patients with ALI [49,50] and persistent elevation of NFκB in patients with sepsis-induced ALI is associated with poor outcome [51,52]. Curcumin has been demonstrated to modulate NFκB activation in cell systems as well as *in vivo* model systems [16,18,53–57]. As an anti-inflammatory agent in association with lung diseases curcumin inhibited pro-inflammatory cytokines including IL-8, IL-1, and TNF through the inhibition of the transcription factors NFκB and AP-1 [26,28]. However, although NFκB plays a major role in regulating expression of cytokines/chemokines, the effects of curcumin in reovirus 1/L-ALI/ARDS cannot solely be attributed to its effect on NFκB since glucocorticoids also inhibit NFκB but do not suppress the development, progression, and mortality associated with reovirus1/L-ALI/ARDS [7,8].

TGFß and its signaling pathways have also been implicated in lung fibrosis [58–60] and TGFß over expression is associated with poorer prognosis in ARDS [61–63] as well as in our model [5,6]. While curcumin has been demonstrated to reduce collagen in experimental pulmonary fibrosis induced by cyclophosphamide, whole-body irradiation, and bleomycin, little mechanistic studies have been performed [20,22–27,64,65]. Here, we demonstrate in reovirus 1/L-ALI/ARDS that while treatment with curcumin did not inhibit the expression of TGFß1 itself, expression of TGFß RII was significantly reduced especially on day 9 post-induction where the transition between inflammation and fibrosis is most evident. Although the precise mechanism remains unclear, in other pulmonary fibrotic models including in bleomycin-induced fibrosis [22,25,66–69], in SiO_2-induced fibrosis [70], and in amiodarone-induced fibrosis [23], curcumin has been shown to reduce either TGFß protein or mRNA expression. In amiodarone-induced fibrosis, this reduction in TGFß is potentially through a decrease in c-Jun expression [23]. Aberrant activation of TGFß signaling has also been implicated in scleroderma fibrosis [20,21,71,72] and in keloid, a fibrotic disease characterized by abnormal accumulation of ECM in the dermis via reduction in TGFß/p-SMAD-2 [73]. Over expression of TGFß has also been implicated in fibrotic kidney disease and curcumin inhibited TGFß signaling and reduced TGFß induced increases in PAI-1, TGFß1, collagen, and fibronectin through a reduction in both TGFß RII and phosphorylation of Smad2/3 in renal cells [74,75]. In hepatic fibrosis curcumin activated PPARγ which contributed to apoptosis and a reduction in extracellular matrix expression in hepatic stellate cells through the interruption of TGFß signaling and suppression of CTGF [76–78].

There is convincing evidence in patients that increased lung epithelial apoptosis is associated with poor outcomes in ALI/ARDS [51,79–81]. Pathways involving both the p38 MAP or Akt kinases are important in PMNs and macrophages, the major infiltrating cells in ALI/ARDS [49,50,82]. Diminished translocation of NFκB and phosphorylation of Akt but not p38 in PMNs of patients with sepsis-induced ALI was associated with improved survival [49]. It has also been demonstrated that activation of p38 MAPK or an increase in caspase-3 activity appears to contribute to the proapoptotic effect of human neutrophil apoptosis by curcumin [83]. Curcumin has been shown to modulate apoptosis in a number of different cell types. In scleroderma, it was shown that scleroderma lung fibroblasts, which are deficient in PKCε, are sensitive to curcumin-induced apoptosis, whereas normal lung fibroblasts are insensitive to curcumin [20,21]. The importance of

PKCε was demonstrated by the observations that increasing PKCε expression in scleroderma lung fibroblasts provides protection against curcumin and decreasing PKCε expression or activity in normal lung fibroblasts causes the cells to become sensitive to curcumin [20,21]. In pleural mesothelioma cells, curcumin was shown to activate p38 MAPK, caspases 9 and 3, caused elevated levels of proapoptotic proteins Bax, stimulated PARP cleavage, and induced apoptosis [84]. Curcumin has also been shown to attenuate gefitinib-induced cell proliferation and enhances apoptosis through altering p38 MAPK activation in intestinal epithelia cell [85]. In the reovirus 1/L-ALI/ARDS model, we have clearly demonstrated a role for apoptosis in reovirus 1/L-ALI/ARDS [9]. Although we demonstrated both apoptosis of the alveolar epithelium via TUNEL analysis and the up regulation of Fas and FasL *in situ* in alveolar epithelium and in cells of the inflammatory infiltrate, modulation of reovirus 1/L-ALI/ARDS was not linked to the inhibition of the Fas/FasL pathway suggesting the involvement of additional apoptosis pathways [9]. Here, we demonstrate in curcumin-treated reovirus 1/L-ALI/ARDS, an increase in P-p38, which has been linked to enhanced PMN apoptosis. While we demonstrated a significant decrease in the total number of infiltrating cells and a decrease in the number of PMN on day 14 in curcumin-treated reovirus 1/L-ALI/ARDS, whether this decrease is reflected in an increase in apoptosis is yet to be determined.

In conclusion, our model provides a very relevant model for infection (viral)-induced ALI/ARDS and for deciphering the mechanism(s) of action of agents that show promising efficacy against ALI/ARDS such as the potent anti-inflammatory agent, curcumin. Our data strongly support the hypothesis in a pre-clinical model that treatment of reovirus 1/L-ALI/ARDS with curcumin inhibits the host inflammatory response potentially through the modulation of cytokine/chemokine expression through the NFκB pathway as well as the host fibrotic response during the regeneration phase of the disease through modulation of the TGFß pathway. Our results also suggest that curcumin may modulate apoptosis pathways mediated through the p38 MAPK pathway. Thus, understanding curcumin's mechanism of action may elucidate compounds that would further improve it's inhibitory activity in an additive or synergistic manner leading to combination studies involving curcumin and other anti-viral agents and/or anti-fibrotic agents. A water soluble curcumin complex has recently been described that attenuated multiple markers of inflammation and injury, including pulmonary edema and neutrophil infiltration in an ALI model [86]. An additional study demonstrated the potential use of curcumin as an adjunct therapy as an anti-inflammatory, immunomodulatory agent along with antibiotics in the case of acute lung infection induced by K. pneumonia [87]. We are currently conducting additional experiments to characterize the mechanism of curcumin's affect on fibrotic lesion development in a therapeutic model. We have preliminary histological data that demonstrates treatment of reovirus 1/L-ALI/ARDS mice with curcumin beginning on day 7 post reovirus 1/L infection (after the onset of inflammation but before significant development of fibrotic lesions) inhibits fibrotic lesion development as evaluated on day 14 (unpublished results). Thus, continued studies of the potent anti-oxidant, anti-microbial, anti-inflammatory agent, curcumin, will likely improve the identification of key study endpoints that may be manipulated to slow or reverse the relentless progression of pulmonary inflammation/fibrosis in acute viral-induced ALI/ARDS, ultimately, leading to new novel treatments to reduce pulmonary dysfunction and improve outcome for critically ill patients.

Acknowledgments

The authors would like to thank Ms. Lindsey Bishop-Jutzeler for assistance with the tenascin-C western.

Author Contributions

Conceived and designed the experiments: SA FZ SDL LL. Performed the experiments: SA FZ RW GL. Analyzed the data: SA FZ GL SDL LL. Wrote the paper: SA FZ LL.

References

1. Ware LB, Matthay MA (2000) The acute respiratory distress syndrome. N Engl J Med 342: 1334–1349.
2. Matthay M, Zimmerman G (2005) Acute lung injury and the acute respiratory distress syndrome: four decades of inquiry into pathogenesis and rational management. Am J Resp Cell Mol Biol 33: 319–327.
3. Ley B, Collard HR, King TE, Jr. (2011) Clinical course and prediction of survival in idiopathic pulmonary fibrosis. Am J Respir Crit Care Med 183: 431–440.
4. Matute-Bello G, Frevert CW, Martin TR (2008) Animal models of acute lung injury. Am J Physiol Lung Cell Mol Physiol 295: L379–399.
5. London L, Majeski EI, Altman-Hamamdzic S, Enockson C, Paintlia MK, et al. (2002) Respiratory reovirus 1/L induction of diffuse alveolar damage: pulmonary fibrosis is not modulated by corticosteroids in acute respiratory distress syndrome in mice. Clin Immunol 103: 284–295.
6. London L, Majeski EI, Paintlia MK, Harley RA, London SD (2002) Respiratory reovirus 1/L induction of diffuse alveolar damage: a model of acute respiratory distress syndrome. Exp Mol Pathol 72: 24–36.
7. Majeski EI, Harley RA, Bellum SC, London SD, London L (2003) Differential role for T cells in the development of fibrotic lesions associated with reovirus 1/L-induced bronchiolitis obliterans organizing pneumonia versus Acute Respiratory Distress Syndrome. Am J Respir Cell Mol Biol 28: 208–217.
8. Majeski EI, Paintlia MK, Lopez AD, Harley RA, London SD, et al. (2003) Respiratory reovirus 1/L induction of intraluminal fibrosis, a model of bronchiolitis obliterans organizing pneumonia, is dependent on T lymphocytes. Am J Pathol 163: 1467–1479.
9. Lopez AD, Avasarala S, Grewal S, Murali AK, London L (2009) Differential role of the Fas/Fas ligand apoptotic pathway in inflammation and lung fibrosis associated with reovirus 1/L-induced bronchiolitis obliterans organizing pneumonia and acute respiratory distress syndrome. J Immunol 183: 8244–8257.
10. Srimal RC, Dhawan BN (1973) Pharmacology of diferuloyl methane (curcumin), a non-steroidal anti-inflammatory agent. J Pharm Pharmacol 25: 447–452.
11. Maheshwari RK, Singh AK, Gaddipati J, Srimal RC (2006) Multiple biological activities of curcumin: a short review. Life Sci 78: 2081–2087.
12. Sharma OP (1976) Antioxidant activity of curcumin and related compounds. Biochem Pharmacol 25: 1811–1812.
13. Stengler M, Balch JF (2002) Natural Physician's Healing Therapies: Prentice Hall Publishers, USA. pgs 444–446.
14. Sharma RA, Gescher AJ, Steward WP (2005) Curcumin: the story so far. Eur J Cancer 41: 1955–1968.
15. Sharma RA, Euden SA, Platton SL, Cooke DN, Shafayat A, et al. (2004) Phase I clinical trial of oral curcumin: biomarkers of systemic activity and compliance. Clin Cancer Res 10: 6847–6854.
16. Aggarwal BB, Harikumar KB (2009) Potential therapeutic effects of curcumin, the anti-inflammatory agent, against neurodegenerative, cardiovascular, pulmonary, metabolic, autoimmune and neoplastic diseases. Int J Biochem Cell Biol 41: 40–59.
17. Anand P, Thomas SG, Kunnumakkara AB, Sundaram C, Harikumar KB, et al. (2008) Biological activities of curcumin and its analogues (Congeners) made by man and Mother Nature. Biochem Pharmacol 76: 1590–1611.
18. Aggarwal BB, Kumar A, Aggarwal MS, et al. (2005) Curcumin derived from turmeric (Curcuma longa): a spice for all seasons;. Preuss PDDBHG, editor. New York: CRC Press pg 350–378.
19. Joe B, Vijaykumar M, Lokesh BR (2004) Biological properties of curcumin-cellular and molecular mechanisms of action. Crit Rev Food Sci Nutr 44: 97–111.
20. Tourkina E, Gooz P, Oates JC, Ludwicka-Bradley A, Silver RM, et al. (2004) Curcumin-induced apoptosis in scleroderma lung fibroblasts: role of protein kinase cepsilon. Am J Respir Cell Mol Biol 31: 28–35.
21. Tourkina E, Hoffman S, Fenton JW, 2nd, Lipsitz S, Silver RW, et al. (2001) Depletion of protein kinase Cepsilon in normal and scleroderma lung fibroblasts has opposite effects on tenascin expression. Arthritis Rheum 44: 1370–1381.
22. Punithavathi D, Venkatesan N, Babu M (2000) Curcumin inhibition of bleomycin-induced pulmonary fibrosis in rats. Br J Pharmacol 131: 169–172.

23. Punithavathi D, Venkatesan N, Babu M (2003) Protective effects of curcumin against amiodarone-induced pulmonary fibrosis in rats. Br J Pharmacol 139: 1342–1350.
24. Venkatesan N, Chandrakasan G (1995) Modulation of cyclophosphamide-induced early lung injury by curcumin, an anti-inflammatory antioxidant. Mol Cell Biochem 142: 79–87.
25. Venkatesan N, Punithavathi V, Chandrakasan G (1997) Curcumin protects bleomycin-induced lung injury in rats. Life Sci 61: PL51–58.
26. Venkatesan N (2000) Pulmonary protective effects of curcumin against paraquat toxicity. Life Sci 66: PL21–28.
27. Literat A, Su F, Norwicki M, Durand M, Ramanathan R, et al. (2001) Regulation of pro-inflammatory cytokine expression by curcumin in hyaline membrane disease (HMD). Life Sci 70: 253–267.
28. Biswas SK, McClure D, Jimenez LA, Megson IL, Rahman I (2005) Curcumin induces glutathione biosynthesis and inhibits NF-kappaB activation and interleukin-8 release in alveolar epithelial cells: mechanism of free radical scavenging activity. Antioxid Redox Signal 7: 32–41.
29. Zhu RF, Zhou M, He JL, Ding FY, Yu SQ, et al. (2008) [Protective effect of curcumin on oleic-induced acute lung injury in rats]. Zhongguo Zhong Yao Za Zhi 33: 2141–2145.
30. Nahra R, Dellinger RP (2008) Targeting the lipopolysaccharides: still a matter of debate? Curr Opin Anaesthesiol 21: 98–104.
31. Tham CL, Lam KW, Rajajendram R, Cheah YK, Sulaiman MR, et al. (2011) The effects of a synthetic curcuminoid analogue, 2,6-bis-(4-hydroxyl-3-methoxybenzylidine)cyclohexanone on proinflammatory signaling pathways and CLP-induced lethal sepsis in mice. Eur J Pharmacol 652: 136–144.
32. Thiemermann C (2006) The spice of life: curcumin reduces the mortality associated with experimental sepsis. Crit Care Med 34: 2009–2011.
33. Vachharajani V, Wang SW, Mishra N, El Gazzar M, Yoza B, et al. (2010) Curcumin modulates leukocyte and platelet adhesion in murine sepsis. Microcirculation 17: 407–416.
34. Sun D, Zhuang X, Xiang X, Liu Y, Zhang S, et al. (2010) A novel nanoparticle drug delivery system: the anti-inflammatory activity of curcumin is enhanced when encapsulated in exosomes. Mol Ther 18: 1606–1614.
35. Guzel A, Kanter M, Aksu B, Basaran UN, Yalcin O, et al. (2009) Preventive effects of curcumin on different aspiration material-induced lung injury in rats. Pediatr Surg Int 25: 83–92.
36. Bellum SC, Dove D, Harley RA, Greene WB, Judson MA, et al. (1997) Respiratory reovirus 1/L induction of intraluminal fibrosis. A model for the study of bronchiolitis obliterans organizing pneumonia. Am J Pathol 150: 2243–2254.
37. Amin K, Ludviksdottir D, Janson C, Nettelbladt O, Bjornsson E, et al. (2000) Inflammation and structural changes in the airways of patients with atopic and nonatopic asthma. BHR Group. Am J Respir Crit Care Med 162: 2295–2301.
38. Laitinen A, Altraja A, Kampe M, Linden M, Virtanen I, et al. (1997) Tenascin is increased in airway basement membrane of asthmatics and decreased by an inhaled steroid. Am J Respir Crit Care Med 156: 951–958.
39. Kaarteenaho-Wiik R, Lakari E, Soini Y, Pollanen R, Kinnula VL, et al. (2000) Tenascin expression and distribution in pleural inflammatory and fibrotic diseases. J Histochem Cytochem 48: 1257–1268.
40. Paakko P, Kaarteenaho-Wiik R, Pollanen R, Soini Y (2000) Tenascin mRNA expression at the foci of recent injury in usual interstitial pneumonia. Am J Respir Crit Care Med 161: 967–972.
41. Del Sorbo L, Slutsky AS (2011) Acute respiratory distress syndrome and multiple organ failure. Curr Opin Crit Care 17: 1–6.
42. Creagh-Brown BC, Griffiths MJ, Evans TW (2009) Bench-to-bedside review: Inhaled nitric oxide therapy in adults. Crit Care 13: 221.
43. Lee PJ (2005) An old spice with new twists: curcumin, p38 mitogen-activated protein kinase, and apoptosis. Crit Care Med 33: 2703–2705.
44. Baldwin AS, Jr. (2001) Series introduction: the transcription factor NF-kappaB and human disease. J Clin Invest 107: 3–6.
45. Tak PP, Firestein GS (2001) NF-kappaB: a key role in inflammatory diseases. J Clin Invest 107: 7–11.
46. Morris GF (2010) An alternative to lung inflammation and fibrosis. Am J Pathol 176: 2595–2598.
47. Han W, Joo M, Everhart MB, Christman JW, Yull FE, et al. (2009) Myeloid cells control termination of lung inflammation through the NF-kappaB pathway. Am J Physiol Lung Cell Mol Physiol 296: L320–327.
48. Tully JE, Nolan JD, Guala AS, Hoffman SM, Roberson EC, et al. (2012) Cooperation between classical and alternative NF-κB pathways regulates proinflammatory responses in epithelial cells. Am J of Resp Cell Mol Biol 47: 497–508.
49. Yang KY, Arcaroli JJ, Abraham E (2003) Early alterations in neutrophil activation are associated with outcome in acute lung injury. Am J Respir Crit Care Med 167: 1567–1574.
50. Moine P, McIntyre R, Schwartz MD, Kaneko D, Shenkar R, et al. (2000) NF-kappaB regulatory mechanisms in alveolar macrophages from patients with acute respiratory distress syndrome. Shock 13: 85–91.
51. Arnalich F, Garcia-Palomero E, Lopez J, Jimenez M, Madero R, et al. (2000) Predictive value of nuclear factor kappaB activity and plasma cytokine levels in patients with sepsis. Infect Immun 68: 1942–1945.
52. Bohrer H, Qiu F, Zimmermann T, Zhang Y, Jllmer T, et al. (1997) Role of NFkappaB in the mortality of sepsis. J Clin Invest 100: 972–985.
53. Singh S, Aggarwal BB (1995) Activation of transcription factor NF-kappa B is suppressed by curcumin (diferuloylmethane) [corrected]. J Biol Chem 270: 24995–25000.
54. Kim GY, Kim KH, Lee SH, Yoon MS, Lee HJ, et al. (2005) Curcumin inhibits immunostimulatory function of dendritic cells: MAPKs and translocation of NF-kappa B as potential targets. J Immunol 174: 8116–8124.
55. Liu K, Chen HL, Huang H, Jing H, Dong GH, et al. (2012) Curcumin Attenuates Cardiopulmonary Bypass-Induced Lung Oxidative Damage in Rats. J Cardiovasc Pharmacol Ther 17: 395–402.
56. Liu K, Shen L, Wang J, Dong G, Wu H, et al. (2012) The preventative role of curcumin on the lung inflammatory response induced by cardiopulmonary bypass in rats. J Surg Res 174: 73–82.
57. Oh SW, Cha JY, Jung JE, Chang BC, Kwon HJ, et al. (2011) Curcumin attenuates allergic airway inflammation and hyper-responsiveness in mice through NF-kappaB inhibition. J Ethnopharmacol 136: 414–421.
58. Prud'homme GJ (2007) Pathobiology of transforming growth factor beta in cancer, fibrosis and immunologic disease, and therapeutic considerations. Lab Invest 87: 1077–1091.
59. Gauldie J, Bonniaud P, Sime P, Ask K, Kolb M (2007) TGF-beta, Smad3 and the process of progressive fibrosis. Biochem Soc Trans 35: 661–664.
60. Scotton CJ, Chambers RC (2007) Molecular targets in pulmonary fibrosis: the myofibroblast in focus. Chest 132: 1311–1321.
61. Dhainaut JF, Charpentier J, Chiche JD (2003) Transforming growth factor-beta: a mediator of cell regulation in acute respiratory distress syndrome. Crit Care Med 31: S258–264.
62. Budinger GR, Chandel NS, Donnelly HK, Eisenbart J, Oberoi M, et al. (2005) Active transforming growth factor-beta1 activates the procollagen I promoter in patients with acute lung injury. Intensive Care Med 31: 121–128.
63. Fahy RJ, Lichtenberger F, McKeegan CB, Nuovo GJ, Marsh CB, et al. (2003) The acute respiratory distress syndrome: a role for transforming growth factor-beta 1. Am J Respir Cell Mol Biol 28: 499–503.
64. Thresiamma KC, George J, Kuttan R (1996) Protective effect of curcumin, ellagic acid and bixin on radiation induced toxicity. Indian J Exp Biol 34: 845–847.
65. Cutroneo KR, White SL, Phan SH, Ehrlich HP (2007) Therapies for bleomycin induced lung fibrosis through regulation of TGF-beta1 induced collagen gene expression. J Cell Physiol 211: 585–589.
66. Xu M, Deng B, Chow YL, Zhao ZZ, Hu B (2007) Effects of curcumin in treatment of experimental pulmonary fibrosis: a comparison with hydrocortisone. J Ethnopharmacol 112: 292–299.
67. Chen B, Zhang DP, Gao W (2008) [Effect of curcumin on the expression of collagen type I protein and transforming growth factor-beta1 mRNA in pulmonary fibrosis rats]. Zhonghua Lao Dong Wei Sheng Zhi Ye Bing Za Zhi 26: 257–261.
68. Zhang DP, Qiu H, Zhuang Y, Meng FQ (2007) [The effect of curcumin on bleomycin-induced pulmonary fibrosis in rats]. Zhonghua Jie He He Hu Xi Za Zhi 30: 197–201.
69. Smith MR, Gangireddy SR, Narala VR, Hogaboam CM, Standiford TJ, et al. (2010) Curcumin inhibits fibrosis-related effects in IPF fibroblasts and in mice following bleomycin-induced lung injury. Am J Physiol Lung Cell Mol Physiol 298: L616–625.
70. Jiang ZY, Zou L, Shi SS, Lu YR, Dong J, et al. (2009) [Effects of curcumin on TNF-alpha and TGF-beta1 in serum and lung tissue of SiO2-induced fibrosis in mice]. Xi Bao Yu Fen Zi Mian Yi Xue Za Zhi 25: 399–401.
71. Song K, Peng S, Sun Z, Li H, Yang R (2011) Curcumin suppresses TGF-beta signaling by inhibition of TGIF degradation in scleroderma fibroblasts. Biochem Biophys Res Commun 411: 821–825.
72. Jimenez SA, Gaidarova S, Saitta B, Sandorfi N, Herrich DJ, et al. (2001) Role of protein kinase C-delta in the regulation of collagen gene expression in scleroderma fibroblasts. J Clin Invest 108: 1395–1403.
73. Hsu YC, Chen MJ, Yu YM, Ko SY, Chang CC (2010) Suppression of TGF-beta1/SMAD pathway and extracellular matrix production in primary keloid fibroblasts by curcuminoids: its potential therapeutic use in the chemoprevention of keloid. Arch Dermatol Res 302: 717–724.
74. Gaedeke J, Noble NA, Border WA (2004) Curcumin blocks multiple sites of the TGF-beta signaling cascade in renal cells. Kidney Int 66: 112–120.
75. Meier M, Menne J, Park JK, Holtz M, Gueler F, et al. (2007) Deletion of protein kinase C-epsilon signaling pathway induces glomerulosclerosis and tubulointerstitial fibrosis in vivo. J Am Soc Nephrol 18: 1190–1198.
76. Zheng S, Chen A (2004) Activation of PPARgamma is required for curcumin to induce apoptosis and to inhibit the expression of extracellular matrix genes in hepatic stellate cells in vitro. Biochem J 384: 149–157.
77. Zheng S, Chen A (2006) Curcumin suppresses the expression of extracellular matrix genes in activated hepatic stellate cells by inhibiting gene expression of connective tissue growth factor. Am J Physiol Gastrointest Liver Physiol 290: G883–893.
78. Zheng S, Chen A (2007) Disruption of transforming growth factor-beta signaling by curcumin induces gene expression of peroxisome proliferator-activated receptor-gamma in rat hepatic stellate cells. Am J Physiol Gastrointest Liver Physiol 292: G113–123.
79. Matute-Bello G, Liles WC, Steinberg KP, Kiener PA, Mongovin S, et al. (1999) Soluble Fas ligand induces epithelial cell apoptosis in humans with acute lung injury (ARDS). J Immunol 163: 2217–2225.

80. Martin TR, Hagimoto N, Nakamura M, Matute-Bello G (2005) Apoptosis and epithelial injury in the lungs. Proc Am Thorac Soc 2: 214–220.
81. Albertine KH, Soulier MF, Wang Z, Ishizaka A, Hashimoto S, et al. (2002) Fas and fas ligand are up-regulated in pulmonary edema fluid and lung tissue of patients with acute lung injury and the acute respiratory distress syndrome. Am J Pathol 161: 1783–1796.
82. Nick JA, Avdi NJ, Young SK, Lehman LA, McDonald PP, et al. (1999) Selective activation and functional significance of p38alpha mitogen-activated protein kinase in lipopolysaccharide-stimulated neutrophils. J Clin Invest 103: 851–858.
83. Hu M, Du Q, Vancurova I, Lin X, Miller EJ, et al. (2005) Proapoptotic effect of curcumin on human neutrophils: activation of the p38 mitogen-activated protein kinase pathway. Crit Care Med 33: 2571–2578.
84. Wang Y, Rishi AK, Wu W, Polin L, Sharma S, et al. (2011) Curcumin suppresses growth of mesothelioma cells in vitro and in vivo, in part, by stimulating apoptosis. Mol Cell Biochem 357: 83–94.
85. Lee JY, Lee YM, Chang GC, Yu SL, Hsieh WY, et al. (2011) Curcumin induces EGFR degradation in lung adenocarcinoma and modulates p38 activation in intestine: the versatile adjuvant for gefitinib therapy. PLoS One 6: e23756.
86. Suresh MV, Wagner MC, Rosania GR, Stringer KA, Min KA, et al. (2012) Pulmonary administration of a water-soluble curcumin complex reduces severity of acute lung injury. Am J Respir Cell Mol Biol 47: 280–287.
87. Bansal S, Chhibber S (2010) Curcumin alone and in combination with augmentin protects against pulmonary inflammation and acute lung injury generated during Klebsiella pneumoniae B5055-induced lung infection in BALB/c mice. J Med Microbiol 59: 429–437.

Mixed Acid-Base Disorders, Hydroelectrolyte Imbalance and Lactate Production in Hypercapnic Respiratory Failure: The Role of Noninvasive Ventilation

Claudio Terzano[1], Fabio Di Stefano[1], Vittoria Conti[1]*, Marta Di Nicola[2], Gregorino Paone[1], Angelo Petroianni[1], Alberto Ricci[1]

1 Fondazione Eleonora Lorillard Spencer Cenci, Sapienza University of Rome, Rome, Italy, **2** Laboratory of Biostatistics, Department of Biomedical Science, University "G. d'Annunzio" of Chieti-Pescara, Chieti, Italy

Abstract

Background: Hypercapnic Chronic Obstructive Pulmonary Disease (COPD) exacerbation in patients with comorbidities and multidrug therapy is complicated by mixed acid-base, hydro-electrolyte and lactate disorders. Aim of this study was to determine the relationships of these disorders with the requirement for and duration of noninvasive ventilation (NIV) when treating hypercapnic respiratory failure.

Methods: Sixty-seven consecutive patients who were hospitalized for hypercapnic COPD exacerbation had their clinical condition, respiratory function, blood chemistry, arterial blood gases, blood lactate and volemic state assessed. Heart and respiratory rates, pH, PaO_2 and $PaCO_2$ and blood lactate were checked at the 1st, 2nd, 6th and 24th hours after starting NIV.

Results: Nine patients were transferred to the intensive care unit. NIV was performed in 11/17 (64.7%) mixed respiratory acidosis–metabolic alkalosis, 10/36 (27.8%) respiratory acidosis and 3/5 (60%) mixed respiratory-metabolic acidosis patients ($p = 0.026$), with durations of 45.1 ± 9.8, 36.2 ± 8.9 and 53.3 ± 4.1 hours, respectively ($p = 0.016$). The duration of ventilation was associated with higher blood lactate ($p < 0.001$), lower pH ($p = 0.016$), lower serum sodium ($p = 0.014$) and lower chloride ($p = 0.038$). Hyponatremia without hypervolemic hypochloremia occurred in 11 respiratory acidosis patients. Hypovolemic hyponatremia with hypochloremia and hypokalemia occurred in 10 mixed respiratory acidosis–metabolic alkalosis patients, and euvolemic hypochloremia occurred in the other 7 patients with this mixed acid-base disorder.

Conclusions: Mixed acid-base and lactate disorders during hypercapnic COPD exacerbations predict the need for and longer duration of NIV. The combination of mixed acid-base disorders and hydro-electrolyte disturbances should be further investigated.

Editor: Mauricio Rojas, University of Pittsburgh, United States of America

Funding: The authors have no support or funding to report.

Competing Interests: The authors have declared that no competing interests exist.

* E-mail: vittoria_conti@hotmail.com

Introduction

Hypercapnic respiratory failure is a complex condition associated with the malfunction of various organs and systems crucial for many physiological processes, leading to an acid-base imbalance.

Carbon dioxide (CO_2) is not the only independent variable that may cause alterations in acid-base status. Total serum protein, albumin in particular, plays an important role, as does the strong ion difference (SID), that is the difference between the strong positive ions in the plasma (sodium (Na^+), potassium (K^+), calcium (Ca^{2+}), and magnesium (Mg^{2+})) and the strong negative ions (chloride (Cl^-) and lactate (Lac^-)):

$$SID = \left[Na^+ + K^+ + Ca^{2+} + Mg^{2+}\right] - \left[Cl^- + Lac^-\right]. \quad (1)$$

At pH 7.4, 37°C and a partial carbon dioxide tension of 40 mmHg, the ideal value of SID is 42 mmol/L . An increased SID causes alkalosis; a reduced SID causes acidosis. Altering SID means altering the water dissociation equilibrium. This provides more/less H^+ for electroneutrality, with a change in $[H^+]$, and so a change in pH.

Acid-base and electrolyte balance are part of the same picture because, for a given increase in CO_2, the only way to minimize the resulting acidemia is to produce compensatory metabolic alkalosis, which is obtained through complex urinary ion excretion mechanisms [2]. Thus, fluid homeostasis depends on the correct relationship between lung and kidney activities because they regulate most of the CO_2 and hydrogen (H^+) concentrations in the extracellular volume, whose total solutes consist almost entirely of Na^+, Cl^- and bicarbonate ions (HCO^{3-}).

In hypoxic and hypercapnic COPD patients, fluid homeostasis is disturbed, with avid retention of sodium and water [3]. The increase in sodium retention by the kidneys during COPD, and the consequent edema, may be explained in part by right heart failure (cor pulmonale) and by other pathophysiological mechanisms involving renal and hormonal abnormalities [3,4].

In hypercapnic COPD exacerbations, the sudden decrease in ventilation causes an acute respiratory acidosis or deteriorates a pre-existing chronic respiratory acidosis. Due to the high prevalence of comorbidities [5] and the associated multidrug therapies in these patients, mixed acid-base and hydro-electrolyte disorders are becoming increasingly common, particularly in the critically ill and elderly populations.

This study had the following aims: to evaluate mixed acid-base, hydro-electrolyte and lactate disorders in patients with hypercapnic COPD exacerbation; to determine the relationship among these disorders, a poor response to pharmacological treatment and the requirement for noninvasive ventilation (NIV); and to analyze the link between these disorders and the duration of NIV in the treatment of hypercapnic respiratory failure.

Methods

Ethics Statement

The institutional review board for human studies (Fondazione Eleonora Lorillard Spencer Cenci Ethics Committee) for human studies approved the protocol, and written consent was obtained from the subjects or their surrogates.

Study design

We investigated patients consecutively hospitalized in our respiratory ward (Respiratory Diseases Unit, Policlinico Umberto I, Rome) for COPD exacerbation and hypercapnic respiratory failure. Between January and April 2010, sixty-seven patients were consecutively hospitalized for COPD exacerbation and hypercapnic respiratory failure. COPD and COPD exacerbation were defined according to the Global Initiative for Chronic Obstructive Lung Disease (GOLD) guidelines [6]. Hypercapnia was defined by a $PaCO_2 \geq 45$ mmHg on arterial blood gas (ABG) analysis [6].

Patients were excluded from this descriptive study if they had concomitant pneumonia, acute lung injury (ALI) or acute respiratory distress syndrome (ARDS), and contraindications to noninvasive ventilation (NIV) [7]. Patients enrolled were not necessarily at the first COPD exacerbation treated with NIV, but those being on chronic NIV treatment at home were excluded. Comorbidities were identified on the basis of clinical records, concomitant therapy, and/or investigations carried out at hospital admission.

Baseline demographic characteristics and clinical parameters, routine blood chemistry and ABG were assessed at admission.

The level of consciousness was assessed using the Glasgow Coma Scale [8]. The severity of the clinical condition was quantified by the Acute Physiology and Chronic Health Evaluation II score [9].

Patients were classified into pure respiratory acidosis or mixed defect (mixed respiratory acidosis–metabolic alkalosis and mixed respiratory-metabolic acidosis) categories [10]. Hypernatremia and hyponatremia were classified as hypovolemic, euvolemic and hypervolemic [11,12], according to the clinical assessment, total body water (TBW), relative body water deficit, serum urea to creatinine ratio, serum sodium (sNa^+), urinary sodium (uNa^+), plasma osmolality (Posm) and urine specific gravity (SG). TBW was expressed as a percentage of body weight (body weight * correction factor, where the correction factor was 0.6 for men, 0.5 for women and elderly men and 0.45 for elderly women). Body water deficit was calculated using the following equation:

$$(TBW) * [1 - (140/Na^+)].$$

Plasma osmolality was calculated using the following equation:

$$2[Na^+] + \frac{[Glucose]}{18} + \frac{[BUN]}{2.8}.$$

Because the patients' clinical conditions did not allow us to conduct reliable pulmonary function tests, the data (FVC and FEV_1) considered for the analysis were those measured subsequently at a stable clinical condition (or rather when vital and gas-exchange parameters improved and stabilized and patients' dyspnea was not severe enough to not allow respiratory manouvres required by lung function testing).

Initially, all patients received controlled oxygen therapy with a Venturi mask, in order to maintain an arterial oxygen saturation (SaO_2) at least $\geq 90\%$, and conventional treatments, including nebulized bronchodilators, intravenous corticosteroids, antibiotics (if necessary) and other drugs, depending on the concomitant comorbidities. NIV was initiated when controlled oxygen therapy and convientional medical treatments failed to improve the clinical conditions, or rather when respiratory distress with accessory muscle use or abdominal paradox and tachypnea (respiratory rate >24/min) were associated with persistent arterial impairment (pH<7.35, $PaCO_2 > 45$ mmHg, and $PaO_2/FiO_2 < 200$) despite optimal pharmacological treatment and oxygen therapy [7,13]. NIV was performed via an oronasal mask using a pressure support turbine ventilator (Polar 2 Hackermann & Bild Ltd., Crespellano, Bologna, Italy) with a bi-tube connection. The pressure support, PEEP and flow-by trigger values were adjusted to obtain a tidal volume of 6–8 ml/kg and to gain the best oxygenation and reduce the respiratory rate. They were modified based on the blood gas data. Heart and respiratory rates, pH, PaO_2 and $PaCO_2$ and blood lactate were checked on the 1st, 2nd, 6th and 24th hours after starting NIV.

NIV was withdrawn when the clinical condition improved and stabilized, as defined by the following objective parameters: respiratory rate <24/min, heart rate <110/min, pH>7.35 and $SaO_2 > 90\%$ on $FiO_2 < 40\%$ [14]. Patients were a priori considered for invasive mechanical ventilation if the following conditions were present: a worsening of arterial pH and carbon dioxide tension despite correct NIV administration, an onset of coma, cardiovascular instability or poor compliance with the NIV device [15].

Statistical analysis

All quantitative variables are summarized as mean and standard deviation (SD), and the qualitative variables are summarized as frequency and percentage. The results are reported separately for each of the two groups (NIV use and no NIV use). The statistical analysis was conducted by parametric or non-parametric test, according to the distribution of variables as assessed by the Shapiro-Wilk test. Student's t-test for unpaired data was used to compare the quantitative variables between the two groups (NIV use and no NIV use), while the chi-squared test was used for qualitative variables. The unadjusted odds ratio (OR) for NIV use vs. no NIV use and its associated 95% confidence interval (95% CI) were calculated for each variable by a logistic regression analysis. One-way ANOVA for repeated measures was used with the clinical parameters, ABG results and lactate values to evaluate the effects of NIV use over 24 h. Contrast analysis, a priori specified, was used for comparisons versus previous time points.

The differences in NIV duration among groups of patients identified according to the ABG analysis values (respiratory acidosis, mixed respiratory acidosis–metabolic alkalosis and mixed respiratory-metabolic acidosis) were evaluated using the Kruskal-Wallis H test. The Mann-Whitney U test with Bonferroni correction was applied to evaluate the differences of various parameters at each time point between respiratory acidosis patients and mixed respiratory acidosis–metabolic alkalosis patients. Linear regression analysis was applied to evaluate the relationships between NIV duration and various parameters.

Statistical analysis was performed using SPSS Advanced Statistical 10.0 software (SPSS Inc., Chicago, Illinois, USA).

Results

Between January and April 2010, 75 patients were consecutively hospitalized for COPD exacerbation and hypercapnic respiratory failure, but 67 were enrolled in the study population (5 patients were excluded for being on chronic NIV treatment at home and the other 3 for the presence of concomitant pneumonia).

We considered 58 of the 67 patients initially enrolled, as 9 were excluded because they were transferred to the intensive care unit for pH<7.1, hypercapnic coma or hemodynamic instability (Figure 1).

The enrolled COPD patients had multiple comorbidities, such as hypertension (27 patients, 46.5%); ischemic heart disease (11, 18.9%); degenerative, hypertensive and valvular heart disease (25 patients, 43.1%); atrial fibrillation and other arrhythmias (18, 31%); cor pulmonale (13, 22.4%); peripheral artery disease (9, 15.5%); diabetes mellitus (17, 29.3%); chronic renal failure (20, 34.5%); and obstructive sleep apnea syndrome (4, 6.9%). Therefore they were on multidrugs treatments including diuretics, ACE inhibitors, angiotensin receptor antagonists, digoxin, anti-arrhythmic drugs (such as propafenone, amiodarone, selective beta-blockers and verapamil), oral hypoglycemic agents, insulin, allopurinol, aspirin, statins and inhaled bronchodilators.

NIV was initiated in 24 patients and succeeded in correcting respiratory acidosis in all of them. The mean duration of NIV was 42.4±10.5 hours, and the mean IPAP employed was 16±4 cmH_2O. Supplementary oxygen was administered during ventilation, which was continuous until clinical conditions were stable with pauses for administration of conventional medications, feeding and general care. None of the patients required the interruption of the ventilatory assistance for discomfort, or refused the treatment. The only complications recorded were 1 case of

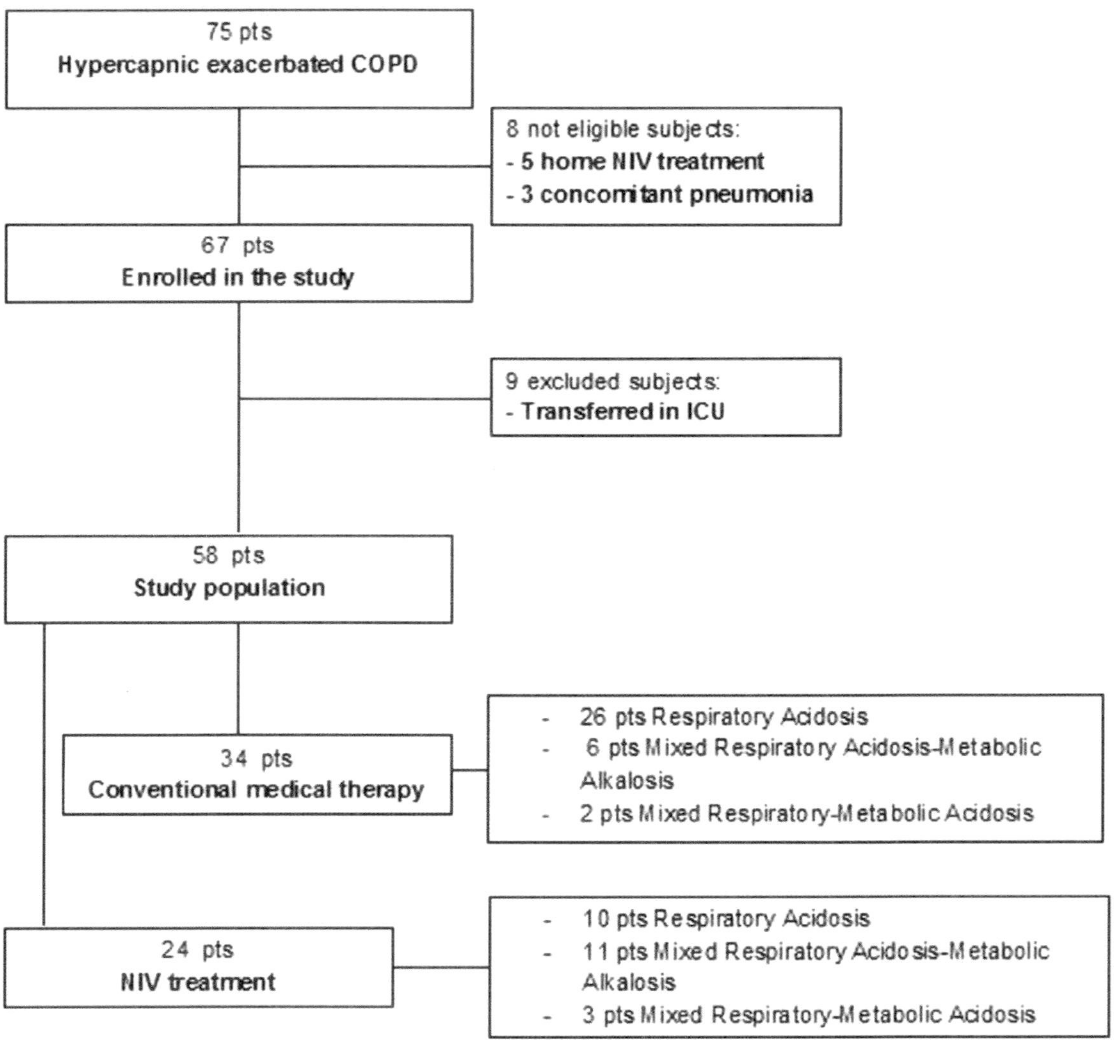

Figure 1. Flow chart of the consecutive COPD patients with acute hypercapnic exhacerbation enrolled in the study.

nasal cutaneous sores and 2 cases of gastric distension, neither of which required interrupting the ventilatory assistance.

Patient demographics and clinical characteristics are shown in table 1. Clinical and metabolic parameters, ABG analysis, electrolyte values, lactate, and urinalysis with electrolytes are shown in table 2.

Compared to patients undergoing standard therapy, subjects requiring NIV had a higher respiratory rate; lower PaO_2, PaO_2/FiO_2, alveolar–arterial PaO_2 gradient, Na^-, Cl^-, pH and serum lactate; and higher $PaCO_2$ and blood lactate (Table 2, figure 2).

The changes in clinical parameters, AEG results and lactate values during the first 24 hours of ventilation are shown in table 3.

Using the ABG data and assessing the SID, we identified 36 patients with pure respiratory acidosis (anion gap 11.4±2.3 mmol/L; SID 40.7±1.2 mmol/L), 17 patients with mixed respiratory acidosis–metabolic alkalosis (anion gap 9.6±1.5 mmol/L; SID 49.1±2.0 mmol/L) and other 5 with mixed respiratory-metabolic acidosis (anion gap 25.9±3.6 mmol/L; SID 29.2±1.8 mmol/L) (Figure 3).

Patients with mixed respiratory acidosis–metabolic alkalosis were more likely to use NIV than those with the pure respiratory acidosis, and their NIV duration was longer (Table 4). NIV was used for 3 of the patients with mixed respiratory-metabolic acidosis, and these patients had the longest ventilation times (Table 4).

NIV duration was significantly associated with higher blood lactate, lower pH and lower serum Na^+ and Cl^- concentrations, as shown by their regression coefficients ($b = 17.038$ and $p<0.001$ for lactate, $b = -111.975$ and $p = 0.016$ for pH, $b = -0.478$ and $p = 0.014$ for Na^+, and $b = -0.660$ and $p = 0.038$ for Cl^-).

In respiratory acidosis and mixed respiratory acidosis–metabolic alkalosis NIV patients, heart rate, respiratory rate, pH, PaO_2, $PaCO_2$ and blood lactate improved in the first 6 hours of NIV (Figure 4), while significant improvements in the same parameters were observed between the 6th and the 24th hour of ventilation in the mixed respiratory-metabolic acidosis patients (data not shown).

We also evaluated hydro-electrolyte balance and identified 11 respiratory acidosis patients who had normochloremic hypervolemic hyponatremia due to chronic renal failure (n = 2), cirrhosis (n = 1), hypothyroidism (n = 1), or chronic congestive heart failure (n = 7).

Of the patients with mixed respiratory acidosis–metabolic alkalosis, 10 had hypovolemic hyponatremia, hypochloremia and hypokalemia due to thiazide or loop diuretic use associated with diarrhea and vomiting during a gastroenteritis episode (n = 2), profuse sweating from febrile influenza syndrome (n = 4) or (probably) poor dietary fluid intake (n = 4). Euvolemic hypochloremia due to thiazide or loop diuretic use not associated with extrarenal hydro-electrolyte loss was detected in 7 patients with mixed respiratory acidosis–metabolic alkalosis.

In mixed respiratory-metabolic acidosis patients, the metabolic acidosis was due to an exacerbation of chronic renal failure (n = 1), rhabdomyolysis (n = 1), ketoacidosis in decompensated insulin-dependent diabetes mellitus (n = 2) or metformin-related lactic acidosis (n = 1 obese diabetic patient).

Discussion

Hypercapnic respiratory failure during acute COPD exacerbation is an alarming event that requires careful management of the resulting respiratory acidosis. The final outcome depends on various factors, such as the patient's overall health status and concomitant comorbidities, the baseline lung function, and the disease severity as judged by the need for assisted ventilation and the degree of acidosis [16]. Our observations provide evidence that mixed acid-base and lactate disorders in patients with hypercapnic respiratory failure due to COPD exacerbation lead to the need for and longer duration of NIV. More data should be provided to evaluate this association with combined mixed acid-base and hydroelectrolyte disorders.

Mixed respiratory acidosis–metabolic alkalosis

We observed that metabolic alkalosis with hyponatremia and/or hypochloremia aggravated the respiratory acidosis due to the COPD exacerbation. Mixed respiratory acidosis–metabolic alkalosis patients were more likely to use NIV and were subjected to longer periods of ventilation compared to those with pure respiratory acidosis. The requirement for and duration of NIV was associated with low serum sodium and chloride, common findings in diuretic-induced metabolic alkalosis. The clinical parameters and ABG analysis indicated more severe ventilatory impairment in the patients with mixed respiratory acidosis–metabolic alkalosis than in those with pure respiratory acidosis,

Table 1. Patients demographics and clinical characteristics.

Variables	Total (n = 58)	NIV use (n = 24)	No NIV use (n = 34)	p-value[a]
Gender: Male (n, %)	43 (74.2)	18 (75)	25 (73.5)	0.028[b]
Gender: Female (n, %)	15 (25.8)	6 (25)	9 (26.5)	
Age (years)	79.3±5.1	79.8±5.4	78.8±4.9	0.511
BMI (Kg/m²)	27.0±2.6	27.3±3.3	26.7±2.1	0.356
SBP (mmHg)	138.8±16.9	135.8±17.7	140.9±16.2	0.256
DBP (mmHg)	76.7±8.2	74.6±9.8	78.2±6.7	0.097
FEV_1 (L)	2.3±0.7	2.4±0.8	2.3±0.7	0.773
FEV_1 (%)	57.9±9.9	58.6±9.6	57.4±10.2	0.654
GCS	12.4±1.6	11.8±1.8	12.8±1.3	0.022
APACHE II score	17.7±6.2	18.4±7.5	17.2±5.1	0.477

Data expressed as Mean ± Standard Deviation.
[a]Student t-test for unpaired data;
[b]Chi-Squared Test. NIV = non invasive ventilation; BMI = Body Mass Index; SBP = Systolic Blood Pressure; DBP = Diastolic Blood Pressure; FEV_1 = Forced Expiratory Volume; GCS = Glasgow Coma Scale; APACHE II score = Acute physiology and chronic health evaluation II score.

Table 2. Patients main clinical and metabolic parameters, ABG analysis, lactate, serum electrolytes and urinalysis.

Variables	Total (n = 58)	NIV use (n = 24)	No NIV use (n = 34)	p-value[a]
Glycemia (mg/dl)	139.5±80.5	150.3±91.2	131.9±72.4	0.396
Serum albumin (g/L)	3.9±0.5	4.0±0.5	3.9±0.4	0.339
Serum uric acid (mg/dl)	5.7±2.1	5.9±2.5	5.6±1.9	0.651
Serum creatinine (mg/dl)	1.3±0.7	1.4±0.7	1.3±0.6	0.798
Heart rate (beats/minute)	116.7±11.7	119.7±12.4	114.6±10.9	0.108
Respiratory rate (breaths/minute)	29.7±4.0	32.2±3.0	27.9±3.6	<0.001
PaO_2 (mmHg)	59.7±6.7	54.5±4.6	63.4±5.4	<0.001
PaO_2/FiO_2	178.6±38.5	160.5±38.2	191.5±33.6	0.002
$P(A\text{-}a)O_2$	20.2±6.1	18.2±5.6	21.6±6.1	0.037
pH	7.31±0.06	7.22±0.04	7.34±0.04	<0.001
$PaCO_2$ (mmHg)	68.6±8.3	75.6±5.5	63.7±6.2	<0.001
Lactate (mmol/L)	1.7±0.2	3.1±0.6	0.7±0.2	<0.001
Serum HCO_3^- (mmol/L)	33.6±7.8	35.6±10.5	32.1±5.0	0.089
sNa^+ (mmol/L)	133.4±9.8	129.4±10.9	136.2±8.0	0.008
sK^+ (mmol/L)	4.0±0.7	3.9±0.9	4.0±0.5	0.683
sCl^- (mmol/L)	98.1±6.1	95.0±6.8	100.2±4.5	0.001
sCa^{2+} (mmol/L)	1.21±0.2	1.19±0.1	1.23±0.1	0.645
sMg^{2+} (mmol/L)	1±0.3	1±0.2	0.9±0.3	0.592
Plasma osmolality (Posm)	304.9±17.9	309.7±21.4	301.4±14.5	0.084
uNa^+ (mmol/L)	141.5±87.2	123.1±82.2	154.5±89.4	0.178
uK^+ (mmol/L)	90.3±28.6	101.3±32.0	85.2±30.0	0.055
uCl^- (mmol/L)	168.2±62.5	176.8±69.8	162.1±57.0	0.384
Urine specific gravity	1025.7±9.1	1025.6±9.1	1025.7±9.2	0.980

Data expressed as Mean ± Standard Deviation.
[a]Student t-test for unpaired data. ABG = arterial blood gases; NIV = non invasive ventilation; FiO_2 = Fraction of inspired O_2; $P(A\text{-}a)O_2$ = alveolar-arterial PO_2 gradient; sNa^+ = serum sodium; sK^+ = serum potassium; sCl^- = serum chloride; sCa^{2+} = serum calcium; sMg^{2+} = serum magnesium; uNa^+ = urine sodium; uK^+ = urine potassium; uCl^- = urine chloride.

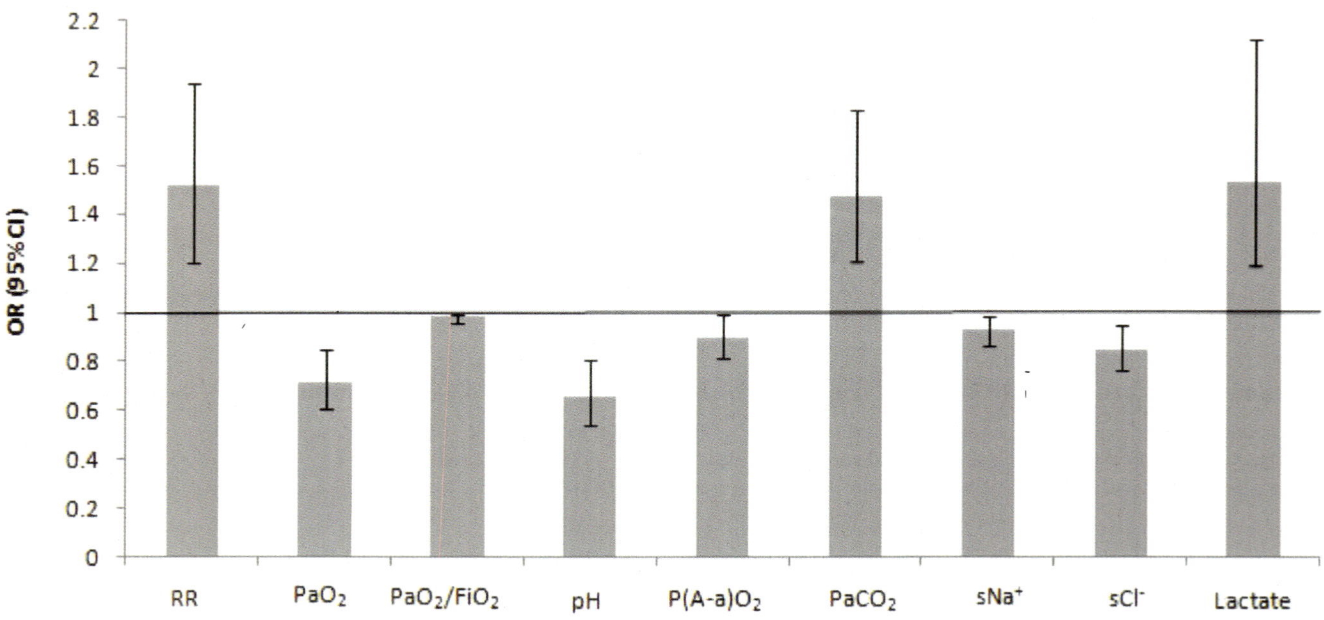

Figure 2. Unadjusted odds ratios (OR) and 95% confidence intervals for NIV use with respect to clinical parameters, ABG results and lactate and electrolyte values that were statistically significant. NIV = noninvasive ventilation; ABG = arterial blood gases; RR = respiratory rate; $P(A\text{-}a)O_2$ = alveolar–arterial PO_2 gradient; sNa^+ = serum sodium; sCl^- = serum chloride.

Table 3. Clinical parameters, ABG analysis and lactate values at different time during NIV.

Variables	1 h	2 h	6 h	24 h	p-value[a]
Heart rate (beats/min)	113.4±14.7	111.3±14.8**	106.9±16.8**	100.3±17.8**	<0.001
Respiratory rate (breaths/min)	29.6±4.9	28.5±4.7**	26.0±5.0**	22.6±4.4**	<0.001
pH	7.26±0.07	7.38±0.07**	7.31±0.07**	7.35±0.06**	<0.001
PaO_2 (mmHg)	59.3±8.9	61.8±9.3*	64.3±10.0**	66.5±10.1*	<0.001
$PaCO_2$ (mmHg)	68.0±12.2	66.5±12.2*	62.7±12.5**	59.5±11.7**	<0.001
Lactate (mmol/L)	2.9±0.6	2.6±0.7**	2.1±0.8**	1.4±0.8**	<0.001

Data expressed as Mean ± Standard Deviation.
[a]ANOVA test for repeated measures;
**p<0.001;
*p<0.01 contrast analysis vs previous time point. ABG = arterial blood gases; NIV = non invasive ventilation.

with the exception of those with an elevated pH due to a simultaneous alkalinizing processes.

In patients with hypercapnic respiratory failure due to COPD exacerbation, the presence of a sufficient metabolic compensation and adequate renal function significantly decreases mortality [17]. In our study, the bicarbonate increase overcame the expected renal compensatory response, reflecting a mixed acid-base disorder with metabolic alkalosis due to various causes in patients with multiple comorbidities and undergoing multidrug treatment. The use of diuretics for cardiovascular comorbidities was the main cause of metabolic alkalosis with hyponatremia and/or hypochloremia.

Metabolic alkalosis causes a direct depression of the respiratory drive, leads to diminished chemoreceptor stimulation and consequently reduces alveolar ventilation to increase $PaCO_2$ and lower pH toward normal levels [18,19,20].

Metabolic alkalosis is usually associated with hypochloremia, which has a relevant inhibitory effect on the ventilatory response to hypercapnia. A reduction of serum chloride is associated with a reduced chloride concentration in the cerebrospinal fluid [21]. Because the cerebrospinal fluid does not contain significant weak acids, a reduction of its chloride level will result in a bicarbonate increase to maintain electroneutrality, which raises the central pH and leads to hypoventilation.

In addition, metabolic alkalosis has been associated with increased airway resistance [22]. In our study, it probably contributed to the increased respiratory impairment in the mixed respiratory acidosis–metabolic alkalosis patients when compared to the subjects with pure respiratory acidosis.

In a study investigating the effects of metabolic acid-base changes on central ventilatory chemoregulation in normocapnic and hypercapnic COPD patients, the ventilatory responsiveness to carbon dioxide was not significantly altered by the induced metabolic state [23]. These results may seem inconsistent with our observations, but we believe that they are not comparable for several reasons. In the van de Ven et al. study [23], chronic metabolic acidosis and alkalosis were experimentally induced by the oral administration of acetazolamide and furosemide, respectively, and were not caused by various comorbidities from their multidrug treatments. The authors evaluated the responses of inspired ventilation (V_I) and mouth occlusion pressure ($P_{0.1}$) to changes in $PaCO_2$, while we investigated the possible deleterious effects of metabolic alkalosis on the ventilatory response to hypercapnia by assessing the requirement and duration of NIV in a real clinical scenario.

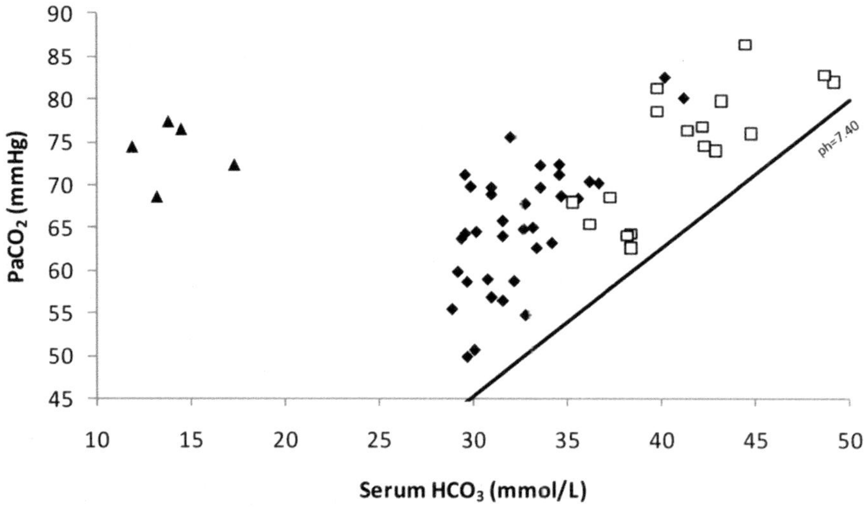

Figure 3. Acid-base balances in patients with hypercapnic COPD exacerbation. *Black lozenge*: Respiratory acidosis. *White square*: Mixed respiratory acidosis–metabolic alkalosis; *Black triangle*: Mixed respiratory-metabolic acidosis.

Table 4. Duration of NIV in groups of patients according to ABG analysis values.

Patients	Overall	NIV use (n, %)[a]	Hours of NIV (Mean ± SD)[b]
Overall	58	24, 41.4	42.4±10.5
Respiratory acidosis	36	10, 27.8	36.2±8.9
Mixed respiratory acidosis - metabolic alkalosis	17	11, 64.7	45.1±9.8
Mixed respiratory - metabolic acidosis	5	3, 60.0	53.3±4.1

NIV = non invasive ventilation; ABG = arterial blood gases.
[a]p = 0.026, Chi-Squared test vs no NIV use.
[b]p = 0.016, Kruskal-Wallis H test.

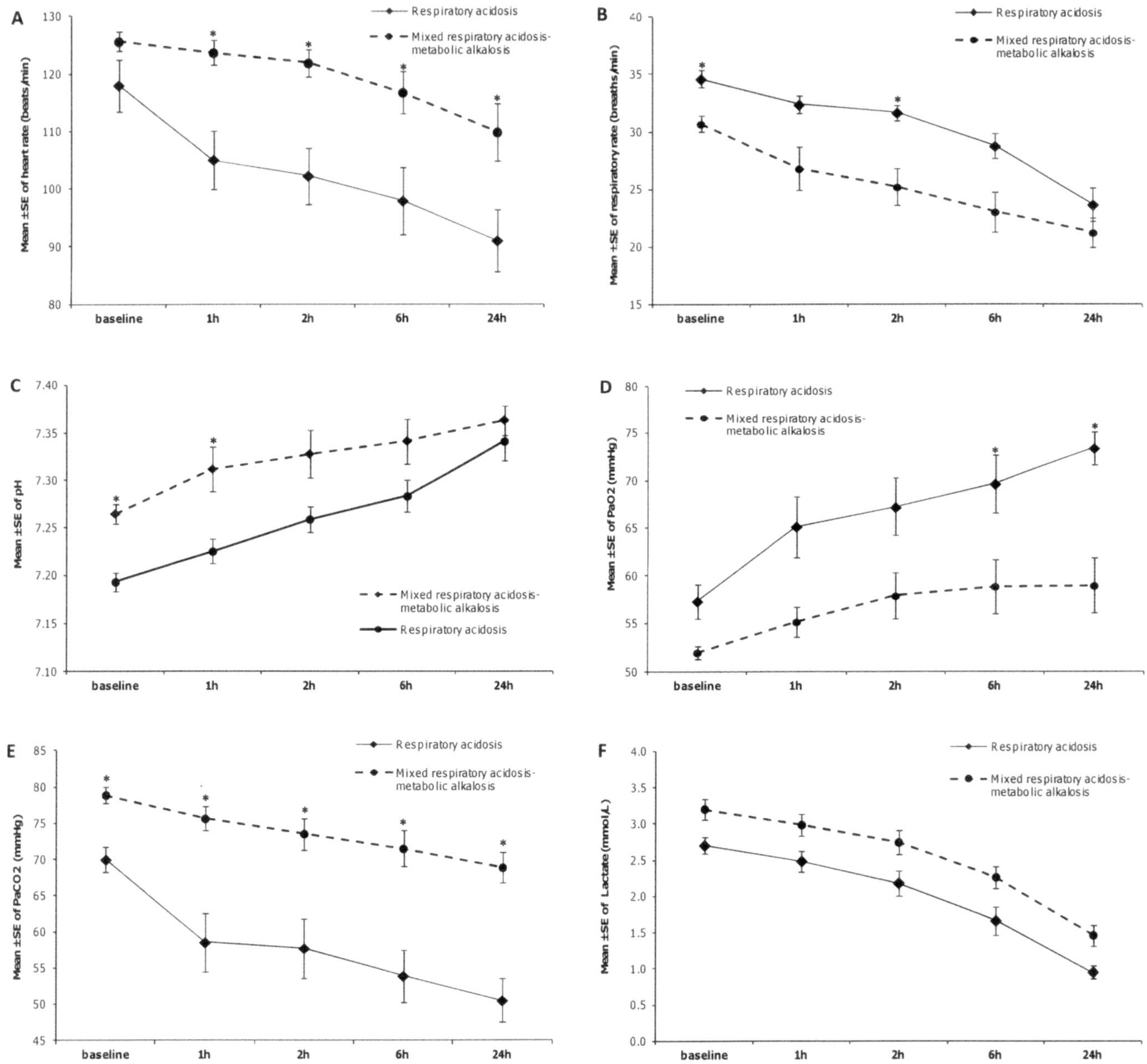

Figure 4. Trends over time in heart rate (panel A), respiratory rate (panel B), pH (panel C), PaO_2 (panel D), $PaCO_2$ (panel E) and blood lactate (panel F) during NIV. * $p<0.0125$, Mann-Whitney U test between groups with Bonferroni correction. NIV = noninvasive ventilation.

The effect of metabolic alkalosis on the clinical outcome of COPD patients was first reported in a study that showed an improvement in gas exchange and clinical symptoms after correcting the coexistent metabolic alkalosis [24].

Discontinuing furosemide, which is prescribed for peripheral edema in patients with stable COPD, increases the minute ventilation and lowers the $PaCO_2$ by correcting metabolic alkalosis [25]. Hypoventilation in response to metabolic alkalosis has serious implications in patients with high $PaCO_2$ and low PaO_2. COPD patients with a tendency toward hypercapnia require extra attention because hypercapnia is believed to be an ominous sign for morbidity and mortality [26,27]. The increased $PaCO_2$ caused by furosemide may lead to fluid retention, which may counteract the diuretic effects of furosemide. This is of clinical relevance, especially considering that loop diuretics are prescribed to a substantial number of COPD patients. Thus, other types of diuretics should be considered when diuretic therapy is indicated in hypercapnic COPD patients. Spironolactone, which causes no acid/base shifts, or acetazolamide, which causes a metabolic acidosis, may be better options. Because loop diuretics are often necessary in COPD patients with cor pulmonale or cardiac comorbidities, acetazolamide could be added to counteract the metabolic alkalosis [28].

Lactate disorders

Lactate clearance, as a surrogate for the magnitude and duration of global tissue hypoxia, is used for diagnostic, therapeutic and prognostic purposes. The normal reference values for lactate are traditionally considered 1±0.5 mmol/l in normal patients and <2 mmol/l in critically ill patients [29].

Increased lactate production indicates increased anaerobic metabolism associated with tissue hypoxia; lactate is one of the intermediate products that increase as a consequence of metabolism derangement during hypoxia [29].

Lactate clearance is a useful prognostic indicator. It reveals improvements in systemic tissue hypoxia and is associated with a decreased mortality rate. Patients with greater early lactate clearance after 6 hours of intensive care treatment have better outcomes than do subjects with lower lactate clearance [30].

In addition, early lactate clearance is significantly associated with decreased levels of inflammatory biomarkers, improvements in organ dysfunction and improved outcomes in severe sepsis and septic shock [31]. In addition, persistently elevated lactate is associated with a higher mortality rate [32,33].

In patients with respiratory failure, the early lactate clearance could be useful to assess the metabolic response to therapy and to identify individuals who are able to reverse the metabolic derangement. Lactate clearance deserves the same diagnostic relevance as other noninvasive markers of delivery/consumption/demand mismatches. While tissue pH, O_2 saturation and PCO_2 can offer a precise "local" picture of cellular oxygen disturbance, lactate does not. Nevertheless, systematically checking lactate clearance could be used to tailor the therapy in many cases of respiratory insufficiency [34,35].

The greatest amounts of lactate are produced by the skin, erythrocytes, skeletal muscles, and leukocytes [36]. Blood lactate concentration may only qualitatively reflect the metabolic phenomena occurring in the tissues. Moreover, lactate production is actually a consequence (and not the cause) of cellular acidosis. Because increased lactate production coincides with acidosis, lactate measurement is an excellent "indirect" marker of the metabolic condition of a cell.

We considered blood lactate as a diagnostic marker of tissue hypoxia and respiratory muscle fatigue (lactate is a valuable energy source within the working muscle), an indirect indicator of hypercapnic COPD exacerbation severity and, as a consequence, an indirect indicator of its response to treatment.

In our study, lactate improved over time once NIV was started. Patients with higher blood lactate were more likely to require NIV and needed longer ventilation times. The effects of hyperlactatemia on pH were attenuated in patients with concomitant hypochloremic metabolic alkalosis. Therefore, acid-base analysis should not only be based on traditional parameters, such as pH, HCO_3^- and the anion gap, but should rely on a more comprehensive evaluation [37]. According to Stewart [1], lactate production modifies the SID and thus influences one of the determinants of H^+ concentration. While there are tissues whose deranged metabolic pathways need lactate as an intermediate metabolite to survive, the production of lactate itself depends on pH [37]. Moreover, the pH controls the rate of lactate uptake from blood by hypoxic skeletal muscles [38].

Mixed respiratory-metabolic acidosis

In this study we identified a few patients with mixed respiratory-metabolic acidosis who required long NIV periods. Metabolic acidosis stimulates hyperventilation, but these patients had impaired ventilation, probably as a result of muscle wasting due to the metabolic academia [39]. Hospitalized patients with acute COPD exacerbations associated with mixed respiratory-metabolic acidosis represent more severe cases with a higher mortality rate than those with the respiratory component of acidemia alone [40].

Preliminary results and further research

In this descriptive study, we did not analyze the subgroups derived from the combinations of mixed acid-base disorders and hydro-electrolyte disturbances because the number of patients was not sufficient to guarantee a significant statistical power for this purpose

Probably the descriptive design of the study does not allow us to obtain definitive conclusions, but we strongly believe to have investigate a field not yet explored, eventually stimulating further prospective multicentric studies in order to completely clarify this topic, which recurs frequently in clinical practice.

Our preliminary results suggest, in fact, that in the clinical respiratory care researchers should address the following questions: a) whether lactate clearance is useful during acute respiratory failure to identify patients at high risk of negative outcomes and, potentially, to increase the intensity of the therapeutic approach; b) whether lactate clearance is predictive of positive outcome and could confirm to physicians that the current therapeutic approach is appropriate; and c) how both the metabolic components of mixed acid-base disorders and the hydroelectrolyte balance alterations may worsen the hypercapnic respiratory failure caused by the COPD exacerbation and may affect its resolution through standard medical therapy, either alone or combined with NIV.

Author Contributions

Conceived and designed the experiments: CT FDS VC AR. Performed the experiments: FDS VC AP GP. Analyzed the data: MDN. Contributed reagents/materials/analysis tools: CT FDS VC GP AP AR. Wrote the paper: CT FDS VC MDN GP AP AR.

References

1. Stewart PA (1981) How to understand acid-base. A quantitative acid-base primer for biology and medicine. New York: Elsevier. pp 1–286.
2. Wooten EW (2004) Quantitative acid-base physiology using the Stewart model. Crit Care 8: 448–452.
3. de Leeuw PW, Dees A (2003) Fluid homeostasis in chronic obstructive lung disease. Eur Respir J Suppl.46: 33s–40s.
4. Baudouin SV (1997) Oedema and cor pulmonale revisited. Thorax 52: 401–402.
5. Terzano C, Conti V, Di Stefano F, Petroianni A, Ceccarelli D, et al. (2010) Comorbidity, hospitalization and mortality in COPD: results from a longitudinal study. Lung 2010;188: 321–329.
6. Global Strategy for the Diagnosis, Management and prevention of Chronic Obstructive Pulmonary Disease 2009 Global Initiative for Chronic obstructive Lung Disease (GOLD) http://www.goldcopd.org Accessed September 2009.
7. British Thoracic Society Standards of Care Committee (2002) Non-invasive ventilation in acute respiratory failure. Thorax 57: 192–211.
8. Teasdale G, Jennett B (1974) Assessment of coma and impaired consciousness. A practical scale. The Lancet 2: 81–84.
9. Knaus WA, Draper EA, Wagner DP, Zimmerman JE (1985) APACHE II: a severity of disease classification system. Crit Care Med 13: 818–829.
10. Stinebaugh BJ, Austin WH (1967) Acid-base balance: common sense approach. Arch Intern Med 119: 182–188.
11. Adrogué HJ, Madias NE (2000) Hypernatremia. N Engl J Med 342: 1493–1499.
12. Adrogué HJ, Madias NE (2000) Hyponatremia. N Engl J Med 342: 1581–1589.
13. Garpestad E, Brennan J, Hill NS (2007) Noninvasive ventilation for critical care. Chest 132: 711–720.
14. Kramer N, Meyer TJ, Meharg J, Cece RD, Hill NS (1995) Randomized, prospective trial of noninvasive positive pressure ventilation in acute respiratory failure. Am J Respir Crit Care Med 151: 1799–1806.
15. Confalonieri M, Garuti G, Cattaruzza MS, Osborn JF, Antonelli M, et al. (2005) Italian noninvasive positive pressure ventilation (NPPV) study group. A chart of failure risk for noninvasive ventilation in patients with COPD exacerbation. Eur Respir J 25: 348–355.
16. Plant PK, Owen JL, Elliott MW (2000) Early use of non-invasive ventilation for acute exacerbations of chronic obstructive pulmonary disease on general respiratory wards: a multicentre randomised controlled trial. Lancet 355: 1931–1935.
17. Ucgun I, Oztuna F, Dagli CE, Yildirim H, Bal C (2008) Relationship of metabolic alkalosis, azotemia and morbidity in patients with chronic obstructive pulmonary disease and hypercapnia. Respiration 76: 270–274.
18. Javaheri S, Kazemi H (1987) Metabolic alkalosis and hypoventilation in humans. Am Rev Respir Dis 136: 1011–1016.
19. Pokorski M, Lahiri S (1982) Inhibition of aortic chemoreceptor responses by metabolic alkalosis in the cat. J Appl Physiol 53: 75–80.
20. Javaheri S, Shore NS, Rose B, Kazemi H (1982) Compensatory hypoventilation in metabolic alkalosis. Chest 81: 296–301.
21. Javaheri S, Kazemi H (1981) Electrolyte composition of cerebrospinal fluid in acute acid-base disorders. Respir Physiol 45: 141–151.
22. Brijker F, van den Elshout FJ, Heijdra YF, Bosch FH, Folgering HT (2001) Effect of acute metabolic acid/base shifts on the human airway calibre. Respir Physiol 124: 151–158.
23. van de Ven MJT, Colier WNJM, van der Sluijs MC, Oeseburg B, Vis P, et al. (2002) Effects of acetazolamide and furosemide on ventilation and cerebral blood volume in normocapnic and hypercapnic patients with COPD. Chest 121: 383–392.
24. Bear R, Goldstein M, Phillipson E, Ho M, Hammekem M, et al. (1977) Effect of metabolic alkalosis on respiratory function in patients with chronic obstructive lung disease. Can Med Assoc J 117: 900–903.
25. Brijker F, Heijdra YF, van den Elshout FJ, Folgering HT (2002) Discontinuation of furosemide decreases $PaCO_2$ in patients with COPD. Chest 121: 377–382.
26. Cooper CB (1994) Life expectancy in severe COPD. Chest 105: 335–337.
27. Foucher P, Baudouin N, Merati M, Pitard A, Bomniaud P, et al. (1998) Relative survival analysis of 252 patients with COPD receiving long-term oxygen therapy. Chest 113: 1580–1587.
28. Dickinson GE, Myers ML, Goldbach M, Sibbald W (1981) Acetazolamide in the treatment of ventilatory failure complicating acute metabolic alkalosis. Anesth Analg 60: 608–610.
29. Mizock BA (1992) Lactic acidosis in critical illness. Crit Care Med 20: 80–93.
30. Nguyen HB, Rivers EP, Knoblich BP, Jacobsen G, Muzzin A, et al. (2004) Early lactate clearance is associated with improved outcome in severe sepsis and septic shock. Crit Care Med 32: 1637–1642.
31. Nguyen HB, Loomba M, Yang JJ, Jacobsen G, Shah K, et al. (2010) Early lactate clearance is associated with biomarkers of inflammation, coagulation, apoptosis, organ dysfunction and mortality in severe sepsis and septic shock. J Inflamm (Lond) 7: 6.
32. Bernardin G, Pradier C, Tiger F, Deloffre P, Mattei M (1996) Blood pressure and arterial lactate level are early indicators of short-term survival in human septic shock. Intensive Care Medicine 22: 17–25.
33. Kaplan LJ, Kellum JA (2004) Initial pH, base deficit, lactate, anion gap, strong ion difference, and strong ion gap predict outcome from major vascular injury. Critical Care Medicine 32: 1120–1124.
34. Scott S, Antonaglia V, Guiotto G, Paladino F, Schiraldi F (2010) Two-hour lactate clearance predicts negative outcome in patients with cardiorespiratory insufficiency. Crit Care Res Pract 2010: 917053. doi:10.1155/2010/917053.
35. Valenza F, Aletti G, Fossali T, Chevallard G, Sacconi F, et al. (2005) Lactate as a marker of energy failure in critically ill patients: hypothesis. Critical Care 9: 588–593.
36. Kreisberg RA (1972) Glucose-lactate interrelations in man. N Engl J Med 287: 132–137.
37. Dubin A, Menises MM, Masevicius FD, Moseinco MC, Kutscherauer DO, et al. (2007) Comparison of three different methods of evaluation of metabolic acid-base disorders. Crit Care Med 35: 1264–1270.
38. Gutierrez LB, Hurtado FJ, Gutierrez AM, Fernandez E (1993) Net uptake of lactate by rabbit hindlimb during hypoxia. Am Rev Respir Dis 148: 1204–1209.
39. Price SR, Du JD, Bailey JL, Mitch WE (2001) Molecular mechanisms regulating protein turn over in muscle. Am J Kidney Dis 37(Suppl. 2): 112s–114s.
40. Roberts CM, Stone RA, Buckingam RJ, Pursey NA, Lowe D (2011) Acidosis, non-invasive ventilation and mortality in hospitalised COPD exacerbations. Thorax 66: 43–48.

Risk of Acute Lung Injury/Acute Respiratory Distress Syndrome in Critically Ill Adult Patients with Pre-Existing Diabetes

Wan-Jie Gu[1,2]☙, You-Dong Wan[2]☙, Hong-Tao Tie[3]☙, Quan-Cheng Kan[4], Tong-Wen Sun[2]*

1 Department of Anaesthesiology, the First Affiliated Hospital, Guangxi Medical University, Nanning, China, **2** Department of Integrated Intensive Care Unit, the First Affiliated Hospital, Zhengzhou University, Zhengzhou, China, **3** The First College of Clinical Medicine, the First Affiliated Hospital, Chongqing Medical University, Chongqing, China, **4** Pharmaceutical Department, the First Affiliated Hospital, Zhengzhou University, Zhengzhou, China

Abstract

Background: The impact of pre-existing diabetes on the development of acute lung injury/acute respiratory distress syndrome (ALI/ARDS) in critically ill patients remains unclear. We performed a meta-analysis of cohort studies to evaluate the risk of ALI/ARDS in critically ill patients with and without pre-existing diabetes.

Materials and Methods: We searched PubMed and Embase from the inception to September 2013 for cohort studies assessing the effect of pre-existing diabetes on ALI/ARDS occurrence. Pooled odds ratio (OR) with 95% confidence interval (CI) was calculated using random- or fixed-effect models when appropriate.

Results: Seven cohort **studies** with a total of 12,794 participants and 2,937 cases of pre-existing diabetes, and 2,457 cases of ALI/ARDS were included in the **meta-analysis**. A fixed-effects model meta-analysis showed that pre-existing diabetes was associated with a reduced risk of ALI/ARDS (OR 0.66; 95% CI, 0.55–0.80; $p<0.001$), with low heterogeneity among the studies ($I^2=18.9\%$; $p=0.286$). However, the asymmetric funnel plot and Egger's test ($p=0.007$) suggested publication bias may exist.

Conclusions: Our meta-analysis suggests that pre-existing diabetes was associated with a decreased risk of ALI/ARDS in critically ill adult patients. However, the result should be interpreted with caution because of the potential bias and confounding in the included studies.

Editor: Xiao Su, Chinese Academy of Sciences, China

Funding: The authors have no support or funding to report.

Competing Interests: The authors have declared that no competing interests exist.

* E-mail: tongwensun1964@sina.com

☙ These authors contributed equally to this work.

Introduction

Acute lung injury (ALI) is a syndrome characterized by hypoxemia, noncardiogenic pulmonary edema, low lung compliance and widespread capillary leakage. When accompanied by more severe hypoxemia ($PaO2/FiO2<200$ mmHg), it is called acute respiratory distress syndrome (ARDS) [1]. Development of ALI/ARDS has been associated with short and long term morbidity, prolonged hospitalization, and high health-care costs [1]. Given the clinical consequences attributable to ALI/ARDS, identifying risk factors for prevention of ALI/ARDS is of great importance and is a priority in intensive care unit (ICU).

Diabetes also is a global health priority. The prevalence of diabetes is expected to dramatically increase by the year 2025 [2]. The proportion of critically ill patients with diabetes is also growing as a result of the worldwide increase in diabetes. However, the association between diabetes and mortality among ICU patients is still debatable. In some studies, pre-existing diabetes has been a risk factor of acute kidney injury in critically ill patients [3,4], and has been associated with an increased mortality of surgical ICU [5], but in some other studies, diabetes does not alter mortality in ICU patients [6,7,8].

The impact of pre-existing diabetes on the development of ALI/ARDS remains unclear in critically ill patients, especially those with one or more predisposing conditions such as sepsis/septic shock, pneumonia, trauma, and aspiration. To our knowledge, the quality and consistency of epidemiological evidence on the topic have not been systematically investigated, which is an important gap in our understanding of the effect of pre-existing diabetes on the development of ALI/ARDS. With recently accumulating evidence, therefore, we performed a meta-analysis of cohort studies to evaluate the risk of ALI/ARDS in critically ill patients with and without pre-existing diabetes.

Materials and Methods

Search strategy

We performed this meta-analysis in accordance with the Meta-analysis of Observational Studies in Epidemiology(MOOSE)

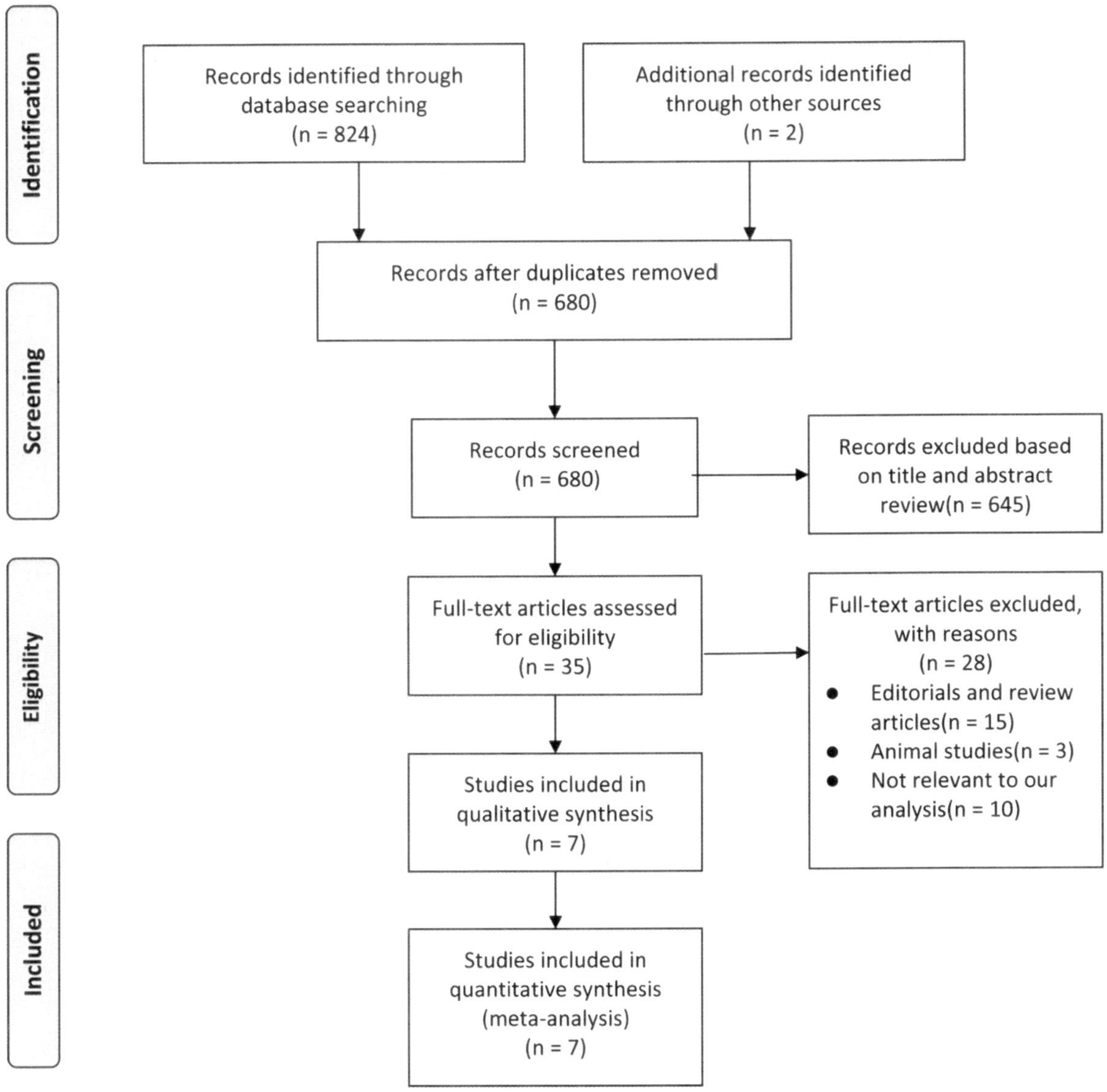

Figure 1. Flow diagram for selection of articles.

statement [9]. PubMed and Embase databases from inception to September 2013 were searched to identify relevant studies, without language restrictions. Search terms included "diabetes", "DM", "acute respiratory distress syndrome", "acute lung injury", "ARDS", "ALI", and "acute respiratory failure". In addition, we reviewed the reference lists of retrieved papers and recent reviews to identify other potentially eligible studies that we had not captured with our primary search.

Study selection

The following inclusive selection criteria were applied: (a) study design: cohort study; (b) study population: critically ill adult patients, it meaned ICU or emergency patients with ALI/ARDS predisposing risk factors, including sepsis, septic shock, pancreatitis, pneumonia, aspiration, trauma, or high-risk surgery; (c) comparison intervention: with and without pre-existing diabetes; and (d) outcome measure: the development of ALI/ARDS. In the case of duplicate data publication (several studies with overlapping samples), we only included the most informative article or complete study to avoid duplication of information.

Data extraction and quality assessment

A standardized data collection form was used to extract the following information from each included article: first author, publication year, sample size, number of diabetes cases, number of ALI/ARDS cases, population characteristics, type of study design, definition of ALI/ARDS, and odds ratios (ORs) with the corresponding 95% confidence intervals (CIs) on multivariable analysis. The supplementary files were also examined for data extraction. Where necessary, we contacted authors of included studies for additional information.

We assessed the methodological quality of each study on 8 items used in the Newcastle-Ottawa Scales (NOS) [10]. We assigned risk of bias categories based on the number of Newcastle–Ottawa Scales (NOS) items judged inadequate in each study, as follows: low risk of bias (0–1 inadequate item); medium risk of bias (2–3

Table 1. Main characteristics of cohort studies included in the meta-analysis.

Author/Year	Study size	Number of diabetes	Number of ALI/ ARDS	Population	Study design	Definition of ALI/ ARDS	OR (95% CI) on multivariate analysis	Adjustment for Covariates
Moss, 2000 [15]	113	32	46	Adult ICU patients with septic shock	PC	American-European Consensus Conference definition	0.33 (0.12–0.90)	Age, source of infection, and history of cirrhosis
Gong, 2005 [16]	688	164	221	Adult ICU patients with>1 predisposing ARDS condition	PC	American-European Consensus Conference definition	0.58 (0.36–0.92)	Predisposing ARDS conditions: Sepsis syndrome, septic shock, direct pulmonary injury; Other: Age, APACHE III, transfusion of PRBCs, number of PRBCs transfused, and hematologic failure
Iscimen, 2008 [17]	160	55	71	Adult ICU patients with septic shock	PC	American-European Consensus Conference definition	0.44 (0.17–1.07)	Predisposing ARDS conditions: Aspiration; Other: Age, APACHE III, alcohol abuse, chemotherapy, delayed goal-directed resuscitation, delayed antibiotics, tachypnea, transfusion of PRBCs
Gajic, 2011 [18]	5584	1295	377	Adult hospitalized patients with sepsis	PC	American-European Consensus Conference definition	0.55 (0.25–1.16)	Predisposing ARDS conditions: Aspiration, high-risk surgery, high-risk trauma, pancreatitis, pneumonia, shock Other: Sex, APACHE II, admission source, acidosis, alcohol abuse, chemotherapy, emergency surgery, hypoalbuminemia, obesity, oxygen supplementation, smoking, tachypnea
Trillo-Alvarez, 2011 [19]	409	87	68	Adult ICU patients with>1 predisposing ARDS condition	RC	American-European Consensus Conference definition	0.16 (0.03–0.77)	Predisposing ARDS conditions: Aspiration, emergent high-risk surgery, sepsis, shock; Other: Alcohol abuse, hypoalbuminemia, oxygen supplementation, smoking, tachypnea
Koh, 2012 [20]	2013	317	720	Adult ICU patients >1 predisposing ARDS condition	RC	American-European Consensus Conference definition	0.76 (0.43–1.33)	Age, sex, BMI, myocardial infarction, medication
Yu, 2013 [21]	3827	987	954	Adult ICU patients with >1 predisposing ARDS condition	PC	American-European Consensus Conference definition	0.75 (0.59–0.94)	Predisposing ARDS conditions: Multiple transfusion, septic shock, trauma Other: Age, APACHE III, BMI, ICU admission hyperglycemia, renal failure, hematologic failure, alcohol use, smoking, medication

ALI/ARDS acute lung injury/acute respiratory distress syndrome, APACHE Acute Physiology and Chronic Health Evaluation, BMI body mass index, ICU intensive care unit, PC prospective cohort, PRBCs packed red blood cells, RC retrospective cohort.

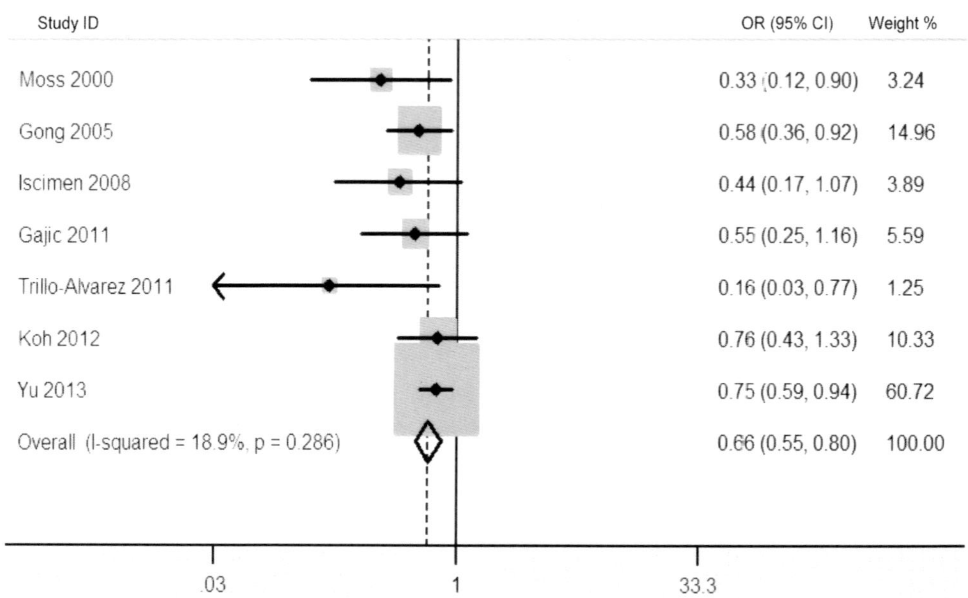

Figure 2. Forest plot showing the risk of ALI/ARDS in critically ill adult patients with pre-existing diabetes.

inadequate items); high risk of bias (over 3 inadequate items); very high risk of bias (no description of methods).

Two investigators (WJ Gu and YD Wan) independently conducted the study selection, data extraction and quality assessment, a third investigator (TW Sun) was consulted to resolve any discrepancies.

Statistical analysis

OR was used as a common measure of the association between pre-existing diabetes and the development of ALI/ARDS across studies. Heterogeneity was tested using the Cochran Q statistic ($p<0.1$) and quantified with the I^2 statistic, which describes the variation of effect size that is attributable to heterogeneity across studies [11–13]. An I^2 value greater than 50% indicates significant heterogeneity. The value of the I^2 statistic was used to select the appropriate pooling method: fixed-effects models were used for $I^2 < 50\%$ and random-effects models for $I^2 \geq 50\%$ [11–13]. To explore the possible source of heterogeneity and to examine the influence of various clinical factors on the overall risk estimate, we further carried out *prior* subgroup analyses according to study design (prospective vs. retrospective), predisposing conditions (sepsis/septic shock vs. >1 predisposing conditions), study center (single-center vs. multicenter), and sample size(≤1000 vs. >1000). We also investigated the influence of a single study on the overall pooled estimate by omitting one study in each turn. Potential publication bias was detected by Begg's funnel plots and Egger's regression test [14,15]. A p value <0.05 was judged as statistically significant, except where otherwise specified. All statistical analyses were performed using STATA, version 11.0 (Stata Corp).

Table 2. Subgroup analyses for ALI/ARDS.

Subgroup	No. of studies	OR (95% CI)	$p_{heterogeneity}$	I^2
Total [15–21]	7	0.66 (0.55–0.80)	0.286	18.9%
Study design				
Prospective cohort [15–18,21]	5	0.67 (0.55–0.81)	0.377	5.2%
Retrospective cohort [19,20]	2	0.64 (0.38–1.09)	0.075	68.4%
Predisposing conditions				
Sepsis/septic shock [15,17,18,31]	4	0.70 (0.57–0.87)	0.246	27.6%
>1 predisposing conditions [16,21–21]	4	0.70 (0.58–0.85)	0.239	28.8%
Study center				
Single-center [16,17,19,20]	4	0.58 (0.42–0.81)	0.302	17.7%
Multicenter [15,18,31]	3	0.70 (0.57–0.88)	0.240	29.9%
Sample size				
≤1000 [15–17,19]	4	0.48 (0.33–0.70)	0.399	0%
>1000 [18,20,31]	3	0.73 (0.60–0.90)	0.744	0%

ALI/ARDS acute lung injury/acute respiratory distress syndrome.

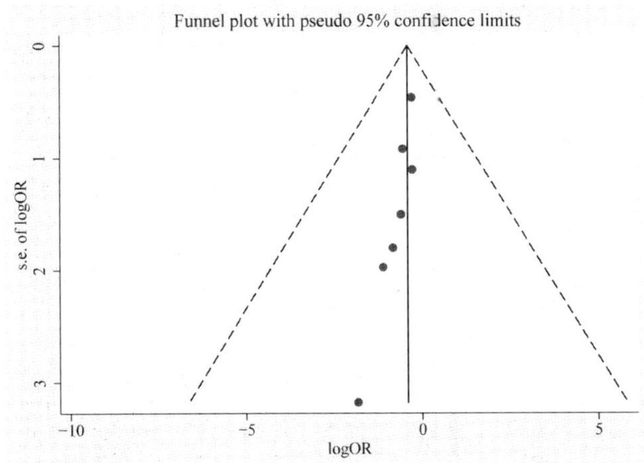

Figure 3. Funnel plot for the risk of ALI/ARDS in critically ill adult patients with pre-existing diabetes.or, risk ratio. s.e., standard error.

Results

Study selection and study characteristics

The initial search yielded 826 relevant publications, of which 819 were excluded for duplicate studies and various reasons (reviews, animal studies, or not relevant to our analysis) on the basis of the title/abstract and full text (see the detail in Figure 1). The remaining seven cohort studies were included in the final analysis [15–21].

The main characteristics of the seven included cohort studies are shown in Table 1. These studies were published between 2000 and 2013. In total, 12,794 participants, 2,937 cases of pre-existing diabetes, and 2,457 cases of ALI/ARDS were enrolled. All the included studies use the same definition of ALI/ARDS (American-European Consensus Conference definition) [22]. The average NOS score of the studies included was 6.7 (range from 6 to 7). An additional file shows this in more detail [see File S1].

Pre-existing diabetes and the risk of ALI/ARDS

Figure 2 shows the pooled results from the fixed-effects model combing the ORs for ALI/ARDS. Overall, 12,794 patients were included in this analysis (2,937 cases of pre-existing diabetes and 2,457 cases of ALI/ARDS). Pre-existing diabetes was associated with a decreased risk of ALI/ARDS in critically ill adult patients (OR 0.66; 95% CI, 0.55–0.80; $p<0.001$), with low heterogeneity among the studies ($I^2 = 18.9\%$; $p = 0.286$). Further exclusion of any single study did not materially alter the overall combined OR, with a range of from 0.55 (95% CI, 0.41–0.74) to 0.63 (95% CI, 0.56–0.83). Table 2 shows the results of subgroup analyses for ALI/ARDS. The finding of decreased risk of ALI/ARDS in critically ill adult patients was consistently found in most subgroup analyses.

Publication bias

Egger's test ($p = 0.007$) suggested that publication bias may exist. Also, there was asymmetry in the lower segments of the funnel plot in which small negative trials were missing (Figure 3), potentially leading to overstatement of the treatment effect. But the low power with only seven studies limited the interpretability of the finding.

Discussion

Main findings

To the best of our knowledge, this is the first meta-analysis to explore the association between pre-existing diabetes and the risk of ALI/ARDS in critically ill adult patients. Our meta-analysis of seven cohort studies suggests that pre-existing diabetes was associated with a decreased risk of ALI/ARDS in critically ill adult patients. In addition, the association was consistently found in most subgroup analyses.

Possible mechanism

Although pre-existing diabetes may decrease the risk of ALI/ARDS, the mechanism remains unclear. Since inflammation plays an important role in the onset and progression of ALI/ARDS [23], several studies have suggested that the protective effect of diabetes for ALI/ARDS may result from the reduced inflammatory response [24,25]. Filgueiras and colleagues [24] reported that in non-diabetic rats with ALI/ARDS secondarily to sepsis, the lung presented edema, leukocyte infiltration, and increased COX2 expression; however, these inflammatory events were less intense in diabetic rats. Similarly, in the diabetic mice with infection, the inflammatory response is lower compared with non-diabetic mice [25]. Decreased inflammatory response may be associated with attenuation of cytokine release and reduction of neutrophil migration [25]. The involved cytokines included PPAR-γ [26], nuclear factor-κB [27], insulin-like growth factor-1 [27,28], leptin, and development of advanced glycation end products [29,30]. For the neutrophil migration, α1-acid glycoprotein is important in the failure of this process after sepsis [31], but the mechanism is not completely understood.

On another note, diabetes therapy modifies some effects that diabetes may have on ALI/ARDS. Insulin is usually the only diabetic treatment that is continued during critical illness. Independent of glycemic control, insulin has been shown to be immunomodulatory Independent of glycemic control [32]. In clinical studies, intensive insulin therapy may decrease mortality for critically ill patients [33], However, it is difficult to know whether insulin may be detrimental or beneficial in ALI/ARDS. According to our study, diabetes is protective in ALI/ARDS, then reversal of the anti-inflammatory effects of diabetes by insulin may negate the beneficial effect of diabetes on ALI/ARDS. Alternatively, if insulin reverses the chronic immunosuppressive effects of diabetes and restores the balance in inflammatory response, then insulin may be potentially beneficial [34]. More studies are needed to determine whether insulin is detrimental or beneficial in ALI/ARDS. Other drug commonly used was metformin, which was recently shown to reduce oxidative injury [35]. But the possible mechanism of diabetes therapy on ALI/ARDS still remains unclear.

Clinical implications

Our findings are of clinical significance to some extent. The most consistent evidence was the decreased risk of ALI/ARDS in critically ill adult patients with pre-existing diabetes. Currently, physicians caring for critically ill patients can not accurately determine which patient will develop ALI/ARDS, since no biological markers have been found to predict it precisely so far [36,37]; however, physicians could roughly predict who was more likely to worsen to ALI/ARDS according to the risk factors in critically ill patients. The following risk factors have been found: alcohol abuse [38], hypoalbuminemia [15,39], transfusions [15], tachypnea [16], high tidal volumes [40], and obesity [41]. Besides, diabetes, as another risk factor of ALI/ARDS has been paid more attention [14–20]. However, to our knowledge, whether pre-existing diabetes will protect patients from converting to ALI/ARDS or facilitate the development of ALI/ARDS remains still unknown. Our meta-analysis suggested pre-existing diabetes was associated with a decreased risk of ALI/ARDS in critically ill adult patients. The findings, for the clinicians, may contribute to the sorting and management of critically ill patients with diabetes, as a protective factor for ALI/ARDS. As a primary prevention strategy, excluding risk factors is equally important to identifying those. Diabetes may be excluded from the high risk factors of ALI/ARDS.

Strengths and limitations

Strengths of this meta-analysis included its exhaustive search without language restrictions and validated systematic review methods following the MOOSE guidelines. Also, all included studies were cohort studies and high-quality, with an average NOS score of 6.7 allowing for the impossibility of randomized controlled trial. High-quality cohort studies may minimize the likelihood of recall bias, which is of particular concern in other epidemiological study designs.

Several limitations of this meta-analysis merit consideration. First, the characteristics of populations, the type of diabetes (type 1 or type 2), the definition of diabetes, severity of the illness, and the adjusted confounding factor were not strictly described in some trials. These factors may result in heterogeneity and have a potential impact on our results. Second, the critically ill patients was really a broad population, in our study, most studies described it as ICU patients with one or more ALI/ARDS predisposing risk factors, including sepsis, septic shock, pancreatitis, pneumonia, aspiration, trauma, or high-risk surgery, etc. So whether the conclusion was suitable for the unselected ICU population remain questionable. Third, both the asymmetric funnel plot and Egger's test suggested publication bias may exist. Small negative trials were missing, potentially resulting in overstatement of the treatment effect. Furthermore, we are unable to assess the impact of pre-existing diabetes on other clinically meaningful end points, such as mortality attributed to ALI/ARDS, because of sparse and inconsistent reporting across studies.

Conclusions

In summary, this meta-analysis of seven cohort studies suggests that pre-existing diabetes decreased the risk of ALI/ARDS in critically ill adult patients; however, the result should be interpreted with caution because of the potential bias and confounding in the included studies.

Author Contributions

Conceived and designed the experiments: WJG YDW HTT QCK TWS. Performed the experiments: WJG YDW HTT. Analyzed the data: WJG YDW HTT QCK TWS. Contributed reagents/materials/analysis tools: WJG YDW HTT QCK TWS. Wrote the paper: WJG YDW.

References

1. Rubenfeld GD, Herridge MS (2007) Epidemiology and outcomes of acute lung injury. Chest 131: 554–562.
2. King H, Aubert RE, Herman WH (1998) Global burden of diabetes, 1995–2025: prevalence, numerical estimates, and projections. Diabetes Care 21: 1414–1431.
3. Cartin-Ceba R, Kashiouris M, Plataki M, Kor DJ, Gajic O, et al. (2012) Risk factors for development of acute kidney injury in critically ill patients: a systematic review and meta-analysis of observational studies. Crit Care Res Pract 2012: 691013.
4. Christiansen CF, Johansen MB, Christensen S, O'Brien JM, Tonnesen E, et al. (2013) Type 2 diabetes and 1-year mortality in intensive care unit patients. Eur J Clin Invest 43: 238–247.
5. Siegelaar SE, Hickmann M, Hoekstra JB, Holleman F, DeVries JH (2011) The effect of diabetes on mortality in critically ill patients: a systematic review and meta-analysis. Crit Care 15: R205.
6. Stegenga ME, Vincent JL, Vail GM, Xie J, Haney DJ, et al. (2010) Diabetes does not alter mortality or hemostatic and inflammatory responses in patients with severe sepsis. Crit Care Med 38: 539–545.
7. Graham BB, Keniston A, Gajic O, Trillo AC, Medvedev S, et al. (2010) Diabetes mellitus does not adversely affect outcomes from a critical illness. Crit Care Med 38: 16–24.
8. Vincent JL, Preiser JC, Sprung CL, Moreno R, Sakr Y (2010) Insulin-treated diabetes is not associated with increased mortality in critically ill patients. Crit Care 14: R12.
9. Stroup DF, Berlin JA, Morton SC, Olkin I, Williamson GD, et al. (2000) Meta-analysis of observational studies in epidemiology: a proposal for reporting. Meta-analysis Of Observational Studies in Epidemiology (MOOSE) group. JAMA 283: 2008–2012.
10. Wells GA SB, O'Connell D, Peterson J, Welch V, Losos M, et al. (2013) The Newcastle-Ottawa Scale (NOS) for assessing the quality of nonrandomized studies in meta-analysis. Available: www.ohri.ca/programs/clinical_epidemiology/oxford.asp.
11. DerSimonian R, Laird N (1986) Meta-analysis in clinical trials. Controlled clinical trials 7: 177–188.
12. Higgins JP, Thompson SG, Deeks JJ, Altman DG (2003) Measuring inconsistency in meta-analyses. BMJ 327: 557–560.
13. Begg CB, Mazumdar M (1994) Operating characteristics of a rank correlation test for publication bias. Biometrics 50: 1088–1101.
14. Egger M, Davey SG, Schneider M, Minder C (1997) Bias in meta-analysis detected by a simple, graphical test. BMJ 315: 629–634.
15. Moss M, Guidot DM, Steinberg KP, Duhon GF, Treece P, et al. (2000) Diabetic patients have a decreased incidence of acute respiratory distress syndrome. Crit Care Med 28: 2187–2192.
16. Gong MN, Thompson BT, Williams P, Pothier L, Boyce PD, et al. (2005) Clinical predictors of and mortality in acute respiratory distress syndrome: potential role of red cell transfusion. Crit Care Med 33: 1191–1198.
17. Iscimen R, Cartin-Ceba R, Yilmaz M, Khan H, Hubmayr RD, et al. (2008) Risk factors for the development of acute lung injury in patients with septic shock: an observational cohort study. Crit Care Med 36: 1518–1522.
18. Gajic O, Dabbagh O, Park PK, Adesanya A, Chang SY, et al. Critical Illness and Injury Trials Group: Lung Injury Prevention Study Investigators (USCIITG-LIPS) (2011) Early identification of patients at risk of acute lung injury: evaluation of lung injury prediction score in a multicenter cohort study. Am J Respir Crit Care Med 183: 462–470.
19. Trillo-Alvarez C, Cartin-Ceba R, Kor DJ, Kojicic M, Kashyap R, et al. (2011) Acute lung injury prediction score: derivation and validation in a population-based sample. Eur Respir J 37: 604–609.
20. Koh GC, Vlaar AP, Hofstra JJ, de Jong HK, van Nierop S, et al. (2012) In the critically ill patient, diabetes predicts mortality independent of statin therapy but is not associated with acute lung injury: a cohort study. Crit Care Med 40: 1835–1843.
21. Yu S, Christiani DC, Thompson BT, Bajwa EK, Gong MN (2013) Role of diabetes in the development of acute respiratory distress syndrome. Crit Care Med 41: 2720–2732.
22. Bernard GR, Artigas A, Brigham KL, Carlet J, Falke K, et al. (1994) The American-European Consensus Conference on ARDS. Definitions, mechanisms, relevant outcomes, and clinical trial coordination. Am J Respir Crit Care Med 149: 818–824.
23. Kollef MH, Schuster DP (1995) The acute respiratory distress syndrome. N Engl J Med 332: 27–37.
24. Filgueiras LJ, Martins JO, Serezani CH, Capelozzi VL, Montes MB, et al. (2012) Sepsis-induced acute lung injury (ALI) is milder in diabetic rats and correlates with impaired NFkB activation. PLoS One 7: e44987.
25. Spiller F, Carlos D, Souto FO, de Freitas A, Soares FS, et al. (2012) α1-Acid glycoprotein decreases neutrophil migration and increases susceptibility to sepsis in diabetic mice. Diabetes 61: 1584–1591.
26. Genovese T, Mazzon E, Di Paola R, Muia C, Crisafulli C, et al. (2005) ROLE OF ENDOGENOUS AND EXOGENOUS LIGANDS FOR THE PEROXISOME PROLIFERATOR-ACTIVATED RECEPTOR alpha IN THE

DEVELOPMENT OF BLEOMYCIN-INDUCED LUNG INJURY. Shock 24: 547–555.

27. Krein PM, Sabatini PJ, Tinmouth W, Green FH, Winston BW (2003) Localization of insulin-like growth factor-I in lung tissues of patients with fibroproliferative acute respiratory distress syndrome. Am J Respir Crit Care Med 167: 83–90.
28. Schnapp LM, Donohoe S, Chen J, Sunde DA, Kelly PM, et al. (2006) Mining the acute respiratory distress syndrome proteome: identification of the insulin-like growth factor (IGF)/IGF-binding protein-3 pathway in acute lung injury. Am J Pathol 169: 86–95.
29. Zhang H, Tasaka S, Shiraishi Y, Fukunaga K, Yamada W, et al. (2008) Role of soluble receptor for advanced glycation end products on endotoxin-induced lung injury. Am J Respir Crit Care Med 178: 356–362.
30. Calfee CS, Ware LB, Eisner MD, Parsons PE, Thompson BT, et al. (2008) Plasma receptor for advanced glycation end products and clinical outcomes in acute lung injury. Thorax 63: 1083–1089.
31. Mestriner FL, Spiller F, Laure HJ, Souto FO, Tavares-Murta BM, et al. (2007) Acute-phase protein alpha-1-acid glycoprotein mediates neutrophil migration failure in sepsis by a nitric oxide-dependent mechanism. Proc Natl Acad Sci U S A 104: 19595–19600.
32. Hansen TK, Thiel S, Wouters PJ, Christiansen JS, Van den Berghe G (2003) Intensive insulin therapy exerts antiinflammatory effects in critically ill patients and counteracts the adverse effect of low mannose-binding lectin levels. J Clin Endocrinol Metab 88: 1082–1088.
33. Van den Berghe G, Wilmer A, Hermans G, Meersseman W, Wouters PJ, et al. (2006) Intensive insulin therapy in the medical ICU. N Engl J Med 354: 449–461.
34. Honiden S, Gong MN (2009) Diabetes, insulin, and development of acute lung injury. Crit Care Med 37: 2455–2464.
35. Zmijewski JW, Lorne E, Zhao X, Tsuruta Y, Sha Y, et al. (2008) Mitochondrial respiratory complex I regulates neutrophil activation and severity of lung injury. Am J Respir Crit Care Med 178: 168–179.
36. Janz DR, Ware LB: Biomarkers of ALI/ARDS (2013) Pathogenesis, Discovery, and Relevance to Clinical Trials. Semin Respir Crit Care Med 34: 537–548.
37. Cepkova M, Brady S, Sapru A, Matthay MA, Church G (2006) Biological markers of lung injury before and after the institution of positive pressure ventilation in patients with acute lung injury. Crit Care 10: R126.
38. Moss M, Bucher B, Moore FA, Moore EE, Parsons PE (1996) The role of chronic alcohol abuse in the development of acute respiratory distress syndrome in adults. JAMA 275: 50–54.
39. Mangialardi RJ, Martin GS, Bernard GR, Wheeler AP, Christman BW, et al. (2000) Hypoproteinemia predicts acute respiratory distress syndrome development, weight gain, and death in patients with sepsis. Ibuprofen in Sepsis Study Group. Crit Care Med 28: 3137–3145.
40. Gajic O, Frutos-Vivar F, Esteban A, Hubmayr RD, Anzueto A (2005) Ventilator settings as a risk factor for acute respiratory distress syndrome in mechanically ventilated patients. Intensive Care Med 31: 922–926.
41. Gong MN, Bajwa EK, Thompson BT, Christiani DC (2010) Body mass index is associated with the development of acute respiratory distress syndrome. Thorax 65: 44–50.

Plasma Adiponectin, Clinical Factors, and Patient Outcomes during the Acute Respiratory Distress Syndrome

Allan J. Walkey[1]*, Serkalem Demissie[2], Dilip Shah[3], Freddy Romero[3], Leah Puklin[3], Ross S. Summer[3]

1 The Pulmonary Center, Boston University School of Medicine, Division of Pulmonary, Allergy and Critical Care Medicine, Boston Medical Center, Boston, Massachusetts, United States of America, **2** Department of Biostatistics, Boston University School of Public Health, Boston, Massachusetts, United States of America, **3** Center for Translational Medicine and Korman Lung Center, Thomas Jefferson University, Philadelphia, Pennsylvania, United States of America

Abstract

Objective: Adiponectin (APN) is an anti-inflammatory hormone derived from adipose tissue that attenuates acute lung injury in rodents. In this study, we investigated the association between circulating APN and outcomes among patients with acute respiratory distress syndrome (ARDS).

Methods: We performed a retrospective cohort study using data and plasma samples from participants in the multicenter ARDS Network Fluid and Catheter Treatment Trial.

Results: Plasma APN concentrations were measured in 816 (81.6%) trial participants at baseline and in 568 (56.8%) subjects at both baseline and day 7 after enrollment. Clinical factors associated with baseline APN levels in multivariable-adjusted models included sex, body mass index, past medical history of cirrhosis, and central venous pressure (model $R^2 = 9.7\%$). We did not observe an association between baseline APN and either severity of illness (APACHE III) or extent of lung injury (Lung Injury Score). Among patients who received right heart catheterization (n = 384), baseline APN was inversely related to mean pulmonary artery pressure ($\beta = -0.015$, R^2 1.5%, p = 0.02); however, this association did not persist in multivariable models ($\beta = -0.009$, R^2 0.5%, p = 0.20). Neither baseline APN levels [HR per quartile1.04 (95% CI 0.91–1.18), p = 0.61], nor change in APN level from baseline to day 7 [HR 1.04 (95% CI 0.89–1.23), p = 0.62)] were associated with 60 day mortality in Cox proportional hazards regression models. However, subgroup analysis identified an association between APN and mortality among patients who developed ARDS from extra-pulmonary etiologies [HR per quartile 1.31 (95% CI 1.08–1.57)]. APN levels did not correlate with mortality among patients developing ARDS in association with direct pulmonary injury [HR 0.96 (95% CI 0.83–1.13)], $p_{interaction} = 0.016$.

Conclusions: Plasma APN levels did not correlate with disease severity or mortality in a large cohort of patients with ARDS. However, higher APN levels were associated with increased mortality among patients developing ARDS from extra-pulmonary etiologies.

Editor: Jörn Karhausen, Duke University Medical Center, United States of America

Funding: This study was supported by National Institutes of Health, National Heart Lung and Blood Institute R21HL112672 (AJW) and R01HL105490 (RSS) (http://www.nhlbi.nih.gov/). The funders had no role in study design, data collection and analysis, decision to publish, or preparation of the manuscript.

Competing Interests: The authors have declared that no competing interests exist.

* Email: alwalkey@bu.edu

Introduction

Adiponectin (APN) is a highly abundant circulating hormone with pleotrophic effects upon diverse pulmonary cell types [1–4] including alveolar macrophages, epithelium, and vascular endothelium [3,5,6]. Though principally derived from adipocytes, circulating APN levels are paradoxically increased in lean individuals and decreased in subjects with higher body mass indexes [7]. In the lung, APN has been shown to have important anti-inflammatory and vascular protective actions, prompting pre-clinical studies examining the role of APN in the pathogenesis of pulmonary disorders including acute respiratory distress syndrome (ARDS) [2–4,8]

ARDS is an acute, life-threatening lung condition involving immune and endothelial cell activation that develops in association with direct (e.g. pneumonia) and indirect pulmonary (e.g., urosepsis) challenges [9]. Although the role of circulating APN in human ARDS has not yet been investigated, animal studies suggest a causal link between hypoadiponectemia and ARDS pathogenesis. For example, APN-deficient mice have a markedly increased susceptibility to developing acute lung injury (the murine equivalent of ARDS) [2,4,6,8] and this susceptibility is attenuated following APN replacement [3]. Further, mice deficient in APN are prone to developing pulmonary vascular abnormalities including elevated pulmonary artery pressures [5], a hemodynamic alteration associated with increased mortality among patients with ARDS [10]. Together, these pre-clinical findings prompted our current investigation into the relationship of circulating APN to outcomes in ARDS.

Materials and Methods

Data Source

We used National Heart, Lung and Blood Institute (NHLBI) ARDS Network Fluid and Catheter Treatment Trial (FACTT) Trial [11,12] research materials obtained from the NHLBI Biologic Specimen and Data Repository Information Coordinating Center (BioLINCC). The ARDS Network is comprised of 42 hospitals across the United States; details regarding protocols of ARDS Network studies can be found at the ARDSNet.org website. The FACTT trial was a 2×2 factorial design, which randomized patients with ARDS to receive either a right heart catheter or a central venous catheter [12] and either conservative or liberal fluid management [11,13]. Patients receiving conservative fluid management had overall fewer days of mechanical ventilation but otherwise outcomes did not differ significantly between groups. For our study, all analyses and procedures were approved by the Boston University School of Medicine, the Thomas Jefferson University School of Medicine Institutional Review Boards and NHLBI BioLINCC.

Covariates and outcomes

Baseline covariates were measured at FACTT enrollment, which was within 48 hours of the development of ARDS. Data obtained from trial participants included demographics (age, race, sex), anthropometrics (body mass index, height, weight), comorbid conditions (HIV/Acquired Immunodeficiency Syndrome, arthritis, chronic pulmonary disease, cirrhosis, dementia, diabetes mellitus, dialysis dependence, alcohol abuse, congestive heart failure, hepatic encephalopathy, hypertension, immunosuppression, leukemia, lymphoma, myocardial infarction, stroke, metastatic solid tumor, peptic ulcer, peripheral vascular disease), vital signs (blood pressure, heart rate, central venous pressure, fluid intake and output, PaO_2/FiO_2, vasopressor requirement), laboratory values (albumin, bicarbonate, blood urea nitrogen, chloride, creatinine, glucose, hemoglobin, platelets, potassium, sodium, protein and white blood cell count), Murray lung injury score (a composite radiographic appearance, oxygenation, PEEP level and lung compliance) [14], and baseline Acute Physiology and Chronic Health Evaluation (APACHE) III score [15]. Among patients randomized to receive a right heart catheterization, recordings of pulmonary artery pressures, pulmonary artery occlusion pressure, cardiac index and transpulmonary pressure gradient (mean pulmonary pressure minus pulmonary artery occlusion pressure) were also utilized. Patients were followed for up to 60 days for outcome of 'death prior to discharge home with unassisted breathing'.

Adiponectin measurements

Plasma APN concentration was measured by enzyme-linked immunosorbent assay using a commercially available kit (R&D Systems, Minneapolis, MN) according to company protocol. All plasma samples were diluted 1:200 in serum diluting buffer prior to assessing APN concentrations.

Statistical Analyses

The distribution of clinical variables among APN quartiles was compared using Kruskal-Wallis testing and Mantel-Haenzel tests, as appropriate. In order to determine clinical factors associated with APN, variables that were nominally associated with APN levels in univariate analyses ($p<0.10$) were entered into multivariable linear regression with backward selection ($p<0.10$). Given *a priori* associations of age with APN levels and clinical outcomes, age was forced into adjusted models that did not include APACHE scores (which are calculated using age). We excluded variables with >15% missing data from inclusion in multivariable models. APN and change in APN were log-transformed and used as dependent variables in multivariable linear regression analyses. We specifically explored the associations between APN and pulmonary hemodynamics, as well as APN and lung injury scores in multivariable models after adjusting for other clinical factors associated with APN. Separate analyses were performed for clinical factors at baseline and for the change in clinical variables from baseline to day 7. We explored the association of APN with 60-day mortality in Cox proportional hazards models using quartiles of APN levels and clinical variables associated with APN as independent variables. We examined the association of APN with 60-day mortality and quartiles of change in APN (among patients surviving to day 7) in a similar manner. Secondary models that included APN and other variables as time-varying covariates in Cox proportional hazards models were also evaluated. Because of the role of APN in attenuating endothelial activation in animal models of acute lung injury [3], we performed an exploratory subgroup analysis investigating the association between APN and mortality stratifying patients by either "direct" pulmonary injury (eg., pneumonia, aspiration) or "indirect" injury from extra-pulmonary etiologies (eg., urosepsis, trauma, transfusion) [16]. We used Kaplan-Meier survival plots with log-rank tests to visually demonstrate the association between APN and mortality and report 60day mortality rates generated from the Kaplan-Meier survival function. Finally, we examined Spearman rank correlations between APN and log-transformed ventilator-free days, a composite outcome of duration of mechanical ventilation and mortality [17]. In order to examine whether multiple hypothesis testing might better explain significant (at $alpha = 0.05$) associations between APN and clinical variables, univariate associations between clinical factors and APN levels were examined in a sensitivity analysis using a Bonferonni-adjusted threshold of $p = 0.001$ (derived from alpha 0.05/50 tests).

Given that a prior study of critically ill patients with respiratory failure demonstrated an odds ratio for 28-day mortality of 1.59 associated for each 5 ug/ml increase in total APN [18], we estimated a power of 82% with $alpha = 0.05$ to detect similar association in the current study. All analyses were performed using SAS 9.1 (Cary, NC, USA), with alpha of 0.05.

Results

Patient characteristics

Of 1000 FACTT trial participants, plasma was available from 827 subjects at baseline, of whom 816 (81.6%) had detectable APN levels, and from 568 (56.8%) subjects at both baseline and day 7 after enrollment. Trial participants were on average 49.8±16 years old, 53% were male, and 64% were white, with 60-day mortality of 26.8% (219/816). Compared to patients from whom plasma was available, the 184 subjects that were not studied had similar distributions of age ($p = 0.92$), sex ($p = 1.0$), race ($p = 0.39$), etiology of ARDS ($p = 0.24$), and APACHE III score ($p = 0.10$). Among the 248 patients who provided baseline but not day 7 plasma samples, 149 (60%) remained hospitalized at day 7, 24 (10%) were discharged home prior to day 7, and 75 (30%) died prior to day 7.

Adiponectin and Clinical Factors

Analysis of plasma APN levels showed that median APN levels increased over the course of hospitalization: baseline [7245 pg/ml (IQR 3610–13288)], day 7 [9451 pg/ml (IQR 5038–15576)] and change from baseline to day 7 [1346 pg/ml (IQR −2194–5879), $p<0.001$]. Demographic and clinical characteristics grouped according to baseline APN quartiles are shown in **Table S1 in File S1**. Factors associated with baseline APN levels after inclusion in multivariable-adjusted models included sex, body mass index, past medical history of cirrhosis, and central venous pressure (**Table 1**, N = 666, model $R^2 = 9.7\%$). Baseline APN levels were not associated with APACHE III critical illness severity scores, Murray lung injury scores, or measures of oxygenation (PaO_2/FiO_2 ratio). Factors associated with change in APN level from baseline to day 7 are shown in **Table S2 in File S1**. In multivariable analysis, only a history of cirrhosis ($\beta = -0.28$, $R^2 = 0.84\%$, $p<0.04$) was associated with change in APN from baseline to day 7.

Table 2 demonstrates the association between baseline APN levels and pulmonary hemodynamic variables among 384 patients who were randomized to receive a pulmonary artery catheter. Baseline APN levels were inversely associated with mean pulmonary arterial pressure ($\beta = -0.015$, $R^2 = 1.5\%$, $p = 0.02$) but not with other measures of pulmonary vascular hemodynamics such as transpulmonary pressure, pulmonary artery occlusion pressure or cardiac index. After adjusting for age, race, sex, body mass index, and relevant clinical factors (ie., PEEP, cirrhosis, HIV) association between mean pulmonary artery pressure and baseline APN was attenuated ($\beta = -0.009$, $R^2 = 0.5\%$, $p = 0.20$).

Adiponectin and Outcomes

When analyzing all subjects, neither baseline APN levels [APN quartile 4: 43% Kaplan-Meier mortality estimate vs. quartile 1: 36% mortality (**Figure 1**); HR per APN quartile1.04 (95% CI 0.91–1.18), p = 0.61;], change in APN from baseline to day 7 [HR 1.04 (0.89–1.23), p = 0.62)] nor analysis of APN as a time-varying covariate [HR for ln APN 1.13 (0.99–1.30) p = 0.07] were significantly associated with 60 day mortality. Further, we did not identify an association between baseline APN and ventilator-free days ($R^2 = 0.14\%$, $p = 0.29$).

To further explore the relationship between APN and mortality we stratified patients based on whether the etiology of ARDS came from direct or indirect lung injury. Patients with indirect lung injury [median 5909 pg/ml (IQR 3332–12127)] had significantly lower baseline APN levels than those with direct lung injury [7784 pg/ml (IQR 4122–14274)] p = 0.004. We observed a significant association between baseline APN levels and mortality among patients with indirect etiologies for ARDS [N = 322, APN quartile 4: 56% Kaplan-Meier mortality vs. quartile 1:34% (**Figure 2**); HR per APN quartile 1.31 (95% CI 1.08–1.57)]. In contrast, we did not identify an association between APN and mortality among patients developing ARDS in association with direct pulmonary injury [N = 494, APN quartile 4:36% Kaplan-Meier mortality vs. quartile 1: 37% (**Figure 3**); HR per APN quartile 0.96 (95% CI 0.83–1.13)], p interaction = 0.016. Among patients with indirect lung injuries, the association between baseline APN and mortality persisted after adjustment for age, race, sex, and body mass index [HR per APN quartile 1.29 (95% CI 1.05–1.58)], but this was attenuated after further adjusting for APACHE III score, central venous pressure and positive end expiratory pressure [HR per APN quartile 1.18(95% CI 0.94–1.49)]. No significant interaction was seen for the association between change in APN levels from baseline to day 7, mortality and mechanism of lung injury (p interaction = 0.63).

Discussion

We investigated the clinical correlates and outcomes associated with plasma APN levels in more than 800 patients with well-classified ARDS. In addition to confirming previously-described associations between APN with sex and body mass index, we identified a novel correlation between APN levels and central venous pressures. We did not find a relationship between plasma APN levels and severity of illness or lung injury as measured by either the APACHE III score or the Murray Lung Injury score. Moreover, associations between APN and mean pulmonary arterial pressure did not persist after adjusting for demographic and clinical variables. Consistent with prior studies of critically ill patients [18,19], we found that plasma APN levels were higher at late time points in ARDS when compared to the onset of disease. Surprisingly, neither baseline nor dynamic changes in APN levels were associated with mortality among all patients with ARDS in the present study. However, subgroup analysis showed an association between baseline APN levels (but not changes in APN) and mortality in patients who developed ARDS with extra-pulmonary etiologies.

Animal studies have demonstrated that hypoadiponectinemia predisposes to the onset of acute lung injury and increases the severity of disease [2–4,8]. However, we are unaware of prior studies examining circulating APN levels, clinical factors, and outcomes in human ARDS. Ahasic et al recently showed that an

Table 1. Multivariable-adjusted model of factors associated with baseline adiponectin levels.

Variable	Beta estimate	Partial R^2	p-value
Age (per year)	0.0045	0.005	0.069
Male sex	−0.3213	0.026	<0.0001
Body mass index	−0.022	0.027	<0.0001
AIDS	0.2626	0.005	0.083
Cirrhosis	0.6903	0.017	0.001
Central venous pressure	−0.0207	0.009	0.015
Positive end expiratory pressure	−0.0191	0.006	0.054

Model N = 666, Model $R^2 = 0.097$.

Table 2. Pulmonary artery catheter hemodynamics and adiponectin levels.

	Baseline Adiponectin Quartile				
Pulmonary artery catheter value	**Quartile 1 (95–3364 pg/ml) N = 96**	**Quartile 2 (3380–7164) N = 96**	**Quartile 3 (7202–13954) N = 96**	**Quartile 4 (13974–60336) N = 96**	**p**
Pulmonary artery systolic pressure (mmHg)	42 (37–51)	40 (34–48)	39 (33–46)	41 (33–49)	0.038
Pulmonary artery diastolic pressure (mmHg)	23 (20–28)	21 (16–26)	22 (17–26)	21 (17–25)	0.013
Mean pulmonary artery pressure (mmHg)	30 (27–35)	27 (23–33)	27 (23–32)	28 (22–33)	0.01*
Pulmonary artery occlusion pressure (mmHg)	16 (12–20)	15 (10–18)	15 (12–18)	15 (11–18)	0.23
Trans-pulmonary pressure gradient (mm Hg)	14.3 (11.3–18)	13.5 (8.8–17)	12.7 (9.3–16.8)	12.7 (8.7–15.7)	0.12
Cardiac Index (l/min/m^2)	4.1 (3.4–4.8)	3.8 (3.2–4.4)	3.7 (3.0–4.8)	4.1 (3.1–5.1)	0.23

Values are medians (Inter-Quartile Range).
Trans-pulmonary pressure gradient: Mean pulmonary artery pressure-Pulmonary artery occlusion pressure.
*$p<0.1$ and selected for inclusion in multivariable models.

APN gene polymorphism rs2082940 was associated with poor outcomes in ARDS, but circulating APN levels were not measured in this study [20]. In a single center cohort of 175 mechanically ventilated patients of diverse diagnoses (21% with ARDS), we previously showed that higher APN levels at study enrollment were associated with increased mortality [18]. Similarly, in a population of 170 critically ill patients Koch et al. reported that higher plasma APN levels measured early in the course disease were predictive of increased mortality [21]. In our current investigation we did not identify an association between plasma APN and mortality among all patients with ARDS, although we observed a positive correlation among patients with extra-pulmonary etiologies for ARDS. Our subgroup analysis may explain why previous studies have reported a positive association between APN and mortality among critically ill subjects, as extra-pulmonary conditions were more prevalent in the general intensive care unit populations in prior studies [18,21].

The clinical observations that *higher* APN levels are associated with poor outcomes appear to conflict with experimental findings in rodents, which have consistently shown a relationship between

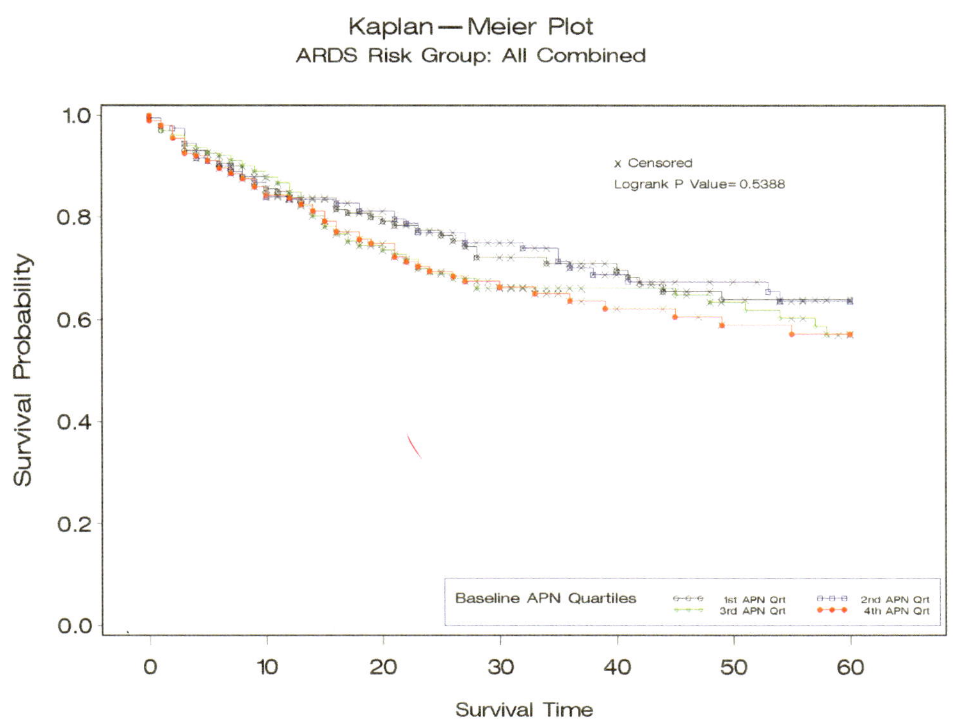

Figure 1. Kaplan-Meier survival plot demonstrating 60-day mortality for patients with acute respiratory distress syndrome stratified by quartile of baseline adiponectin (APN) level for full cohort (N = 816). APN Quartile 1: 95–3589 pg/ml; Quartile 2: 3630–7241 pg/ml; Quartile 3: 7248–13212; Quartile 4: 7243–13212.

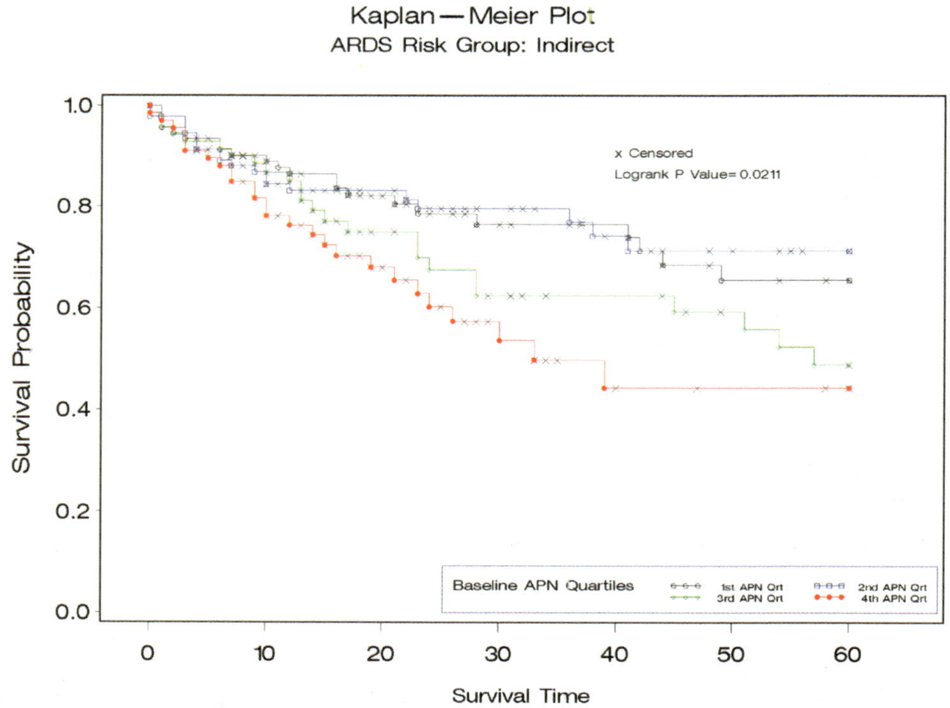

Figure 2. Kaplan-Meier survival plots demonstrating 60-day mortality for patients with acute respiratory distress syndrome stratified by quartile of baseline adiponectin (APN) level for patients with indirect lung injury (N = 322). A significant interaction was demonstrated (p = 0.016) for the association between baseline APN levels and mortality based on whether the mechanism of acute respiratory distress syndrome was presumed to be from "direct" pulmonary injury (eg., pneumonia, aspiration) or "indirect" injury from extra-pulmonary etiologies (eg., urosepsis, trauma, transfusion).

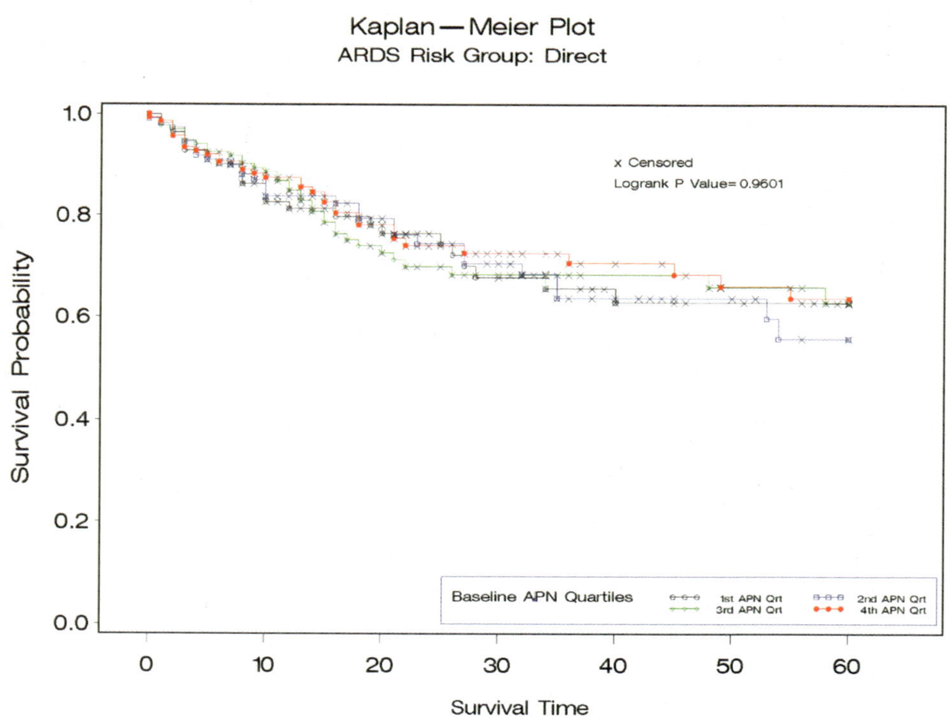

Figure 3. Kaplan-Meier survival plots demonstrating 60-day mortality for patients with acute respiratory distress syndrome stratified by quartile of baseline adiponectin (APN) level for patients with direct lung injury (N = 494).

low adiponectin states (ie, knockout mice) and poor outcomes in acute lung injury [2,4,6,8]. However, in pre-clinical rodent studies (e.g. knock-out mice) changes in APN levels occur prior to the onset of disease, whereas in human studies APN levels are examined after disease onset. Thus, we postulate that higher APN levels in patients early after onset of an acute illness may represent a dysregulated immune response. We propose that future studies exploring this hypothesis focus on patients with extrapulmonary etiologies of ARDS, in whom APN-endothelial [3,16] interactions may be of greater importance.

Our study confirmed prior associations of plasma APN levels with female sex, low body mass index, and cirrhosis [18,21]. Additionally, we identified a novel association between plasma APN levels and central venous pressure. Although this observation was unanticipated, results are consistent with findings in other studies showing that APN acts on systemic blood vessels to increase nitric oxide production and decrease vascular tone [22]. We hypothesize that increased nitric oxide production might partly explain why lower central venous pressures were observed in patients with higher APN levels in our study.

This study has a number of strengths and several limitations. The most obvious strengths are that analyses were performed on a large number of samples and that detailed clinical characteristics were available for all subjects enrolled in our study. While a robust database provided us with sufficient power to detect moderate associations between APN and clinical factors, we recognize that more subtle associations might have been missed by our analyses. We also acknowledge that when testing multiple clinical factors to identify associations there is a greater risk of type I errors. However, our results would not have significantly changed with use of p-values corrected for multiple hypothesis tests. In addition, our analysis of the association between patient outcomes and changes in APN levels over time may have been affected by selection bias; patients without APN levels available on day 7 were more likely to have died prior to day 7 than patients available for sample collection. Measurement of daily APN may better demonstrate associations between temporal changes in APN and clinical outcomes in future studies. One other limitation of our study is that only total APN levels were measured in our samples. Since APN is known to circulate in at least three functionally distinct isoforms [23,24] it is plausible that changes in individual APN isoforms may have more strongly correlated with outcomes in our study. In addition, analyses among subgroups of ARDS etiology were exploratory and should be considered hypothesis-generating. Lastly, as with all observational studies, causal inference for associations between clinical factors and APN levels is limited.

In conclusion, our study fills multiple knowledge gaps regarding the relationship between APN, clinical factors and clinical outcomes in ARDS. Although we did not observe significant associations between plasma APN and mortality in the entire cohort of patients, we identified novel clinical correlates of APN. Our analysis demonstrates an interaction between the mechanism of lung injury and the association of APN with mortality, a finding that is supported by experimental evidence and argues for further clinical investigation examining the role of APN in patients with indirect causes of ARDS.

Acknowledgments

This manuscript was prepared using ARDS Network FACTT research materials obtained from the National Heart, Lung and Blood Institute's Biologic Specimen and Data Repository Information Coordinating Center and does not necessarily reflect the opinions or views of the ARDSNet, FACTT or the NHLBI. We thank the ARDS Network investigators and the ARDS Network study participants for their contributions to this work.

Author Contributions

Conceived and designed the experiments: AJW SD RSS. Performed the experiments: AJW SD DS FR LP RSS. Analyzed the data: AJW SD RSS. Contributed reagents/materials/analysis tools: DS FR LP RSS. Wrote the paper: AJW SD RSS.

References

1. Nigro E, Scudiero O, Sarnataro D, Mazzarella G, Sofia M, et al. (2013) Adiponectin affects lung epithelial A549 cell viability counteracting TNFalpha and IL-1ss toxicity through AdipoR1. Int J Biochem Cell Biol 45: 1145–1153. 10.1016/j.biocel.2013.03.003; 10.1016/j.biocel.2013.03.003.
2. Xu L, Bao HG, Si YN, Han L, Zhang R, et al. (2013) Effects of adiponectin on acute lung injury in cecal ligation and puncture-induced sepsis rats. J Surg Res 183: 752–759. 10.1016/j.jss.2013.01.055; 10.1016/j.jss.2013.01.055.
3. Konter JM, Parker JL, Baez E, Li SZ, Ranscht B, et al. (2012) Adiponectin attenuates lipopolysaccharide-induced acute lung injury through suppression of endothelial cell activation. J Immunol 188: 854–863 10.4049/jimmunol.1100426; 10.4049/jimmunol.1100426.
4. van Meurs M, Castro P, Shapiro NI, Lu S, Yano M, et al. (2012) Adiponectin diminishes organ-specific microvascular endothelial cell activation associated with sepsis. Shock 37: 392–398. 10.1097/SHK.0b013e318248225e; 10.1097/SHK.0b013e318248225e.
5. Summer R, Fiack CA, Ikeda Y, Sato K, Dwyer D, et al. (2009) Adiponectin deficiency: A model of pulmonary hypertension associated with pulmonary vascular disease. Am J Physiol Lung Cell Mol Physiol 297: L432–8. 10.1152/ajplung.90599.2008.
6. Teoh H, Quan A, Bang KW, Wang G, Lovren F, et al. (2008) Adiponectin deficiency promotes endothelial activation and profoundly exacerbates sepsis-related mortality. Am J Physiol Endocrinol Metab 295: E658–64. 10.1152/ajpendo.90384.2008.
7. Arita Y, Kihara S, Ouchi N, Takahashi M, Maeda K, et al. (1999) Paradoxical decrease of an adipose-specific protein, adiponectin, in obesity. Biochem Biophys Res Commun 257: 79–83.
8. Li S, Bao HG, Han L, Liu L, Wang X (2012) Effects of adiponectin on mortality and its mechanism in a sepsis mouse model. J Invest Surg 25: 214–219. 10.3109/08941939.2011.624257; 10.3109/08941939.2011.624257.
9. Ware LB, Matthay MA (2000) The acute respiratory distress syndrome. N Engl J Med 342: 1334–1349. 10.1056/NEJM200005043421806.
10. Bull TM, Clark B, McFann K, Moss M, National Institutes of Health/National Heart, Lung, and Blood Institute ARDS Network (2010) Pulmonary vascular dysfunction is associated with poor outcomes in patients with acute lung injury. Am J Respir Crit Care Med 182: 1123–1128. 10.1164/rccm.201002-0250OC.
11. Wiedemann HP, Wheeler AP, Bernard GR, Thompson BT, Hayden D, et al. (2006) Comparison of two fluid-management strategies in acute lung injury. N Engl J Med 354: 2564–75. NEJMoa062200 [pii] 10.1056/NEJMoa062200 [doi].
12. Wheeler AP, Bernard GR, Thompson BT, Schoenfeld D, Wiedemann HP, et al. (2006) Pulmonary-artery versus central venous catheter to guide treatment of acute lung injury. N Engl J Med 354: 2213–24. NEJMoa061895 [pii] 10.1056/NEJMoa061895 [doi].
13. Wiedemann HP (2008) A perspective on the fluids and catheters treatment trial (FACTT). fluid restriction is superior in acute lung injury and ARDS. Cleve Clin J Med 75: 42–48.
14. Murray JF, Matthay MA, Luce JM, Flick MR (1988) An expanded definition of the adult respiratory distress syndrome. Am Rev Respir Dis 138: 720–723.
15. Knaus WA, Wagner DP, Draper EA, Zimmerman JE, Bergner M, et al. (1991) The APACHE III prognostic system. risk prediction of hospital mortality for critically ill hospitalized adults. Chest 100: 1619–1636.
16. Pelosi P, D'Onofrio D, Chiumello D, Paolo S, Chiara G, et al. (2003) Pulmonary and extrapulmonary acute respiratory distress syndrome are different. Eur Respir J Suppl 42: 48s–56s.

17. Schoenfeld DA, Bernard GR, ARDS Network (2002) Statistical evaluation of ventilator-free days as an efficacy measure in clinical trials of treatments for acute respiratory distress syndrome. Crit Care Med 30: 1772–1777.
18. Walkey AJ, Rice TW, Konter J, Ouchi N, Shibata R, et al. (2010) Plasma adiponectin and mortality in critically ill subjects with acute respiratory failure. Crit Care Med 38: 2329–2334. 10.1097/CCM.0b013e3181fa0561; 10.1097/CCM.0b013e3181fa0561.
19. Langouche L, Vander Perre S, Frystyk J, Flyvbjerg A, Hansen TK, et al. (2009) Adiponectin, retinol-binding protein 4, and leptin in protracted critical illness of pulmonary origin. Crit Care 13: R112. 10.1186/cc7956.
20. Ahasic AM, Zhao Y, Su L, Sheu CC, Thompson BT, et al. (2014) Adiponectin gene polymorphisms and acute respiratory distress syndrome susceptibility and mortality. PLoS One 9: e89170. 10.1371/journal.pone.0089170; 10.1371/journal.pone.0089170.
21. Koch A, Sanson E, Voigt S, Helm A, Trautwein C, et al. (2010) Serum adiponectin upon admission to the intensive care unit may predict mortality in critically ill patients. J Crit Care. 10.1016/j.jcrc.2010.07.015.
22. Chen H, Montagnani M, Funahashi T, Shimomura I, Quon MJ (2003) Adiponectin stimulates production of nitric oxide in vascular endothelial cells. J Biol Chem 278: 45021–45026. 10.1074/jbc.M307878200.
23. Kobayashi H, Ouchi N, Kihara S, Walsh K, Kumada M, et al. (2004) Selective suppression of endothelial cell apoptosis by the high molecular weight form of adiponectin. Circ Res 94: e27–31. 10.1161/01.RES.0000119921.86460.37.
24. Neumeier M, Weigert J, Schaffler A, Wehrwein G, Muller-Ladner U, et al. (2005) Different effects of adiponectin isoforms in human monocytic cells. J Leukoc Biol 79: 803–808. 10.1189/jlb.0905521.

Association of Radiologic Findings with Mortality in Patients with Avian Influenza H7N9 Pneumonia

Feng Feng[1,8], Yebin Jiang[1,7], Min Yuan[1], Jie Shen[1], Huabin Yin[2], Daoying Geng[3], Jianrong Xu[4], Yanqing Hua[5], Jingyun Shi[6], Yuxin Shi[1]*, Zhiyong Zhang[1]*

1 Department of Radiology, Shanghai Public Health Clinical Center, Fudan University, Shanghai, China, **2** Department of Radiology, The Fifth People's Hospital of Shanghai, Fudan University, Shanghai, China, **3** Department of Radiology, Huashan Hospital, Fudan University, Shanghai, China, **4** Department of Radiology, Renji Hospital, Shanghai Jiaotong University, Shanghai, China, **5** Department of Radiology, Huadong Hospital, Fudan University, Shanghai, China, **6** Department of Radiology, Shanghai Pulmonary Hospital, Tongji University, Shanghai, China, **7** Cancer Center, University of Michigan, Ann Arbor, Michigan, United States of America, **8** Department of Radiology, Nantong Tumor Hospital, Nantong University, Nantong, China

Abstract

Background: The novel H7N9 virus causes severe illness, including pneumonia and acute respiratory distress syndrome, with high rates of mortality. We investigated the association of initial radiologic characteristics obtained at admission with clinical outcomes in patients with avian influenza H7N9 pneumonia.

Methods: Demographics, comorbidities, clinical findings, radiologic appearance and scores of the affected lung parenchyma were compared between survivor group (n = 15) and mortality group (n = 7). Two radiologic scores were calculated, one using chest radiography and one using CT. Follow-up CT scans at discharge were analyzed in 12 patients of the survival group.

Results: All the patients in mortality group developed acute respiratory distress syndrome and required mechanical ventilation, while in the survival group 33% (5/15) developed acute respiratory distress syndrome ($P<0.05$) and 27% (4/15) required mechanical ventilation ($P<0.05$). The mean radiographic and CT scores of the mortality group were 50% higher compared to the survival group ($P<0.05$). ROC analysis revealed an area under curve of 0.738 for the radiographic score with an optimal cutoff value of a score of 19 for prediction of mortality, with a sensitivity of 71% and a specificity of 67%, and an area under curve of 0.833 for the CT score with an optimal cutoff value of a CT score of 21 for prediction of mortality, with a sensitivity of 86% and a specificity of 73%. The mean CT score of the affected lung parenchyma at discharge was 30% lower than the initial CT examination ($P<0.05$).

Conclusion: High initial radiologic score is associated with mortality in patients with avian influenza H7N9 pneumonia.

Editor: Steven J. Drews, University of Calgary & ProvLab Alberta, Canada

Funding: The authors have no support or funding to report.

Competing Interests: The authors have declared that no competing interests exist.

* E-mail: shiyx828288@163.com (YS); zhangzy@shaphc.org (ZZ)

Introduction

Influenza is a highly contagious disease of global importance. The virus infects a variety of animals including birds, and infects humans. Three subtypes of influenza A were previously reported to infect humans, i.e., H1N1, H1N2, and H3N2 [1]. During the past few years, several subtypes of avian influenza A have been shown to cross the species barrier and infect humans. In the spring of 2013, a novel avian-origin influenza A virus, H7N9, emerged and spread among humans in China. The first documented case of human infection with the influenza H7N9 virus occurred in Shanghai in March [2]. As of May 9, the World Health Organization (WHO) reported 131 laboratory-confirmed cases, including 32 deaths [3]. Of the 111 patients with the H7N9 virus infection has been reported recently, 76.6% were admitted to an intensive care unit (ICU) [4]. On admission, 108 patients (97.3%) had findings consistent with pneumonia. The clinical features, blood cell counts, and laboratory and biochemical findings in patients with H7N9 virus infection have been described [5–7]. Patients usually presented with fever and cough, and with early sputum production. The illness progressed rapidly to severe pneumonia, with moderate-to-severe acute respiratory distress syndrome [5].

During the outbreak of avian flu, imaging studies provided important information for diagnosis, management, and control of H7N9 infection [6]. On chest radiographs or computed tomographic (CT) scans, bilateral ground glass opacities and consolidation were the typical radiologic findings [4,8].

Because H7N9 virus infection is potentially fatal disease and extremely contagious with mortality rate of 27% [4], it is important during the current influenza outbreak to identify initial imaging findings as potential risk stratification to help triage patient, guide treatment, and monitor disease progression and treatment response. We therefore investigated the association of initial chest radiographic findings and CT characteristics obtained at admission with clinical outcomes in patients with avian influenza H7N9 pneumonia.

Methods

Patients

This study was approved by the Institutional Review Boards of Shanghai Public Health Clinical Center, the Fifth People's Hospital of Shanghai, Huashan Hospital, Renji Hospital, Huadong Hospital, and Shanghai Pulmonary Hospital. The requirement of informed consent was waived. Between March 2013 and May 2013, 22 patients who fulfilled the clinical criteria for H7N9 influenza infection established by the National Centers for Disease Control and Prevention (CDC) were hospitalized in the above 6 different institutions. Diagnosis of H7N9 infection was made by positive test for H7N9 viral RNA, in throat-swab specimens collected from patients by real-time reverse transcription polymerase chain reaction (RT-PCR) using standard RT-PCR protocol at Shanghai CDC. All patients were in-hospital and had undergone chest radiographs and CT scans. Two radiologic scores were calculated, one using chest radiography and one using CT.

The 22 patients were treated with oral oseltamivir 75 mg, twice daily. Patients were also given antibiotics, included moxifloxacin, sulbactam and cefoperazone, levofloxacin, meropenem, piperacillin, imipenem, and cilastatin, when there was positive test in blood and/or throat-swab for specific bacterial infection. Some patients also received glucocorticoid, or intravenous immunoglobulin administration.

Chest radiographs

Chest radiographs were obtained using conventional radiography with posteroanterior projection, or portable computed radiography at bedside with anteroposterior projection.

CT scans

The types of scanners and protocols used for the CT scans varied since they were from 6 different institutions. The technical parameters included 0.75 mm or 1 mm collimation at 5–7 mm intervals. Follow-up scans were obtained at discharge from 12 patients. All examinations were performed with the patient in the supine position and with breath-holding following inspiration, without administration of contrast material.

Images were obtained with both mediastinal (width 350–450 HU; level 20–40 HU) and parenchymal (width 1200–1600 HU; level −500 to −700 HU) window settings.

Imaging evaluation

Three chest radiologists reviewed the images independently initially, with a final finding reached by consensus when there was a discrepancy. They were blinded to the clinical information or clinical progress of the patients, except for the knowledge that these were cases of H7N9 virus infection.

Chest radiographic and CT findings included ground glass opacity, consolidation, and nodular opacities. Ground glass opacities were defined as hazy areas of increased opacity or attenuation without concealing the underlying vessels. Consolidation was defined as homogeneous opacification of the parenchyma obscuring the underlying vessels. Nodular opacities were defined as focal round opacities (diameter <2 cm). The presence of lymphadenopathy defined as a lymph node ≥1 cm in short-axis diameter.

The extent of involvement of each abnormality was assessed independently for each of 3 zones: upper (above the carina), middle (below the carina and above the inferior pulmonary vein), and lower (below the inferior pulmonary vein). The location of the lesion was defined as peripheral if it was in the outer one-third of the lung, or as central otherwise. The radiographic and CT findings were graded on a 3-point scale: 1 as normal attenuation, 2 as ground-glass attenuation, and 3 as consolidation. The CT scans were scored on the axial images. The ground-glass attenuation and consolidation areas were determined using the method described by Grieser et al [9]. The Hounsfield Units (HU) of normal attenuation, ground-glass attenuation and consolidation areas were measured. Each lung zone, with a total of six lung zones in each patient, was assigned a following scale according to distribution of the affected lung parenchyma using a method modified from a previously described protocol [10]: 0 as normal, 1 as <25% abnormality, 2 as 25–50% abnormality, 3 as 50–75% abnormality, and 4 as >75% abnormality. The four-point scale of the lung parenchyma distribution was then multiplied by the radiologic scale described above (Figure 1). Points from all zones were added for a final total cumulative score, with value ranging from 0 to 72.

Statistical analysis

All data were expressed as mean ± standard deviation (SD), or median and interquartile range (IQR) for the continuous variables and as a number of individuals with percentage in each group for the categoric variables. The comparison of continuous variables between groups was performed using the Mann-Whitney U test. Frequencies of categoric variables were compared by the Fisher exact test. A receiver operating characteristic curve was plotted to determine the appropriate cut-off value with maximum sensitivity and specificity for the endpoint of death. All analyses were considered significant at p values of less than 0.05 (two-tailed).

Results

The 22 patients included 5 women and 17 men, with median age of 67 years (interquartile range, IQR, 56–75 years). Of the 22 patients, 20 (91%) were admitted to an intensive care unit (ICU), including 14 directly admitted to ICU and 6 transferred to ICU during hospitalization. The main adverse outcome measure was in-hospital death. As of July 10, a total of 7 patients had died in hospital, and 15 patients were discharged in recovered condition. The median time from the onset of illness to death was 18 days (IQR, 12 to 54 days). All the patients were devided into mortality (n = 7) and survival (n = 15) groups.

Table 1 shows the comparison of patient age, sex, comorbid illnesses, outcomes as resulting in required mechanical ventilation or developing acute respiratory distress syndrome, and clinical symptoms, between mortality and survival groups. The mortality rate in this study was 32% (7 of 22 patients). There were no significant differences between the two groups with respect to patient age, sex, comorbidities, and clinical manifestations. All the patients in mortality group developed acute respiratory distress syndrome and all of them required mechanical ventilation, while in survival group 33% (5/15) developed acute respiratory distress syndrome ($P = 0.004$) and 27% (4/15) required mechanical ventilation ($P = 0.005$). Only two patients in mortality group required invasive mechanical ventilation, while others required non-invasive mechanical ventilation.

Table 2 compares the frequency of chest radiographic findings, distribution patterns, and chest radiographic score of the affected lung parenchyma between the survival group and the mortality

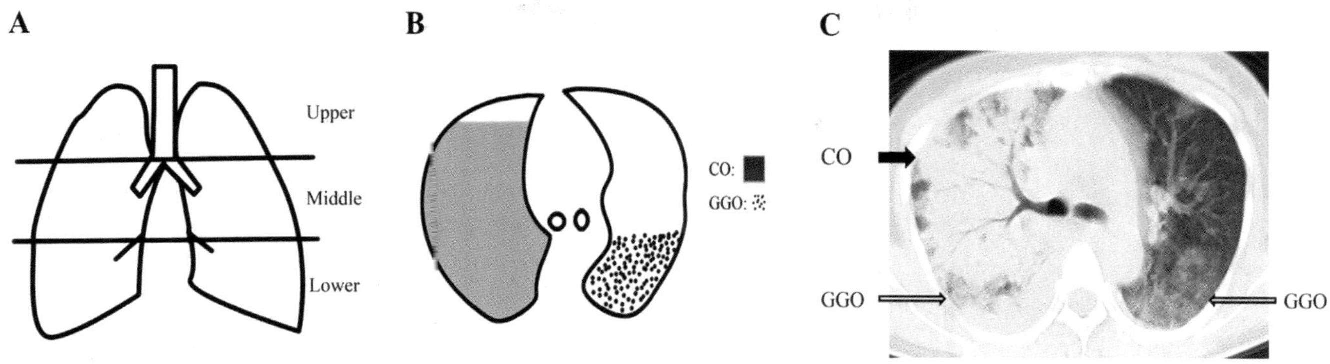

Figure 1. The schematic of CT scoring system. Schematic coronal representations of zones, extent of ground-glass opacity and consolidation on an axial image, and a sample scoring on an axial CT image. Schematic coronal representation of zones (A) evaluated in the lungs of patients with H7N9 infection shows upper zones which are above the carina, middle zones between the carina and the inferior pulmonary vein, and lower zones which are below the inferior pulmonary vein. Schematic representation of the extent of ground-glass opacity (GGO) and consolidation (CO) on an axial image (B) which were determined using the modified Grieser system. Points from all zones were added for a cumulative score, with value ranging from 0 to 72. A sample scoring on an axial CT image (C) of a 52-year-old woman from mortality group demonstrates a total score of 18, calculated as 3 (consolidation, solid arrow) ×4 (>75% distribution in middle zone of the right lung) +2 (ground-glass opacity, open arrow) ×1 (<25% distribution in middle zone of the right lung) +2 (ground-glass opacity, open arrow) ×2 (25–50% distribution in middle zone of the left lung).

group. The predominant chest radiographic findings at presentation consisted of a bilateral mixed pattern of ground glass opacity and areas of consolidation in 18 patients (82%), air bronchograms in 11 patients (50%), and both central and peripheral distributions in 21 patients (95%). A small pleural effusion was found in 9 patients (41%). The mediastinal lymphadenopathies, pneumothorax and pneumomediastinum were not seen on chest radiographs.

The mean chest radiographic score of the mortality group (Figure 2) was 50% higher compared to survival group (Figure 3) ($P = 0.035$). In the receiver operating characteristic curve analysis (Figure 4), an optimal cutoff value of a chest radiographic score of 19 had a sensitivity of 71% and a specificity of 67% for the prediction of mortality. The area under the receiver operating characteristic curve was 0.738 (95% confidence interval: 0.568, 0.985). There was no statistically significant difference in the

Table 1. Demorgraphics, comorbidities, and clinical presentations in mortality and survival groups.

Variable	All patients	Survival Group	Mortality Group
	N = 22	N = 15	N = 7
Age, median(*IQR*), years	67(56–75)	67(56–78)	67(52–86)
Sex: men, women	17,5	12,3	5,2
Exposure to live poultry	2(9)	1(7)	1(14)
Coexisting medical condition			
Any	15(68)	10(67)	5(71)
Hypertension	9(41)	7(47)	2(29)
Diabetes	4(18)	3(20)	1(14)
Coronary heart disease	4(18)	3(20)	1(14)
Chronic obstructive pulmonary disease	2(9)	2(13)	0
Brest cancer	1(5)	1(7)	0
Hepatitis B infection	1(5)	0	1(14)
Outcome			
Acute respiratory distress syndrome	12(55)	5(33)	7(100) **
Requiring mechanical ventilation	11(50)	4(27)	7(100) **
Symptoms			
Fever >38°C	22(100)	15(100)	7(100)
Cough	20(91)	14(93)	6(86)
Dyspnea	16(73)	10(67)	6(86)
Expectoration	4(18)	3(20)	1(14)

**$P < 0.01$ versus survival group.
Percentages are in parentheses, unless indicated as IQR (interquartile range).

Table 2. Chest radiographic features in mortality and survival groups.

Chest radiographic features	All patients N=22	Survival Group N=15	Mortality Group N=7
Symptom onset before chest radiograph, median(*IQR*), days	7(4–8)	7(3–9)	6(4–7)
GGO	2(9)	2(13)	0
Consolidation	1(5)	0	1(14)
Both of GGO and consolidation	19(86)	13(87)	6(86)
Radiographic score, median(*IQR*)	18(16–24)	18(11–24)	27(18–31) *
Air bronchogram	11(50)	7(47)	4(57)
Nodular opacities	0	0	0
Lymphadenopathy	0	0	0
Pleural effusions	9(41)	6(40)	3(43)
Unilateral	5(23)	3(20)	2(29)
Bilateral	4(18)	3(20)	1(14)
Anatomic sides involved			
Unilateral	3(14)	2(13)	1(14)
Bilateral	19(86)	13(87)	6(86)
Predominant distribution			
Central	0	0	0
Peripheral	1(5)	1(7)	0
Both central and peripheral	21(95)	14(93)	7(100)
Involved zone			
Upper	17(77)	11(73)	6(86)
Middle	22(100)	15(100)	7(100)
Lower	22(100)	15(100)	7(100)

$^*P<0.05$ versus survival group.
Percentages are in parentheses, unless indicated as IQR (interquartile range).
GGO: ground grass opacity.

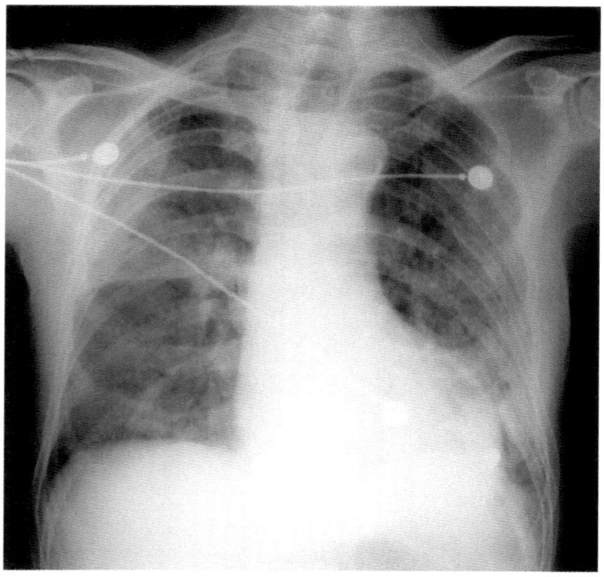

Figure 2. A 74 year old male patient with H7N9 pneumonia from mortality group. Chest radiograph with score of 28 shows bilateral patchy consolidations and ground glass opacities.

frequency and distribution of the chest radiographic findings between the survival and mortality groups.

Table 3 compares the frequency of CT findings, distribution patterns, and CT score of the affected lung parenchyma between the survival group and the mortality group. The predominant CT findings at presentation consisted of a bilateral mixed pattern of ground glass opacity and areas of consolidation in 20 patients (91%), air bronchograms in 15 patients (68%), and both central and peripheral distributions in 21 patients (95%). A small pleural effusion was found in 12 patients (55%). The mediastinal lymphadenopathies were observed in 2 patients (9%) with coexistent chronic obstructive pulmonary disease. Pneumothorax and pneumomediastinum were not seen on CT.

The mean CT score of the mortality group (Figure 5) was 50% higher compared to survival group (Figure 6) ($P=0.013$). In the receiver operating characteristic curve analysis (Figure 7), an optimal cutoff value of a CT score of 21 had a sensitivity of 86% and a specificity of 73% for the prediction of mortality. The area under the receiver operating characteristic curve was 0.833 (95% confidence interval: 0.659, 1). There was no statistically significant difference in the frequency and distribution of the CT findings between the survival and mortality groups.

Table 4 presents the frequency of CT findings, distribution patterns, and CT score of the affected lung parenchyma among 12 patients of the survival group who underwent follow up CT scans at discharge. The mean score of the affected lung parenchyma at discharge was 30% lower than the initial CT examination

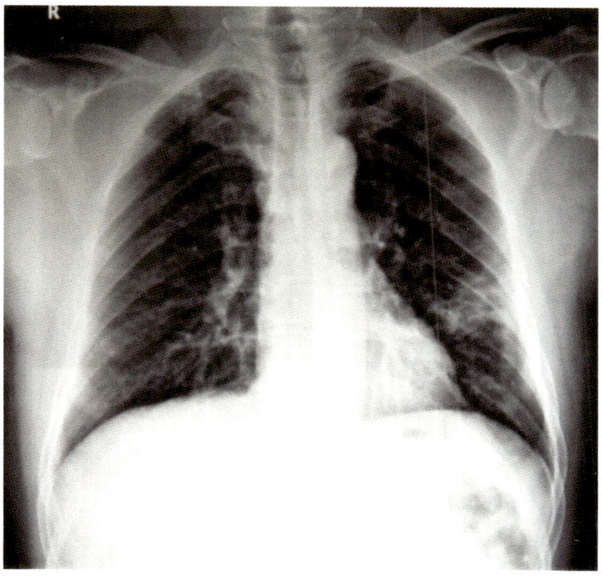

Figure 3. A 67 year old male patient with H7N9 pneumonia from survival group. Chest radiograph with score of 4 shows patchy consolidations and ground glass opacities in the left middle and lower zones.

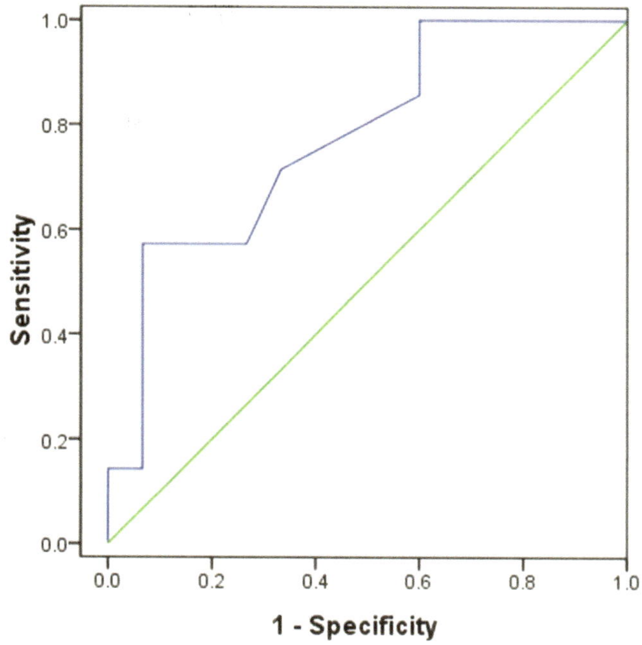

Figure 4. ROC analysis of the chest radiographic score for prediction of mortality. N = 22; AUC = 0.738.

(P = 0.029). There was no statistically significant difference in CT findings and distribution patterns between the initial and follow-up examination.

Discussion

In this study, patients who were hospitalized with H7N9 virus infection tended to be older. Among all patients, 68% had one or more coexisting medical conditions such as hypertension, cardiac disease, and chronic obstructive pulmonary disease. This finding that H7N9 virus infection appears to attach older adults with coexisting chronic diseases is consistent with prior study [4]. Indeed, a proportion of elderly people have some level of sensitized immune system following exposure to the 1918 virus or related strains that circulated until 1957 [11], and elderly and immunocompromised persons are at increased risk for the development of fulminant influenza virus pneumonia [12]. Of note, 56% (62/111) patients with H7N9 infection provided a clear history and reported close contact with live poultry in previous 14 days before the onset of illness [4]. In our study, however, only 9% (2/22) patients had the same history.

In the present series, frequencies of mechanical ventilation and acute respiratory distress syndrome was higher in mortality group than in survival group, while survival and mortality groups showed no significant differences with respect to patient age, sex, coexisting medical condition, and clinical findings. This is different from H1N1 pneumonia or severe acute respiratory syndrome (SARS). In the previous reports, patients with H1N1 pneumonia or SARS who died were significantly older than those who survived [9,13]. A possible explanation is the predominance of elderly patients in this outbreak of H7N9 virus infection. However, patients who died had significantly higher frequencies of mechanical ventilation and acute respiratory distress syndrome than those who survived. Acute respiratory distress syndrome is a strong predictor of mortality, which reflects the severity of respiratory failure [14]. Furthermore, for patients with H7N9 virus infection, mechanical ventilation is an important treatment when patients experience respiratory failure [15].

In our study, the overall initial chest radiographic and CT scores were 50% higher in mortality group than in survivors. For the survivors at discharge, their CT score is 30% lower compared with score at admission. Regarding the prediction of mortality, we found an optimal cutoff value of a chest radiographic score of 19 (sensitivity of 71% and specificity of 67%), and a CT score of 21 (sensitivity of 86% and specificity of 73%). The overall radiologic score was based on the severity of air-space disease and its distribution. The more extensive consolidations were observed in the mortality patients than in the survivors. This can be probably explained by the report that main cause of death is hypoxemia [4]. The previous studies stated that patients of viral pneumonias with consolidations on CT have a more severe clinical course than those who present with ground glass opacities [16,17]. These abnormalities can be pathologically correlated with diffuse alveolar damage [18]. Patients who died tended to have more consolidation and asymmetric disease, while patients of viral pneumonias with bilateral consolidations had a more protracted clinical course [17]. Because H7N9 virus infection is an extremely contagious and potentially fatal disease, risk stratification in our study using the simple scoring method may help triage patient, and may indicate that more aggressive treatment and closely monitoring of disease progression should be applied to the patient with higher overall radiologic scores. However, the efficacy of such approaches to decrease mortality remains to be validated in future study.

Our study demonstrated that a mixture pattern of ground glass opacities and consolidation, air bronchogram, and small pleural effusion were of consistent common radiographic and CT features in both survival and mortality group, distributing in bilateral and central and peripheral locations in the early course of the disease. Our finding of a mixed pattern are consistent with the first report indicating that all three patients had coexisting ground glass opacities and consolidation on radiographs or CT on day 7 after the onset of illness [15], and consistent with a recent report in 111 cases [4]. However, this finding was different from the CT findings

Table 3. CT features in mortality and survival groups.

CT features	All patients N=22	Survival Group N=15	Mortality Group N=7
Symptom onset before CT, median(*IQR*), days	7(3–9)	7(4–9)	6(4–8)
GGO	1(5)	1(7)	0
Consolidation	1(5)	0	1(14)
Both of GGO and consolidation	20(91)	14(93)	6(86)
CT score, median(*IQR*)	21(15–24)	18(11–23)	27(21–33) *
Air bronchogram	15(68)	10(67)	5(71)
Nodular opacities	2(9)	2(13)	0
Lymphadenopathy	2(9)	2(13)	0
Pleural effusions	12(55)	8(53)	4(57)
Unilateral	6(27)	4(27)	2(29)
Bilateral	6(27)	4(27)	2(29)
Anatomic sides involved			
Unilateral	2(9)	1(7)	1(14)
Bilateral	20(91)	14(93)	6(86)
Predominant distribution			
Central	0	0	0
Peripheral	1(5)	1(7)	0
Both central and peripheral	21(95)	14(93)	7(100)
Involved zone			
Upper	18(82)	12(80)	6(86)
Middle	22(100)	15(100)	7(100)
Lower	22(100)	15(100)	7(100)

*$P<0.05$ versus survival group.
Percentages are in parentheses, unless indicated as IQR (interquartile range).
GGO: ground grass opacity.

in H1N1 influenza A (H1N1) virus-associated pneumonia by Marchiori et al. [19] who noted that ground glass opacity (12/20, 60%) was the most common CT finding and that a mixed pattern (6/20,30%) was the second most common finding 4–9 days after the onset of symptoms. Studies on the CT findings of pneumonia due to H5N1 infection are limited and do not distinguish between ground glass opacity and consolidation [20]. In addition, mediastinal or hilar lymphadenopathy was rare. This finding is similar to the CT appearance of pneumonia caused by H1N1 and H5N1 virus infections, which have been consistently reported in other studies [21–23]. A small pleural effusion was observed in 12 cases (55%), including bilateral effusion in 6 patients and unilateral effusion in 6 patients. Pleural effusions are generally considered rare with human influenza A infection [20]. However, these

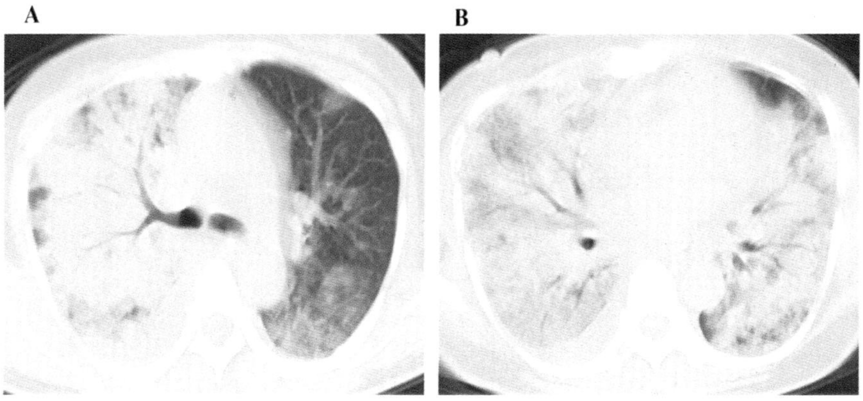

Figure 5. A 52 year old female patient with H7N9 pneumonia from mortality group. CT images with score of 38 show ground glass opacity and consolidation in the middle (A) and the lower zones (B). There is a small amount of right pleural effusion.

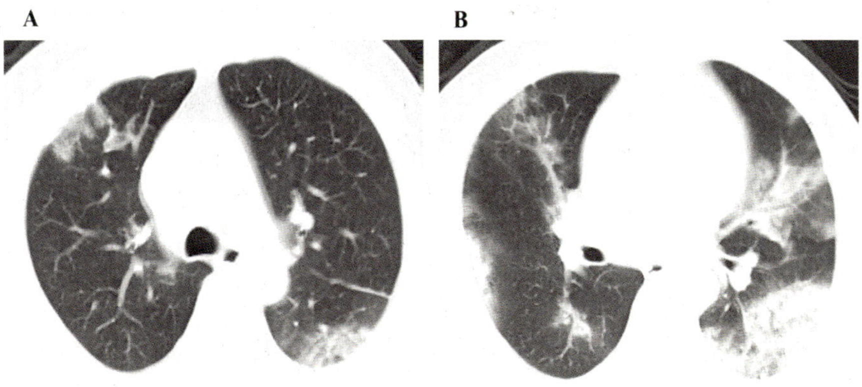

Figure 6. A 53 year old male patient with H7N9 pneumonia from survival group. CT images with CT score of 18 show ground glass opacity mostly in the upper zones (A) and consolidation in the lower zones (B).

occurred relatively frequently in our patients. A previous study also reported pleural effusions with often severe coexisting consolidation observed in one third of 178 patients infected by H5N1 avian influenza virus, and the effusions were bilateral in nearly all patients during the course of the disease [23]. In addition, a small pleural effusion was previously observed in 5 patients (25%) with H1N1 infection using CT [19].

In this study, we evaluated the prognostic implication of both chest radiographic and CT scores assessed by determining the extent of patchy areas of ground-glass attenuation mixed with consolidation. The chest radiographic and CT scores could help perform risk stratification. In our study, CT attention as HU was −313.2 (±123.8) for ground-glass attenuation, and 11.8 (±79.7) for consolidation areas. We found that the CT attention was helpful to determine ground-glass attenuation and consolidation areas. Using the grading method, the scores at initial chest radiographs and CT images have significance in the prediction of clinical outcomes. Extensive involvement of both lungs was associated with adverse prognosis. Further investigations are warranted to apply this semi-quantitative approach of grading system to calculate or predict ultimate outcome, evaluate disease phenotypes, monitor disease progression, and evaluate treatment

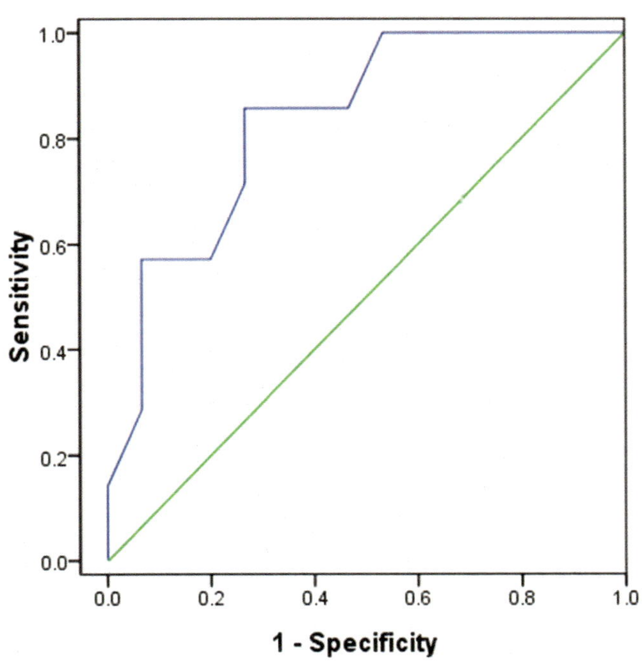

Figure 7. ROC analysis of the CT score for prediction of mortality. N = 22; AUC = 0.833.

Table 4. Initial and follow-up CT features of 12 patients in survival group.

CT features	Initial CT Scan N = 12	CT Scan at Discharge N = 12
Symptom onset before CT, median(*IQR*), days	5(7–9)	29(26–32)
GGO	1(8)	2(17)
Consolidation	0	0
Both of GGO and consolidation	11(92)	10(83)
CT score, median(*IQR*)	19(11–24)	11(9–16)*
Air bronchogram	8(67)	6(50)
Nodular opacities	1(8)	0
Lymphadenopathy	1(8)	1(8)
Pleural effusions	7(58)	9(75)
Unilateral	4(33)	8(67)
Bilateral	3(25)	1(8)
Anatomic sides involved		
Unilateral	1(8)	2(17)
Bilateral	11(92)	10(83)
Predominant distribution		
Central	0	0
Peripheral	0	2(17)
Both central and peripheral	12(100)	10(83)
Involved zone		
Upper	10(83)	8(67)
Middle	12(100)	11(92)
Lower	12(100)	12(100)

*$P<0.05$ versus survival group.
Percentages are in parentheses, unless indicated as IQR (interquartile range).
GGO: ground grass opacity.

response and efficacy for other viral pneumonia or other air space diseases in genetic studies, clinical researches, epidemiological investigations, and clinical trials.

There were several limitations in this study. First, it was retrospective and included only relatively small number of cases. All of the patients in our current study were reported to the CDC from March 2013 to May 2013 and required hospitalization. Therefore, the analysis was biased toward patients with more severe forms of the disease. Second, despite the use of a standardized data-collection form, not all information was collected for all patients. Because none of the mortality patients performed follow-up CT scans, the follow-up CT images included only patients of the survival group with available follow-up CT examination at discharge. Finally, there was a lack of information regarding interobserver agreement, because the study design placed a greater emphasis on the final consensus interpretation rather than independent reading.

In conclusion, we have evaluated the prognostic implication of both chest radiographic and CT score assessed by determining the extent of patchy areas of ground glass attenuation mixed with consolidation in patients with H7N9 infection. High initial chest radiographic or CT score in patients with avian influenza H7N9 pneumonia is associated with mortality, especially in patients with acute respiratory distress syndrome and requiring mechanical ventilation. Since H7N9 virus infection is potentially fatal and highly contagious, risk stratification based on the air-space disease may help triage patients, guide treatment, and monitor disease progression and treatment response.

Author Contributions

Conceived and designed the experiments: YS ZZ. Performed the experiments: FF MY J. Shen HY DG YH JX J. Shi YJ YS ZZ. Analyzed the data: FF HY DG YH JX J. Shi YJ YS ZZ. Contributed reagents/materials/analysis tools: FF HY DG YH JX J. Shi YJ YS ZZ. Wrote the paper: FF YJ YS ZZ.

References

1. Tran TH, Nguyen TL, Nguyen TD, Luong TS, Pham PM, et al. (2004) Avian influenza A (H5N1) in 10 patients in Vietnam. N Engl J Med 350: 1179–1188.
2. Parry J (2013) H7N9 avian flu kills seven and infects 23 in China. BMJ 346:f2222.
3. Number of confirmed human cases of avian influenza A (H7N9) reported to WHO. Geneva: World Health Organization, May 2013. Available: http://www.who.int/influenza/human_animal_interface/influenza_ih7n9/05_Report-WebH7N9Number.pdf. Accessed 2013 June 3.
4. Gao HN, Lu HZ, Cao B, Du B, Shang H, et al. (2013) Clinical findings in 111 cases of influenza A (H7N9) virus infection. N Engl J Med 368: 2277–2285.
5. Lu SH, Xi XH, Zheng YF, Cao Y, Liu XN, et al. (2013) Analysis of the clinical characteristics and treatment of two patients with avian influenza virus (H7N9). Biosci Trends 7: 109–112.
6. Chen Y, Liang W, Yang S, Wu N, Gao H, et al. (2013) Human infections with the emerging avian influenza A H7N9 virus from wet market poultry: clinical analysis and characterisation of viral genome. Lancet 381: 1916–1925.
7. Uyeki TM, Cox NJ (2013) Global concerns regarding novel influenza A (H7N9) virus infections. N Engl J Med 368: 1862–1864.
8. Wang Q, Zhang Z, Shi Y, Jiang Y (2013) Emerging H7N9 influenza A (novel reassortant avian-origin) pneumonia: Radiologic findings. Radiology 268:882–889.
9. Grieser C, Goldmann A, Steffen IG, Kastrup M, Fernandez CM, et al. (2012) Computed tomography findings from patients with ARDS due to Influenza A (H1N1) virus-associated pneumonia. Eur J Radiol 81: 389–394.
10. Chang YC, Yu CJ, Chang SC, Galvin JR, Liu HM, et al. (2005) Pulmonary sequelae in convalescent patients after severe acute respiratory syndrome: evaluation with thin-section CT. Radiology 236: 1067–1075.
11. Bautista E, Chotpitayasunondh T, Gao Z, Harper SA, Shaw M, et al. (2010) Clinical aspects of pandemic 2009 influenza A (H1N1) virus infection. N Engl J Med 362: 1708–1719.
12. Kim EA, Lee KS, Primack SL, Yoon HK, Byun HS, et al. (2002) Viral pneumonias in adults: radiologic and pathologic findings. Radiographics 22 Spec No: S137–S149.
13. Ko SF, Lee TY, Huang CC, Cheng YF, Ng SH, et al. (2004) Severe acute respiratory syndrome: prognostic implications of chest radiographic findings in 52 patients. Radiology 233: 173–181.
14. So LK, Lau AC, Yam LY, Cheung TM, Poon E, et al. (2003) Development of a standard treatment protocol for severe acute respiratory syndrome. Lancet 361: 1615–1617.
15. Gao R, Cao B, Hu Y, Feng Z, Wang D, et al. (2013) Human infection with a novel avian-origin influenza A (H7N9) virus. N Engl J Med 368: 1888–1897.
16. Grinblat L, Shulman H, Glickman A, Matukas L, Paul N (2003) Severe acute respiratory syndrome: radiographic review of 40 probable cases in Toronto, Canada. Radiology 228: 802–809.
17. Marchiori E, Zanetti G, D'Ippolito G, Verrastro CG, Meirelles GS, et al. (2011) Swine-origin influenza A (H1N1) viral infection: thoracic findings on CT. AJR Am J Roentgenol 196: W723–W728.
18. Marchiori E, Zanetti G, Fontes CA, Santos ML, Valiante PM, et al. (2011) Influenza A (H1N1) virus-associated pneumonia: high-resolution computed tomography-pathologic correlation. Eur J Radiol 80: e500–e504.
19. Marchiori E, Zanetti G, Hochhegger B, Rodrigues RS, Fontes CA, et al. (2010) High-resolution computed tomography findings from adult patients with Influenza A (H1N1) virus-associated pneumonia. Eur J Radiol 74: 93–98.
20. Bay A, Etlik O, Oner AF, Unal O, Arslan H, et al. (2007) Radiological and clinical course of pneumonia in patients with avian influenza H5N1. Eur J Radiol 61: 245–250.
21. Li P, Su DJ, Zhang JF, Xia XD, Sui H, et al. (2011) Pneumonia in novel swine-origin influenza A (H1N1) virus infection: high-resolution CT findings. Eur J Radiol 80: e146–e152.
22. Franquet T (2011) Imaging of pulmonary viral pneumonia. Radiology 260: 18–39.
23. Qureshi NR, Hien TT, Farrar J, Gleeson FV (2006) The radiologic manifestations of H5N1 avian influenza. J Thorac Imaging 21: 259–264.

Retrospective Cohort Analysis of Chest Injury Characteristics and Concurrent Injuries

Xi Zheng[9], **Yang Hu**[9], **Yong Yuan**, **Yong-Fan Zhao***

Department of Thoracic Surgery, West China Hospital, Sichuan University, Chengdu, Sichuan Province, China

Abstract

Background: The aim of this study was to compare retrospectively the characteristics of chest injuries and frequencies of other, concurrent injuries in patients after earthquakes of different seismic intensity.

Methods: We compared the cause, type, and body location of chest injuries as well as the frequencies of other, concurrent injuries in patients admitted to our hospital after the Wenchuan and Lushan earthquakes in Sichuan, China. We explored possible relationships between seismic intensity and the causes and types of injuries, and we assessed the ability of the Injury Severity Score, New Injury Severity Score, and Chest Injury Index to predict respiratory failure in chest injury patients.

Results: The incidence of chest injuries was 9.9% in the stronger Wenchuan earthquake and 22.2% in the less intensive Lushan earthquake. The most frequent cause of chest injuries in both earthquakes was being accidentally struck. Injuries due to falls were less prevalent in the stronger Wenchuan earthquake, while injuries due to burial were more prevalent. The distribution of types of chest injury did not vary significantly between the two earthquakes, with rib fractures and pulmonary contusions the most frequent types. Spinal and head injuries concurrent with chest injuries were more prevalent in the less violent Lushan earthquake. All three trauma scoring systems showed poor ability to predict respiratory failure in patients with earthquake-related chest injuries.

Conclusions: Previous studies may have underestimated the incidence of chest injury in violent earthquakes. The distributions of types of chest injury did not differ between these two earthquakes of different seismic intensity. Earthquake severity and interval between rescue and treatment may influence the prevalence and types of injuries that co-occur with the chest injury. Trauma evaluation scores on their own are inadequate predictors of respiratory failure in patients with earthquake-related chest injuries.

Editor: Qinghua Sun, The Ohio State University, United States of America

Funding: The authors have no support or funding to report.

Competing Interests: The authors have declared that no competing interests exist.

* E-mail: doctorzhaoyongfan@hotmail.com

[9] These authors contributed equally to this work.

Introduction

In 2008, the devastating Wenchuan earthquake hit China's Sichuan province and led to 69,181 deaths, 18,522 missing and 374,171 injured. Five years later, another violent earthquake hit Sichuan, this time in the Lushan area, leading to at least 196 deaths, 21 missing, and 11,470 injured. The Wenchuan earthquake was rated as 8.0 on the Richter scale, with a maximum intensity of XI on a seismic intensity scale of I–XII defined by the Chinese State Bureau of Quality and Technical Supervision. The Lushan earthquake was rated as 7.0 on the Richter scale with a maximum intensity of IX. Both earthquakes occurred in geologically and demographically similar areas, providing an unusual opportunity to compare the prevalence and types of casualties in two earthquakes differing primarily in seismic intensity.

Previous studies have reported that chest injuries account for only a small proportion of all earthquake-related injuries, and that most patients with chest injuries present with other, concurrent types of injuries that can significantly affect clinical outcomes [1–3]. These studies have not, however, addressed the question of whether the characteristics of chest injuries or co-occurring injuries vary with earthquake intensity. Addressing this question ideally requires examining two earthquakes that differ in intensity but that affect similar geologic areas with similar types of populations and distributions, and in which the casualties were treated at similar medical facilities. West China Hospital of Sichuan University is roughly equidistant from the epicenters of both earthquakes and was unaffected; it provided medical treatment to more trauma patients in both disasters than other hospitals, altogether 4,092 patients in the Wenchuan earthquake and 400 in the Lushan earthquake. Thus the data collected at West China Hospital on patients treated in both earthquakes provide a unique opportunity to examine the effects of seismic intensity on injury characteristics. Such comparisons may help predict the types of injuries likely to occur in earthquakes of given severity and help administrators allocate limited medical resources appropriately.

We also hoped to take advantage of our data set from two earthquakes in order to verify the efficacy of three types of trauma scoring systems for predicting respiratory failure in patients with chest injuries, all based on the the Abbreviated Injury Scale 2005 (AIS2005): the Injury Severity Score (ISS), the New Injury Severity Score (NISS) and the Chest Injury Index (CII). Our analysis of patients in the Wenchuan earthquake suggested that NISS was superior to the other indices [1,4], so we wished to verify that finding using data from the Lushan earthquake.

Materials and Methods

The Institutional Review Board of West China Hospital approved the protocol for this retrospective study before it was undertaken; informed consent from participants was ruled unnecessary because we retrospectively analyzed data routinely collected from all inpatients and we analyzed the data anonymously.

Patients from earthquake-affected areas were transported either directly by helicopter from the scene to West China Hospital, or by car or helicopter from field hospitals. All patients admitted to our hospital with possible chest disorders were examined by two thoracic surgeons. Diagnosis of chest injury was made based on physical examination, chest X-ray, computed tomography (CT), fibrobronchoscopy or diagnostic pleuracentesis. All patients with chest injuries were included in our study. Since injuries of the thoracic vertebrae, scapula, and clavicle were treated by orthopedic surgeons, patients with only these injuries but no concurrent chest injury were excluded from our study. Simple contusion of the chest wall and injuries unrelated to the earthquakes, such as spontaneous pneumothorax, were also excluded.

Several items of information were collected from all patients after admission, including age, sex, location where the injury occurred, whether the injury occurred during the primary shock or during aftershocks, the cause and type of injury, diagnosis, duration of mechanical ventilation, and treatment outcome (recovery, deterioration or death). The procedures used to collect these data and update them after the Wenchuan earthquake have been described [4]; the data from patients in the Lushan earthquake were up-dated through 20 July 2013.

Causes of injuries were categorized based on previous studies of earthquakes and reports from the U.S. Centers for Disease Control and Prevention [5]: injuries due to falls, being buried, or being accidentally struck, or other injuries, such as burns, cuts, motor vehicle crashes, and delayed effects of injuries. The cause of injury of patients with multiple injuries were classified based on the cause of the clinically most important injury; for example, patients with multiple injuries due primarily to prolonged burial were classified as having injury due to burial.

In order to estimate the seismic intensity experienced by patients at the time of injury, we used Richter scale data and intensity distribution maps of both earthquakes generated based on Xu et al. [6] and data from the China Earthquake Networks Center. Seismic intensity assesses the intensity of ground shaking and consequences of an earthquake. Seismic intensity usually weakens with increasing distance from the epicenter, except for certain locations where this relationship does not hold. The locations where patients sustained injuries were located on this map and used to explore possible relationships between seismic intensity and the causes and types of injuries. We included in this analysis only patients for whom we obtained reliable information about where they had sustained their injuries.

Chest injuries were assessed using the ISS, NISS, and CII scales as described [4]. Patients who were mechanically ventilated for more than 24 h, either invasively or noninvasively, were diagnosed with respiratory failure.

Data on causes and types of injury in patients from both earthquakes were analyzed using SPSS 17.0 (IBM, Chicago, IL). Differences in continuous variables between patients from the two earthquakes were assessed for statistical significance using Student's t test or the Mann-Whitney U test. Differences in dichotomous variables were analyzed using the chi-squared test or Fisher's exact test. In order to compare the accuracy with which ISS, NISS and CII predict respiratory failure, we calculated receiver operating characteristics (ROC) curves and cut-off values using Medcalc 11.4.2.0 software. A two-sided $p<0.05$ was considered significant.

Results

In the Wenchuan earthquake, 1,856 patients were admitted to West China Hospital, and 184 (9.9%) were diagnosed with chest injuries [4,7]. All these patients were admitted after the primary shock; unfortunately patient data were not collected in the wake of the aftershocks. After excluding one woman diagnosed with spontaneous diaphragmatic hernia, we retained 183 in the final analysis. Of these, 165 (90.16%) showed improved and were discharged from our hospital within two months after the quake. A total of 28 patients (15.3%) were diagnosed with chest injuries without concurrent injuries. Thoracic surgical procedures, including closed thoracic drainage, were performed in 69 patients (37.7%). Six of the 183 (3.28%) died, accounting for 18.18% of all the 33 deaths in our hospital in the Wenchuan earthquake [7]. In the Lushan earthquake, 81 of 325 inpatients (24.9%) were diagnosed with chest injuries. Of these, we excluded 7 patients whose injuries were not earthquake-related and 2 patients with simple contusion of the chest wall, leaving 72 patients (22.2%) in the final analysis. None of the patients in our cohort presented with chest injuries exclusively; all had at least one additional injury on admission. Of the total 72 chest injury patients, 67 were injured during the primary shock, and 5 during aftershocks. By 20 July 2013, 60 (83.3%) had shown improvement and had been discharged from our hospital. By this date, no deaths among the patients admitted to our hospital were declared after the earthquake. A total of 15 patients (20.83%) received thoracic surgical procedures.

The trauma patients from both earthquakes had a similar age ($p = 0.316$) and gender composition ($p = 0.397$). We categorized each patient by his or her principal type of injury, and found that the frequencies of most types of injury differed significantly between the two earthquakes (Table 1). The frequency of "other" injuries could not be compared because of inadequate sample size. Injuries due to being accidentally struck were among the most frequent injuries in both earthquakes; other frequent causes of injury were being buried (Wenchuan) or falling (Lushan).

Among patients with chest injuries in both earthquakes, the most frequent diagnoses were rib fractures and pulmonary contusions (Table 2). Rib fracture was more frequent in the Wenchuan earthquake, while pulmonary contusion predominated

Table 1. Comparison of the causes of chest injury in patients admitted to our hospital in the Wenchuan and Lushan earthquakes.

Cause of injury[a]	Wenchuan, n (%)	Lushan, n (%)	p*
Being buried	21 (11.5)	1 (1.4)	0.010
Being accidentally struck	143 (78.1)	39 (54.2)	<0.001
Falling	18 (9.8)	30 (41.7)	<0.001
Other	1 (0.5)	2 (2.8)	0.193

[a]Patients with injuries reflecting multiple causes were classified according to the cause of their principal injury.
*Based on the Pearson chi-squared test or Fisher's exact test.

in the Lushan disaster. The frequencies of hemothorax, pneumothorax and sternum fracture differed significantly between the two earthquakes.

Injuries co-occurring with chest injuries were classified into 1 of 6 regions and compared between the two earthquakes (Table 3). Patients with chest injuries presented with concurrent head and spine injuries more often in the Lushan earthquake than in the Wenchuan earthquake.

Next we explored whether chest injury frequency and characteristics were associated with earthquake severity based on data from both earthquakes. We could perform this analysis on only 177 patients because we did not have reliable information about where other patients sustained their injuries. Given this limited sample size, and given the fact that structures in the areas affected by both earthquakes were built to withstand earthquakes up to an intensity of VII (Ministry of Housing and Urban-Rural Development of the People's Republic of China, code of aseismic design of buildings), we divided seismic intensities into two categories, IV–VII and VIII–XI. Types of injury varied with seismic intensity (Table 4): the frequency of being unintentionally struck increased with greater intensity, whereas the frequency of falling decreased. In contrast, the frequencies of different types of chest injury were similar for the two intensity categories (Table 5).

In the Wenchuan earthquake, 38 inpatients with chest injuries (20.7%) suffered from respiratory failure [4]. In the Lushan disaster, 18 of the 72 inpatients with chest injuries (25.0%) developed respiratory failure. Building on our previous work assessing the ability of the ISS, NISS and CII scales to predict respiratory failure in chest injury patients in the Wenchuan earthquake, we performed the same analysis on Lushan patients. We calculated the area under ROC curves and estimated 95% confidence intervals (95%CI) for all scales (Figure 1 and Table 6). Although NISS was significantly more accurate than the two other scales in our analysis of Wenchuan chest injury patients [4], all three scales performed similarly poorly for Lushan chest injury patients.

Discussion

Earthquakes are major geological disasters that cause tremendous human and economic losses around the world [8,9]. However, relatively little is known about how earthquake factors such as seismic intensity affect the prevalence and types of casualties. Here we examine the prevalence and causes of different types of chest injury between the more violent Wenchuan earthquake and less violent Lushan earthquake, which affected similar regions of Sichuan province. Our analysis suggests that chest injuries occur more frequently in earthquake victims than previously thought, and that seismic intensity affects causes of chest injury. On the other hand, seismic intensity may not affect types of chest injury. These results may help emergency response centers predict the kinds of patients that they will need to treat and thereby lead to more rational allocation of limited medical resources.

The fact that our hospital was the major provider of medical services to patients in both the Wenchuan and Lushan

Table 2. Comparison of the prevalence of types of chest injury among patients admitted to our hospital in the Wenchuan and Lushan earthquakes.

Chest injury type	Wenchuan, n (%)	Lushan, n (%)	p*
Rib fracture	161 (88.0)	39 (54.2)	<0.001
Pulmonary contusion	117 (63.9)	57 (79.2)	0.019
Hemopneumothorax	39 (21.3)	9 (12.5)	0.105
Hemothorax	33 (18.0)	1 (1.4)	<0.001
Pneumothorax	19 (10.4)	2 (2.8)	0.047
Fracture of sternum	4 (2.2)	7 (9.7)	0.020
Diaphragmatic hernia	2 (1.1)	0 (0.0)	1.000
Thoracic duct injury	1 (0.5)	0 (0.0)	1.000
Traumatic asphyxia	1 (0.5)	0 (0.0)	1.000
Mediastinal emphysema	0 (0.0)	2 (2.8)	0.079
Mediastinal effusion	0 (0.0)	1 (1.4)	0.282

*Based on the Pearson chi-squared test, continuity-corrected chi-squared test or Fisher's exact test.

Table 3. Comparison of the prevalence and types of injuries co-occurring with chest injury in patients admitted to our hospital after the Wenchuan and Lushan earthquakes.

Concurrent injury type[a]	Wenchuan, n (%)	Lushan, n (%)	p*
Brain and skull	33 (18.0)	23 (31.9)	0.016
Face and neck	8 (4.4)	5 (6.9)	0.600
Abdomen	19 (10.4)	13 (18.1)	0.096
Spine and spinal cord	51 (27.9)	39 (54.2)	<0.001
Extremities[b]	113 (61.7)	35 (48.6)	0.056
External injuries	64 (35.0)	34 (47.2)	0.070

[a]Some patients contained concurrent injuries of multiple types; those patients therefore appear multiple times in the table.
[b]Extremities include the upper and lower limbs, clavicle, scapula, bony pelvis and hip.
*Based on the Pearson chi-squared test or continuity-corrected chi-squared test.

earthquakes gives us a unique opportunity to examine how seismic intensity may affect the prevalence and characteristics of different types of injuries. Normally such comparisons are difficult because the earthquakes being compared differ in numerous respects. In this case, however, both Lushan and Wenchuan counties have similar geologic features and are located at the Longmenshan Fault Zone [10]. Other factors known to affect earthquake losses, such as demographic structure, population density, outbreak time, architectural features and local medical infrastructure, are also similar between the two affected areas [11]. Our hospital is approximately equidistant (100 km) from both epicenters. Thus, the major difference between the two earthquakes in our analysis is seismic intensity, allowing us to draw conclusions about how this parameter may affect casualties admitted to hospital.

Chest injuries were diagnosed in 9.9% of the patients admitted to our hospital in the Wenchuan earthquake [4] and 22.2% in the Lushan earthquake. These incidences are consistent with reports suggesting a 10–15% incidence of chest injuries among trauma patients [12,13]. At the same time, most chest injuries in our patients were minor or moderate and resolved after conservative treatment, as reported in other major earthquakes [2,3,14]. The exception to this, both in our study and previous work, is severe chest injury, especially crushing injuries of the chest, which are associated with high mortality [15–18].

Contrary to our expectations, the incidence of chest injury was higher among patients in the less violent Lushan earthquake than in the more violent Wenchuan disaster, as was the incidence of crushing and other severe chest injuries. In fact, the incidence of chest injury in Lushan is higher than that reported in previous studies of chest injuries in several major earthquakes [1,3,19–21]. We speculate that all these findings reflect the fact that major transportation networks were more severely disrupted in the Wenchuan disaster, significantly delaying the arrival of patients at our hospital and leading to a larger number of pre-admission deaths due to severe chest trauma. In the Lushan earthquake, in contrast, most transportation networks remained open, facilitating prompt rescue and delivery to our hospital. Therefore we suspect that the data on severe chest injury in our Lushan cohort more accurately reflect what happens in a major earthquake. Previous studies of severe chest injury and other types of severe injury in earthquakes should be interpreted with caution given the risk of underestimating prevalence as a result of missing individuals and pre-admission deaths. Our findings further suggest that prompt rescue and medical attention after destructive earthquakes may save the lives of many patients with severe chest injuries.

Our comparison of the two earthquakes identified several other informative differences. While injuries due to being accidentally struck were the most common type of injury in both earthquakes, injuries due to falls were more frequent in the less intense Lushan earthquake, while injuries due to being buried were more frequent in the more intense Wenchuan disaster. These results can be attributed to seismic intensity since more intense earthquakes like the Wenchuan disaster involve more extensive structural damage, leading to building collapse and increasing the risk of burial. In less intense earthquakes such as Lushan, fewer buildings collapse, so a greater proportion of injuries are due to falls. Only 4 aftershocks at >5.0 on the Richter scale were recorded in the Lushan earthquake, and all were nondestructive. This may explain why only 5 patients in our Lushan cohort (6.9% of the total admitted) were injured during aftershocks; most of these injuries were due to falling or being accidentally struck. These individuals may have been engaging in unsafe behaviors during the disaster, perhaps as

Table 4. Relationships between seismic intensity and cause of injury in patients admitted to our hospital after the Wenchuan and Lushan earthquakes.

Cause of injury, n (%)	Seismic intensity		p*
	IV–VII	VIII–XI	
Being buried	3 (4.1)	6 (5.8)	<0.001
Being accidentally struck	38 (51.4)	86 (83.5)	
Falling	31 (41.9)	10 (9.7)	
Other	2 (2.7)	1 (1.0)	

*Based on the likelihood ratio of the chi-squared test.

Table 5. Relationships between seismic intensity and the prevalence of types of chest injury in patients admitted to our hospital after the Wenchuan and Lushan earthquakes.

Chest injury type, n (%)[a]	Seismic intensity		p*
	IV–VII	VIII–XI	
Rib fracture	52 (39.1)	86 (46.2)	0.267
Pulmonary contusion	55 (41.4)	61 (32.8)	
Hemopneumothorax	11 (8.3)	21 (11.3)	
Hemothorax	4 (3.0)	4 (2.2)	
Pneumothorax	5 (3.8)	11 (5.9)	
Fracture of sternum	6 (4.5)	3 (1.6)	

[a]Some patients suffered from more than one type of chest injury and therefore appear multiple times in this table. One patient with diaphragmatic hernia, one with thoracic duct injury, two with mediastinal emphysema and one with mediatinal effusion were not included in the analysis.
*Based on the likelihood ratio chi-squared test.

a result of psychological or physical trauma after the primary shocks [22].

Our findings lead us to recommend the deployment of emergency responders trained in dealing with such critical conditions as crush syndrome, severe infection and brain injuries in the wake of violent earthquakes, where the risk of burial-related injuries is high. In less intense earthquakes, rapid response of psychologists may be particularly important for preventing avoidable injuries due to shock and disorientation.

The most frequent types of chest injury in both earthquakes were rib fractures and pulmonary contusions, similar to the causes of chest injuries in other medical emergencies [23]. Comparing the two earthquakes showed that greater seismic intensity was associated with greater prevalence of rib fractures but lower prevalence of pulmonary contusion. Greater intensity was also associated with higher frequencies of severe injuries like hemothorax and pneumothorax. These findings should be interpreted with caution given the limited sample size, due to lack of reliable data on where most patients sustained their injuries within the earthquake-affected areas. In fact, combining the results of Tables 2 and 5 suggests that seismic intensity may not affect the overall distribution of chest injury types. However, this analysis is based on a crude stratification of intensities into only two categories. Future work should involve many more patients and more detailed stratification of intensity. Despite these limitations, the data suggest that greater proportions of patients in more violent earthquakes may require closed drainage of the pleural cavity. Our lack of statistical power prevents us from drawing any conclusions about a possible relationship between seismic intensity and rare injuries such as diaphragmatic hernia and thoracic duct injury.

In earthquakes, patients presenting only with chest injury are rare; most chest injuries occur simultaneously with other types of injury [1,3]. Similarly we found that 84.7% of Wenchuan chest injury patients and all Lushan chest injury patients presented concurrently with other types of injury. Since injuries that occur together with chest injuries can affect patient outcomes, we compared the prevalence and types of such concurrent injuries between the two earthquakes. In both disasters, injuries of the face, neck and abdomen were uncommon, and external injuries were frequent but usually mild (Table 3). More than 50% of Wenchuan patients admitted to our hospital [7] and more than 70% of Lushan patients were treated in the orthopedic department, similar to what has been reported in other earthquakes [24]. Injuries of the spine and extremities were the most frequent injuries concurrent with chest injuries. We were surprised to find that the prevalence of concurrent injuries affecting the brain, skull, spine or spinal cord was higher in the less violent Lushan earthquake. Again, the explanation may reflect the fact that many patients with severe injuries of the brain and spinal cord die rapidly, so a greater proportion of such patients in the Wenchuan earthquake may have died before they could be rescued and transported to our hospital. Therefore we recommend the deployment of adequate numbers of orthopedic and neurological specialists to attend to patients with chest injuries in violent earthquakes.

Accurately predicting which earthquake casualties are likely to suffer respiratory failure would significantly aid in emergency triage and allocation of limited medical resources. The three injury

Table 6. Comparison of the ability of conventional injury severity scores to predict respiratory failure in patients admitted to our hospital from the Lushan earthquake.

Scoring system	Cut-off value	Sensitivity (%)	Specificity (%)	AUC	95%CI
ISS	14	100.0	40.7	0.713[a]	0.594–0.813
NISS	28	55.6	81.5	0.720	0.601–0.819
CII	18	44.4	75.9	0.590[b]	0.468–0.705

Abbreviations: AUC, area under the ROC curve; CII, chest injury index; ISS, injury severity score; NISS, new injury severity score; 95%CI, 95% confidence interval.
[a]NISS vs. ISS, $p = 0.880$.
[b]NISS vs. CII, $p = 0.136$.

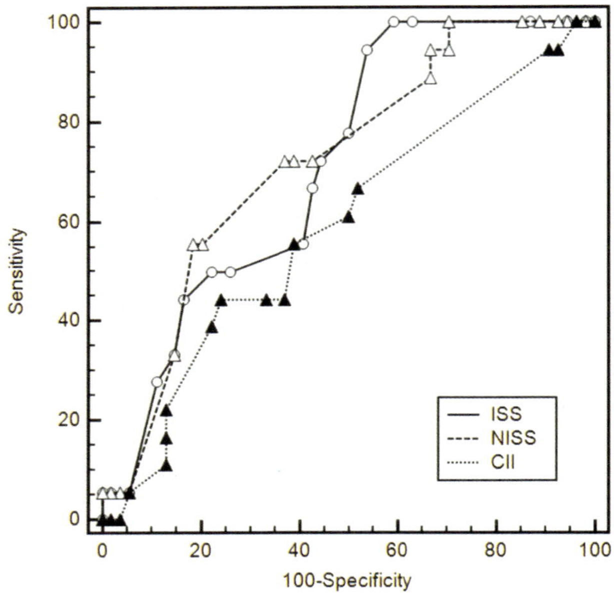

Figure 1. Receiver operating characteristic (ROC) curves of different trauma scoring systems for predicting respiratory failure in patients admitted to our hospital in the Lushan earthquake. The solid line indicates the ROC curve for the Injury Severity Score (ISS); the dashed line, the curve for the New Injury Severity Score (NISS); and the dotted line, the curve for the Chest Injury Index (CII) [4].

scales ISS, NISS, and CII, all based on the AIS2005 scale, are widely used to predict survival in disasters, and we recently applied them to the prediction of respiratory failure among Wenchuan chest injury patients [4]. Our results in that study suggested that the NISS was superior to the other scales. When we examined the Lushan cohort, however, all three scales showed unsatisfactory AUC values ranging from 0.590–0.720, compared to values of 0.837–0.893 in the Wenchuan earthquake [4]. While the high sensitivity of ISS may make it useful as a screening method, NISS and CII show poor sensitivity and moderate specificity, limiting their diagnostic usefulness. The AIS2005 scale assesses only injury severity, regardless of how long the patient has had the injury and what treatments have been administered [25]. Nevertheless, clinicians often use it to predict trauma progression [1,26–28], even though many factors other than injury severity affect such progression. In earthquake-related trauma in particular, factors such as pre-admission treatments, the delay between injury and treatment, and the presence of comorbidities may also affect trauma progression. All these factors may therefore influence the risk of respiratory failure, so we recommend combining conventional injury severity scales with more comprehensive trauma assessment in order to predict respiratory failure in chest injury patients.

Our analysis of patients admitted to our hospital in the Wenchuan and Lushan earthquakes leads us to several conclusions. Previous studies may have underestimated the true incidence of chest injuries in violent earthquakes, and these injuries most frequently involve rib fractures or pulmonary contusions due to being accidentally struck. Greater seismic intensity is associated with lower prevalence of injuries due to falling and higher prevalence of injuries due to being buried. However, seismic intensity does not appear to affect the prevalence and types of chest injury. Earthquake-related chest injuries usually occur together with other injuries, most frequently with orthopedic injuries. The prevalence and types of concurrent injuries may be affected by the delay between rescue and treatment as well as the severity of the earthquake. Injury severity scales by themselves are inadequate for predicting respiratory failure in chest injury patients in earthquakes; more factors should be taken into account when evaluating such trauma.

Acknowledgments

We thank the public relations department of West China Hospital for help in acquiring data. We would also like to express our gratitude to all doctors and nurses who were involved in rescue work in the two earthquakes.

Author Contributions

Conceived and designed the experiments: YFZ YH XZ YY. Performed the experiments: XZ YH YY. Analyzed the data: YH XZ YY YFZ. Contributed reagents/materials/analysis tools: XZ YY. Wrote the paper: YH XZ. Revised the manuscript according to the comments of reviewers: XZ YH YY.

References

1. Toker A, Isitmangil T, Erdik O, Sancakli I, Sebit S (2002) Analysis of chest injuries sustained during the 1999 Marmara earthquake. Surg Today 32: 769–771.
2. Hu J, Guo YQ, Zhang EY, Tan J, Shi YK (2010) Chest injuries associated with earthquakes: an analysis of injuries sustained during the 2008 Wen-Chuan earthquake in China. Surg Today 40: 729–733. doi:10.1007/s00595-009-4130-6.
3. Sato K, Kobayashi M, Ishibashi S, Ueda S, Suzuki S (2013) Chest injuries and the 2011 Great East Japan Earthquake. Respir Investig 51: 24–27. doi:10.1016/j.resinv.2012.11.002.
4. Hu Y, Tang Y, Yuan Y, Xie TP, Zhao YF (2010) Trauma evaluation of patients with chest injury in the 2008 earthquake of Wenchuan, Sechuan, China. World J Surg 34: 728–732. doi:10.1007/s00268-010-0427-2.
5. LeMier M, Cummings P, West TA (2001) Accuracy of external cause of injury codes reported in Washington State hospital discharge records. Inj Prev 7: 334–338.
6. Xu C, Xu X, Zhou B, Yu G (2013) Revisions of the M 8.0 Wenchuan earthquake seismic intensity map based on co-seismic landslide abundance. Nat Hazards: 1–18. doi:10.1007/s11069-013-0757-0.
7. Xie J, Du L, Xia T, Wang M, Diao X, et al. (2008) Analysis of 1856 inpatients and 33 deaths in the West China Hospital of Sichuan University from the Wenchuan earthquake. J Evid Based Med 1: 20–26. doi:10.1111/j.1756-5391.2008.00010.x.
8. Doocy S, Daniels A, Packer C, Dick A, Kirsch TD (2013) The human impact of earthquakes: a historical review of events 1980–2009 and systematic literature review. PLoS Curr 5. Available: http://www.ncbi.nlm.nih.gov/pmc/articles/PMC3644288/. Accessed 8 January 2014. doi:10.1371/currents.dis.67bd14fe457f1db0b5433a8ee20fb833.
9. Ratnapradipa D, Conder J, Ruffing A, White V (2012) The 2011 Japanese earthquake: an overview of environmental health impacts. J Environ Health 74: 42–50.
10. Zheng Y, Ge C, Xie Z, Yang Y, Xiong X, et al. (2013) Crustal and upper mantle structure and the deep seismogenic environment in the source regions of the Lushan earthquake and the Wenchuan earthquake. Sci China Earth Sci 56: 1158–1168. doi:10.1007/s11430-013-4641-2.
11. Whitman RV, Anagnos T, Kircher CA, Lagorio HJ, Lawson RS, et al. (1997) Development of a National Earthquake Loss Estimation Methodology. Earthquake Spectra 13: 643–661. doi:http://dx.doi.org/10.1193/1.1585973.
12. Al-Koudmani I, Darwish B, Al-Kateb K, Taifour Y (2012) Chest trauma experience over eleven-year period at al-mouassat university teaching hospital-Damascus: a retrospective review of 888 cases. J Cardiothorac Surg 7: 35.

13. LoCicero J 3rd, Mattox KL (1989) Epidemiology of chest trauma. Surg Clin North Am 69: 15–19.
14. Yoshimura N, Nakayama S, Nakagiri K, Azami T, Ataka K, et al. (1996) Profile of chest injuries arising from the 1995 southern Hyogo Prefecture earthquake. Chest 110: 759–761. doi:10.1378/chest.110.3.759.
15. Gaillard M, Herve C, Mandin L, Raynaud P (1990) Mortality prognostic factors in chest injury. J Trauma 30: 93–96.
16. Demirhan R, Onan B, Oz K, Halezeroglu S (2009) Comprehensive analysis of 4205 patients with chest trauma: a 10-year experience. Interact Cardiovasc Thorac Surg 9: 450–453. doi:10.1510/icvts.2009.206599.
17. Conn JH, Hardy JD, Fain WR, Netterville RE (1963) Thoracic trauma: analysis of 1022 cases. J Trauma 3: 22–40.
18. Shorr RM, Crittenden M, Indeck M, Hartunian SL, Rodriguez A (1987) Blunt thoracic trauma. Analysis of 515 patients. Ann Surg 206: 200–205.
19. Yi-Szu W, Chung-Ping H, Tzu-Chieh L, Dar-Yu Y, Tain-Cheng W (2000) Chest injuries transferred to trauma centers after the 1999 Taiwan earthquake. Am J Emerg Med 18: 825–827. doi:10.1053/ajem.2000.18132.
20. Ghodsi SM, Zargar M, Khaji A, Karbakhsh M (2005) Chest injury in victims of Bam earthquake. Chin J Traumatol 9: 345–348.
21. Ozdogan S, Hocaoglu A, Caglayan B, Imamoglu OU, Aydin D (2001) Thorax and lung injuries arising from the two earthquakes in Turkey in 1999. Chest 120: 1163–1166. doi:10.1590/S1807-59322011000500013.
22. Honma M, Endo N, Osada Y, Kim Y, Kuriyama K (2012) Disturbances in equilibrium function after major earthquake. Sci Rep 2: 749. doi:10.1038/srep00749.
23. Veysi VT, Nikolaou VS, Paliobeis C, Efstathopoulos N, Giannoudis PV (2009) Prevalence of chest trauma, associated injuries and mortality: a level I trauma centre experience. Int Orthop 33: 1425–1433. doi:10.1007/s00264-009-0746-9.
24. Mulvey JM, Awan SU, Qadri AA, Maqsood MA (2008) Profile of injuries arising from the 2005 Kashmir earthquake: the first 72 h. Injury 39: 554–560. doi:10.1016/j.injury.2007.07.025.
25. Baker SP, O'Neill B, Haddon W Jr, Long WB (1974) The injury severity score: a method for describing patients with multiple injuries and evaluating emergency care. J Trauma 14: 187–196.
26. Osler T, Baker SP, Long W (1997) A modification of the injury severity score that both improves accuracy and simplifies scoring. J Trauma 43: 922–925; discussion 925–926.
27. Kimura A, Chadbunchachai W, Nakahara S (2012) Modification of the Trauma and Injury Severity Score (TRISS) method provides better survival prediction in Asian blunt trauma victims. World J Surg 36: 813–818. doi:10.1007/s00268-012-1498-z.
28. Liman ST, Kuzucu A, Tastepe AI, Ulasan GN, Topcu S (2003) Chest injury due to blunt trauma. Eur J Cardiothorac Surg 23: 374–378. doi:10.1016/s1010-7940(02)00813-8.

18

Epidemiology and Outcome of Severe Sepsis and Septic Shock

Jianfang Zhou[1], Chuanyun Qian[2], Mingyan Zhao[3], Xiangyou Yu[4], Yan Kang[5], Xiaochun Ma[6], Yuhang Ai[7], Yuan Xu[8], Dexin Liu[9], Youzhong An[10], Dawei Wu[11], Renhua Sun[12], Shusheng Li[13], Zhenjie Hu[14], Xiangyuan Cao[15], Fachun Zhou[16], Li Jiang[17], Jiandong Lin[18], Enqiang Mao[19], Tiehe Qin[20], Zhenyang He[21], Lihua Zhou[22], Bin Du[1]*, for the China Critical Care Clinical Trials Group (CCCCTG)

1 Medical ICU, Peking Union Medical College Hospital, Peking Union Medical College & Chinese Academy of Medical Sciences, Beijing, China, **2** Department of Emergency Medicine and Medical ICU, The First Affiliated Hospital of Kunming Medical University, Kunming, China, **3** Department of Critical Care Medicine, The First Affiliated Hospital of Harbin Medical University, Harbin, China, **4** Department of Critical Care Medicine, First Affiliated Hospital, Xinjiang Medical University, Urumqi, China, **5** Department of Critical Care Medicine, West China Hospital, Sichuan University, Chengdu, China, **6** Department of Critical Care Medicine, The First Affiliated Hospital of China Medical University, Shenyang, China, **7** Department of Critical Care Medicine, Xiangya Hospital, Central South University, Changsha, China, **8** Department of Critical Care Medicine, Beijing Tongren Hospital, Capital Medical University, Beijing, China, **9** Department of Critical Care Medicine, The Second Hospital of Jilin University, Changchun, China, **10** Department of Critical Care Medicine, Peking University People's Hospital, Beijing, China, **11** Department of Critical Care Medicine, Qilu Hospital of Shandong University, Jinan, China, **12** Department of Critical Care Medicine, Zhejiang Provincial People's Hospital, Hangzhou, China, **13** Department of Critical Care Medicine, Tongji Hospital of Tongji Medical College, Huazhong University of Science & Technology, Wuhan, China, **14** Department of Critical Care Medicine, Hebei Medical University Fourth Hospital, Shijiazhuang, China, **15** Department of Critical Care Medicine, General Hospital of Ningxia Medical University, Yinchuan, China, **16** Department of Emergency and Intensive Care Medicine, The First Affiliated Hospital of Chongqing Medical University, Chongqing, China, **17** Department of Critical Care Medicine, Fuxing Hospital, Capital Medical University, Beijing, China, **18** Department of Critical Care Medicine, The First Affiliated Hospital of Fujian Medical University, Fuzhou, China, **19** Emergency ICU, Ruijin Hospital, Shanghai Jiao Tong University, Shanghai, China, **20** Department of Critical Care Medicine, Guangdong General Hospital, Guangzhou, China, **21** Department of Critical Care Medicine, Hainan Provincial People's Hospital, Haikou, China, **22** Department of Critical Care Medicine, The Affiliated Hospital of Inner Mongolia Medical University, Huhhot, China

Abstract

Introduction: Information about sepsis in mainland China remains scarce and incomplete. The purpose of this study was to describe the epidemiology and outcome of severe sepsis and septic shock in mixed ICU in mainland China, as well as the independent predictors of mortality.

Methods: We performed a 2-month prospective, observational cohort study in 22 closed multi-disciplinary intensive care units (ICUs). All admissions into those ICUs during the study period were screened and patients with severe sepsis or septic shock were included.

Results: A total of 484 patients, 37.3 per 100 ICU admissions were diagnosed with severe sepsis (n = 365) or septic shock (n = 119) according to clinical criteria and included into this study. The most frequent sites of infection were the lung and abdomen. The overall ICU and hospital mortality rates were 28.7% (n = 139) and 33.5% (n = 162), respectively. In multivariate analyses, APACHE II score (odds ratio[OR], 1.068; 95% confidential interval[CI], 1.027–1.109), presence of ARDS (OR, 2.676; 95%CI, 1.691–4.235), bloodstream infection (OR, 2.520; 95%CI, 1.142–5.564) and comorbidity of cancer (OR, 2.246; 95%CI, 1.141–4.420) were significantly associated with mortality.

Conclusions: Our results indicated that severe sepsis and septic shock were common complications in ICU patients and with high mortality in China, and can be of help to know more about severe sepsis and septic shock in China and to improve characterization and risk stratification in these patients.

Editor: Jorge I. F. Salluh, D'or Institute of Research and Education, Brazil

Funding: This research was supported in part, by the Capital Clinical Application Research grant (Number: Z131107002213112) from the Science and Technology Commission of Beijing, and the funders had no role in study design, data collection and analysis, decision to publish, or preparation of the manuscript.

Competing Interests: The authors have declared that no competing interests exist.

* Email: dubin98@gmail.com

Introduction

Severe sepsis and septic shock are among the main factors contributing to mortality in intensive care units (ICUs), and exhibit a significant disease burden and negative economic impact [1–3].

The incidence of sepsis varies among different racial and ethnic groups [4–7]. Between 6 and 54% of patients admitted to ICUs have severe sepsis [2,3,6,8–10], and the mortality rate for these patients varies from 20 to 60% [6,10–12], which will increase stepwise with increasing disease severity [13]. Although the mortality rate may have decreased in recent years [5,7], the incidence of severe sepsis and septic shock is increasing, so that overall deaths are increasing [2,4,7]. Even death has been avoided, the patient who survives sepsis would have a significantly compromised long-term health-related quality of life than general population [1,14].

There have been a number of studies describing the epidemiology, risk factor and outcome of severe sepsis and septic shock in different countries [2,4,7,10,11]. Yet, information about sepsis in mainland China remains scarce and incomplete. Cheng et al [3] have described the epidemiology of severe sepsis in surgical ICUs, but data concerning the epidemiology of severe sepsis/septic shock in mixed ICUs are limited. So the China Critical Care Clinical Trials Group (CCCCTG) conducted an inception cohort study to investigate the epidemiology and outcome of severe sepsis and septic shock in mixed ICUs in China.

Patients and Methods

Study development

This was a secondary analysis of a prospective cohort study aiming to describe the demographics, case mix, interventions, and clinical outcome of critically ill patients admitted to ICUs in Mainland China and performed from 1 July 2009 to 31 August 2009 in 22 ICUs [15], so the data in the current study were collected prospectively but the analysis was done retrospectively. The participating ICUs were members of the CCCCTG and located in different provinces of China. The detailed characteristics of those ICUs, such as number of ICU beds, types of ICU, number of intensivists and nurses, and number of admissions in 2009 are showed in table 1. This study was approved by the institutional review board of Fuxing hospital (Number: 2009FXHEC-KY032), and the need for informed consent was waived. The ethical approval of Fuxing hospital was endorsed by the institutional review boards of all other participating centers (see the Appendix S1 for the full names and affiliation of participating hospitals) before data collection.

We used a case report form (CRF) to collect data. Every participating ICU nominated a study coordinator who was responsible for screening and enrollment of patients and data collection. The CCCCTG data monitoring team was responsible for auditing the integrity of data.

Selection of participants, data collection, and definitions

During the study period, all admissions of participating ICUs were screened for eligibility. Patients less than 15 years old or with an ICU length of stay (LOS) less than 24 hours were excluded. Patients with severe sepsis/septic shock at ICU admission or during ICU hospitalization were included in the study cohort, and only the first episode of severe sepsis or septic shock was counted. Patients readmitted into ICU during the same hospitalization were not screened again. The following information was recorded: demographic characteristics, admission category, comorbidities and preexisting organ insufficiency. The Acute Physiology and Chronic Health Evaluation (APACHE) II score [16] and Sequential Organ Failure Assessment (SOFA) score [17] on the first day of ICU were recorded to evaluate the severity of illness. Severe sepsis and septic shock were defined according to the American College of Chest Physicians/Society of Critical Care Medicine consensus conference definitions [18]. Acute respiratory distress syndrome (ARDS) were defined according to the American-European Consensus Conference criteria [19]. Acute kidney injury (AKI) was defined based on the Risk of renal dysfunction, Injury to the kidney, Failure of kidney function, Loss of kidney function and End-stage kidney disease(RIFLE) criteria [20]. Chronic organ failure and immunocompromise were diagnosed according to the criteria in APACHE II score. ICU-acquired infection was defined as the infection identified at least 48 hours after ICU admission, and ICU-acquired severe sepsis was defined as one occurring at least 48 hours following ICU admission. The reasons for ICU admission were based on disease categories of APACHE II scores.

Outcome measures

All enrolled patients were followed up till death in the hospital or hospital discharge or until November 30, 2009, whichever occurred earlier. The primary outcome measure was incidence and crude hospital mortality of severe sepsis and septic shock, as well as the risk factors for death. ICU mortality, ICU LOS and hospital LOS were also assessed. Patients who were still in hospital on November 30, 2009 were deemed survivors.

Statistical analysis

Data were analyzed using the SPSS 16.0 software program. Data are presented as mean and standard deviation (SD) for variables that exhibited normal distributions. On rejection of the normality hypothesis, we used median and interquartile range (IQR). Student's t-test for independent groups was applied to data with a normal distribution. When normality was rejected, the Mann–Whitney U-test was used for independent groups. For categorical variables the chi-square or Fisher's exact test was applied as appropriate. For determination of independent predictors for hospital mortality in severe sepsis patients, odds ratios (OR) and respective 95% confidence intervals (CIs) were estimated by means of multivariate logistic regression analysis. Variables including demographics, underlying diseases, severity of illness, admission status, and complications were entered into the model if $p<0.2$ in univariate analysis. The Hosmer-Lemeshow test was used to assess the calibration of the regression model. All comparisons were unpaired and all tests of significance were two-tailed. A p value <0.05 was considered statistically significant.

Results

Population characteristics and incidence of severe sepsis and septic shock

We screened 3063 admissions during the study period and 1297 patients (42.3%) were enrolled (Figure 1). A total of 484 patients developed severe sepsis or septic shock, including 336 males (69.4%), and their median age was 66 (interquartile range [IQR], 51–77) years. More than half of the patients were admitted into ICU because of respiratory diseases (53.5%), and two-thirds (67.4%) had at least one underlying disease or chronic organ system dysfunction. The median APACHE II score was 21 (IQR, 16–27), and the median SOFA score on ICU day 1 was 7.5 (IQR, 5–10). Further baseline characteristics are shown in Table 2.The incidence of severe sepsis and septic shock was 37.3 per 100 ICU admissions.

Table 1. Characteristics of participating ICUs.

*	Participating ICUs (n = 22)
Type of hospital	
University affiliated	19
Public	3
Number of hospital beds (median, IQR)	1730 (1402–2100)
Type of ICU	
Medical/Surgical	18
Surgical	3
Medical	1
Number of ICU beds (median, IQR)	20.5 (12.0–28.0)
Total number of intensivists	12.0 (8.5–13.8)
Total number of nurses	33.5 (26.3–45.0)
Total ICU admissions in 2009 (median, IQR)	791 (446–1353)
Hospital mortality (%)	12.1 (8.2–18.7)

ICU, intensive care unit; IQR, interquartile range.

Sources of infection and microbiology

The lung (85.7%) and the abdomen (18.0%) were the most common sites of infection (Table 3). One hundred and sixty-seven patients (34.5%) had two or more infection sites. Only 37 patients (7.6%) had bloodstream infection.

Only half of the ICU (11/22) reported the microbiology, and 148 patients (30.6%) had microbiological documentations associated with severe sepsis and septic shock. Out of these 148 patients with microbiological results, Gram-negative bacilli were isolated in 111 patients (75.0%), and Gram-positive organisms were isolated in 32 patients (21.6%). Only six patients were diagnosed as invasive fungal infection or fungemia (4.1%). Forty-nine patients (33.1%) had polymicrobial (≥2 infection agents) infections. The most prevalent species were *Acinetobacter baumannii*, *Pseudomonas aeruginosa*, *Escherichia coli*, *Klebsiella pneumoniae*, methicillin-resistant *Staphylococcus aureus*, and *Stenotrophomonas maltophilia* (Table 4).

Outcome of patients

Among the 484 patients included in the cohort, 139 died in ICU, and 23 died during hospitalization after transfer to general wards. Twenty patients (4.1%) were still in hospital at the end of follow-up (i.e. November 30, 2009) and were deemed survivors. The crude ICU and hospital mortality rates were 28.7% and 33.5%, respectively. The median ICU LOS was 7 days (IQR, 4–15) and hospital LOS was 18 days (IQR, 10–38). About three fourths (72.3%) of patients had stayed in ICU for less than 2 weeks, while 9.5% of patients had an ICU LOS of more than 4 weeks. Compared with patients without shock, patients with septic shock were more likely to receive mechanical ventilation (78.2% vs.

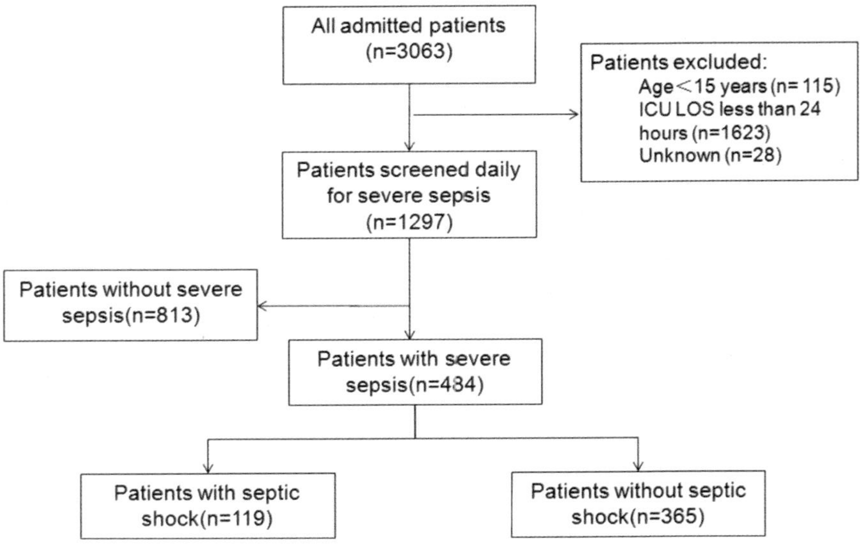

Figure 1. Flow diagram of enrolled patients and their outcome. ICU, intensive care unit; LOS, length of stay.

Table 2. Characteristics and outcome of patients with severe sepsis.

Variables	All patients (n = 484)	Survivors (n = 322)	Non-survivors (n = 162)	*P* Value
Age, median (IQR)	66 (51–77)	62 (47–74)	71 (56–80)	<0.001
Male sex	336 (69.4%)	216 (67.1%)	120 (74.1%)	0.115
ICU admission categories				
Medical	371 (76.7%)	239 (74.2%)	132 (81.5%)	0.075
Scheduled surgery	39 (8.1%)	27 (8.4%)	12 (7.4%)	0.709
Emergency surgery	74 (15.3%)	56 (17.4%)	18 (11.1%)	0.070
Reasons for ICU admission				
Respiratory disease	259 (53.5%)	163 (50.6%)	96 (59.3%)	0.072
Gastrointestinal disease	59 (12.2%)	46 (14.3%)	13 (8.0%)	0.047
Neurological disease	49 (10.1%)	35 (10.9%)	14 (8.6%)	0.443
Cardiovascular disease	46 (9.5%)	27 (8.4%)	19 (11.7%)	0.237
Trauma	34 (7.0%)	28 (8.7%)	6 (3.7%)	0.043
Renal disease	26 (5.4%)	14 (4.3%)	12 (7.4%)	0.159
Miscellaneous	11 (2.3%)	9 (2.8%)	2 (3.7%)	0.277
Comorbidities				
No comorbidity	158(32.6%)	119(37.0%)	39(24.1%)	0.004
Hypertension	166(34.3%)	102(31.7%)	64(39.5%)	0.087
Diabetes mellitus	85(17.6%)	53(16.5%)	32(19.8%)	0.369
Coronary artery disease	83(17.1%)	53(16.5%)	30(18.5%)	0.571
COPD	80(16.5%)	48(14.9%)	32(19.8%)	0.176
Cancer	55(11.4%)	27(8.4%)	28(17.3%)	0.004
Hematologic malignancy	10(2.1%)	7(2.2%)	3(1.9%)	1.000
Organ transplantation	9(1.9%)	4(1.2%)	5(3.1%)	0.169
Chronic respiratory failure	73(15.1%)	44(13.7%)	29(17.9%)	0.219
Chronic heart failure	56(11.6%)	23(7.1%)	33(20.4%)	<0.001
Immunocompromise	48(9.9%)	25(7.8%)	23(14.2%)	0.025
Chronic renal failure	13(2.7%)	6(1.9%)	7(4.3%)	0.138
Chronic liver dysfunction	11(2.3%)	7(2.2%)	4(2.5%)	1.000
APACHE II, median (IQR)	21(16–27)	18(14–24)	25(19–32)	<0.001
SOFA on ICU day1, median (IQR)	7.5(5–10)	7(5–9)	9(6.75–12)	<0.001
Complications				
Septic shock	119(24.6%)	68(21.1%)	51(31.5%)	0.012
Acute kidney injury	201(41.5%)	119(37.0%)	82(50.6%)	0.004
ARDS	265(54.8%)	150(46.6%)	115(71.0%)	<0.001
ICU stay, days, median (IQR)	7(4–15)	7(4–14)	9(4–17)	0.067

APACHE II, Acute Physiology and Chronic Health Evaluation II; ARDS, acute respiratory distress syndrome; COPD, Chronic obstructive pulmonary disease; ICU, Intensive care unit; IQR, interquartile range; SOFA, Sequential Organ Failure Assessment.

63.3%, p = 0.003), and had a longer ICU LOS (9 [IQR, 4–17.5] vs. 7 [IQR, 4–15], p = 0.011).

Prognostic factors

Variables added into the multivariate model included age, sex, comorbidity of cancer, hypertension, COPD, and organ transplantation, chronic heart failure, immune-compromised status, type of ICU admission (respiratory disease, gastrointestinal disease, renal disease and trauma), ICU admission categories (medical, scheduled surgery and emergency surgery), APACHE II score, SOFA score of day1 in ICU, presence of septic shock, ARDS and AKI, bloodstream infection, soft tissue infection, central nervous system infection. As shown in Table 5, APACHE II score, presence of ARDS, bloodstream infection and comorbidity of cancer were independent risk factors for hospital mortality. The Chi-square value of Hosmer-Lemeshow test was 4.868, and the p value was 0.772.

Discussion

The incidence of severe sepsis in the present study was 37.3 cases per 100 ICU admissions, and 9.2% (n = 119) of the patients admitted into ICU developed septic shock. The lung and abdomen were the most frequent sites of infection. The ICU and hospital mortality rates of severe sepsis were 28.7% and 33.5%, respectively. Patients with shock had a much higher mortality rate (42.9%) than those without shock (30.4%). Patients with

Table 3. The source of infection of patients with severe sepsis (total >100% because 167 patients had more than one infection sites).

Variables	All patients (n = 484)	Survivors (n = 322)	Non-survivors (n = 162)	*P* Value
Pneumonia	419 (86.6%)	276 (85.7%)	143 (88.3%)	0.436
Intra-abdominal infection	80 (16.5%)	58 (18.0%)	22 (13.6%)	0.215
Gastroenteritis	41 (8.5%)	27 (8.4%)	14 (8.6%)	0.924
Urinary tract infection	37 (7.6%)	25 (7.8%)	12 (7.4%)	0.889
Bloodstream infection	37 (7.6%)	16 (5%)	21 (13%)	0.002
Soft tissue infection	34 (7.0%)	19 (5.9%)	15 (9.3%)	0.172
Central nervous system infection	23 (4.8%)	19 (5.9%)	4 (2.5%)	0.094
Multiple-site infection (≥2)	167 (34.5%)	111 (34.5%)	56 (34.6%)	0.983

higher APACHE II score, presence of ARDS, bloodstream infection and comorbidity of cancer may have higher risk of death.

In comparison with previous studies [3,6,7,21], the treated incidence of severe sepsis in the study ICUs is very high. This difference may be due to the increasing trend of severe sepsis [4,5], as our study was conducted much later. However, secular trend may not be the only cause of incidence variation, because even higher incidence of severe sepsis has been reported in previous studies [9]. Different inclusion criteria may also explain the reported discrepancy. For example, Adrie et al included patients with ICU LOS of at least 48 hours [9], while Padkin et al only screened patients for severe sepsis within the first 24 hours of ICU admission [21]. In order to include cases with early recovery from or late onset of severe sepsis, we screened all ICU admissions with ICU LOS no less than 24 hours. Second, patient population in different studies may be quite different. Cheng et al only studied patients admitted to surgical ICUs [3], while, in the current study, 18 out of the 22 participating ICUs were general ICUs, and 76.7% of our cohort were medical patients. Another possible reason is the relative lack of ICU beds in China compared to other countries, which might have led to admission of sicker patients into the study ICUs [22,23]. Finally, definitions of severe sepsis employed in various studies may be also different [21].

The outcome of severe sepsis patients varies considerably in different studies. In SOAP study, ICU mortality rate was 32.2% for severe sepsis and 54.1% for septic shock [24]. In France, patients with severe sepsis had a hospital mortality rate of 59% [8], whereas patients with septic shock had a hospital mortality of

Table 4. Distribution of microorganisms isolated from 148 patients.

Microorganism	Total (n = 269)	ICU-acquired (n = 221)	Non-ICU-acquired (n = 48)
Gram positives	39 (14.5%)	34 (15.4%)	5 (10.4%)
Methicillin-resistant *Staphylococcus aureus*	17 (6.3%)	14 (6.3%)	3 (6.3%)
Coagulase-negative *Staphylococcus*	10 (3.7%)	8 (3.6%)	2 (4.2%)
Enterococcus faecium	8 (3.0%)	8 (3.6%)	0
Enterococcus faecalis	3 (1.1%)	3 (1.4%)	0
Streptococcus viridans	1 (0.4%)	1 (0.5%)	0
Gram negatives	168 (62.5%)	137 (62.0%)	31 (64.6%)
Acinetobacterbaumannii	38 (14.1%)	30 (13.6%)	8 (16.7%)
Pseudomonas aeruginosa	33 (12.3%)	27 (12.2%)	6 (12.5%)
Escherichia coli	26 (9.7%)	24 (10.9%)	2 (4.2%)
Klebsiellapneumoniae	25 (9.3%)	21 (9.5%)	4 (8.3%)
Stenotrophomonasmaltophilia	16 (5.9%)	12 (5.4%)	4 (8.3%)
Proteus mirabilis	5 (1.9%)	3 (1.4%)	2 (4.2%)
Serratiamarcescens	4 (1.5%)	3 (1.4%)	1 (2.1%)
Other Gram negatives*	21 (7.8%)	17 (7.7%)	4 (8.3%)
Fungi**	6 (2.2%)	6 (2.7%)	0
Candida albicans	1 (0.4%)	1 (0.5%)	0
Aspergillus spp.	4 (1.5%)	4 (1.8%)	0
Pneumocystis	1 (0.4%)	1 (0.5%)	0

*including Burkholderia cepacia, Chryseobacter iumindologenes, Enterobacter cloacae, Enterobacteraerogenes, and Serratialiquefaciens.
**fungal infection here refers to the invasive fungal infection and fungemia.

Table 5. Multivariate logistic regression analysis of independent predictors of hospital mortality in patients with severe sepsis and septic shock.

Risk factor	OR (95% CI)		P value	
	Univariate	Multivariate	Univariate	Multivariate
APACHE II	1.113(1.083–1.144)	1.068(1.027–1.109)	<0.001	0.001
ARDS	3.173(2.129–4.730)	2.676(1.691–4.235)	<0.001	<0.001
Bloodstream infection	2.848(1.443–5.624)	2.520(1.142–5.564)	0.002	0.022
Cancer	2.283(1.295–4.024)	2.246(1.141–4.420)	0.004	0.019

APACHE II, Acute Physiology and Chronic Health Evaluation II; ARDS, Acute respiratory distress syndrome; CI, confidence interval; OR, odds ratio.

61.2% [4]. Finfer et al reported that overall ICU and hospital mortality rates were 26.5% and 37.5% for patients with severe sepsis in Australia and New Zealand [6]. In comparison, the mortality rates of patients with severe sepsis (30.4%) and septic shock (42.9%) in the current study were lower than that in most studies [6,12,25]. Many factors can explain the difference. First, the severity of acute illness might be different. For example, patients included in the study of Khwannimit et al [12] were more severely ill, as suggested by a higher APACHE II score (26.8 vs. 21), and were more likely to die than our cohort (49.7% vs. 33.5%). Second, previous studies found that, compared with patients who developed sepsis outside ICU, patients with ICU-acquired sepsis had a higher mortality [24,26]. Only 12.6% of patients in the current study developed ICU-acquired severe sepsis or septic shock, while 25% episodes of severe sepsis in France were ICU-acquired [8]. Despite the fact that hospital mortality rate in the current study was lower than that in many studies, it was still higher with a median APACHE II score of only 21. This was possibly attributable to the very low compliance with sepsis resuscitation and management bundles, although not reported in the current study but consistently observed in other studies involving Chinese patients [27]. There should be no doubt that clinical outcome of severe sepsis/septic shock could be improved significantly by better understanding of pathogenesis, as well as increasing the uniform compliance with standard therapy and other treatments proven effective for severe sepsis in the future. Due to the high mortality rate in patients with septic shock, patients with risk factors [28,29], such as higher SOFA score should be observed closely.

Similar to other studies [4,6,8], we found that lung and abdomen were the most common source of infection. The potential implication of this finding is that, when the source of infection remains unknown in a patient with severe sepsis/septic shock, clinicians should consider pulmonary and intra-abdominal sources. Furthermore, majority of our patients had pneumonia, indicating the importance of implementing effective strategies to prevent both community-acquired pneumonia (such as public education, and vaccination against influenza and pneumococcus in high risk population) and hospital-acquired pneumonia (such as hand hygiene, and selective digestive decontamination). In accordance with other studies [3,12], most isolated pathogens in our study were Gram-negative bacilli, although some studies in developed countries reported predominance of Gram-positive bacteria [2,6,24]. Many factors, including geographic variation, case mix, and antibiotic prescription habits, may explain the observed difference. Moreover, clinical significance of the same pathogens may vary in different studies. Cheng et al reported that *Acinetobacter baumannii* (25.8%) and *Escherichia coli* (13.8%) were the most common pathogens, while only 13.8% of the infections were caused by *Pseudomonas aeruginosa*. Despite a similar frequency of *Acinetobacter baumannii* (25.7%), *Pseudomonas aeruginosa* and *Klebsiella pneumonia* were much more common in our study. The dramatic increase in the incidence of *Pseudomonas aeruginosa* is worth mentioning as *Pseudomonas* species may be associated with increased mortality rates [24]. There might be bias in the results of microorganisms distribution as not all units reported microbiology results. Furthermore, we cannot rule out the possibility that many patients included in our study were nosocomial cases of sepsis, which might have resulted in the high frequency of *Acinetobacter baumannii*.

Independent risk factors associated with increased mortality in severe sepsis include higher APACHE II score [12,27], presence of ARDS [12,30], bloodstream infection [8] and comorbid cancer [2,3,24,31], which was a consistent finding across literatures. Although patients with shock had a higher mortality, the presence of shock was not an independent risk factor for death in our study.

As we know, there are few data about the epidemiology of severe sepsis and septic shock in mixed ICU in China. Our report may add some valuable information. Nonetheless, some limitations merit discussion. First, there may have been bias only concerning ICU admissions. In general, patients with severe sepsis would be treated in ICU in those participating hospitals, unless they responded to simple measures such as fluid resuscitation and antibiotics. Some patients may not be admitted into ICU because of personal willingness. However, most Chinese people tend to reject advance directives, and prefer family-centered decision making than other ethnic and cultural groups. Even if the illness is irreversible, families may strongly advocate aggressive treatment, as they endorse the cultural belief that withdrawing or withholding support of their family member with critical illness is disgraceful or not filial piety [32]. Chinese doctors seldom advise families to withdraw treatment because of the possibility of involvement in medical disputes and undertaking legal liability [33]. Second, the results of the present study might not be able to generalize to ICUs in small local hospitals. Although about 10% (47/484) of our cohort are transferred from other hospitals, we believe that even more patients with severe sepsis/septic shock are treated in local hospitals, possibly with higher mortality rate. Third, only a minority of patients had microbiological documentation, and the rest were with negative or unreported positive culture results. But the distribution of pathogens obtained in this research was similar to the result of Cheng and colleagues' research [3], and there was no significant difference in patient demographics and mortality rate (38% vs. 31.3%, $p=0.144$) between those ICUs with and without microbiological results. Zahar et al have also found that microbiological characteristics of infection did not influence the outcome of patients with severe sepsis [34]. Fourth, the exclusion criterion of ICU LOS<24 hours would have the effect of excluding the sickest patients who died early and might have bias the study results. Finally, the data were not collected for the primary purpose of identifying severe sepsis. Some important information related to severe sepsis was not reported, such as the compliance with sepsis bundle which might affect the clinical outcome of severe sepsis and the results of multivariate regression analysis. Further studies focusing on the rate of compliance with the resuscitation bundle and its influence factors should be conducted in China.

Conclusions

Severe sepsis is an important public health problem and a frequent cause of ICU admission with a high mortality rate. Higher APACHE II score, presence of ARDS, bloodstream infection and comorbidity of cancer are risk factors contributing to fatal outcome. This argues that severe sepsis/septic shock represents a major disease burden in mainland China. Future clinical research is warranted to ensure early identification of high risk patient population, prompt implementation of validated treatment, and significant improvement of clinical outcome.

Acknowledgments

The China Critical Care Clinical Trials Group (CCCCTG) is composed of 24 ICUs in different hospitals in China, and the individual authors (their affiliations) within this group are listed as follows: Bin Du, Li Weng (Medical ICU, Peking Union Medical College Hospital, Peking Union Medical College & Chinese Academy of Medical Sciences, Beijing, China); Chuanyun Qian, Wei Zhang (Department of Emergency Medicine and Medical ICU, The First Affiliated Hospital of Kunming Medical University, Kunming, China); Mingyan Zhao, Dongsheng Fei (Department of Critical Care Medicine, The First Affiliated Hospital of Harbin Medical University, Harbin, China); Xiangyou Yu, Yi Wang (Department of Critical Care Medicine, First Affiliated Hospital, Xinjiang Medical University, Urumqi, China); Yan Kang, Xuelian Liao (Department of Critical Care Medicine, West China Hospital, Sichuan University, Chengdu, China); Xiaochun Ma, Yini Sun (Department of Critical Care Medicine, The First Affiliated Hospital of China Medical University, Shenyang, China); Yuhang Ai, Li Huang (Department of Critical Care Medicine, Xiangya Hospital, Central South University, Changsha, China); Yuan Xu, Wei He (Department of Critical Care Medicine, Beijing Tongren Hospital, Capital Medical University, Beijing, China); Yongjie Yin, Dexin Liu (Department of Critical Care Medicine, The Second Hospital of Jilin University, Changchun, China); Youzhong An, Huiying Zhao (Department of Critical Care Medicine, Peking University People's Hospital, Beijing, China); Dawei Wu, Chen Li (Department of Critical Care Medicine, Qilu Hospital of Shandong University, Jinan, China); Renhua Sun, Qian Li (Department of Critical Care Medicine, Zhejiang Provincial People's Hospital, Hangzhou, China); Shusheng Li, Xiao Ran (Department of Critical Care Medicine, Tongji Hospital of Tongji Medical College, Huazhong University of Science & Technology, Wuhan, China); Zhenjie Hu, Yan Huo (Department of Critical Care Medicine, Hebei Medical University Fourth Hospital, Shijiazhuang, China); Xiangyuan Cao, Xigang Ma (Department of Critical Care Medicine, General Hospital of Ningxia Medical University, Yinchuan, China); Fachun Zhou, Fang Xu (Department of Emergency and Intensive Care Medicine, The First Affiliated Hospital of Chongqing Medical University, Chongqing, China); Li Jiang, Qi Zhang (Department of Critical Care Medicine, Fuxing Hospital, Capital Medical University, Beijing, China); Jiandong Lin, Xiongjian Xiao (Department of Critical Care Medicine, The First Affiliated Hospital of Fujian Medical University, Fuzhou, China); Enqiang Mao, Cheng Zhu (Emergency ICU, Ruijin Hospital, Shanghai Jiao Tong University, Shanghai, China); Tiehe Qin, Shouhong Wang (Department of Critical Care Medicine, Guangdong General Hospital, Guangzhou, China); Zhenyang He, Rui Li (Department of Critical Care Medicine, Hainan Provincial People's Hospital, Haikou, China); Lihua Zhou, Lipeng Zhang (Department of Critical Care Medicine, The Affiliated Hospital of Inner Mongolia Medical University, Huhhot, China); Rongqing Sun, Yuexia Li (Intensive Care Unit, The First Affiliated Hospital, Zhengzhou University); Xijing Zhang, Binxiao Su (Surgical Intensive Care Unit, Xijing Hospital). The lead author for this group is Bin Du, and his contact email address is dubin98@gmail.com.

We would like to thank persons listed above but not designated as the author of this article in those 22 participating ICUs for their help with data collection.

Author Contributions

Conceived and designed the experiments: BD. Performed the experiments: CQ MZ XY YK XM Y. Ai YX DL Y. An DW RS SL Z. Hu XC FZ LJ JL EM Z. He LZ TQ. Analyzed the data: BD JZ. Contributed reagents/materials/analysis tools: JZ BD. Wrote the paper: JZ.

References

1. Heyland DK, Hopman W, Coo H, Tranmer J, McColl MA (2000) Long-term health-related quality of life in survivors of sepsis. Short Form 36: a valid and reliable measure of health-related quality of life. Crit Care Med 28: 3599–3605.
2. Angus DC, Linde-Zwirble WT, Lidicker J, Clermont G, Carcillo J, et al. (2001) Epidemiology of severe sepsis in the United States: analysis of incidence, outcome, and associated costs of care. Crit Care Med 29: 1303–1310.
3. Cheng B, Xie G, Yao S, Wu X, Guo Q, et al. (2007) Epidemiology of severe sepsis in critically ill surgical patients in ten university hospitals in China. Crit Care Med 35: 2538–2546.
4. Annane D, Aegerter P, Jars-Guincestre MC, Guidet B (2003) Current epidemiology of septic shock: the CUB-Rea Network. Am J Respir Crit Care Med 168: 165–172.
5. Martin GS, Mannino DM, Eaton S, Moss M (2003) The epidemiology of sepsis in the United States from 1979 through 2000. N Engl J Med 348: 1546–1554.
6. Finfer S, Bellomo R, Lipman J, French C, Dobb G, et al. (2004) Adult-population incidence of severe sepsis in Australian and New Zealand intensive care units. Intensive Care Med 30: 589–596.
7. Harrison DA, Welch CA, Eddleston JM (2006) The epidemiology of severe sepsis in England, Wales and Northern Ireland, 1996 to 2004: secondary analysis of a high quality clinical database, the ICNARC Case Mix Programme Database. Crit Care 10: R42.
8. Brun-Buisson C, Doyon F, Carlet J, Dellamonica P, Gouin F, et al. (1995) Incidence, risk factors, and outcome of severe sepsis and septic shock in adults. A multicenter prospective study in intensive care units. French ICU Group for Severe Sepsis. Jama 274: 968–974.
9. Adrie C, Alberti C, Chaix-Couturier C, Azoulay E, De Lassence A, et al. (2005) Epidemiology and economic evaluation of severe sepsis in France: age, severity, infection site, and place of acquisition (community, hospital, or intensive care unit) as determinants of workload and cost. J Crit Care 20: 46–58.
10. Blanco J, Muriel-Bombin A, Sagredo V, Taboada F, Gandia F, et al. (2008) Incidence, organ dysfunction and mortality in severe sepsis: a Spanish multicentre study. Crit Care 12: R158.
11. Rodriguez F, Barrera L, De La Rosa G, Dennis R, Duenas C, et al. (2011) The epidemiology of sepsis in Colombia: a prospective multicenter cohort study in ten university hospitals. Crit Care Med 39: 1675–1682.
12. Khwannimit B, Bhurayanontachai R (2009) The epidemiology of, and risk factors for, mortality from severe sepsis and septic shock in a tertiary-care university hospital setting. Epidemiol Infect 137: 1333–1341.
13. Rangel-Frausto MS, Pittet D, Costigan M, Hwang T, Davis CS, et al. (1995) The natural history of the systemic inflammatory response syndrome (SIRS). A prospective study. Jama 273: 117–123.
14. Perl TM, Dvorak L, Hwang T, Wenzel RP (1995) Long-term survival and function after suspected gram-negative sepsis. Jama 274: 338–345.
15. Du B, An Y, Kang Y, Yu X, Zhao M, et al. (2013) Characteristics of critically ill patients in ICUs in Mainland China. Crit Care Med 41: 84–92.
16. Knaus WA, Draper EA, Wagner DP, Zimmerman JE (1985) APACHE II: a severity of disease classification system. Crit Care Med 13: 818–829.
17. Vincent JL, de Mendonca A, Cantraine F, Moreno R, Takala J, et al. (1998) Use of the SOFA score to assess the incidence of organ dysfunction/failure in intensive care units: results of a multicenter, prospective study. Working group on "sepsis-related problems" of the European Society of Intensive Care Medicine. Crit Care Med 26: 1793–1800.
18. Bone RC, Balk RA, Cerra FB, Dellinger RP, Fein AM, et al. (1992) Definitions for sepsis and organ failure and guidelines for the use of innovative therapies in

sepsis. The ACCP/SCCM Consensus Conference Committee. American College of Chest Physicians/Society of Critical Care Medicine. Chest 101: 1644–1655.
19. Bernard GR, Artigas A, Brigham KL, Carlet J, Falke K, et al. (1994) The American-European Consensus Conference on ARDS. Definitions, mechanisms, relevant outcomes, and clinical trial coordination. Am J Respir Crit Care Med 149: 818–824.
20. Bellomo R, Ronco C, Kellum JA, Mehta RL, Palevsky P (2004) Acute renal failure - definition, outcome measures, animal models, fluid therapy and information technology needs: the Second International Consensus Conference of the Acute Dialysis Quality Initiative (ADQI) Group. Crit Care 8: R204–212.
21. Padkin A, Goldfrad C, Brady AR, Young D, Black N, et al. (2003) Epidemiology of severe sepsis occurring in the first 24 hrs in intensive care units in England, Wales, and Northern Ireland. Crit Care Med 31: 2332–2338.
22. Austin S, Murthy S, Wunsch H, Adhikari NK, Karir V, et al. (2014) Access to urban acute care services in high- vs. middle-income countries: an analysis of seven cities. Intensive Care Med 40: 342–352.
23. Du B, Xi X, Chen D, Peng J (2010) Clinical review: critical care medicine in mainland China. Crit Care 14: 206.
24. Vincent JL, Sakr Y, Sprung CL, Ranieri VM, Reinhart K, et al. (2006) Sepsis in European intensive care units: results of the SOAP study. Crit Care Med 34: 344–353.
25. Silva E, Pedro Mde A, Sogayar AC, Mohovic T, Silva CL, et al. (2004) Brazilian Sepsis Epidemiological Study (BASES study). Crit Care 8: R251–260.
26. Sakr Y, Elia C, Mascia L, Barberis B, Cardellino S, et al. (2013) Epidemiology and outcome of sepsis syndromes in Italian ICUs: a muticentre, observational cohort study in the region of Piedmont. Minerva Anestesiol 79: 993–1002.
27. Phua J, Koh Y, Du B, Tang YQ, Divatia JV, et al. (2011) Management of severe sepsis in patients admitted to Asian intensive care units: prospective cohort study. BMJ 342: d3245.
28. Glickman SW, Cairns CB, Otero RM, Woods CW, Tsalik EL, et al. (2010) Disease progression in hemodynamically stable patients presenting to the emergency department with sepsis. Acad Emerg Med 17: 383–390.
29. Song YH, Shin TG, Kang MJ, Sim MS, Jo IJ, et al. (2012) Predicting factors associated with clinical deterioration of sepsis patients with intermediate levels of serum lactate. Shock 38: 249–254.
30. Mikkelsen ME, Shah CV, Meyer NJ, Gaieski DF, Lyon S, et al. (2013) The Epidemiology of Acute Respiratory Distress Syndrome in Patients Presenting to the Emergency Department With Severe Sepsis. Shock.
31. de Montmollin E, Tandjaoui-Lambiotte Y, Legrand M, Lambert J, Mokart D, et al. (2013) Outcomes in critically ill cancer patients with septic shock of pulmonary origin. Shock 39: 250–254.
32. Blumenthal D, Hsiao W (2005) Privatization and its discontents–the evolving Chinese health care system. N Engl J Med 353: 1165–1170.
33. Li LB (2013) Clinical review: Ethics and end-of-life care for critically ill patients in China. Crit Care 17: 244.
34. Zahar JR, Timsit JF, Garrouste-Orgeas M, Francais A, Vesim A, et al. (2011) Outcomes in severe sepsis and patients with septic shock: pathogen species and infection sites are not associated with mortality. Crit Care Med 39: 1886–1895.

Changes in Positive End-Expiratory Pressure Alter the Distribution of Ventilation within the Lung Immediately after Birth in Newborn Rabbits

Marcus J. Kitchen[1], Melissa L. Siew[2], Megan J. Wallace[2], Andreas Fouras[4], Robert A. Lewis[5,6], Naoto Yagi[7], Kentaro Uesugi[7], Arjan B. te Pas[3¶], Stuart B. Hooper[2*¶]

1 School of Physics, Monash Institute of Medical Research, Clayton, Victoria, Australia, **2** The Ritchie Centre, Monash Institute of Medical Research, Clayton, Victoria, Australia, **3** Department of Pediatrics, Leiden University Medical Centre, Leiden, Netherlands, **4** Department of Mechanical and Aerospace Engineering, Monash University, Clayton, Victoria, Australia, **5** Department of Medical Imaging and Radiation Science, Monash University, Clayton, Victoria, Australia, **6** Biomedical Engineering, University of Saskatchewan, Saskatoon, Canada, **7** SPring-8/Japan Synchrotron Radiation Research Institute, Sayo, Hyogo, Japan

Abstract

Current recommendations suggest the use of positive end-expiratory pressures (PEEP) to assist very preterm infants to develop a functional residual capacity (FRC) and establish gas exchange at birth. However, maintaining a consistent PEEP is difficult and so the lungs are exposed to changing distending pressures after birth, which can affect respiratory function. Our aim was to determine how changing PEEP levels alters the distribution of ventilation within the lung. Preterm rabbit pups (28 days gestation) were delivered and mechanically ventilated with one of three strategies, whereby PEEP was changed in sequence; 0-5-10-5-0 cmH_2O, 5-10-0-5-0 cmH_2O or 10-5-0-10-0 cmH_2O. Phase contrast X-ray imaging was used to analyse the distribution of ventilation in the upper left (UL), upper right (UR), lower left (LL) and lower right (LR) quadrants of the lung. Initiating ventilation with 10PEEP resulted in a uniform increase in FRC throughout the lung whereas initiating ventilation with 5PEEP or 0PEEP preferentially aerated the UR than both lower quadrants ($p<0.05$). Consequently, the relative distribution of incoming V_T was preferentially directed into the lower lobes at low PEEP, primarily due to the loss of FRC in those lobes. Following ventilation at 10PEEP, the distribution of air at end-inflation was uniform across all quadrants and remained so regardless of the PEEP level. Uniform distribution of ventilation can be achieved by initiating ventilation with a high PEEP. After the lungs have aerated, small and stepped reductions in PEEP result in more uniform changes in ventilation.

Editor: Edgardo Szyld, Icahn School of Medicine at Mount Sinai, United States of America

Funding: This research was supported by the Australian Research Council (http://www.arc.gov.au), the Australian National Health and Medical Research Council (http://www.nhmrc.gov.au) and the Victorian Government's Operational Infrastructure Support Program (http://www.business.vic.gov.au). The authors acknowledge financial support from the Access to Major Research Facilities Programme (http://www.ansto.gov.au/) which is a component of the International Science Linkages Programme established under the Australian Government's innovation statement, Backing Australia's Ability. The authors also gratefully acknowledge the support provided by the SPring-8 synchrotron facility (http://www.spring8.or.jp) which was granted by the SPring-8 Program Review Committee. Marcus J. Kitchen and Andreas Fouras are the recipients of ARC Australian Research Fellowship and NHMRC Career Development Fellowships respectively. Arjan B. te Pas is recipient of a Veni-grant, The Netherlands Organisation for Health Research and Development (http://www.zonmw.nl/en), part of the Innovational Research Incentives Scheme Veni-Vidi-Vici (project nos. 91612027). The funders had no role in study design, data collection and analysis, decision to publish, or preparation of the manuscript.

Competing Interests: The authors have declared that no competing interests exist.

* E-mail: stuart.hooper@monash.edu

MJK and MLS are joint first authors on this work.

¶ ABtP and SBH are joint senior authors on this work.

Introduction

The lungs of premature newborns are structurally and functionally immature and so have a greater tendency to collapse than the adult lung [1–3]. Specifically, the lung tissue is inelastic and the distal airways lack surfactant [4], which is required to reduce surface tension and promote uniform lung aeration [5,6]. In addition, as their chest walls are highly compliant [7], the premature newborn's ability to oppose lung recoil and maintain functional residual capacity (FRC) is reduced, which may contribute to a lower FRC [8].

Positive end-expiratory pressure (PEEP) and continuous positive airway pressure (CPAP) oppose lung atelectasis by applying an internal distending pressure on the airways, which keeps them aerated at end-expiration [9]. As a result, end-expiratory pressures improve FRC development, gas exchange, lung compliance and reduce lung injury and inflammation [9–11]. However, providing consistent end-expiratory pressure support in the delivery room can be difficult and changing levels often cannot be avoided. Indeed, face mask leak is common [12,13] and assisted ventilation is often interrupted by mask repositioning, suctioning or intubation, which can rapidly decrease lung gas volumes [14]. Little is known about how these pressure changes alter the distribution of ventilation within the immature lung.

In adults with a non-uniform pattern of acute respiratory distress syndrome (ARDS), increasing PEEP levels recruits lung volume preferentially in the apical lobes, which increases compliance to a greater extent in the apical than basal lobes

[15,16]. Similar observations have been made in children with ARDS [17] and a preference for the distribution of air into apical lung regions has also been observed in vertically positioned dead newborn fetal rabbits following consecutive pressure/volume loops applied using air [18]. At birth, as the immature lung lacks surfactant [4] and incompletely clears airway liquid [19], the resulting large regional differences in lung compliance likely contributes to the heterogenous ventilation commonly observed in preterm infants. Thus, it is likely that regional differences in lung compliance, which influence the distribution of ventilation within the lung at FRC, will likely change with different PEEP levels.

We have used phase contrast X-ray imaging [9,18–20] to examine how changing PEEP levels alter the distribution of ventilation within the lung in preterm rabbits ventilated from birth. We hypothesized that air will preferentially enter the apical lobes at low PEEP levels and that once apical regions have aerated, higher PEEP levels mainly affect the distribution of air towards the basal lobes of the lungs.

Methods

Animal Procedures

Experiments were performed in the Biomedical Imaging Centre at the SPring-8 synchrotron in Japan. All experiments were approved by Animal Ethics Committees at SPring-8 in Japan and at the School of Biomedical Science, Monash University. Pregnant near-term New Zealand white rabbits (28 days of gestation; term = 32 days) were initially anaesthetised with propofol (Rapinovet; i.v.; 12 mg/kg bolus), intubated and then maintained by isoflourane inhalation (1.5–4%). Pups were delivered by caesarean section, sedated with pentobarbital (Nembutal; 0.1 mg, i.p.) and intubated with an endotracheal (ET) tube (18G). The ET tube was occluded to prevent spontaneous breathing before ventilation onset. Pups were positioned upright in a pre-warmed (40°C) water-filled, plethysmograph (head out) located in the path of the X-ray beam within the imaging hutch, as previously described [19,21]. The ET tube was connected to the ventilator.

Mechanical Ventilation

Pups were randomised into groups and ventilated with one of three PEEP strategies (Figure 1).

Strategy A: The initial PEEP was set at 0 cmH_2O and was changed to 5, to 10, to 5 and to 0 cmH_2O (0-5-10-5-0PEEP). This strategy was designed to examine the effect of gradually increasing and decreasing PEEP on lung aeration and the distribution of ventilation.

Strategy B: PEEP was initially set at 5 cmH_2O and was then changed to 10, to 0, to 5 and to 0 cmH_2O (5-10-0-5-0PEEP). This strategy was designed to examine the effect of PEEP recruitment (from 5 cmH_2O) on the distribution of ventilation and the ability of 5 cmH_2O of PEEP to re-recruit the lung following a loss of PEEP.

Strategy C: PEEP was initially set at 10 cmH_2O and was then changed to 5, to 0 to 10 and to 0 cmH_2O, (10-5-0-10-0PEEP). This strategy was designed to assess the ability of an initial high PEEP strategy, followed by a normal PEEP level, to aerate the lung and to assess the ability of high PEEP to re-recruit the lung following a loss of PEEP.

Phase contrast X-ray movies, found in the Supporting Information, demonstrate the effect of changing PEEP on lung aeration. Movie S1 shows a representative example of Strategy A, Movie S2 is an example of Strategy B and Movie S3 is an example of Strategy C. Pups were ventilated at each PEEP until FRC and tidal volume (V_T) had reached a plateau; this required ~2–3 minutes. Pups were ventilated using a SAR-830/AP (CWE Inc, Ardmore, Pennsylvania, USA) flow restrictor ventilator, which utilises a pressure-limited system and a variable bias gas flow through the ventilator circuit; in this mode, the pressure wave is triangular in shape. The peak inflation pressure (PIP) was set at 35 cmH_2O and the PEEP was controlled by raising and lowering the expiratory tube outlet in a water-filled PEEP trap; i.e. submerging the tube 5 cm generated a PEEP of 5 cmH_2O. Inspiratory and expiratory times were 1.0 and 1.5 sec, respectively. Changes in

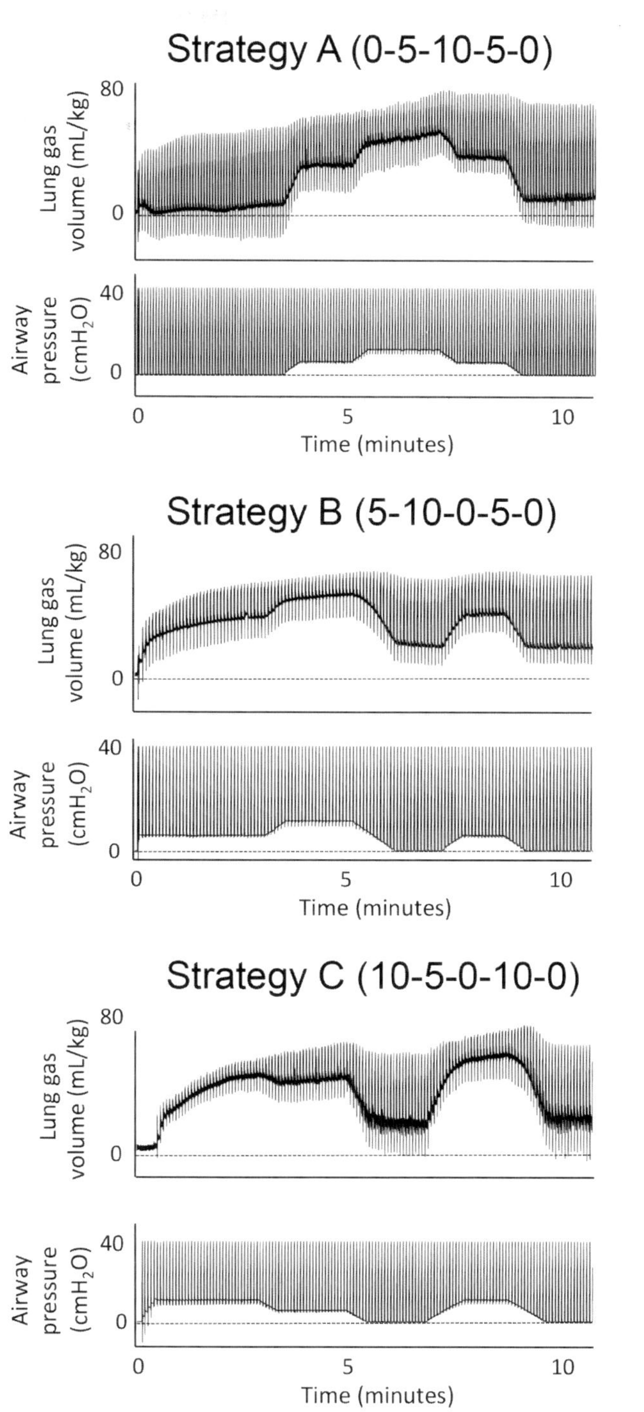

Figure 1. Diagram of ventilation Strategies A, B and C. Plethysmograph and airway pressure recordings of pups that were ventilated from birth using each of the PEEP Strategies A, B or C.

airway pressures were recorded digitally (Powerlab, ADInstruments; Sydney, Australia). At the conclusion of the experiment, pups were euthanized with sodium pentobarbital (Nembutal; 100 mg/kg; i.p.).

Image Acquisition

Phase contrast images were acquired using a monochromatic X-ray beam (24 keV) with the detectors placed 2.0 m downstream from the pups (see [18]). X-rays were converted to visible light and images acquired using an electron multiplying charge-coupled device (EMCCD) camera (Hamamatsu, C9100-02). The effective pixel size was 31.82 µm and the field of view was 32(H) × 32(V) mm^2, which captured the entire pup's chest in a single exposure. Image acquisition was synchronised with ventilation whereby inflation onset triggered the camera to acquire a sequence of six images, 300 ms apart using an exposure time of 80 ms. Three images were acquired during inspiration and three during expiration.

Image Processing and Analysis

The first 4 lung inflations at the onset of lung ventilation and the 4 inflations immediately preceding and following a change in PEEP were used for analysis. Regional lung air volumes were calculated using the image processing technique developed by [18]. This technique utilises differences in X-ray attenuation between air and water to determine changes in gas volume within the image. Despite the images being two-dimensional (2D) projections, this technique enables very small (25 µL) changes in air volumes to be measured without having to reconstruct the three-dimensional (3D) structure using computed tomography [18].

To assess the uniformity of lung aeration, images were partitioned into quadrants using the vertebral column and the 7th rib as landmarks [18]. The four quadrants were labelled upper right (UR), upper left (UL), lower right (LR) and lower left (LL) and are in reference to the image as observed. The position of the regions of interest was held constant within consecutive image by tracking the displacement of the skeleton for each pup using a cross-correlation analysis [18]. Volumetric information extracted from the lung quadrants were used to assess changes in the lung's regional functional residual capacity (FRC), V_T and air volumes at peak inspiratory pressure (V_{PIP}). As the lung volume in each quadrant differs between quadrants and between animals within the same quadrant, lung gas volumes (FRC, V_T and V_{PIP}) were normalised to the maximum lung gas volume obtained in each lung quadrant for each animal within a given imaging sequence. Regional dynamic lung compliance was measured as the change in lung volume in one quadrant divided by the change in airway pressure (PIP-PEEP).

Statistical Analysis

Statistical analysis was performed using Sigmastat (Systat software Inc., USA). Results were presented as mean ± standard error of the mean (SEM) and all data were checked for normality and tested for equal variance. Changes in the distribution of ventilation at FRC, V_T and V_{PIP} were analysed using a 2-way repeated measures ANOVA. Changes in FRC and V_T in response to decreasing or increasing PEEP levels were analysed using a 2-way ANOVA. All statistical tests were followed by a Tukey post hoc test. A $p<0.05$ was considered statistically significant.

Results

Animal data

16 newborn preterm rabbit pups were ventilated from birth and the distribution of air within the lung determined using PC X-ray imaging. 6 pups were ventilated according to PEEP Strategy A, 5 according to PEEP Strategy B and 5 according to PEEP Strategy C. There were no significant differences in mean pup weight between any of the groups ($p>0.05$) and no pups developed a pneumothorax.

Lung air volume distribution between quadrants

Irrespective of the strategy, the lower quadrants had significantly greater maximal lung air volumes (at end inflation) than the upper quadrants ($p<0.05$), which mainly reflects the size differences. The LR and LL quadrants were not significantly different from each other (20.4±1.3 mL/kg vs 17.5±1.7 mL/kg, $p>0.05$) and the UR and UL were also not statistically different from each other (11.7±0.6 mL/kg vs 7.7±0.6 mL/kg, $p>0.05$).

Changes in gas distribution: Strategy A

Air distribution at FRC (Fig 2A). Ventilation with 0PEEP initially resulted in poor aeration of the lung at FRC (<6%) in all quadrants and, although the air volume at FRC gradually increased with time, it was substantially less than with both other strategies by the end of the first ventilation period (Strategy B, Fig 3A and Strategy C, Fig 4A). Furthermore, the relative increase in air volume was unequal and was significantly greater in the UR (28.2±7.3%) than in both LL (13.7±3.0%) and LR (10.3±1.9%) quadrants ($p<0.05$). Subsequent ventilation at 5PEEP, improved aeration in all quadrants but the unequal distribution between quadrants at FRC remained. At 10PEEP, both upper quadrants remained better aerated at FRC than both lower quadrants ($p< 0.05$). Following the return to 0PEEP, only the UR quadrant was significantly better aerated than both lower quadrants (UR 42.9±5.3% vs LR 29.1±5.5% and LL 26.1±5.2%, $p<0.05$).

Distribution of incoming V_T (Fig 2B). Following initial lung aeration with 0PEEP, ventilation with 5PEEP and then with 10PEEP did not alter the size of the incoming V_T, which contributed to 20–30% of total lung air volumes at end-inflation (V_{PIF}). However, by the end of the 10PEEP period, the lower quadrants started to receive a significantly ($p<0.05$) greater proportion of this volume than the upper quadrants. With the onset of subsequent 5PEEP ventilation, both lower quadrants persisted in receiving a significantly larger proportion of the incoming V_T than both upper quadrants (~43% vs ~30%; $p< 0.05$). This non-uniform distribution of incoming V_T persisted during the subsequent 5PEEP and 0PEEP periods, despite a significant increase in V_T.

Air distribution at end-inflation (V_{PIP}) (Fig 2c). At the initiation of ventilation with 0PEEP, the distribution of air in the lung at V_{PIP} was preferentially directed towards both upper quadrants. By the end of the 0PEEP period, the proportion of air in the upper quadrants at V_{PIP} (range 43–54% of maximal lung gas volume) was significantly greater than the lower quadrants (~33% of maximal lung gas volume; $p<0.05$). During the subsequent 10PEEP ventilation period, when the lung had fully aerated, all quadrants were similarly ventilated at V_{PIP} (>90%, $p>0.05$) and remained so for the rest of the experiment.

Changes in ventilation distribution: Strategy B

Air distribution at FRC (Fig 3A). During ventilation at 5PEEP and then at 10PEEP, the distribution of air in the lungs at FRC was greater in both upper than in both lower quadrants ($p<$

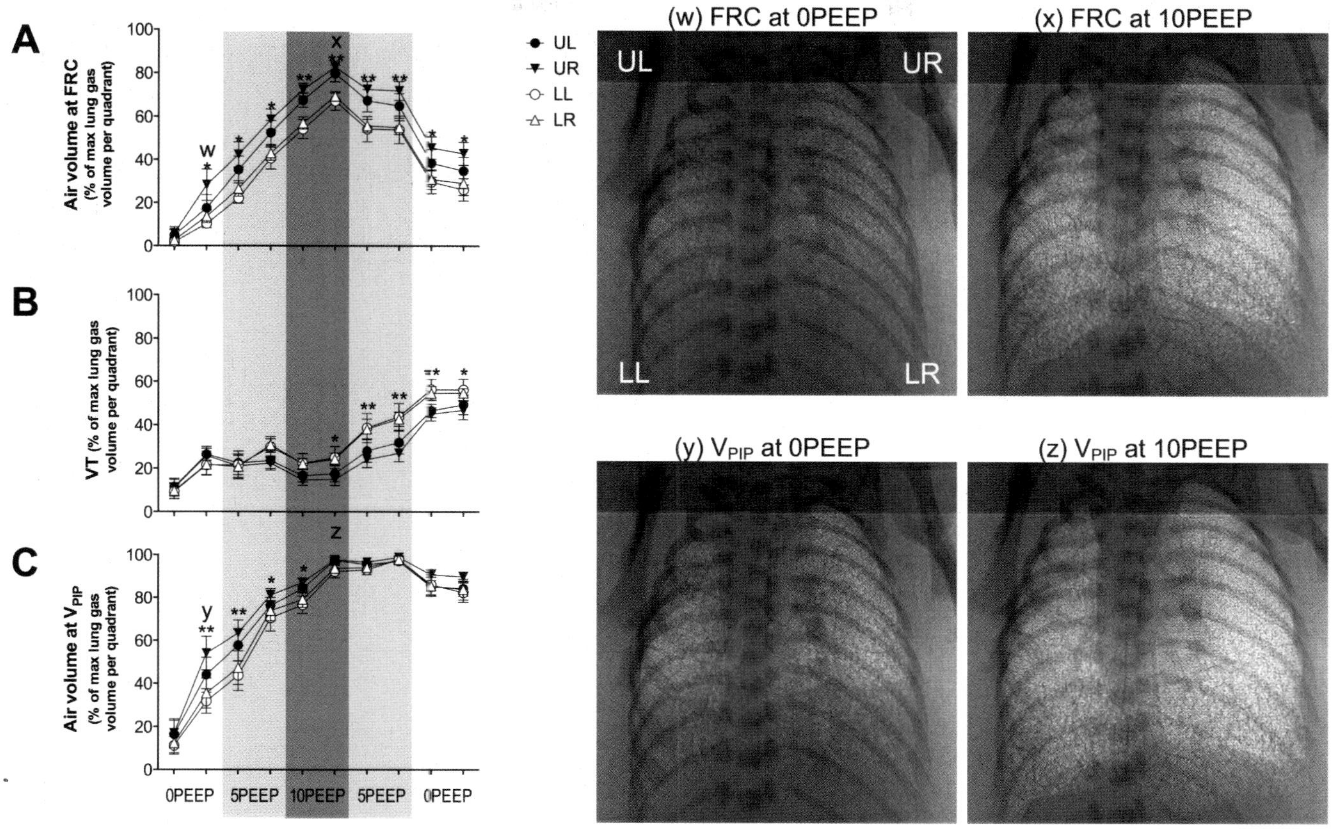

Figure 2. Changes in FRC, V_T and V_{PIP} during ventilation with Strategy A. Distribution of ventilation (A) at functional residual capacity (FRC), (B) of the incoming tidal volume (V_T) and (C) volume at peak inflation pressure (V_{PIP}) in the upper right (open triangles), upper left (closed triangles), lower right (open circles) and lower left (closed circles) regions of the lung during ventilation with Strategy A. Asterisks (*) indicate that UR quadrant is significantly different to the lower quadrants. Double asterisks (**) indicate that the upper quadrants are significantly different to the lower quadrants. Values are significantly different if $p<0.05$. Lower case letters (w-z) correspond to when phase contrast X-ray images of lung aeration at FRC and at V_{PIP} were acquired.

0.05). Reducing PEEP to 0PEEP increased the air volumes in the UR quadrant at FRC and reduced the amount in the LL quadrant (UR 36.3±5.1% and UL 30.6±3.6% vs LL 18.7±3.9% and LR 24.8±5.0%; $p<0.05$). This non-uniform distribution of air in the lungs at FRC persisted during the remainder of the experimental period; relative air volumes in the UR and LL quadrants at FRC remained greater and lower, respectively, than the other quadrants ($p<0.05$).

Distribution of incoming V_T (Fig 3B). Initially at 5PEEP, the distribution of incoming air with each inflation was relatively even across all quadrants, increasing from ~10% to 30% of total volume at end-inspiration. However, following ventilation at 10PEEP, decreasing the PEEP to 0PEEP resulted in a significantly smaller proportion of the V_T entering the UR quadrant ($p<0.05$), compared with the other quadrants, despite the UR quadrant having the highest proportional air volume at FRC. This indicates that some airway closure and gas trapping may have resulted from the sudden reduction in PEEP. Importantly, subsequent ventilation at 5PEEP did not alter this pattern, with the majority of incoming V_T being distributed towards the lower quadrants (~44%; $p<0.05$) rather than upper quadrants (~30%).

Air distribution at V_{PIP} (Fig 3C). During the initial 5PEEP and 10PEEP recruitment periods, the distribution of air in the lung at V_{PIP} predominantly occurred in the upper quadrants, whereas the LL quadrant aerated the least ($p<0.05$). Following ventilation at 10PEEP, all quadrants were similarly aerated at V_{PIP} and subsequent PEEP changes maintained this uniform distribution of air ($p>0.05$).

Changes in ventilation distribution: Strategy C

Air distribution at FRC (Fig 4A). Initiating ventilation with 10PEEP rapidly increased FRC and this air was uniformly distributed across all 4 quadrants of the lung ($p<0.05$). Decreasing the PEEP to 5PEEP, significantly decreased relative air volumes at FRC within the lower quadrants compared with the UR quadrant, which did not change ($p<0.05$). When PEEP was decreased further to 0PEEP, the air volume at FRC in all quadrants rapidly decreased, but the retention of air in the UR quadrant was better than in all other quadrants ($p<0.05$). This pattern of non-uniform air distribution at FRC was abolished by subsequent ventilation with 10PEEP, but returned during the second period of ventilation with 0PEEP.

Distribution of incoming V_T (Fig 4B). Initiating ventilation at birth with 10PEEP resulted in a relatively uniform distribution of the V_T across all quadrants ($p>0.05$). Reducing PEEP to 5PEEP increased V_T in all quadrants, but there was less V_T entering the UR compared to the lower quadrants ($p<0.05$); the UL was not significantly different to any quadrant ($p>0.05$). This non-uniform pattern of incoming V_T distribution was also observed during both 0PEEP ventilation periods but was not observed at the end of the second 10PEEP ventilation period.

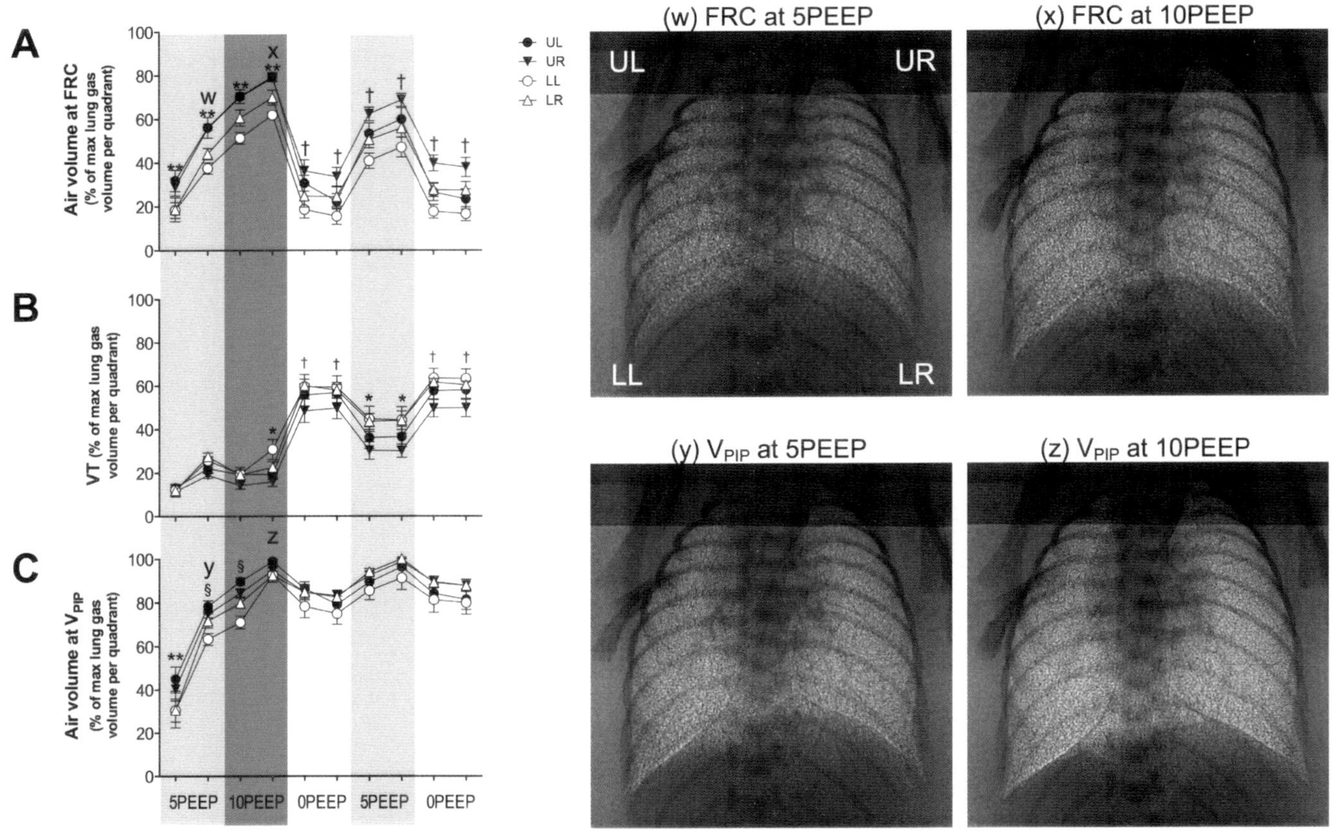

Figure 3. Changes in FRC, V_T and V_{PIP} during ventilation with Strategy B. Distribution of ventilation (A) at functional residual capacity (FRC), (B) of the incoming tidal volume (V_T) and (C) volume at peak inflation pressure (V_{PIP}) in the upper right (open triangles), upper left (closed triangles), lower right (open circles) and lower left (closed circles) regions of the lung during ventilation with Strategy B. Asterisks (*) indicate that UR quadrant is significantly different to the lower quadrants. Double asterisks (**) indicate that the upper quadrants are significantly different to the lower quadrants. Daggers (†) indicate that UR quadrant is significantly different to all other quadrants. Section symbol (§) indicates that the LL quadrant is significantly different to all other quadrants. Values are significantly different if $p<0.05$. Lower case letters (w-z) correspond to when phase contrast X-ray images of lung aeration at FRC and at V_{PIP} were acquired.

During this time, the distribution of V_T was again relatively uniform across all quadrants ($p>0.05$).

Air distribution at V_{PIP} (Fig 4C). Ventilation with 10PEEP rapidly increased lung air volumes at V_{PIP}, which were remarkably uniform across all 4 quadrants. Importantly, this uniform distribution of air between quadrants at V_{PIP} persisted even during both periods of ventilation with 0PEEP, indicating that the initial ventilation with 10PEEP has persisting benefits on the uniformity of ventilation at V_{PIP}.

V_T and FRC changes in response to decreasing PEEP in a ventilated lung

During ventilation strategies A and B, decreasing the PEEP by 5 cmH_2O steps to 0PEEP, (ie from 10 to 5 to 0PEEP during Strategy A or from 5 to 0PEEP during Strategy B) caused a small reduction in FRC and an increase in V_T, with the relative changes in both V_T and FRC being similar in all quadrants (Fig 5). In contrast, a large and continuous decrease in PEEP (ie from 10 to 0PEEP during Strategy C), resulted in changes in V_T and FRC that were not evenly distributed across all quadrants. Indeed, compared to PEEP reductions of only $5cmH_2O$, continuous PEEP reductions of $10cmH_2O$ caused larger reductions in FRC and increases in V_T in both lower quadrants ($p<0.05$; Fig. 5). For instance in the LL quadrant the increase in V_T was markedly greater following the change from 10 to 0PEEP compared with the 10-5-0PEEP change ($42.8\pm3.9\%$ vs $31.1\pm5.5\%$, $p<0.05$, Fig. 6A).

Changes in regional dynamic lung compliance (C_L)

During all PEEP strategies, dynamic lung compliance was higher in the lower than in the upper quadrants, primarily due to size differences between quadrants, and increased with increasing lung aeration. However, this increase was markedly greater in pups that commenced ventilation with PEEP. The gradual time-related increase in dynamic lung compliance for all strategies was associated with both increasing and decreasing PEEP levels (Fig 6). Initiating ventilation with either 5 or 10PEEP resulted in much greater lung compliances, particularly in the lower lobes, irrespective of the PEEP level. Indeed, at the midway point of the experiment, when pups in strategy A were ventilated with 10PEEP and pups in both other strategies were ventilated with 0PEEP, dynamic compliances were markedly higher in all quadrants in pups ventilated with Strategies B and C, compared to Strategy A. Similarly, during the last ventilation phase, when all pups were ventilated with 0PEEP, dynamic lung compliances were higher if ventilation commenced with PEEP, particularly within both lower quadrants.

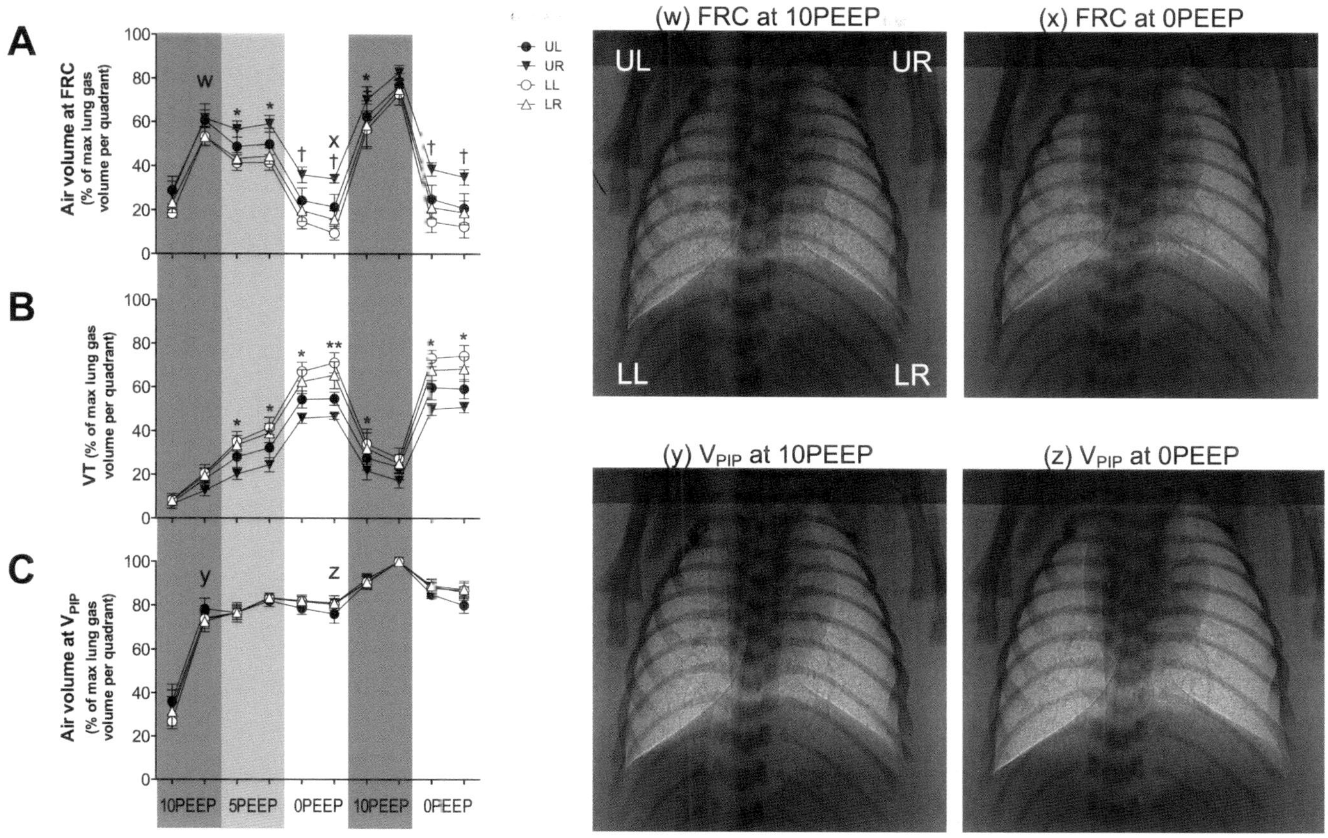

Figure 4. Changes in FRC, V_T and V_{PIP} during ventilation with Strategy C. Distribution of ventilation (A) at functional residual capacity (FRC), (B) of the incoming tidal volume (V_T) and (C) volume at peak inflation pressure (V_{PIP}) in the upper right (open triangles), upper left (closed triangles), lower right (open circles) and lower left (closed circles) regions of the lung during ventilation with Strategy C. Asterisks (*) indicate that UR quadrant is significantly different to the lower quadrants. Double asterisks (**) indicate that the upper quadrants are significantly different to the lower quadrants. Daggers (†) indicate that UR quadrant is different to all other quadrants. Values are significantly different if $p<0.05$. Lower case letters (w-z) correspond to when phase contrast X-ray images of lung aeration at FRC and at V_{PIP} were acquired.

Discussion

Our findings indicate that ventilating preterm rabbits with different and changing PEEP levels markedly effects the distribution of ventilation within the lung and on lung compliance during the immediate newborn period. We have used the quantitative capability [18] and high spatial resolution of phase contrast X-ray imaging to measure the distribution of air in the lung at both FRC and end-inspiration (V_{PIP}) as well as the relative distribution of the incoming V_T with each inflation. We found that, in preterm rabbit pups, changes in PEEP rapidly changed the distribution of air in the lung at FRC and the relative spatial distribution of the incoming V_T. Initiating ventilation at birth with 0PEEP, not only resulted in the lowest air volumes in all quadrants, the relative distribution of air between quadrants was not uniform, resulting in a significantly greater distribution of air towards the upper compared to the lower quadrants at FRC. Importantly, this unequal distribution of air at FRC persisted throughout the experiment even after subsequent ventilation at 5 and 10PEEP. Similarly, although initiating ventilation with 5PEEP increased lung air volumes compared to 0PEEP, the relative distribution of air was again unequal, being significantly greater in the upper compared to the lower quadrants, and persisted throughout the experimental period, even after ventilation with 10PEEP. In contrast, initiating ventilation with 10PEEP resulted in rapid FRC accumulation, which was uniformly distributed across all quadrants at both FRC and V_{PIP}. Although subsequent ventilation with 5PEEP and 0PEEP resulted in the preferential distribution of air into the upper quadrants at FRC, the distribution of air at V_{PIP} remained remarkably uniform across all quadrants. As a result, during ventilation with 5 and 0PEEP in this group, the incoming V_T was preferentially directed into the lower lung quadrants. These data indicate that initiating ventilation at birth with higher PEEP levels has effects on the distribution of ventilation in the lung at both FRC and V_{PIP} that temporarily persist even at different subsequent PEEP levels.

The immature lung is prone to collapse at end-expiration because of its low tissue compliance, high surface tension and a highly compliant chest wall. PEEP or CPAP can prevent atelectasis by acting as an internal "splint" to promote FRC maintenance (see [21–24]. Our results also demonstrate that initiating ventilation with high PEEP levels (i.e. 10PEEP) promoted uniform air distribution at both FRC and V_{PIP} (Fig. 4A) whereas lower PEEPs demonstrated a more non-uniform air distribution, with lower quadrants less ventilated than upper quadrants (Fig. 2A and 3A). It is possible that the momentum of deflating lung tissue during expiration influences the distribution of air in the lung at FRC. As momentum is the product of an object's mass and velocity, the larger mass of lung tissue in the lower quadrants may generate greater momentum during expiration and be more prone to collapse than the upper quadrants, which have a smaller mass. Thus, medium PEEP levels (5PEEP) are able to

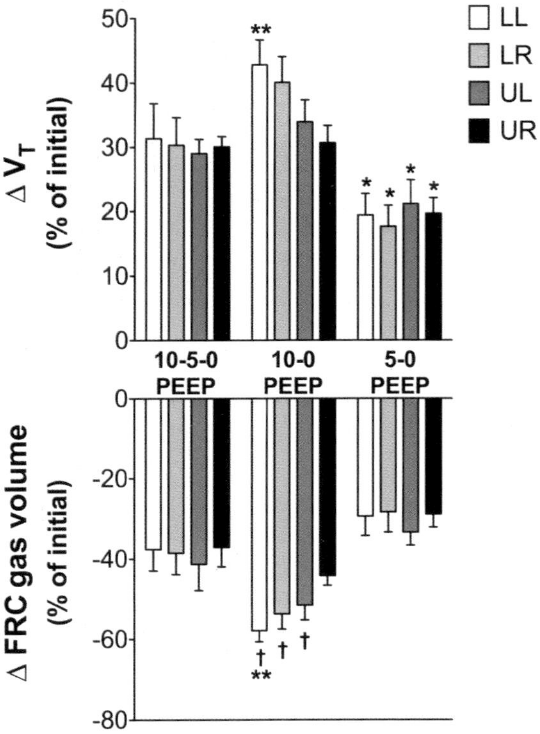

Figure 5. Changes in V_T and FRC during decreasing PEEP. The increase in tidal volume (V_T) and decrease in functional residual capacity (FRC) when positive end-expiratory pressure (PEEP) is decreased in 5 cmH_2O stepwise decrements (10-5-0PEEP), large steps (10-0PEEP) and from a small step (5-0PEEP) in the ventilated lung. Asterisks (*) indicate that values during 5-0PEEP are significantly different to their corresponding quadrant during 10-5-0PEEP and 10-0PEEP. Double asterisks (**) indicate that values during 10-5-0PEEP are significantly different to their corresponding quadrant during 10-0PEEP. Daggers (†) indicate that values during 5-0PEEP are significantly different to their corresponding quadrant during 10-0PEEP. Values are significantly different if $p<0.05$. There was no significant difference between quadrants within any group.

oppose lung collapse in the upper lung quadrants, which have a smaller mass, whereas higher PEEP levels are required to oppose lung collapse in regions with a greater mass. Alternatively, regional differences in chest wall compliance, with the upper chest being less compliant, may account for the regional differences in FRC across the lung.

The persisting effects that the initial PEEP level had on the distribution of air within the lung at FRC during the experiment, despite subsequent changes in PEEP, are difficult to explain. When ventilation was initiated with 0 or 5PEEP, the non-uniform distribution of air at FRC persisted at all PEEP levels throughout the experiment, even during ventilation with 10PEEP. However, when ventilation was initiated with 10PEEP, the distribution of air at FRC was uniform and although the uniformity decreased with decreasing PEEP, it was restored by ventilation with 10PEEP. This indicates that the initial distribution of lung aeration may define the subsequent mechanical behaviour of localised lung regions, with regions that do not initially aerate persisting with lower compliances and lower air volumes at FRC no matter what the subsequent PEEP setting. Further studies are required to determine whether this effect PEEP extends for longer than the duration of this experiment.

In contrast to many studies that investigate the distribution of lung ventilation in supine patients [15–17,25,26], our study imaged newborn rabbit pups positioned upright in a water-filled plethysmograph. It is possible that the upright positioning of the pups during ventilation contributed to the greater distribution of air in the upper compared to the lower quadrants, although we would expect this to have been more apparent if the pups were supine due to the effect of the abdominal contents pushing the diaphragm. In this experiment, the overall influence of gravity on the lung is likely to be minimal as the pups were ventilated whilst suspended in a water-filled plethysmograph. This alleviates the weight of the more vertical lungs regions and the heart on the lower regions thus reducing the dependent/non-dependent lung effect. It also removes the influence of the abdominal contents and the upward displacement of the diaphragm on the lung that would occur if the pup were positioned horizontally. As such, the position of the pup is not expected to significantly influence the distribution of ventilation. As neonates are normally positioned supine or prone, the non-uniform ventilation distributions we observed may exist and be amplified in infants. Ventilation heterogeneity would be expected due to the effects of gravity between non-dependent and dependent lung regions [17,25] and the pressure applied by abdominal contents on the diaphragm, which displaces it into the thorax. Ventilation inhomogeneity has been observed in ventilated infants lying supine, prone and quarter prone, but the authors suggest that ventilation distribution is minimally impacted by gravity [26].

Previous studies have cautioned against the use of high PEEP levels because it can reduce pulmonary blood flow (PBF) [27,28], overexpand alveoli and increase the risk of lung injury [29]. As such, PEEP levels as high as 10 cmH_2O are not recommended for neonates, but in those studies, the newborn lungs were aerated before the high PEEP level was applied. Thus, it is not known whether high PEEP levels during lung aeration at birth cause similar effects. A recent study has shown that an initial sustained inflation of ~1 min (to 35 cmH_2O) induces a greater increase in PBF than conventional ventilation [30]. This indicates that a sustained increase in airway pressure during lung aeration does not have the same negative impact on PBF as it does once the lung has aerated. In our study, none of the rabbit pups developed a pneumothorax, despite appearing maximally aerated at V_{PIP} during ventilation with 10PEEP (see Movies S1–S3, during the period of 10PEEP ventilation). More specifically, when ventilation commenced with 10PEEP, the lungs did not maximally aerate at V_{PIP} during the initial 10PEEP period. This suggests that the lungs were not over-expanded, either globally or in any one region by initiating ventilation with a temporary period of 10PEEP. Furthermore, a short period of ventilation with 10PEEP at birth was found to confer considerable benefit resulting in a remarkably uniform distribution of air across the lung during subsequent ventilation. While there are more familiar methods to promote uniform lung ventilation at birth, such as sustained inflations [23] and prophylactic surfactant [5], initial ventilation with a high PEEP level may be a more practical alternative.

There are many studies demonstrating multiple advantages of PEEP/CPAP on lung aeration and gas exchange in newborns, however, it is difficult to deliver these pressures uninterrupted in the delivery room. Not all positive pressure ventilation devices deliver a set PEEP reliably [31,32] and face mask leak is common [33] and if large (>60%) substantially reduces the effective PEEP level [12]. Our results suggest that if the loss of PEEP is gradual (i.e. 10-5-0PEEP), or if the reduction in PEEP is small (i.e. 5-0PEEP), the changes in V_T and FRC are relatively uniform throughout the lung. (Fig. 5). However, large and continuous reductions in PEEP (i.e. 10-0PEEP) caused large changes in V_T and FRC predominantly within in the lower lung quadrants

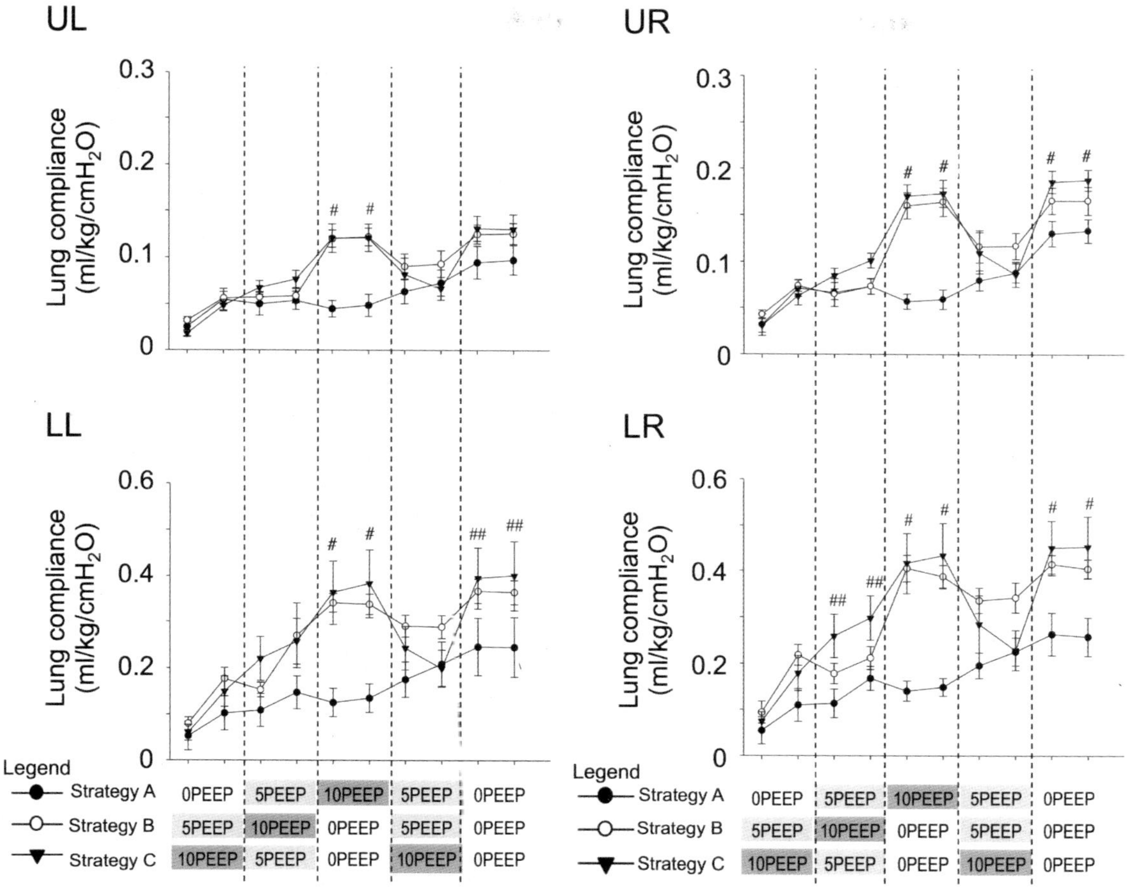

Figure 6. Changes in lung compliance in ventilation strategies A, B and C. Lung compliance of each quadrant (upper left (UL), upper right (UR), lower left (LL) and lower right (LR)) compared between Strategy A (closed circles), Strategy B (open circles) and Strategy C (closed triangles). The x-axis demonstrates the timing and sequence of PEEP change for each strategy. Hashes (#) indicate that Strategy A was significantly different to Strategy B and C. Double hashes (##) indicate that Strategy A was different only to Strategy C. Values are significantly different if $p<0.05$.

(Fig. 5). In the delivery room, respiratory support is often interrupted to reposition the facemask, perform suction, to change mask size, to change the interface for transport and during transfer of the infant to a transportation crib. Previous studies in preterm infants at 7 days of postnatal age have shown that such a rapid reduction in PEEP reduces FRC by as much as 30% within a minute of removing the PEEP [34]. Based on our results, sudden and large losses in PEEP would alter the distribution of ventilation within the lungs, causing marked reductions in FRC and greater V_T changes in the dependent lobes thereby increasing the risk of shear stress injury in these regions. While such interruptions in respiratory support are often necessary, the risks could be minimised by 1) reducing the PEEP gradually and 2) reducing the size of the dependent lung by placing the infant on its side, preferably the left.

It is unclear why the degree of continuous PEEP decrease affected the distribution of air at FRC and the incoming V_T, as the total changes in lung air volumes at 0PEEP were the same between 10-0PEEP and 10-5-0PEEP (data not shown). It is unlikely to be due to the rate of PEEP decrease, because the maximum rate of PEEP decrease was ~1 cmH_2O per inflation, such that a 5 cmH_2O decrease required ~5 inflations and a 10 cmH_2O decrease required ~10 inflations. It is possible that a large continuous decrease in PEEP generates momentum within the lung tissue, particularly in the lower quadrants with larger masses, resulting in larger decreases in FRC with each expiration. However, when the decrease in PEEP was interrupted by a period of ventilation at 5PEEP, the distribution of ventilation between quadrants remained relatively even despite the reduction to 0PEEP, again indicating that previous PEEP history can impact on the distribution of ventilation within the lung.

It is likely that the lower lung quadrants had greater volume changes in response to changes in PEEP because these lung regions are larger and are thus more compliant (Fig. 6). It may appear counter intuitive that dynamic lung compliance in all quadrants gradually increased during ventilation with both an increasing (Strategy A) and decreasing (Strategy B) PEEP strategy. Increasing PEEP and PEEP recruitment strategies are known to increase lung compliance by allowing tidal expansion to occur within a more compliant region of the pressure volume curve [11,35]. However, these pups were premature and surfactant deficient and the initial dynamic compliance measurements are dominated by the presence of airway liquid, which increases airway resistance ~100 fold [20]. Thus, the gradual increase in lung compliance mainly reflects the gradual increase in lung aeration. As such, our findings indicate that the presence of airway liquid is the dominant determinant of dynamic lung compliance during lung aeration. However, following complete lung aeration (usually after ventilation with 10PEEP), increasing PEEP from 0PEEP (Strategies B & C) mostly reduced measures of dynamic lung compliance, whereas decreasing PEEP to 0PEEP increased dynamic lung compliance. Furthermore, during the final 0PEEP ventilation period in all strategies, regional lung compliance, particularly in the lower quadrants, was markedly greater if ventilation had commenced with PEEP (either 5 or 10 cmH_2O) compared with 0PEEP. Although the mechanism is unknown, our study demonstrates that initiating ventilation with PEEP effects subsequent ventilation. These effects were observed for 10 minutes in our experiment but, as lung aeration continues to increase, these affects will likely persist beyond the experimental period.

After the lungs had fully aerated (ie after ventilation with 10PEEP in all strategies), as all pups were ventilated with a set PIP of 35 cmH_2O, the air volumes and the distribution of air at V_{PIP} remained relatively stable at all subsequent PEEP levels. Thus, although V_{PIP} tended to decrease at 0PEEP, the increase and decrease in V_T associated with decreases and increases in PEEP, respectively, mainly resulted from decreases and increases in FRC. This indicates that the effect of PEEP on the pressure-volume (P-V) relationship of the aerating lung immediately after birth is substantially different than it is following complete lung aeration. We found that altering the PEEP level had little or no effect on lung air volumes at V_{PIP}, resulting in a lower V_T when the FRC increased in response to a higher PEEP. How this effects CO_2 clearance is unclear as, although V_T is reduced which would normally increase CO_2 retention, our previous study has shown that V_{PIP} is a primary determinant of CO_2 clearance during lung aeration [36].

At birth, as the lungs make their transition from a liquid-filled to an air-filled organ, changes in PEEP have a marked influence on the distribution of ventilation. Our results demonstrate that when initiating ventilation at birth, the uniformity of ventilation depends on the level of PEEP, with higher PEEPs promoting more uniform ventilation. As such, it is possible that starting infant resuscitation with higher PEEP levels and then gradually reducing the PEEP to currently recommended levels after a few minutes may increase the distribution of ventilation in preterm infants. Furthermore, after the lungs were fully aerated, larger continuous changes in PEEP reduced ventilation within the lower lung quadrants to a greater extent than in the upper lung quadrants. Since providing consistent assisted ventilation at birth is difficult, due to face mask leak or the need to temporarily remove pressure support, it is important to acknowledge that changes in PEEP, even brief, are not without impact on lung volumes and ventilation distribution that can persist. These effects may impair gas exchange or increase the risk of lung damage.

Supporting Information

Movie S1 Phase contrast X-ray movie of a preterm rabbit pup ventilated with Strategy A (0-5-10-5-10PEEP).

Movie S2 Phase contrast X-ray movie of a preterm rabbit pup ventilated with Strategy B (5-10-0-5-0PEEP).

Movie S3 Phase contrast X-ray movie of a preterm rabbit pup ventilated with Strategy C (10-5-0-10-0PEEP).

Author Contributions

Conceived and designed the experiments: ABtP SBH MJK MLS. Performed the experiments: MJK MLS MJW AF RAL NY KU ABtP SBH. Analyzed the data: MJK MLS. Contributed reagents/materials/analysis tools: MJK. Wrote the paper: MJK MLS ABtP SBH MJW AF RAL NY KU.

References

1. Hooper SB, Harding R (2005) Role of aeration in the physiological adaptation of the lung to air-breathing at birth. Current Respiratory Medicine Reviews 1: 185–195.
2. te Pas AB, Davis PG, Kamlin CO, Dawson J, O'Donnell CP, et al. (2008) Spontaneous breathing patterns of very preterm infants treated with continuous positive airway pressure at birth. Pediatric Research 64: 281–285.
3. Mortola JP (1984) Breathing pattern in newborns. J Appl Physiol 56: 1533–1540.
4. Jobe AH, Ikegami M (2000) Lung development and function in preterm infants in the surfactant treatment era. AnnuRevPhysiol 62 825–846.
5. Siew ML, te Pas AB, Wallace MJ, Kitchen MJ, Islam M, et al. (2011) Surfactant increases the uniformity of lung aeration at birth in ventilated preterm rabbits. Pediatr Res 70: 50–55.
6. Enhorning G, Robertson B, Milne E, Wagner R (1975) Radiologic evaluation of the premature newborn rabbit after pharyngeal deposition of surfactant. Am J Obstet Gynecol 121: 475–480.
7. Gerhardt T, Bancalari E (1980) Chestwall compliance in full-term and premature infants. Acta Paediatrica Scandinavica 69: 359–364.
8. Hjalmarson O, Sandberg K (2002) Abnormal lung function in healthy preterm infants. Am J Respir Crit Care Med 165: 83–87.
9. Siew ML, te Pas AB, Wallace MJ, Kitchen MJ, Lewis RA, et al. (2009) Positive end expiratory pressure enhances development of a functional residual capacity in preterm rabbits ventilated from birth. J Appl Physiol 106: 1487–1493.
10. Probyn ME, Hooper SB, Dargaville PA, McCallion N, Crossley K, et al. (2004) Positive end expiratory pressure during resuscitation of premature lambs rapidly improves blood gases without adversely affecting arterial pressure. Pediatric Research 56: 198–204.
11. Nilsson R, Grossmann G, Robertson B (1980) Artificial ventilation of premature newborn rabbits: effects of positive end-expiratory pressure on lung mechanics and lung morphology. Acta Paediatrica Scandinavica 69: 597–602.
12. te Pas AB, Schilleman K, Klein M, Witlox RS, Morley CJ, et al. (2011) Low versus high gas flow rate for respiratory support of infants at birth: a manikin study. Neonatology 99: 266–271.
13. Schilleman K, Schmolzer GM, Kamlin OC, Morley CJ, te Pas AB, et al. (2011) Changing gas flow during neonatal resuscitation: a manikin study. Resuscitation 82: 920–924.
14. Tingay DG, Copnell B, Grant CA, Dargaville PA, Dunster KR, et al. (2010) The effect of endotracheal suction on regional tidal ventilation and end-expiratory lung volume. Intensive Care Med 36: 888–896.
15. Puybasset L, Gusman P, Muller JC, Cluzel P, Coriat P, et al. (2000) Regional distribution of gas and tissue in acute respiratory distress syndrome. III. Consequences for the effects of positive end-expiratory pressure. Intensive Care Medicine 26: 1215–1227.
16. Nieszkowska A, Lu Q, Vieira S, Elman M, Fetita C, et al. (2004) Incidence and regional distribution of lung overinflation during mechanical ventilation with positive end-expiratory pressure. Critical Care Medicine 32: 1496–1503.
17. Wolf GK, Grychtol B, Frerichs I, van Genderingen HR, Zurakowski D, et al. (2007) Regional lung volume changes in children with acute respiratory distress syndrome during a derecruitment maneuver. Crit Care Med 35: 1972–1978.
18. Kitchen MJ, Lewis RA, Morgan MJ, Wallace MJ, Siew MLL, et al. (2008) Dynamic measures of lung air volume using phase contrast X-ray imaging. Phys Med Biol 53: 6065–6077.
19. Hooper SB, Kitchen MJ, Wallace MJ, Yagi N, Uesugi K, et al. (2007) Imaging lung aeration and lung liquid clearance at birth. FASEB J 21: 3329–3337.
20. te Pas AB, Siew M, Wallace MJ, Kitchen MJ, Fouras A, et al. (2009) Effect of sustained inflation length on establishing functional residual capacity at birth in ventilated premature rabbits. Pediatric Research 66: 295–300.
21. Siew ML, Wallace MJ, Kitchen MJ, Lewis RA, Fouras A, et al. (2009) Inspiration regulates the rate and temporal pattern of lung liquid clearance and lung aeration at birth. J Appl Physiol 106: 1888–1895.
22. Dinger J, Topfer A, Schaller P, Schwarze R (2001) Effect of positive end expiratory pressure on functional residual capacity and compliance in surfactant-treated preterm infants. Journal of Perinatal Medicine 29: 137–143.
23. te Pas AB, Siew M, Wallace MJ, Kitchen MJ, Fouras A, et al. (2009) Establishing functional residual capacity at birth: the effect of sustained inflation and positive end expiratory pressure in a preterm rabbit model. Pediatr Res 65: 537–541.
24. Thome U, Topfer A, Schaller P, Pohlandt F (1998) The effect of positive endexpiratory pressure, peak inspiratory pressure, and inspiratory time on functional residual capacity in mechanically ventilated preterm infants. European Journal of Pediatrics 157: 831–837.
25. Frerichs I, Schiffmann H, Oehler R, Dudykevych T, Hahn G, et al. (2003) Distribution of lung ventilation in spontaneously breathing neonates lying in different body positions. Intensive Care Med 29: 787–794.
26. Hough JL, Johnston L, Brauer S, Woodgate P, Schibler A (2013) Effect of body position on ventilation distribution in ventilated preterm infants. Pediatr Crit Care Med 14: 171–177.
27. Polglase GR, Morley CJ, Crossley KJ, Dargaville P, Harding R, et al. (2005) Positive end-expiratory pressure differentially alters pulmonary hemodynamics

and oxygenation in ventilated, very premature lambs. J ApplPhysiol 99: 1453–1461.
28. Schlessel JS, Susskind H, Joel DD, Bossuyt A, Harrold WH, et al. (1989) Effect of PEEP on regional ventilation and perfusion in the mechanically ventilated preterm lamb. JNuclMed 30: 1342–1350.
29. Naik AS, Kallapur SG, Bachurski CJ, Jobe AH, Michna J, et al. (2001) Effects of ventilation with different positive end-expiratory pressures on cytokine expression in the preterm lamb lung. AmJRespirCrit Care Med 164: 494–498.
30. Sobotka KS, Hooper SB, Allison BJ, Pas ABT, Davis PG, et al. (2011) An Initial Sustained Inflation Improves the Respiratory and Cardiovascular Transition at Birth in Preterm Lambs. Pediatric Research 70: 56–60.
31. Dawson JA, Gerber A, Kamlin COF, Davis PG, Morley CJ (2011) Providing PEEP during neonatal resuscitation: Which device is best? Journal of Paediatrics and Child Health 47: 698–703.
32. Morley CJ, Dawson JA, Stewart MJ, Hussain F, Davis PG (2010) The effect of a PEEP valve on a Laerdal neonatal self-inflating resuscitation bag. Journal of Paediatrics and Child Health 46: 51–56.
33. Schmolzer GM, Kamlin OC, O'Donnell CP, Dawson JA, Morley CJ, et al. (2010) Assessment of tidal volume and gas leak during mask ventilation of preterm infants in the delivery room. ArchDisChildFetal Neonatal Ed 95: F393–F397.
34. Vilstrup CT, Bjorklund LJ, Larsson A, Lachmann B, Werner O (1992) Functional residual capacity and ventilation homogeneity in mechanically ventilated small neonates. JApplPhysiol 73: 276–283.
35. Kelly E, Bryan H, Possmayer F, Frndova H, Bryan C (1993) Compliance of the respiratory system in newborn infants pre- and postsurfactant replacement therapy. Pediatric Pulmonology 15: 225–230.
36. Hooper SB, Fouras A, Siew ML, Wallace MJ, Kitchen MJ, et al. (2013) Expired CO2 levels indicate degree of lung aeration at birth. PLoS One 8: e70895.

Association between Different Indexations of Extravascular Lung Water (EVLW) and PaO_2/FiO_2

Wolfgang Huber[1]*, Josef Höllthaler[1], Tibor Schuster[2], Andreas Umgelter[1], Michael Franzen[1], Bernd Saugel[1], Colin Cordemans[3], Roland M. Schmid[1], Manu L. N. G. Malbrain[3]

1 II. Medizinische Klinik und Poliklinik, Klinikum rechts der Isar der Technischen Universität München, München, Germany, **2** Institut für Medizinische Epidemiologie und Statistik, Klinikum rechts der Isar der Technischen Universität München, München, Germany, **3** Department of Intensive Care, Ziekenhuis Netwerk Antwerpen, Antwerpen, Belgium

Abstract

Background: Variability of body weight (BW) and height calls for indexation of volumetric hemodynamic parameters. Extravascular lung water (EVLW) has formerly been indexed to *actual* BW (BW_{act}) termed EVLW-index (EVLWI). In overweight patients indexation to BW_{act} might inappropriately lower indexed $EVLWI_{act}$. Several studies suggest indexation of EVLWI to *predicted* BW ($EVLWI_{pred}$). However, data regarding association of $EVLWI_{act}$ and $EVLW_{pred}$ to mortality and PaO_2/FiO_2 are inconsistent. Two recent studies based on biometric database-analyses suggest indexation of EVLWI to height ($EVLWI_{height}$). Therefore, our study compared the association of un-indexed EVLW, $EVLWI_{height}$, $EVLW_{pred}$ and $EVLWI_{act}$ to PaO_2/FiO_2 and Oxygenation index (OI = mean airway pressure*FiO_2*/PaO_2).

Methods: A total of 2119 triplicate transpulmonary thermodilutions (TPTDs; PiCCO; Pulsion Medical-Systems, Germany) were performed in 50 patients from the evaluation, and 181 patients from the validation groups. Correlations of EVLW and EVLWI to PaO_2/FiO_2, OI and ROC-AUC-analyses regarding $PaO_2/FiO_2<200$ mmHg (primary endpoint) and OI>10 were performed.

Results: In the evaluation group, un-indexed EVLW (AUC 0.758; 95%-CI: 0.637-0.880) and $EVLWI_{height}$ (AUC 0.746; 95%-CI: 0.622-0.869) provided the largest ROC-AUCs regarding $PaO_2/FiO_2<200$ mmHg. The AUC for $EVLWI_{pred}$ was smaller (0.713). $EVLWI_{act}$ provided the smallest AUC (0.685). This was confirmed in the validation group: $EVLWI_{height}$ provided the largest AUC (0.735), $EVLWI_{act}$ (0.710) the smallest. In the merged data-pool, AUC was significantly greater for $EVLWI_{height}$ (0.729; 95%-CI: 0.674–0.784) compared to all other indexations including $EVLWI_{act}$ (ROC-AUC 0.683, p = 0.007) and $EVLWI_{pred}$ (ROC-AUC 0.707, p = 0.015). The association of EVLW(I) was even stronger to OI compared to PaO_2/FiO_2. In the merged data-pool, $EVLWI_{height}$ provided the largest AUC regarding "OI>10" (0.778; 95%-CI: 0.713–0.842) compared to 0.739 (95%-CI: 0.669–0.810) for $EVLWI_{act}$ and 0.756 (95%-CI: 0.688–0.824) for $EVLWI_{pred}$.

Conclusions: Indexation of EVLW to height ($EVLWI_{height}$) improves the association of EVLW(I) to PaO_2/FiO_2 and OI compared to all other indexations including $EVLWI_{pred}$ and $EVLWI_{act}$. Also considering two recent biometric database analyses, EVLWI should be indexed to height.

Editor: Jörn Karhausen, Duke University Medical Center, United States of America

Funding: The authors have no support or funding to report.

Competing Interests: Wolfgang Huber, Bernd Saugel and Manu LNG Malbrain received lecture fees and are members of the Medical Advisory Board of Pulsion Medical Systems, Feldkirchen, Germany. All other authors have no conflict of interest.

* Email: wolfgang.huber@lrz.tum.de

Introduction

Extravascular lung water (EVLW) is a measure of the interstitial, alveolar and lymphatic fluid content of the lungs. EVLW and its indexation to body weight (EVLWI) became routinely available after the introduction of single-indicator transpulmonary thermodilution (TPTD) [1–5]. A number of animal and clinical studies demonstrated an association of EVLW(I) to mortality and to parameters of pulmonary function such as PaO_2/FiO_2 [5–19]. Variability of body weight (BW) and height strongly calls for biometric adjustment and indexation. *Ideally*, appropriate indexation should be based on a limited number of routinely available biometric data, and it should result in consistent normal values for patients with different height, weight, age, gender and race [20–21]. Originally actual body weight (BW_{act}) was used for indexation of EVLW. However, triggered by a rapidly increasing number of obese patients [22, 23], the question arose as to *which* weight to choose for EVLW indexation since indexation to BW_{act} might inappropriately decrease $EVLWI_{act}$ in obese patients. Based on a better correlation to mortality, a number of studies have suggested indexation of EVLW to predicted BW ($EVLWI_{pred}$) (see Table 1) [12: 14]. However, data are inconsistent regarding other endpoints: e.g. if available data provide worse [12], similar [14, 16] or slightly better correlation of $EVLWI_{pred}$ to PaO_2/FiO_2 than $EVLWI_{act}$ [13]. In one of the most recent studies [15], "Chew et al. found that EVLW indexed to absolute body weight resulted in a stronger association with outcome" including mortality compared to $EVLWI_{pred}$ [24]. Despite the overall strong predictive capacity of EVLWI in this and other recent trials [12–19], these inconsistencies demonstrate the need to optimize indexation of EVLW. Therefore, we recently analyzed a prospectively maintained database regarding the association of EVLW to biometric data [18]. This study demonstrated that height was the only biometric parameter independently associated to EVLW. These data were recently confirmed by Wolf et al., using a similar approach in a surgical group [19]. Despite these conclusive data, both studies did not investigate, if indexation of EVLW to height ($EVLWI_{height}$) provides better association to pulmonary function and outcome. Furthermore, all these trials were mono-centric.

Therefore, this two-center study compared the association of PaO_2/FiO_2 (and other outcome markers) to EVLW (un-indexed), $EVLWI_{act}$, $EVLWI_{pred}$, $EVLWI_{height}$ and EVLWI indexed to other biometric indices. To provide sufficient balance of biometric data, we investigated a group with a representative distribution of body mass index (BMI) [22], as well as an unselected second group from a second center.

Materials and Methods

Munich-evaluation-group

The institutional ethics committee approved the study (Ethikkommission Technische Universität München; Fakultät für Medizin; No. 3049/11). Patients on mechanical ventilation monitored using TPTD regardless of the study were included in the prospectively maintained database. The need for informed consent was waived due to the non-interventional design of the study. The patients included in this study completely distinct to the group previously analysed regarding the association of EVLW to biometric data [18].

To provide a representative distribution regarding bodyweight [22], we included 15 consecutive patients with BMI≥30 kg/m², 15 consecutive patients with 25≤BMI<30 kg/m² and 20 consecutive patients with a normal BMI (<25 kg/m²) irrespective of fulfilling the criteria of acute respiratory distress syndrome (ARDS). Conscious patients were asked for actual biometric data. In unconscious patients body weight and height were extracted from the patients records. In case of doubt height was verified using a flexible tape measure in the supine position.

A 5-F thermistor-tipped femoral arterial line (PV2025L20, Pulsiocath, Pulsion Medical Systems, Munich, Germany) connected to the PiCCO monitor device (PiCCO-Plus; Pulsion Medical Systems) was used for TPTD measurements. The mean EVLW was measured based on TPTD performed in triplicate with 15 ml cold saline 0.9%.

Antwerp-validation-group

Retrospective analysis of data from a prospectively developed independent cohort was performed for the first 7 days of ICU admission. Data of 181 critically ill patients requiring mechanical ventilation and TPTD-hemodynamic monitoring treated in two ICU's in ZNA Campus Stuivenberg, Antwerp, Belgium were collected prospectively. Ethics approval had been obtained and due to the retrospective analysis and non-intervention-nature of the study the need for informed consent was waived (project number EC 3765; Commisie voor Medische Ethiek, Ziekenhuisnetwerk Antwerpen 2020). Parts of the data not related to EVLW-indexation have already been published in Annals of Intensive Care [25, 26].

The measuring technique was identical to the Munich-evaluation-group, with the only difference being that three 20 ml boluses of cooled saline were used for TPTD.

Mean length of the ICU-stay in the Munich group was 27.2±21.4 days with a range of 3 to 120 days. In the Antwerp group the mean ICU stay was 25.9±41.7 days with a range of 1to 429 days.

Table 1. Indexations of extravascular lung water (index) EVLW/EVLWI.

$EVLWI_{act}$ = $EVLW/BW_{act}$		
$ELWI_{pred}$ = $EVLW/BW_{pred}$	BW_{pred} = Predicted body weight [kg]:	Male: 50+0.91 ×(height − 152.4)
		Female: 45.5+0.91 ×(height − 152.4)
$EVLWI_{id}$ = $EVLW/BW_{id}$	BW_{id} = Ideal body weight [kg]:	Male: (height − 100) ×0.9
		Female: (height − 100) ×0.85
$EVLWI_{adj}$ = $EVLW/BW_{adj}$	Adjusted body weight [kg]:	Male: $ideal_{male}BW$ + (actual BW − $ideal_{male}BW$) ×0.4
		Female: $ideal_{female}BW$ + (actual BW − $ideal_{female}BW$) ×0.4
$EVLWI_{height}$ = EVLW/height [cm]		
$EVLWI_{BMI}$ = EVLWI/BMI	BMI = Body Mass Index [kg/m²]:	BW_{act} [kg]/(height[m])²
$EVLWI_{BSA}$ = $EVLW/BSA_{Dubois}$	BSA_{Dubois} [m²] =0.007184*weight [kg]$^{0.425}$*height [cm]$^{0.725}$	
$EVLWI_{TLC}$ = EVLW/TLC	TLC = Total Lung Capacity TLC [L]:	Male: 7.99*height [m] −7.08
		Female: 6.60*height [m] − 5.79

Endpoints and Statistics

1) **Weight and weight-correction formula based indexations.** To compare the distribution of normal (EVLWI< 7 ml/kg), slightly elevated (7≤EVLWI<10 ml/kg) and markedly elevated EVLWI (EVLWI≥10 ml/kg) in dependency of the indexation, un-indexed EVLW was indexed according to actual ($EVLWI_{act}$), predicted ($EVLWI_{pred}$), ideal ($EVLWI_{id}$) and adjusted BW ($EVLWI_{adj}$) using the formulas mentioned in Table 1. The cut-offs of 10 ml/kg and 14 ml/kg have been demonstrated to be associated with ARDS [15] and mortality [5].

- *Intra-group comparisons*: For the weight-related indexations, intragroup comparisons of weight-correction based $EVLWI_{pred}$, $EVLWI_{id}$ and $EVLWI_{adj}$ to $EVLWI_{act}$ were performed for all patients and the subgroups with BMI<25 kg/m^2, 25≤BMI<30 kg/m^2 and BMI≥30 kg/m^2 (Wilcoxon-test for paired samples; Table 2).

- *Inter-group comparisons*: Furthermore, we compared EVLWI according to all investigated indexations (also including $EVLWI_{height}$, $EVLWI_{BMI}$, $EVLWI_{BSA}$ and $EVLWI_{TLC}$) between patients with BMI<25 kg/m^2 and patients with BMI≥30 kg/m^2 (Wilcoxon-test for unpaired samples; Table 2).

2) **Association of EVLW(I) to PaO_2/FiO_2 and oxygenation index (OI= mean airway pressure * F_iO_2 * PaO_2^{-1}).** For appropriate analysis of multiple serial measurements in 231 patients from the two groups several statistical analyses were performed:

  2a.) Prediction of critical thresholds of PaO_2/FiO_2 and oxygenation index: The clinically relevant prediction of critical thresholds of "PaO_2/FiO_2<200 mmHg" (primary endpoint) and "OI>10" by EVLW(I) was investigated using receiver operating characteristics area under the curve (ROC-AUC) analyses of all measurements.

  2b.) Inter-individual ("between-subject") correlations: Furthermore, correlations of EVLW and differently indexed EVLWI to PaO_2/FiO_2 and oxygenation index (OI= mean airway pressure * F_iO_2 * PaO_2^{-1}) were calculated. Since multiple serial measurements within 241 different patients were available, we analysed *inter-* and *intra-*individual correlations.

To correct for different numbers of measurements for each patient, the means of EVLW(I), PaO_2/FiO_2 and OI were calculated for each individual patient ("one point per patient"). Subsequently the correlations between EVLW(I) and PaO_2/FiO_2 and between EVLWI and OI were calculated.

  2c.) Intra-individual ("within subject") correlations: The above-mentioned "one point per patient" analyses reflect the *inter-individual* association of EVLW(I) to PaO_2/FiO_2 and OI. However, in cases of multiple serial measurements within different patients, *between-subject heterogeneity* may obscure correlations *on an individual level (within subject correlation)* which might be even more interesting than the inter-individual association. The effect of the confounder (between-subject heterogeneity) can be removed by calculating "partial" correlation between EVLW(I) and PaO_2/FiO_2 (or OI) adjusting for heterogeneity of different patients (individual patient number/identifier as the adjustment factor).

3) **Mortality analysis.** Better prediction of mortality by EVLWI according to any indexation might be related to the direct association of the indexation to mortality. To overcome this problem, multiple binary logistic regression analysis regarding mortality included the first and last values of *unindexed* EVLW as well as BW_{act}, height, gender and acute physiology and chronic health evaluation (version 2, APACHE-II).

All analyses were performed separately in both groups and in the merged data, with the only exceptions being intergroup-comparisons and mortality analyses which were restricted to the BMI-representative Munich-evaluation-group. Results of merged data were considered superior to those derived from sub-groups. No correction of p-values was applied to adjust for multiple testing. However, results of all statistical tests being conducted were thoroughly reported so that an informal adjustment of p-values can be performed while reviewing the data [27].

All statistical tests were conducted 2-sided and a p-value <0.05 was considered to indicate statistical significance. The software used was IBM SPSS statistics, version 20.

Results

Patients' characteristics

A total of 2119 TPTDs (each with triplicate TPTD) were performed in 231 patients from both groups.

Table 2 summarizes the patients' characteristics of both groups.

1) **Weight and weight-correction formula based indexations.** *Comparison of $EVLWI_{act}$, $EVLWI_{pred}$, $EVLWI_{id}$ and $EVLWI_{adj}$*: Table 2 demonstrates that in the Munich-evaluation-group mean values of $EVLWI_{pred}$, $EVLWI_{adj}$ and $EVLWI_{id}$ were significantly *higher* than $EVLWI_{act}$ in the subgroups of patients with BMI≥30 kg/m^2 and with 25≤ BMI<30 kg/m^2 as well as for the totality of patients (*intra*-BMI-group-comparison). By contrast, $EVLWI_{pred}$ and $EVLWI_{adj}$ were significantly *lower* than $EVLWI_{act}$ in the subgroup of patients with a *normal* BMI.

Similarly, in the Antwerp-validation-group mean values of $EVLWI_{pred}$, $EVLWI_{adj}$ and $EVLWI_{id}$ were higher than mean the $EVLWI_{act}$.

Impact of indexation according to different weight correction-formulas for the classification of EVLWI: Distribution of EVLWI-values classified as normal (EVLWI<7 ml/kg), moderately elevated (7 ml/kg≤EVLWI<10 ml/kg) and markedly elevated EVLWI (EVLWI≥10 ml/kg) significantly varied among the patients with a BMI≥30 kg/m^2 as well as in the total patient groups depending on the weight used for indexation of EVLWI (Fig. 1). For example in patients with a BMI≥30 kg/m^2, 51% (133/263) of $EVLWI_{act}$ measurements were within the normal range (EVLWI<7 ml/kg). By contrast only 16% (43/263; p< 0.001 vs. $EVLWI_{act}$), 14%, (38/263; p<0.001) and 30% of the measurements (79/263; p<0.001) were within the normal range if EVLWI was indexed according to predicted, ideal and adjusted BW, respectively. In addition to the different distributions of EVLWI classifications, different indexations obviously had an impact on the coefficient of variation (COV), in particular in patients with a BMI≥30 kg/m^2 (Table 2). COV amongst these

Table 2. Patients' characteristics.

	Munich-Evaluation-Group								Antwerp-Validation-Group	
	All patients		**BMI<25 kg/m²**		**25≤BMI<30 kg/m²**		**BMI≥30 kg/m²**		**All patients from Antwerp**	
Gender	22 female, 28 male		6 female, 14 male		7 female, 8 male		9 female, 6 male		62 female, 119 male	
Age	64.1±14.8 years		67.6±14.3		62.5±18.7		63.3±11.2		62.4±16.4	
Weight	82.0±23.5		63.9±9.2		78.7±12.2		105.1±29.2		74.5±17.6	
Height	169±10.1		169±9.0		172±13.0		169±8.9		170.1±11.6	
Body mass index	28.3±6.7		22.0±1.9		27.4±1.3		35.9±6.3		25.6±5.5	
APACHE II-Score	24.9±9.8		25.7±8.6		23.2±7.8		24.6±9.2		22.9±10.3	
Etiology									Respiratory failure:	
Sepsis	21		11		3		7		- acute on chronic 11/181	
Pneumonia/ARDS	11		3		3		5		- acute 152/181	
Liver cirrhosis	7		3		3		1		- coma 18/181	
Pancreatitis	4		1		2		1		Medical patients 158	
Other etiology	7		2		4		1		Surgical patients 23	
Parameter	**Mean ± SD**	**Median; COV**	**Mean ± SD**	**Median; COV**	**Mean ± SD**	**Median; COV**	**Mean ± SD**	**Median; COV**	**Mean ± SD**	**Median; COV**
EVLWI unindex.	716±363	637; 0.51	711±266	700; 0.37	618±270	560;0.44	783±469§	660; 0.60	773±346	683; 0.45
$EVLWI_{act}$	8.9±3.8	8; 0.43	11.2±3.7	11; 0.33	7.7±3.1	7; 0.40	7.4±3.0‡	6; 0.41	10.6±4.7	10; 0.44
$EVLWI_{pred}$	10.8±5.2†	9; 0.48	10.7±3.9†	10; 0.36	9.3±4.4†	8; 0.47	11.7±6.3†§	10; 0.54	11.9±5.7†	11; 0.48
$EVLWI_{id}$	11.2±5.4†	10; 0.48	11.2±4.1	11; 0.37	9.6±4.5†	8; 0.47	12.3±6.6†§	10; 0.54	12.3±5.9†	11; 0.48
$EVLWI_{ad}$	9.7±4.2†	9; 0.43	11.0±3.8†	11; 0.35	8.4±3.8†	7; 0.45	9.3±4.3†‡	8; 0.46	11.4±5.5†	10; 0.48
$EVLWI_{BMI}$	26.3±11.9	24.2; 0.45	32.9±11.7	31.4; 0.36	22.8±9.8	21.0; 0.43	22.0±10.4‡	20.0; 0.47	30.6±13.3	28.2; 0.43
$EVLWI_{BSA}$	370±155	329; 0.42	410±140	400; 0.34	322±132	283.8; 0.41	361±171‡	298.7; 0.47	415±178	372.1; 0.43
$EVLWI_{height}$	4.20±2.02	3.75; 0.48	4.19±1.50	4.06; 0.36	3.60±1.51	3.17; 0.42	4.6±2.6§	3.84; 0.57	4.52±2.00	4.00; 0.44
$EVLWI_{TLC}$	120±56	102; 0.47	119±43	111; 0.36	103±47	88; 0.46	132±69§	113; 0.52	124±62	110; 0.50
PaO_2	92.9±20.7	90.9; 0.22	94.5±20.1	91.6; 0.21	86.5±16.7	83.0; 0.19	95.1±22.1	96.0; 0.23	121.7±70	102; 0.58
FiO_2	0.47±0.16	0.45; 0.34	0.44±0.14	0.40; 0.32	0.51±0.17	0.50; 0.33	0.46±0.16	0.40; 0.35	59.6±24.9	50; 0.42
P_{aw}	13.5±4.4	13.0; 0.33	12.4±3.4	12.0; 0.27	13.5±4.4	13.0; 0.33	14.7±5.1	13.0; 0.35	15.7±4.3	15.6; 0.27
PaO_2/F_iO_2	219±82	211; 0.37	230±70	226; 0.30	182±76	170; 0.42	188±71	225; 0.38	242±115	229; 0.48
P_{aw}*PaO2/FiO2	7.05±5.95	5.9; 0.84	5.7±3.5	5.0; 0.61	8.1±5.9	7.0; 0.73	7.8±7.5	6.0; 0.96	8.8±0.64	6.8; 0.73
PEEP	8.6±3.0	8.0; 0.35	7.9±2.6	8.0; 0.33	8.9±3.3	8.0;0.37	9.1±3.0	8.0; 0.33	8.8±3.4	9.0; 0.39
Measurements	693		263		167		263		1426	

Intra-group comparison † $p<0.001$ vs. $EVLWI_{act}$ (for $EVLWI_{pred}$, $EVLWI_{id}$ and $EVLWI_{adj}$) within the same BMI-group.
Inter-group comparison ‡ $p<0.001$ group with BMI≥30 kg/m² vs. group with normal BMI (BMI<25 kg/m²).
(BMI≥30 kg/m² vs. BMI<25 kg/m²) § $p>0.05$ group with BMI≥30 kg/m² vs. group with normal BMI (BMI<25 kg/m²).

patients was markedly lower for $EVLWI_{act}$ (0.41) than for $EVLWI_{height}$ (0.57) or un-indexed EVLW (0.60). *Inter*-BMI-group-comparison demonstrated significantly lower values in patients with a BMI≥30 kg/m^2 for $EVLWI_{act}$, $EVLWI_{BMI}$, $EVLWI_{BSA}$ and $EVLWI_{adj}$, whereas there was no inter-group difference for EVLW, $EVLWI_{pred}$, $EVLWI_{id}$, $EVLWI_{height}$ and $EVLWI_{TLC}$. In conclusion, significant inter-BMI-group-differences were found only for $EVLWI_{act}$ and indexations including BW_{act} in their formulas (BW_{adj}, BMI and BSA) (Table 2).

2) **Association of EVLW(I) to parameters of pulmonary function.** *2a.) Prediction of "PaO_2/FiO_2<200 mmHg" (primary endpoint) and "OI>10"*: As demonstrated in Table 3, in the Munich-evaluation-group the greatest ROC-AUCs regarding *"PaO_2/FiO_2<200 mmHg"* were found for un-indexed EVLW (ROC-AUC 0.758; 95%-CI: 0.637–0.880) and $EVLWI_{height}$ (ROC-AUC 0.746; 95%-CI: 0.622–0.869). $EVLWI_{act}$ provided the lowest ROC-AUC (0.685, 95%-CI: 0.554–0.817)

In general, these observations were confirmed in the Antwerp-validation-group: $EVLWI_{height}$ had the highest predictive capability (ROC-AUC 0.735; 95%-CI: 0.674–0.796), whereas weight-indexed $EVLWI_{act}$ (ROC-AUC 0.710; 95%-CI: 0.648–0.773) and $EVLWI_{BMI}$ (ROC-AUC 0.704; 95%-CI: 0.641–0.767) provided the smallest ROC-AUCs.

Statistical analysis of the merged data of both groups demonstrated a number of significant differences between different indexations, summarized as follows:

1) The greatest ROC-AUC regarding *"PaO_2/FiO_2 < 200 mmHg"* was found for $EVLWI_{height}$ (ROC-AUC 0.729; 95%-CI: 0.674–0.784; primary endpoint)
2) The ROC-AUC was significantly greater for $EVLWI_{height}$ compared to all other indexations including $EVLWI_{act}$ (ROC-AUC 0.683; 95%-CI: 0.626–0.741; p = 0.007) and $EVLWI_{pred}$ (ROC-AUC 0.707; 95%-CI: 0.650–0.763; p = 0.015). Only un-indexed EVLW (ROC-AUC 0.728; 95%-CI: 0.673–0.783) and $EVLWI_{BSA}$ (ROC-AUC 0.718; 95%-CI: 0.663–0.774; p = 0.137) were not significantly inferior compared to $EVLW_{height}$.

Regarding the prediction of the threshold "OI>10", in both collectives as well as in the merged data, the largest ROC-AUCs were obtained for $EVLWI_{height}$ and EVLW, with the lowest for $EVLWI_{act}$ (Table 4): 0.737 (0.589–0.885), 0.732 (0.583–0.881) and 0.669 (0.502–0.835) in the Munich-evaluation-group, 0.778 (0.713–0.842), 0.771 (0.705–0.836), and 0.739 (0.669–0.810) in the

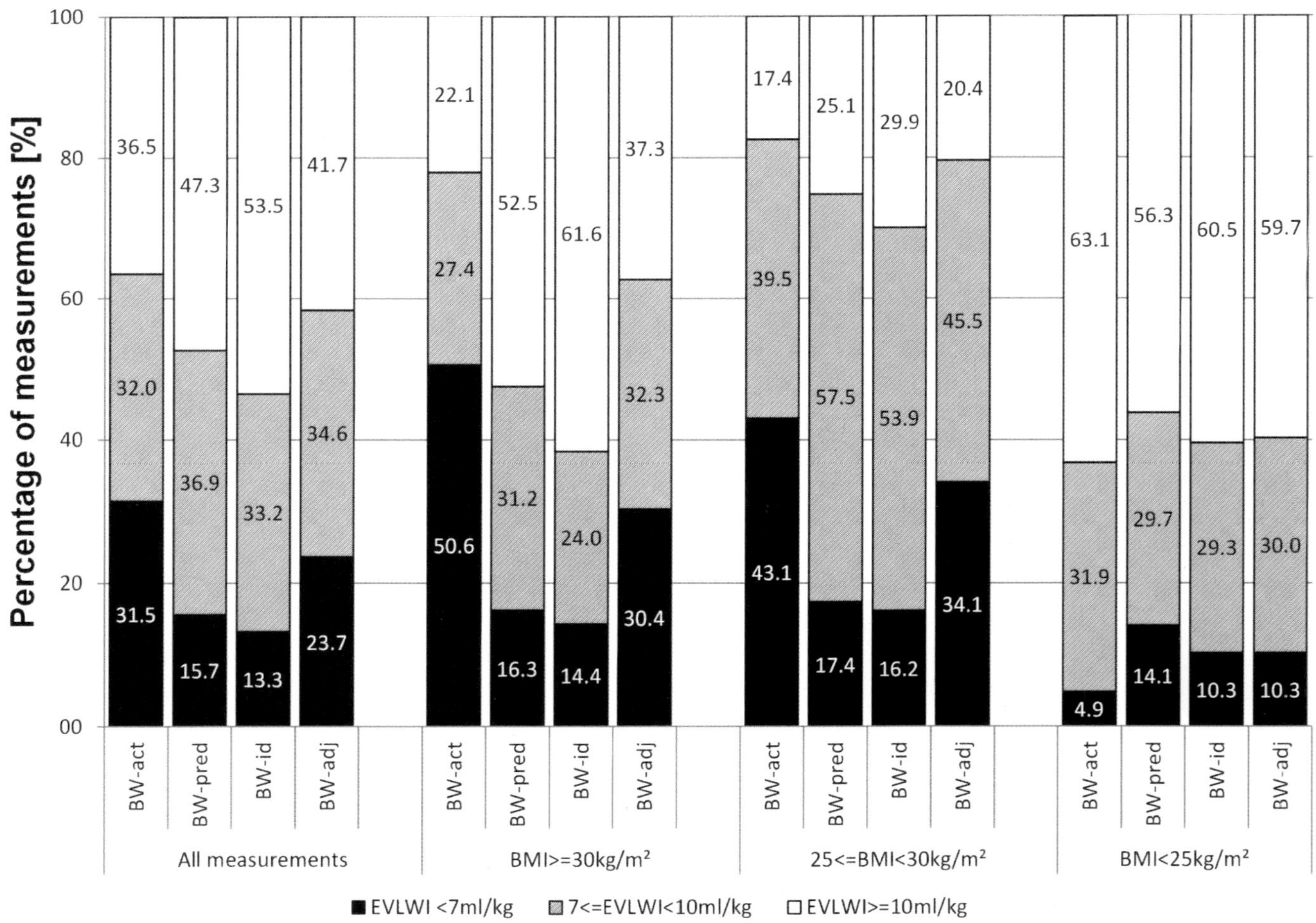

Figure 1. Distribution of measurements classified as "normal" (EVLWI<7 mL/kg), "moderately elevated" (7≤EVLWI<10 mL/kg) and "markedly elevated" (EVLWI≥10 mL/kg) depending on the indexation of EVLWI according to weight-based indexations to BW_{act}, BW_{pred}, BW_{id} and BW_{adj}. Numbers in the columns indicate the percentage of measurements within this classification (*p<0.05 and ** p<0.001 vs. percentage of normal measurements of $EVLWI_{act}$<7 mL/kg within the same BMI-category).

Table 3. Comparison of receiver operating characteristics area under the curve (ROC-AUC) regarding "$PaO_2/FiO_2<200$" and "Oxygenation-Index (OI)>10" depending on indexation of extravascular lung water (index) EVLW(I): ROC-AUCs for different indexations of EVLW(I) regarding "$PaO_2/FiO_2<200$" (left side of the table) and "OI>10" (right side of the table).

"ROC-AUCs regarding $PaO_2/FiO_2<200$ mmHg"				p-values for comparison of ROC-AUCs									ROC-AUCs regarding "OI>10"		
Patients		AUC	95%-CI	EVLW	$EVLWI_{act}$	$EVLWI_{pred}$	$EVLWI_{id}$	$EVLWI_{adj}$	$EVLW_{BMI}$	$EVLWI_{BSA}$	$EVLWI_{height}$	$EVLWI_{TLC}$		AUC	95%-CI
Total	EVLW	0.728	0.673–0.783		0.055	0.331	0.336	0.183	0.034*	0.377	0.215	0.304	EVLW	0.756	0.695–0.817
Total	$EVLWI_{act}$	0.683	0.626–0.741	0.017*		0.104	0.094	0.054	0.382	0.001*	0.017*	0.157	$EVLWI_{act}$	0.716	0.649–0.782
Total	$EVLWI_{pred}$	0.707	0.650–0.763	0.085	0.158		0.386	0.263	0.160	0.370	0.138	0.319	$EVLWI_{pred}$	0.748	0.686–0.810
Total	$EVLWI_{id}$	0.707	0.650–0.763	0.069	0.155	0.399		0.235	0.145	0.377	0.128	0.295	$EVLWI_{id}$	0.749	0.686–0.811
Total	$EVLWI_{adj}$	0.699	0.643–0.756	0.027*	0.109	0.284	0.279		0.141	0.070	0.050*	0.353	$EVLWI_{adj}$	0.739	0.675–0.802
Total	$EVLW_{BMI}$	0.693	0.636–0.750	0.021*	0.227	0.227	0.300	0.343		0.012*	0.019*	0.216	$EVLW_{BMI}$	0.719	0.653–0.785
Total	$EVLWI_{BSA}$	0.718	0.663–0.774	0.249	0.000*	0.215	0.201	0.005*	0.026*		0.198	0.342	$EVLWI_{BSA}$	0.752	0.691–0.814
Total	$EVLWI_{height}$	0.729	0.674–0.784	0.388	0.007*	0.015*	0.008*	0.005*	0.024*	0.137		0.136	$EVLWI_{height}$	0.762	0.702–0.822
Total	$EVLWI_{TLC}$	0.706	0.650–0.763	0.116	0.187	0.396	0.397	0.327	0.321	0.245	0.038*		$EVLWI_{TLC}$	0.745	0.682–0.807
				EVLW	$EVLWI_{act}$	$EVLWI_{pred}$	$EVLWI_{id}$	$EVLWI_{adj}$	$EVLW_{BMI}$	$EVLWI_{BSA}$	$EVLWI_{height}$	$EVLWI_{TLC}$			
Munich	EVLW	0.758	0.637–0.880		0.180	0.398	0.398	0.352	0.184	0.323	0.370	0.397	EVLW	0.732	0.583–0.881
Munich	$EVLWI_{act}$	0.685	0.554–0.817	0.076		0.184	0.175	0.101	0.351	0.109	0.135	0.169	$EVLWI_{act}$	0.669	0.502–0.835
Munich	$EVLWI_{pred}$	0.713	0.585–0.841	0.131	0.313		0.399	0.335	0.273	0.354	0.382	0.325	$EVLWI_{pred}$	0.729	0.580–0.879
Munich	$EVLWI_{id}$	0.710	0.581–0.839	0.091	0.328	0.373		0.324	0.264	0.345	0.379	0.350	$EVLWI_{id}$	0.730	0.580–0.880
Munich	$EVLWI_{adj}$	0.711	0.582–0.840	0.114	0.200	0.397	0.398		0.269	0.396	0.285	0.297	$EVLWI_{adj}$	0.714	0.560–0.869
Munich	$EVLW_{BMI}$	0.716	0.588–0.844	0.168	0.114	0.398	0.395	0.394		0.213	0.170	0.257	$EVLW_{BMI}$	0.681	0.517–0.845
Munich	$EVLWI_{BSA}$	0.728	0.602–0.855	0.137	0.072	0.319	0.272	0.156	0.349		0.213	0.327	$EVLWI_{BSA}$	0.716	0.562–0.870
Munich	$EVLWI_{height}$	0.746	0.622–0.869	0.180	0.107	0.130	0.070	0.129	0.271	0.212		0.399	$EVLWI_{height}$	0.737	0.589–0.885
Munich	$EVLWI_{TLC}$	0.707	0.577–0.836	0.123	0.351	0.305	0.382	0.392	0.392	0.285	0.121		$EVLWI_{TLC}$	0.736	0.588–0.884
				EVLW	$EVLWI_{act}$	$EVLWI_{pred}$	$EVLWI_{id}$	$EVLWI_{adj}$	$EVLW_{BMI}$	$EVLWI_{BSA}$	$EVLWI_{height}$	$EVLWI_{TLC}$			
Antwerp	EVLW	0.725	0.664–0.787		0.147	0.225	0.228	0.164	0.077	0.390	0.187	0.173	EVLW	0.771	0.705–0.836
Antwerp	$EVLWI_{act}$	0.710	0.648–0.773	0.301		0.296	0.286	0.256	0.395	0.003*	0.060	0.359	$EVLWI_{act}$	0.739	0.669–0.810
Antwerp	$EVLWI_{pred}$	0.723	0.661–0.784	0.390	0.326		0.294	0.366	0.290	0.173	0.036*	0.110	$EVLWI_{pred}$	0.756	0.688–0.824
Antwerp	$EVLWI_{id}$	0.724	0.662–0.785	0.395	0.315	0.225		0.353	0.280	0.177	0.033*	0.126	$EVLWI_{id}$	0.757	0.689–0.825
Antwerp	$EVLWI_{adj}$	0.722	0.660–0.783	0.383	0.250	0.397	0.391		0.251	0.013*	0.035*	0.394	$EVLWI_{adj}$	0.752	0.683–0.821
Antwerp	$EVLW_{BMI}$	0.704	0.641–0.767	0.173	0.337	0.268	0.254	0.165		0.016*	0.044*	0.353	$EVLW_{BMI}$	0.738	0.667–0.809
Antwerp	$EVLWI_{BSA}$	0.734	0.673–0.795	0.307	0.022*	0.264	0.275	0.100	0.024*		0.356	0.126	$EVLWI_{BSA}$	0.773	0.708–0.839
Antwerp	$EVLWI_{height}$	0.735	0.674–0.796	0.074	0.151	0.151	0.156	0.176	0.078	0.393		0.033*	$EVLWI_{height}$	0.778	0.713–0.842
Antwerp	$EVLWI_{TLC}$	0.716	0.654–0.778	0.329	0.383	0.069	0.079	0.353	0.345	0.183	0.098		$EVLWI_{TLC}$	0.750	0.681–0.819
				EVLW	$EVLWI_{act}$	$EVLWI_{pred}$	$EVLWI_{id}$	$EVLWI_{adj}$	$EVLW_{BMI}$	$EVLWI_{BSA}$	$EVLWI_{height}$				

*$p<0.05$.
In the middle of the table p-values for the comparison of ROC-AUCs according to different indexations are given.

Table 4. Intra- and inter-individual correlations of extravascular lung water (index) EVLW(I) to PaO_2/FiO_2.

Group	Parameter	Comparison to PaO_2/FiO_2				Comparison to oxygenation index(mean airway pressure* FiO_2*/PaO_2)			
		correlation of patient means (between-subject correlation; Spearman)		partial correlation: all measurements (within-subject correlation)		correlation of patient means (between-subject correlation; Spearman)		partial correlation: all measurements (within-subject correlation)	
		r-value	r^2-value	r-value	r^2-value	r-value	r^2-value	r-value	r^2-value
Munich	EVLW	−0.34*	0.12*	−0.74**	0.55**	0.44*	0.19**	0.80**	0.64**
Munich	$EVLWI_{act}$	−0.21	0.04	−0.66**	0.44**	0.32*	0.10**	0.57**	0.32**
Munich	$EVLWI_{pred}$	−0.27	0.07	−0.69**	0.48**	0.47*	0.22**	0.76**	0.58**
Munich	$EVLWI_{ideal}$	−0.26	0.07	−0.69**	0.48**	0.48**	0.23**	0.76**	0.58**
Munich	$EVLWI_{adj}$	−0.29*	0.08*	−0.68**	0.46**	0.46*	0.21**	0.68**	0.46**
Munich	$EVLW_{BMI}$	−0.26	0.07	−0.72**	0.52**	0.31*	0.10**	0.65**	0.42**
Munich	$EVLWI_{BSA}$	−0.28	0.08	−0.71**	0.50**	0.42*	0.18**	0.71**	0.50**
Munich	$EVLWI_{height}$	−0.32*	0.10*	−0.73**	0.53**	0.45*	0.20**	0.78**	0.61**
Munich	$EVLWI_{TLC}$	−0.26	0.07	−0.69**	0.48**	0.48**	0.23**	0.76**	0.58**
Antwerp	EVLW	−0.43**	0.18**	−0.68**	0.46**	0.45**	0.20**	0.76**	0.58**
Antwerp	$EVLWI_{act}$	−0.42**	0.18**	−0.63**	0.40**	0.40**	0.16**	0.72**	0.52**
Antwerp	$EVLWI_{pred}$	−0.43**	0.18**	−0.65**	0.42**	0.44**	0.19**	0.73**	0.53**
Antwerp	$EVLWI_{ideal}$	−0.43**	0.18**	−0.65**	0.42**	0.44**	0.19**	0.73**	0.53**
Antwerp	$EVLWI_{adj}$	−0.43**	0.18**	−0.62**	0.38**	0.43**	0.18**	0.70**	0.49**
Antwerp	$EVLW_{BMI}$	−0.38**	0.14**	−0.62**	0.38**	0.37**	0.14**	0.70**	0.49**
Antwerp	$EVLWI_{BSA}$	−0.46**	0.21**	−0.66**	0.44**	0.46**	0.21**	0.75**	0.56**
Antwerp	$EVLWI_{height}$	−0.45**	0.20**	−0.68**	0.46**	0.47**	0.22**	0.76**	0.58**
Antwerp	$EVLWI_{TLC}$	−0.41**	0.17**	−0.63**	0.40**	0.42**	0.18**	0.72**	0.52**
All Patients	EVLW	−0.39**	0.15**	−0.68**	0.46**	0.46**	0.21**	0.78**	0.61**
All Patients	$EVLWI_{act}$	−0.36**	0.13**	−0.60**	0.36**	0.39**	0.15**	0.69**	0.48**
All Patients	$EVLWI_{pred}$	−0.38**	0.14**	−0.63**	0.40**	0.46**	0.21**	0.75**	0.56**
All Patients	$EVLWI_{ideal}$	−0.37**	0.14**	−0.60**	0.36**	0.47**	0.22**	0.75**	0.56**
All Patients	$EVLWI_{adj}$	−0.38**	0.14**	−0.63**	0.40**	0.44**	0.19**	0.71**	0.50**
All Patients	$EVLW_{BMI}$	−0.34**	0.12**	−0.61**	0.37**	0.38**	0.14**	0.70**	0.49**
All Patients	$EVLWI_{BSA}$	−0.41**	0.17**	−0.65**	0.42**	0.47**	0.22**	0.74**	0.55**
All Patients	$EVLWI_{height}$	−0.41**	0.17**	−0.67**	0.45**	0.48**	0.23**	0.77**	0.59**
All Patients	$EVLWI_{TLC}$	−0.38**	0.14**	−0.63**	0.40**	0.44**	0.19**	0.74**	0.55**

Partial correlations were calculated with the individual patient as the controlling adjustment variable. *$p<0.05$ **$p<0.001$.

Antwerp-validation group and 0.762 (0.702–0.822), 0.756 (0.695–0.817) and 0.716 (0.649–0.782) for the merged data, respectively.

For the merged data, the AUC was significantly higher for $EVLWI_{height}$ (0.762) compared to $EVLWI_{act}$ (0.716; p = 0.017), $EVLWI_{adj}$ (0.739; p = 0.05) and $EVLWI_{BMI}$ (0.719; p = 0.019).

2b.), 2.c) Inter-individual and intra-individual correlations of EVLW(I)to PaO_2/FiO_2 and to oxygenation index: In general, the *inter*-individual association (represented by patients' means) of EVLW(I) to PaO_2/FiO_2 and OI was not as strong as the *intra*-individual association represented by partial correlations. Means of EVLW(I) and PaO_2/FiO_2 moderately correlated with r-values between −0.21 and −0.46. By contrast, *intra*-individual correlations represented by partial correlations provided r-values between −0.6 and −0.74 (Table 4).

Within the Munich-evaluation-group only the patients' means of EVLW, $EVLWI_{height}$ and $EVLWI_{adj}$ significantly correlated with PaO_2/FiO_2 (r = −0.34; p = 0.017, r = −0.32, p = 0.026 and r = −0.29; p = 0.041, respectively). In contrast, the patients' mean EVLWI according to all other indexations including $EVLWI_{pred}$ and $EVLWI_{act}$ did not correlate to PaO_2/FiO_2. Overall, the lowest r-values were found for $EVLWI_{act}$. The highest coefficients of correlations to PaO_2/FiO_2 were found for un-indexed EVLW and $EVLWI_{height}$ (Table 4).

However, in the same group all *partial* correlations of EVLW(I) and PaO_2/FiO_2 were highly significant (p<0.001) and provided coefficients of partial correlation between −0 66 and −0.74.

Similar data were obtained for the correlation between OI and EVLW and its indexations (Table 3). Intra-individual partial correlations with r-values between 0.57 and 0.80 were more pronounced than inter-individual correlations represented by r-values between 0.31 and 0.48 for correlations of patients' means. All these correlations were significant. In both groups as well as in the merged data the highest coefficients of correlation to OI were found for $EVLWI_{height}$ and EVLW, the lowest for $EVLWI_{act}$ (r-values for merged data 0.77, 0.78 and 0.69, respectively) (Table 4; partial correlation).

3) **Mortality analysis.** Univariable logistic regression analysis of the Munich-evaluation-group demonstrated a significant association between mortality with APACHE-II-Score (p = 0.005; 95%-CI: 1.063–1.422; β-coefficient of regression 0.207), but not with age (p = 0.262), height (p = 0.265) and BW_{act} (p = 0.123). The strongest association to mortality was found for the *last* EVLW (p = 0.001; 95%-CI: 1.185–2.035; β-coefficient of regression 0.440 for increments in EVLW of 100 ml). The *first* EVLW was associated with mortality with borderline significance (p = 0.054; 95%-CI: 0.098–1.350; β-coefficient of regression 0.149).

Subsequently, a multivariable logistic regression analysis regarding mortality was performed. A model including APACHE-II, the first and the last EVLW provided high predictive capabilities regarding mortality (Nagelkerkes $R^2 = 0.697$). First (p = 0.021) and last (p = 0.004) EVLW were independently associated to mortality. The APACHE-II score slightly failed to reach significance (p = 0.064), but markedly contributed to the R^2-value of the total model ($R^2 = 0.628$ without APACHE-II).

ROC-analysis (Figure 2) regarding mortality demonstrated high predictive capabilities of the model including APACHE-II as well as first and last EVLW (AUC 0.936; 95%-CI: 0.868–1.000; p< 0.001), which provided a markedly larger ROC-AUC than each of the included single parameters. Among single parameters, the last EVLW (AUC 0.868; 95%-CI: 0.765–0.970; p<0.001) and APACHE-II (AUC 0.779; 95%-CI: 0.636–0.923; p = 0.002) provided high predictive capabilities compared to the first EVLW (AUC 0.603; 95%-CI: 0.424–0.782; p = 0.244).

Discussion

Data regarding EVLW-indexation are contradictory. Therefore, our study investigated the association between different indexations of EVLW(I) to PaO_2/FiO_2 and OI in two groups with mechanical ventilation and representative distribution of BMI. Our study demonstrated that

1) indexation of EVLWI to BW_{act} is inferior to no indexation at all,
2) indexation to BW_{pred} might provide a certain improvement compared to indexation to BW_{act} and
3) indexation according to height or no indexation at all (EVLW) are superior to indexation to BW_{act} or BW_{pred}.

These results are – at first glance – surprising, as several studies have suggested BW_{pred} as the appropriate indexation factor [12–14].

Historically, different techniques have been established to quantify pulmonary edema termed as "EVLW" which was originally determined without indexation. Early studies frequently used animal models with post-mortem gravimetric determination of EVLW as the gold-standard [1, 2, 4, 10]. Regarding investigations in different species, indexation to BW_{act} provided "basic" indexation allowing *interspecies* comparisons between different animal and human data.

However, in obese patients indexation to BW_{act} might inappropriately diminish indexed $EVLWI_{act}$. Based on a better prediction of *mortality* rather than on a better correlation to PaO_2/FiO_2, superiority of $EVLWI_{pred}$ to $EVLWI_{act}$ has been suggested: In the study by Phillips et al. [12] including 19 patients, $EVLWI_{act}$ was not related to mortality. By contrast, mortality of the seven out of 19 patients was univariately associated to $EVLWI_{pred}$. However, $EVLWI_{act}$ obviously provided a better correlation to PaO_2/FiO_2 than $EVLWI_{pred}$ (coefficient of correlation: −0.525 for $EVLWI_{pred}$ and −0.773 for $EVLWI_{act}$). With only 19 patients included, this study did not approach a multivariate mortality-analysis. Another study that included 44 patients (225 measurements) demonstrated better discrimination of ARDS- and non-ARDS-patients by $EVLWI_{pred}$ compared to $EVLWI_{act}$ [13]. A third study (44 patients; 44 measurements) showed the improved association of mortality by $EVLWI_{pred}$ compared to $EVLWI_{act}$ in a multivariate model [14]. However, similarly to the data of Phillips et al. this study did not demonstrate a better correlation of $EVLWI_{pred}$ to PaO_2/FiO_2 compared to $EVLWI_{act}$ (coefficients of correlation −0.57 vs. −0.55). This is in accordance with two more recent studies suggesting a comparable [16] or even stronger [15] association of $EVLWI_{act}$ compared to $EVLWI_{pred}$ with mortality.

Nevertheless, mortality is multifactorial, also depending on "do-not-resuscitate" statements and might be directly associated to some of the components of indexation (weight, BMI) [28-36]. E.g. further analysis of the data by Phillips et al. demonstrates that mean EVLW and BMI were increased to a similar degree in the non-survivors compared to survivors (45% and 31%, respectively). Therefore, mortality is not an obvious endpoint to compare the appropriateness of different indexations of EVLWI, particularly when applied in small mono-centric collectives.

In our study-groups un-indexed EVLW - next to $EVLWI_{height}$ - provided the highest predictive capability regarding PaO_2/FiO_2 and OI. This indicates that particularly *weight*-based indexation

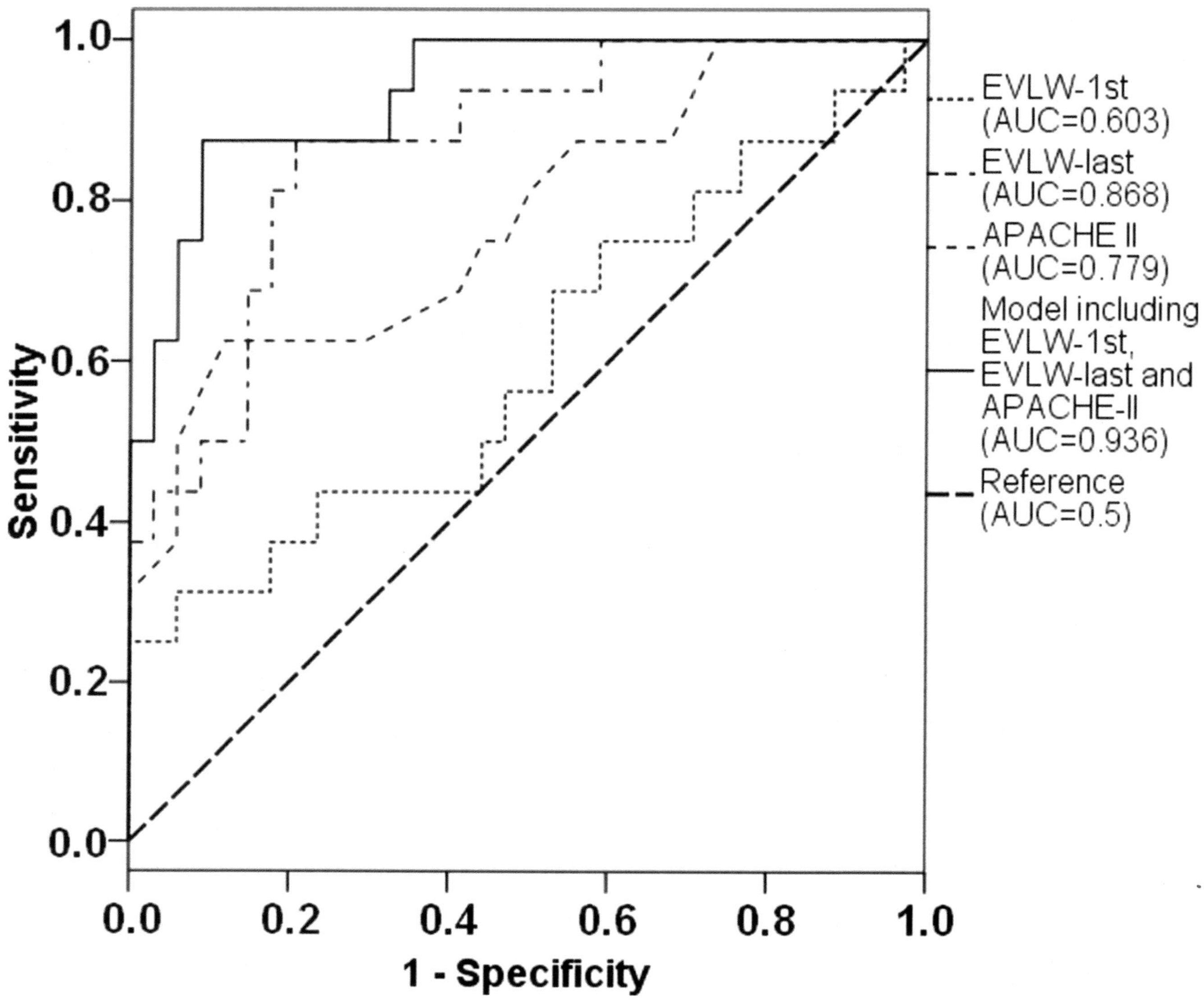

Figure 2. ROC curve regarding the prediction of mortality provided by first EVLW, last EVLW, APACHE-II and regression model combining first EVLW, last EVLW and APACHE-II.

might be a confounder rather than an improvement of the inter-individual comparison of EVLW(I) in an adult population. In the analysis of patients' means, PaO_2/FiO_2 was significantly associated to unindexed EVLW, $EVLWI_{height}$ and $EVLWI_{adj}$, whereas the correlation was not significant for all other indexations. These findings suggest that the association of EVLW(I) to PaO_2/FiO_2 might be obscured by inappropriate indexation. In general, the association of EVLW(I) was closer to OI compared to PaO_2/FiO_2. Including mean airway pressure in addition to PaO_2/FiO_2, OI also reflects the Positive End Expiratory Pressure (PEEP), peek and plateau pressure, ventilation mode (there is a usually higher mean airway pressure in controlled compared to assisted ventilation) as well as I:E ratio. Since the association of EVLW(I) to OI was not extensively investigated in the previous studies, the close association in our study might even strengthen the role of EVLW(I) as a parameter of pulmonary (patho)physiology.

With regard to indexation of other pulmonary parameters, the strong performance of height as an indexation for EVLWI is not surprising. As stated in recent consensus guidelines "lung volumes are related to body size, with standing height being the most important factor" [21].

Furthermore, a look at the "weight correction-formulas" demonstrates that BW_{pred} and BW_{id} (Table 1) do not contain any weight at all, but simply adjust height for gender and subtract a length-constant [20, 21, 28].

In addition to weight and height, the third major determinant of most indexation formulas is *gender*, which has impact on BW_{pred}, BW_{id}, BW_{adj} and TLC. With regard to the above-mentioned formulas, indexation according to BW_{id} increases EVLWI by 5.5% for women. $EVLWI_{pred}$ of women with a height between 150 and 190 cm is increased by 5–10% compared to men with the same height. However, this marked impact of gender on EVLW is not substantiated by our data: Multiple regression analysis regarding EVLW in our merged data including the variables age, height, weight, PaO_2/FiO_2 and gender demonstrated that gender was not independently associated to EVLW.

Finally, the question remains, whether in adults "no indexation at all" is the answer. Regarding our data in two adult groups with a high variability in body weight and BMI, but lower variability in height, this might be a reasonable option. However, it must be kept in mind that the variability in height was low in these groups: e.g. mean height in the Munich-evaluation-group was 170 ± 10 cm (median 171 cm, range 150–190 cm).

On the other hand it is self-evident that indexation will improve the predictive capabilities in a group with a higher variability of parameters closely associated to EVLW such as height. There is elaborate data on the pulmonary function parameters in children and adolescents: Normal values in these groups with high variability in height and weight are mainly adjusted to height [20, 21].

Limitations of the study

Despite the inclusion of two different groups and the large sample size compared to the previous data, our study has several limitations. Our Munich-evaluation-group was a preselected group of non-operative mechanically ventilated patients with a prolonged ICU-stay. Although this drawback might be - at least in part - outweighed by a re-evaluation in a large group of non-selected anesthesiology patients, the data of both groups might not apply to patients without pulmonary impairment. On the other hand, the significance of modest correlations with r-values as low as -0.29 require cautious interpretation, since large numbers of patients promote significance of modest associations. Furthermore, these data are mainly derived from Caucasians. Despite a "considerable lack of data on lung-volumes in non-Caucasians" [20, 37] at least two studies give hints on differences regarding TLC between whites and blacks [38], Polynesians, Northern Indians and Pakistanis [39–41]. Finally, we cannot extrapolate our results to a pediatric population in which indexation to height may be much more appropriate than unindexed EVLW which was comparable to $EVLW_{height}$ in our adult groups.

Conclusions

EVLW is a marker significantly associated to pulmonary function and mortality. Regarding the prediction of PaO_2/FiO_2 and OI, indexation of $EVLWI_{act}$ is inappropriate. $EVLWI_{pred}$ provides a slight improvement. The highest predictive capabilities in an adult population were found for $EVLWI_{height}$ and unindexed EVLW. Therefore, our data suggest that EVLW should be indexed to height ($EVLWI_{height}$) or remain unindexed in adults.

Acknowledgments

The authors would like to thank Analena Beitz and Benedikt Henschel for language revision.

Author Contributions

Conceived and designed the experiments: WH JH TS CC MM RS. Performed the experiments: WH JH AU MF BS CC MM. Analyzed the data: WH JH TS BS CC MM RS. Contributed to the writing of the manuscript: WH JH TS BS CC MM RS.

References

1. Neumann P (1999) Extravascular lung water and intrathoracic blood volume: double versus single indicator dilution technique. Intensive Care Med 25(2):216–219.
2. Rossi P, Wanecek M, Rudehill A, Konrad D, Weitzberg E, et al. (2006) Comparison of a single indicator and gravimetric technique for estimation of extravascular lung water in endotoxemic pigs. Crit Care Med 34(5):1437–1443.
3. Tagami T, Kushimoto S, Yamamoto Y, Atsumi T Tosa R, et al. (2010) Validation of extravascular lung water measurement by single transpulmonary thermodilution: human autopsy study. Crit Care 14(5) R162.
4. Kuzkov VV, Kirov MY, Sovershaev MA, Kuklin VN, Suborov EV, et al. (2006) Extravascular lung water determined with single transpulmonary thermodilution correlates with the severity of sepsis-induced acute lung injury. Crit Care Med 34(6):1647–1653.
5. Sakka SG, Klein M, Reinhart K, Meier-Hellmann A (2002) Prognostic value of extravascular lung water in critically ill patients. Chest 122(6):2080–2086.
6. Eisenberg PR, Hansbrough JR, Anderson D, Schuster DP (1987) A prospective study of lung water measurements during patient management in an intensive care unit. Am Rev Respir Dis 136(3):662–668.
7. Mitchell JP, Schuller D, Calandrino FS, Schuster DP (1992) Improved outcome based on fluid management in critically ill patients requiring pulmonary artery catheterization. Am Rev Respir Dis 145(5):990–998.
8. Fernandez-Mondejar E, Castano-Perez J, Rivera-Fernandez R, Colmenero-Ruiz M, Manzano F, et al. (2003) Quantification of lung water by transpulmonary thermodilution in normal and edematous lung. J Crit Care 18(4):253–258.
9. Groeneveld AB, Verheij J (2006) Extravascular lung water to blood volume ratios as measures of permeability in sepsis-induced ALI/ARDS. Intensive Care Med 32(9):1315–1321.
10. Kirov MY, Kuzkov VV, Kuklin VN, Waerhaug K, Bjertnaes LJ (2004) Extravascular lung water assessed by transpulmonary single thermodilution and postmortem gravimetry in sheep. Crit Care 8(6):R451–458.
11. Martin GS, Eaton S, Mealer M, Moss M (2005) Extravascular lung water in patients with severe sepsis: a prospective cohort study. Crit Care 9(2):R74–82.
12. Phillips CR, Chesnutt MS, Smith SM (2008) Extravascular lung water in sepsis-associated acute respiratory distress syndrome: indexing with predicted body weight improves correlation with severity of illness and survival. Crit Care Med 36(1):69–73.
13. Berkowitz DM, Danai PA, Eaton S, Moss M, Martin GS (2008) Accurate characterization of extravascular lung water in acute respiratory distress syndrome. Crit Care Med 36(6):1803–1809.
14. Craig TR, Duffy MJ, Shyamsundar M, McDowell C, McLaughlin B, et al. (2010) Extravascular lung water indexed to predicted body weight is a novel predictor of intensive care unit mortality in patients with acute lung injury. Crit Care Med 38(1):114–120.
15. Chew MS, Ihrman L, During J, Bergenzaun L, Ersson A, et al. (2012) Extravascular lung water index improves the diagnostic accuracy of lung injury in patients with shock. Crit Care 16(1):R1.
16. Mallat J, Pepy F, Lemyze M, Barrailler S, Gasan G, et al. (2012) Extravascular lung water indexed or not to predicted body weight is a predictor of mortality in septic shock patients. J Crit Care 27(4):376–83.
17. Jozwiak M, Silva S, Persichini R, Anguel N, Osman D, et al. (2013) Extravascular lung water is an independent prognostic factor in patients with acute respiratory distress syndrome. Crit Care Med 41(2):472–80.
18. Huber W, Mair S, Götz SQ, Tschirdewahn J, Siegel J, et al. (2013) Extravascular lung water and its association with weight, height, age, and gender: a study in intensive care unit patients. Intensive Care Med 39(1):146–50.
19. Wolf S, Riess A, Landscheidt JF, Lumenta CB, Schürer L, et al. (2013) How to perform indexing of extravascular lung water: a validation study. Crit Care Med 41(4):990–8.
20. Stocks J, Quanjer PH (1995) Reference values for residual volume, functional residual capacity and total lung capacity. ATS Workshop on Lung Volume Measurements. Official Statement of The European Respiratory Society. Eur Respir J 8(3):492–506.
21. Wanger J, Clausen JL, Coates A, Pedersen OF, Brusasco V, et al. (2005) Standardisation of the measurement of lung volumes. Eur Respir J 26(3):511–522.
22. Ogden CL, Carroll MD, Curtin LR, McDowell MA, Tabak CJ, et al. (2006) Prevalence of overweight and obesity in the United States, 1999–2004. JAMA: the journal of the American Medical Association 295(13):1549–1555.
23. Beutler S, Schmidt U, Michard F (2004) Hemodynamic monitoring in obese patients: a big issue. Crit Care Med 32(9):1981.
24. Camporota L, De Neef M, Beale R (2012) Extravascular lung water in acute respiratory distress syndrome: potential clinical value, assumptions and limitations. Crit Care 16(1):114.
25. Cordemans C, De laet I, Van Regenmortel N, Schoonheydt K, Dits H, et al. (2012) Aiming for negative fluid balance in patients with acute lung injury and increased intra-abdominal pressure: A pilot study looking at the effects of PAL treatment. Ann Intensive Care 2(Supplem 1):S15.
26. Cordemans C, De laet I, Van Regenmortel N, Schoonheydt K, Dits H, et al. (2012) Fluid management in critically ill patients: The role of extravascular lung water, abdominal hypertension, capillary leak and fluid balance. AnnIntensive Care 2(Supplem 1):S1.
27. Saville DJ (1990) Multiple comparison procedures—the practical solution. Am Statistician 44:174–180.
28. Pai MP, Paloucek FP (2000) The origin of the "ideal" body weight equations. Ann Pharmacother 34(9):1066–1069.
29. Akinnusi ME, Pineda LA, El Solh AA (2008) Effect of obesity on intensive care morbidity and mortality: a meta-analysis. Crit Care Med 36(1):151–158.

30. Sakr Y, Madl C, Filipescu D, Moreno R, Groeneveld J, et al. (2008) Obesity is associated with increased morbidity but not mortality in critically ill patients. Intensive Care Med 34(11):1999–2009.
31. Naimark A, Cherniack RM (1960) Compliance of the respiratory system and its components in health and obesity. J Appl Physiol 15:377–382.
32. Bedell GN, Wilson WR, Seebohm PM (1958) Pulmonary function in obese persons. J Clin Invest 37(7):1049–1060.
33. Ray CS, Sue DY, Bray G, Hansen JE, Wasserman K (1983) Effects of obesity on respiratory function. Am Rev Respir Dis 128(3):501–506.
34. Jones RL, Nzekwu MM (2006) The effects of body mass index on lung volumes. Chest 130(3):827–833.
35. Brivet FG (2012) Pulmonary vascular permeability index should not be called extravascular lung water pulmonary blood volume ratio. Crit Care 16(2):417.
36. O'Brien JM Jr, Phillips GS, Ali NA, Lucarelli M, Marsh CB, et al. (2006) Body mass index is independently associated with hospital mortality in mechanically ventilated adults with acute lung injury. Crit Care Med 34(3):738–744.
37. Cook CD, Hamann JF (1961) Relation of lung volumes to height in healthy persons between the ages of 5 and 38 years. J Pediatr 59:710–714.
38. O'Brien RJ, Drizd TA (1983) Roentgenographic determination of total lung capacity: normal values from a National Population Survey. Am Rev Respir Dis 1983, 128(5):949–952.
39. Miller GJ, Saunders MJ, Gilson RJ, Ashcroft MT (1977) Lung function of healthy boys and girls in Jamaica in relation to ethnic composition, test exercise performance, and habitual physical activity. Thorax 32(4):486–496.
40. Pool JB, Greenough A (1989) Ethnic variation in respiratory function in young children. Respir Med 83(2):123–125.
41. Rahman MA, Ullah MB, Begum A (1990) Lung function in teenage Bangladeshi boys and girls. Respir Med 84(1):47–55.

Proteomic Profiles in Acute Respiratory Distress Syndrome Differentiates Survivors from Non-Survivors

Maneesh Bhargava[1]*, Trisha L. Becker[1], Kevin J. Viken[1], Pratik D. Jagtap[2], Sanjoy Dey[3], Michael S. Steinbach[3], Baolin Wu[4], Vipin Kumar[3], Peter B. Bitterman[1], David H. Ingbar[1], Christine H. Wendt[1,5]

1 Department of Medicine, University of Minnesota, Minneapolis, Minnesota, United States of America, **2** Minnesota Supercomputer Institute, University of Minnesota, Minneapolis, Minnesota, United States of America, **3** Department of Computer Science and Engineering, University of Minnesota, Minneapolis, Minnesota, United States of America, **4** School of Public Health, University of Minnesota, Minneapolis, Minnesota, United States of America, **5** Minneapolis VA Medical Center, University of Minnesota, Minneapolis, Minnesota, United States of America

Abstract

Acute Respiratory Distress Syndrome (ARDS) continues to have a high mortality. Currently, there are no biomarkers that provide reliable prognostic information to guide clinical management or stratify risk among clinical trial participants. The objective of this study was to probe the bronchoalveolar lavage fluid (BALF) proteome to identify proteins that differentiate survivors from non-survivors of ARDS. Patients were divided into early-phase (1 to 7 days) and late-phase (8 to 35 days) groups based on time after initiation of mechanical ventilation for ARDS (Day 1). Isobaric tags for absolute and relative quantitation (iTRAQ) with LC MS/MS was performed on pooled BALF enriched for medium and low abundance proteins from early-phase survivors (n = 7), early-phase non-survivors (n = 8), and late-phase survivors (n = 7). Of the 724 proteins identified at a global false discovery rate of 1%, quantitative information was available for 499. In early-phase ARDS, proteins more abundant in survivors mapped to ontologies indicating a coordinated compensatory response to injury and stress. These included coagulation and fibrinolysis; immune system activation; and cation and iron homeostasis. Proteins more abundant in early-phase non-survivors participate in carbohydrate catabolism and collagen synthesis, with no activation of compensatory responses. The compensatory immune activation and ion homeostatic response seen in early-phase survivors transitioned to cell migration and actin filament based processes in late-phase survivors, revealing dynamic changes in the BALF proteome as the lung heals. Early phase proteins differentiating survivors from non-survivors are candidate biomarkers for predicting survival in ARDS.

Editor: Nades Palaniyar, The Hospital for Sick Children and The University of Toronto, Canada

Funding: 12SDG8160000 American Heart Association Scientist Development Grant (MB PI). 1UL1RR033183-01 and 8UL1TR000114-02 UMN KL2 Scholars Award (MB, Blazar-PI). MFN MED FDN/3899-9238-09 Minnesota Medical Foundation Research Grant (MB PI). The funders had no role in study design, data collection and analysis, decision to publish, or preparation of the manuscript.

Competing Interests: The authors have declared that no competing interests exist.

* Email: bharg005@umn.edu

Introduction

Acute Respiratory Distress Syndrome (ARDS) is characterized by the abrupt onset of tachypnea, hypoxia and loss of lung compliance in response to infectious or inflammatory triggers [1]. Extensive research has improved our understanding of ARDS pathophysiology [2], epidemiology [3,4], treatment options [5–7], and outcomes [3,8], yet ARDS patients continue to have a high mortality rate. There is strong interest in identifying biomarkers to predict the development of ARDS in at-risk subjects [9–11], assist in diagnosis [12–15], and inform prognosis [13,16–20]. Biomarkers enabling risk stratification would not only be useful in the clinical care setting, but also in clinical trials of new therapeutic interventions to phenotype clinical trial subjects and serve as surrogate endpoints.

Development of ARDS is associated with the activation of a large number of inflammatory mediators that damage the alveolar epithelium, endothelium, and basement membrane. Biomarkers based on the tissue of origin have been studied in both single center studies [11,21,22] and in NHLBI ARDS network cohorts [13,16,21]. Most studies have focused on investigating an individual biomarker in blood, bronchoalveolar lavage fluid (BALF), or urine. Markers of inflammation such as interleukin-1β [23], interleukin 6 [7], and soluble TNF receptor I and II [24] are associated with poor prognosis in ARDS. Markers of endothelial damage including ICAM-1 [7,21], Angiopoeitin (Ang) [13], and Von Willibrand Factor (vWF) [25] correlate with higher mortality from ARDS. Poorer outcomes are also associated with higher plasma levels of SP-D (but not SP-A), a marker of type 2 alveolar epithelial cell damage [19], and receptor of advance glycation end products (RAGE), a marker of type 1 alveolar epithelial cell damage. Several other molecules, such as those involved in coagulation [26], damage to extracellular matrix [20], and oxidative stress (urine NO) [20], correlate with ARDS outcomes. A combination of biomarkers and clinical predictors was found to be superior to clinical predictors or biomarkers alone for predicting mortality in ARDS [27]. However, the identification of a single biomarker or a combination of biomarkers that could be widely used has remained elusive [28] due to lack of correlation between the biochemical marker, pathophysiological variables and clinical outcomes.

The primary aim of this study was to identify pathways of survival and stimulate new biomarker discovery by characterizing the BALF protein expression profile of ARDS survivors and non-survivors at different stages (early versus late) of disease progression. We analyzed medium and low abundant protein fractions in BALF samples by using contemporary high-resolution mass spectrometry (MS)-based proteomics techniques, along with quantitative labeling methodology. Our hypothesis was that patients who are able to survive ARDS would exhibit a distinct BALF protein profile during the early phase of mechanical ventilator support. Here, we show distinct differences in the BALF proteome between patients who survive ARDS from those who die. Moreover, the ontologies of differentially expressed proteins in late-phase survivors (cell migration and actin cytoskeleton organization) differ markedly from those in early-phase survivors, suggesting a critical role for these processes during lung repair. Enhancing these processes may provide new directions for therapy in ARDS.

Methods

Study population

The University of Minnesota Institutional Review Board Human Subjects Committee approved this study. Patients were recruited at the University of Minnesota Medical Center. Informed consent for study participation was obtained from either the patient or the patient's legal representative. The early-phase ARDS BALF samples were available from clinically indicated bronchoscopies with excess supernatant made available for these studies. The late-phase ARDS samples were excess supernatant BALF obtained from research bronchoscopies with consent from the patient or the surrogate. BAL (100 mls normal saline) was performed using standard protocol in either the right middle lobe or left upper lobe (lingual)

For this study, patients were grouped based on the timing of the bronchoscopy – conducted in either the early phase of ARDS (Day 1–7) or the late phase (Day 8–35), referenced to the initiation of mechanical ventilation (designated Day 1) – and the outcome at the time of discharge (non-survivor or survivor). We thus studied patients in the early phase who were grouped into survivors or non-survivors and late-phase survivors. Late phase non-survivors were not included in this study as not enough BALF was available to perform the protein expression profile. The APAHCHEE-II score was calculated to assess the severity of illness on the day of bronchoscopy for patients in early phase of ARDS as previously described [29].

Sample preparation

BALF samples were processed as previously described [30] with some modifications. BALF containing equal amounts of protein from individual patients were pooled to collect a total of 4 mg protein for each group (early-phase survivors, early-phase non-survivors, and late-phase survivors). Pooled BALF was concentrated and desalted by centrifugation with an Amicon 3-MWCO spin filter (Millipore, catalog number UFC800396). To decrease the dynamic range, we enriched the medium and low abundance proteins by selectively immunodepleting the fourteen most abundant proteins in the concentrated samples on Seppro IgY 14 spin columns (Sigma-Aldrich, cat # SEP010). The Seppro IgY 14 spin columns deplete albumin, IgG, α_1-antitrypsin, IgA, IgM, transferrin, haptoglobin, α_2-macroglobulin, fibrinogen, complement C3, α_1-acid glycoprotein, aplopoproteins A-1, A-II and B. Per the manufacturer's instructions, each sample was mixed in the dilution buffer to a final volume of 500 µl, loaded onto the immunoaffinity depletion column, and incubated for 15 minutes at room temperature. To prevent saturation of the column, 250 µg of protein was depleted at a time. The unbound medium and low abundance proteins were collected in the flow through. Pooled samples from each representative group was required to have adequate protein concentrations since immunodepletion results in >90% of the proteins being removed. An additional wash was performed with 0.5 ml of the dilution buffer. The depleted samples were then concentrated with an Amicon filter. A buffer exchange with 0.5 M triethylammonium bicarbonate (TEAB) was performed to remove TRIS, and the sample was concentrated with an Amicon filter. A Bradford protein assay was performed to quantify the enriched low abundant proteins.

iTRAQ labeling and 2D LC-Orbitrap MS

Enriched medium and low abundance proteins (50 µg from early-phase survivors and non-survivors, 25 µg from late phase survivors) were digested by trypsin and labeled with iTRAQ reagent (AB Sciex, Foster City, CA) [30] for mass spectrometric analysis. The total peptide mixture was purified with an MCX Oasis cartridge (Waters, Milford, MA) before separation via two-dimensional liquid chromatography-mass spectrometry (2D LC-MS). LC and MS experimental details were previously reported [30]. Proteins were separated and concentrated offline in the 1st dimension into 15 peptide-containing fractions, collected in 2-minute intervals on a C18 Gemini column (Phenomenex, Torrance, CA) at pH 10, and in the 2nd dimension by a C18 reversed phase capillary LC with a nano LC system (Eksigent, Dublin, CA). Data-dependent acquisition of the 6 most intense peaks per LC fraction was performed on an Orbitrap Velos system, with HCD (higher energy collision induced dissociation) as the activation type for peptide tandem MS.

Database search for protein identification and quantification

Each of the 15.RAW files generated from the Orbitrap Velos MS system were converted to mzML files by using msconvert, then converted to a ProteinPilot compatible Mascot Generic Format (MGF) with preselected iTRAQ reporter ions. The MGF files were searched against the Human UniProt database along with contaminant protein sequences (84,838 sequences in total; December 2012) using ProteinPilot version 4.5 and the following search parameters: Sample Type: iTRAQ 4-plex (peptide labeled); Cys-alkylation: MMTS; Instrument: Orbi MS, Orbi MS/MS; Run Quant; Use bias correction; Search focus on biological modifications and amino-acid substitutions; Thorough search and with a Detected Protein Threshold (Unused Protscore (Conf)): 10%. The ProteinPilot searches and subsequent generation of PSPEP (FDR) reports and protein and peptide-level summaries were generated within Galaxy-P [31]. Because MS data acquisition was performed on BALF samples after depletion of 14 high abundance plasma proteins, the high abundance proteins (or their fragment) were manually removed if they were present in the list of inferred proteins generated by ProteinPilot. Protein Summary with iTRAQ ratios (with early-phase survivors as the denominator for determining fold change) was processed through a workflow built within Galaxy-P so that it yielded UniProt accession numbers and gene names of differentially expressed proteins. The mass

Table 1. Demographic and Clinical Characteristics of Subjects by Study Group.

Variable	Early-phase ARDS survivors (N = 7)	Early-phase ARDS non-survivors (N = 8)	Late phase ARDS survivors (N = 7)	p-value*
Age	42.29±11.43	58.13±20.49	47.86±10.07	0.16
Gender	M = 5, F = 2	M = 6, F = 2	M = 5, F = 2	
Immunocompromised/Immunecompetent	4/3	3/5	2/5	
APACHEE-II score	19.14±7.4	19.75±4.7		0.85
ARDS Day of BALF collection	2.0±1.15	3.25±2.19	18.6±13.3	<0.001#
PF Ratio on day of bronchoscopy	143.7±34.1	150±71.1	161.5±83.7	0.137
BALF WBC count (cells/μl)	496±342.6	364.4±408.7	451.1±471.5	0.75
BALF Neutrophils (%)	56.0±33.3	49.0±38.1	40.6±38.5	0.9327

*One-way analysis of variance (ANOVA) with Tukey post-test.
#Statistically significant difference between late-phase survivors and early-phase survivors ($p<0.05$) and between late-phase survivors and early-phase non-survivors ($p<0.05$), but no difference between early-phase survivors and early-phase non-survivors.
PF ratio- PaO_2 to FiO_2 ratio.

spectrometry proteomics data have been deposited to theProteomeXchange Consortium [32] via the PRIDE partner repository with the dataset identifier PXD001095.

Statistical analysis

Differences in the clinical characteristics of the three participant groups were calculated by using ANOVA and, when appropriate, a post hoc Tukey test. For protein identification and quantification, multiple hypothesis correction was performed by controlling for false discovery rate (FDR), which measures the expected proportion of false positives among the statistically significant findings. The FDR cutoff was set at ≤1% (global) for protein identification in ProteinPilot. For quantification of protein abundance, each ratio (obtained by comparison of early-phase non-survivors to survivors or late-phase survivors to early- phase survivors) was compared to one; multiple hypothesis correction was performed by controlling the FDR set at ≤5% [33] and computing q-values with the *mafdr* routine in Matlab. Proteins with q-values less than 0.05 were retained for further analysis.

Gene Ontology (GO) Enrichment Analysis

To gain insight into the biological significance of differentially expressed proteins, we used the Database for Annotation, Visualization, and Integrated Discovery (DAVID, http://david.abcc.ncifcrf.gov, search date 7/11/13) [34]. DAVID provides batch annotations to highlight the most relevant GO term associated with a gene (or protein) list. Of the three GO terms annotated to a gene (molecular function, biological process, and

Table 2. Pulmonary history and clinical risk factors for ARDS in the study subjects.

Past Pulmonary History	Early-phase ARDS survivors (n = 7)	Early-phase ARDS Non-survivors (n = 8)	Late phase ARDS survivors (n = 7)
None	3	6	1
VTE	1	0	0
Smoker (prior or current)	1	0	3
Lung infection	2	0	0
COPD	0	0	1
NSCLC	0	2	1
Prior ARDS	0	0	1
Risk factor for ARDS			
Disseminated candidiasis	1	0	0
Sepsis	4	2	0
Pneumonia, not specified	0	1	
Pneumonia, gram negative	0	1	2
Pneumonia, gram positive	0	2	0
Pneumonia, fungal	0	1	0
Pneumonia, viral	0	0	1
Pneumonia, aspiration	2	0	3
Pancreatitis	0	1	0
Unknown	0	0	1

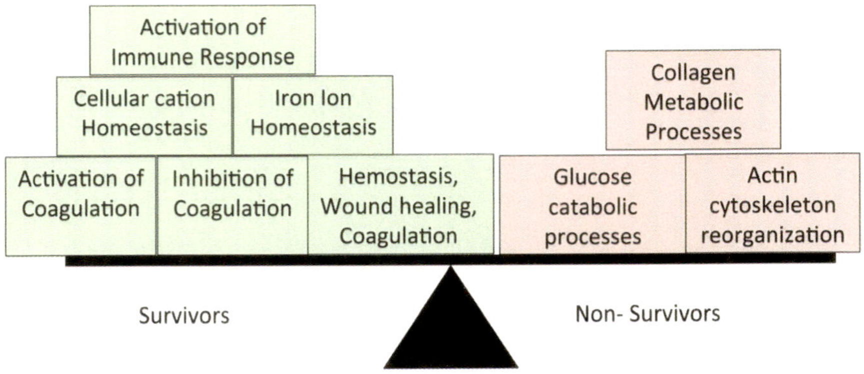

Figure 1. Biological processes represented by 165 proteins that are differentially expressed when early-phase non-survivors are compared to early-phase survivors. GO enrichment analysis was performed using the universe of identified BALF proteins as a background. A Functional Annotation Clustering tool was used to group related biological processes. Annotation clusters with an enrichment score >1.3 are shown. In the functional annotation-clustering tool, an enrichment score of 1.3 that corresponds to a non-log scale p-value of 0.05 was used as the cutoff for significance.

cell compartment), we limited the biological process annotation to differentially expressed proteins. Functional annotation clustering analysis in DAVID was used to identify the combinations of genes according to common biological function. DAVID generates an enrichment score for a group of genes indicating annotation term member associations in a given experiment. An enrichment score of 1.3 is equivalent to a non-log scale p-value of 0.05.

Individual Protein Quantification

Levels for selected proteins were measured by ELISA with commercially available kits (BlueGene Life Science Advance (MUC5AC), R and D Systems, (MMP9 and SP-D), APC Biomaterials LLC (club cell secretory protein), Abcam (Kiniongen, Antithrombin III, Ceruplasmin, Plasminogen, Prothrombin), MyBioSource Inc (decay-accelerating factor, thoredoxin), AssyPro (Factor 12), Cloud-Clone Corp (Moesin), CusaBio (CD9), MBL International (S100A9) and CusaBio (Ezirin).

Results

Characteristics of study participants

We analyzed BALF samples from 22 unique ARDS patients (Table 1 and Table 2): 7 in the early-phase survivor group (mean ARDS day of sample collection $=2.0\pm1.15$ days), 8 in the early phase non-survivor group (mean ARDS day of sample collection $=3.25\pm2.19$ days), and 7 in the late-phase survivor group (mean ARDS day of sample collection $=18.6\pm13.3$ days). Although the mean age of patients in the early-phase non-survivor group was higher than in the other two groups, this difference was not statistically significant (ANOVA p-value $=0.16$). The three groups did not differ in the severity of gas exchange on the day of the bronchoscopy, APACHEE-II score, BALF leukocyte count, or BALF neutrophil count. The average time from onset of ARDS to death in the early phase non-survivor group was 19.9 ± 14.5 days.

Proteins identified by peptide spectral matching and database searching

The ProteinPilot PSPEP FDR Summary reported 20,601 spectra matched to 10,355 distinct peptides at ≤1% global FDR for a total of 792 inferred proteins (Table S1, Protein Pilot PSPEP summary and protein identified at 1% FDR tab). High abundance proteins or their fragments (Table S1, High abundance/contaminants tab) that were incompletely removed by the depletion column were removed manually from the protein list. Suspected contaminants or misidentified proteins such as trypsin, bovine albumin, and the reverse matches that occurred from use of the target decoy strategy for peptide identification were also manually removed. After exclusion of these proteins, the number of inferred proteins was 724 (Table S1, BALF proteome tab). These724 proteins were used as the background for GO enrichment analysis (i.e. the "universe of identified BALF proteome"). Of these 724 proteins, quantitative spectral data were available on 499 to allow determination of the bias corrected relative abundance in the two comparison groups for this study (Table S1, BALF with quantification tab). All but three proteins had at least two peptides used for identification. Bias factors for the two comparison groups were 2.8 for the early phase non-survivors to survivors and 0.64 for early phase survivor to late phase survivor group. Bias factors were used for normalization of the protein quantification within ProteinPilot.

Proteins differentiating early-phase survivors and early-phase non-survivors

Controlling for an FDR of ≤5%, we identified 161 proteins that were differentially expressed in the BALF of early-phase survivors compared with early-phase non-survivors (Table S2, proteins with q-values ≤5%). Eighty-six of these proteins were more abundant in non-survivors (Table S2, high in non-survivors tab) and 75 were more abundant in survivors (Table S2, high in survivors tab). Gene ontology enrichment analysis demonstrated significant differences in the biological processes represented by these differentially expressed proteins (Figure 1). The differentially expressed proteins represented six ontologies in survivors (Table 3): three involved in coagulation (fibrinolysis and coagulation and wound healing), two representing cellular ion homeostasis, and one involved in immune activation. In contrast, differentially expressed proteins mapped to three ontologies in non-survivors (Table 4, Table S2, GO non-survivors tab). Non-survivors showed disruption of bioenergetics with evidence of carbohydrate catabolism and cellular damage as evidenced by disorganization of actin filament based processes. In addition, there was evidence of collagen biosynthesis in non-survivors early in ARDS.

Changes in the proteome among late-phase survivors

We identified 172 proteins (FDR at ≤5%) that demonstrated differential expression between early-phase and late-phase survi-

Table 3. Early-phase ARDS Survivor Ontology Groups and Associated Proteins.

GO Biological Process	Official Gene Symbol	Protein Name	Fold change*
Positive Regulation of blood coagulation	AHSG	Alpha-2-HS-glycoprotein	0.21
	APOH	Apolipoprotein H	0.21
	HRG	Histidine-rich glycoprotein	0.34
	PLG	Plasminogen	0.35
	F12	Coagulation factor XII	0.36
	F2	Coagulation factor II	0.57
	SERPINF2	Serpin peptidase inhibitor, member 2	0.38
Negative regulation of blood coagulation	AHSG	Alpha-2-HS-glycoprotein	0.21
	APOH	Apolipoprotein H	0.21
	KNG1	Kininogen 1	0.24
	PLG	Plasminogen	0.35
	F12	Coagulation factor XII	0.36
	APOE	Apolipoprotein E	0.44
	ANXA5	Annexin A5	0.45
	F2	Coagulation factor II	0.57
	ANXA2	Annexin A2	0.81
Regulation of body fluid levels	SERPINC1	Antithrombin III	0.16
	APOH	Apolipoprotein H	0.21
	KNG1	Kininogen 1	0.24
	PLG	Plasminogen	0.35
	F12	Coagulation factor XII	0.36
	ANXA5	Annexin A5	0.45
	F2	Coagulation factor II	0.57
	ANXA2	Annexin A2	0.81
Cellular cation homeostasis	KNG1	Kininogen 1	0.24
	HPX	Hemopexin	0.30
	SFTPD	Surfactant protein D	0.38
	APOE	Apolipoprotein E	0.44
	F2	Coagulation factor II	0.57
	FTL	Ferritin, light polypeptide	0.62
	FTH1	Ferritin, heavy polypeptide 1	0.62
	55	Decay accelerating factor	0.78
	CP	Ceruloplasmin	0.84
Iron ion homeostasis	HPX	Hemopexin	0.30
	FTH1	Ferritin, heavy polypeptide 1	0.62
	FTL	Ferritin, light polypeptide	0.62
	CP	Ceruloplasmin	0.84
Positive regulation of immune response	C4BPA	Complement component 4 binding protein, alpha	0.09
	PLG	Plasminogen	0.35
	F12	Coagulation factor XII	0.36
	CFH	Complement factor H-related 2	0.45
	C1RL	Complement component 1r	0.56
	F2	Coagulation factor II	0.57
	CLU	Histone cluster 1,	0.65
	C5	Complement component 5	0.66
	KRT1	Keratin 1	0.67

Table 3. Cont.

GO Biological Process	Official Gene Symbol	Protein Name	Fold change*
	CD55	Decay accelerating factor	0.78
	C8A	Complement component 8, alpha	0.79
	C6	Complement component 6	0.80
	APOH	Apolipoprotein H	0.21

*Fold change is relative to survivors, therefore a fold change <1represents proteins more abundant in survivors.

vors of ARDS (Table S3, FDR q-values tab). Of these 172 proteins, 91 were more abundant in early-phase ARDS survivors (Table S3, high in early phase tab) and 81 were more abundant in late-phase ARDS survivors (Table S3, high in late phase tab). Gene ontology enrichment analysis employing the functional annotation-clustering tool in DAVID identified three ontology annotations that were over represented in early-phase survivors: lymphocyte and leukocyte immune response, cellular cation homeostasis, and iron ion homeostasis (Table S3, GO early phase tab). In contrast, proteins that were more abundant in late-phase survivors represented two clusters of ontologies involved in lung repair: cell migration and actin cytoskeleton organization (Figure 2 and Table S2, GO late phase tab).

Changes in key proteins concentrations in individual samples

As we used pooled samples for our proteomic studies, we measured protein concentration from individual BALF samples by ELISA. Similar to the MS data, the level of club cell secretory protein was significantly higher in early phase non-survivors when compared to early phase survivors (2458±1409 vs. 922±534 ng/mL, p-value =0.048, figure 3a). Moesin (1.02±0.52 vs. 2.63±1.76 ng/ml, p-value 0.055, Figure 3b) and MMP 9 (93.51±133.1 vs. 10±11.87 ng/mL, p-value =0.19, figure 3c) demonstrated a non-significant increase in early phase non-survivors compared to survivors. Although MUC5A was higher in survivors, it did not reach statistical significance (10.74±14.16 vs. 4.499±3.48, p-value =0.29 whereas SP-D was not different.

To develop a panel of candidate proteins that could discriminate early phase survivors from non-survivors, we measured BALF levels of several key proteins that were higher in survivors

Table 4. Early-phase ARDS Non-Survivor Ontology Groups and Associated Proteins.

GO Biological Process	Official Gene Symbol	Protein Name	Fold change
Actin filament-based process	TMSB4X	Thymosin-like 2	2.65
	EZR	Ezrin	2.15
	PFN1	Profilin 1	1.93
	VASP	Vasodilator-stimulated phosphoprotein	1.81
	CAP1	Adenylate cyclase-associated protein 1	1.58
	ARHGDIB	Rho GDP dissociation inhibitor (GDI) beta	1.52
	S100A9	S100 calcium binding protein A9	1.51
	FLNA	Filamin A, alpha	1.31
	MYH9	Non-muscle myosin, heavy chain 9	1.27
	STMN1	Stathmin 1	1.20
Glycolysis	GAPDHL6	Glyceraldehyde-3-phosphate dehydrogenase-like 6	2.01
	TXN	Thioredoxin	1.82
	PGK1	Phosphoglycerate kinase 1	1.73
	TPI1	Triosephosphate isomerase 1	1.63
	GPI	Glucose phosphate isomerase	1.63
	ENO1	Enolase 1, (alpha)	1.51
	PGAM1	Phosphoglycerate mutase 1	1.42
Collagen metabolic process	COL5A1	Type V collagen, alpha 1	2.33
	MUC5AC	Mucin 5AC	2.04
	COL3A1	Type III collagen alpha 1	1.99
	MMP9	Matrix metallopeptidase 9	1.84
	COL1A1	Type I collagen, alpha 1	1.75

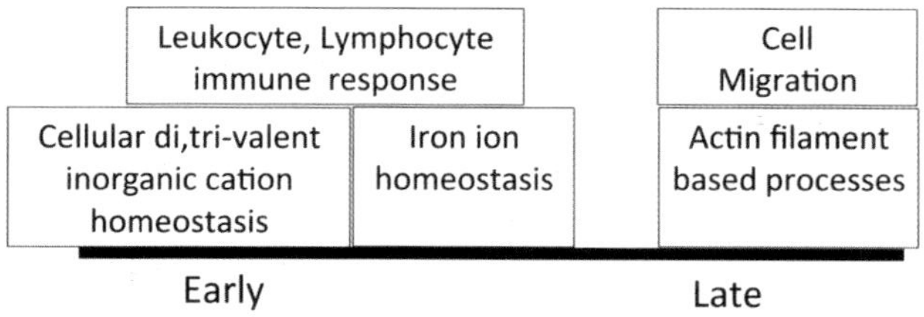

Figure 2. Biological processes represented by 175 proteins that are differentially expressed when late-phase survivors are compared to early-phase survivors. GO enrichment analysis was performed using the universe of identified BALF proteins as a background. A Functional Annotation Clustering tool was used to group related biological processes. Annotation clusters with an enrichment score >1.3 are shown. In the functional annotation-clustering tool, an enrichment score of 1.3 that corresponds to a non-log scale p-value of 0.05 was used as the cutoff for significance.

and participated in biological processes listed in Table 3. BALF levels of Plasminogen, Factor 12, Antithrombin and Cerulopasmin were consistent with our iTRAQ MS/MS findings (Figure 4). However, BALF levels of kininogen and Prothrombin (Factor 2) did not mirror the quantitative iTRAQ MS/MS data. We also measured levels of key proteins that participated in biological processes in early phase non-survivors listed in Table 4. S100A9 and Thioredoxin levels measured by ELISA mirrored the iTRAQ data (figure 5). Similar to the iTRAQ MS data, Ezrin level measured by ELISA in pooled BA was higher in non-survivors compared to survivors (2.45 ng/ml vs. 0.737 ng/ml.) We were not able to detect decay accelerating factor and CD9 by ELISA in our BALF samples.

Discussion

In this study we achieved deep coverage of the BALF proteome through the use of high-resolution mass spectrometry based proteomics and an optimized sample preparation designed to enrich medium and low abundance protein fractions. This extent of proteome coverage has not been previously reported in human BALF from normal or diseased lungs [35–40]. The semi-quantitative techniques used in this study reveal dynamic changes in the distal airspace of patients with ARDS. Differences in the BALF protein expression profile are seen early in the course of ARDS in patients who die compared with those who live. Further, GO enrichment analysis demonstrates highly informative, biologically coherent differences in the ontologies represented by the differentially expressed proteins when early-phase survivors are compared to late-phase survivors or early-phase non-survivors.

The BALF protein expression profile for patients early in ARDS was different comparing survivors to non-survivors. Patients who died had evidence of aberrant lung repair early on in the disease process, as evidenced by approximately a two-fold differential expression of type I, III and V collagen, a signature of activated fibroblasts, and newly synthesized collagen deposition. This is in line with previous reports that higher levels of collagen I and III in ARDS [41] reflect matrix remodeling locally in the lung. Increased levels of BALF type III procollagen also correlated with fatal outcomes in ARDS [42]. In contrast, survivors early in the disease course demonstrated a more coordinated response that includes coagulation as the focal point, including plasminogen-mediated fibrinolysis. The balance of activation of coagulation and fibrinolysis is an important determination of the extent of fibrin deposition. In previous studies, tissue factor mediated pro-coagulant [43], protein C mediated anti-coagulant [44], and plasminogen mediated fibrinolysis pathways appeared to be important in ARDS [45]. Up-regulation of plasminogen activator inhibitor in BALF suggests a shift from a pro-fibrinolytic to an anti-fibrinolytic phenotype being associated with poorer outcomes [46]. In our study, a similar pattern of active collagen deposition suggesting an anti-fibrinolytic milieu even in the exudative phase in ARDS non-survivors is seen, while ARDS survivors have a more prominent fibrinolytic milieu. This indicates a profound difference in response to alveolar injury in survivors compared to non-survivors.

In addition to abnormal repair, non-survivors also have evidence of increased catabolism and cellular disruptions. In contrast, survivors demonstrate a coordinated activation of cation and iron homeostasis. Prior studies have shown the importance of iron in the development of ARDS [47,48]. Cell and tissue damage resulting from inflammatory/oxidative stress can ultimately be a consequence of disruption of normal iron metabolism. Patients with ARDS have increased concentrations of heme and non-heme iron that could lead to generation of oxidative stress and resultant lung damage [49]. Polymorphisms in ferritin light chain and heme-oxygenase have also been associated with increased susceptibility to ARDS [50]. In survivors, higher levels of several proteins involved in iron regulation such as ferritin heavy and light chain, hemopexin, and cerruloplasmin indicate better capacity to counteract the redox stress mediated by iron or other reactive oxygen species in the lungs.

In addition to giving insight into mechanisms of disease, differentially expressed proteins in the early phase of ARDS can be used to discern non-survivors from survivors for prognostication. The ideal biomarker would have biological significance related to lung injury and repair. Alternatively, a panel of proteins that represent the divergent biological processes in the two groups

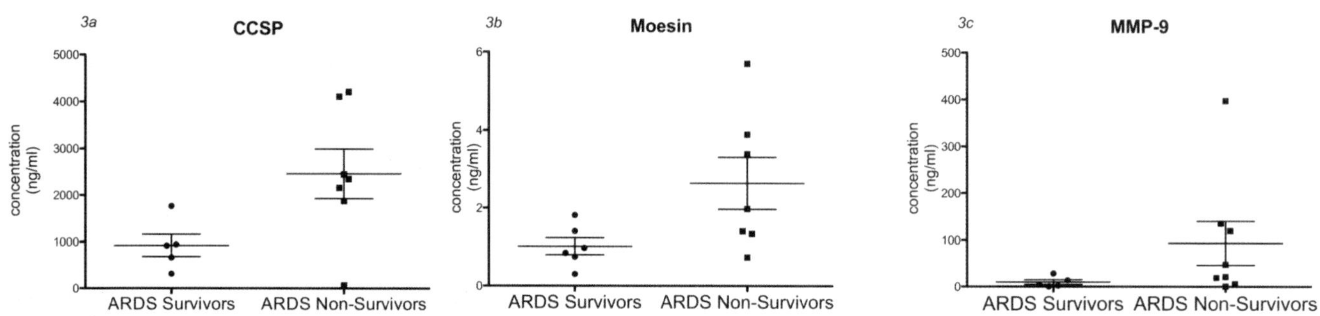

Figure 3. Protein levels of selected candidates. ELISA was performed to quantify CCSP, Moesin and MMP9. Levels of these proteins were higher in early phase non-survivors in comparison to survivor (p-value <0.05 t-test) for CCSP and <0.1 for Moesin.

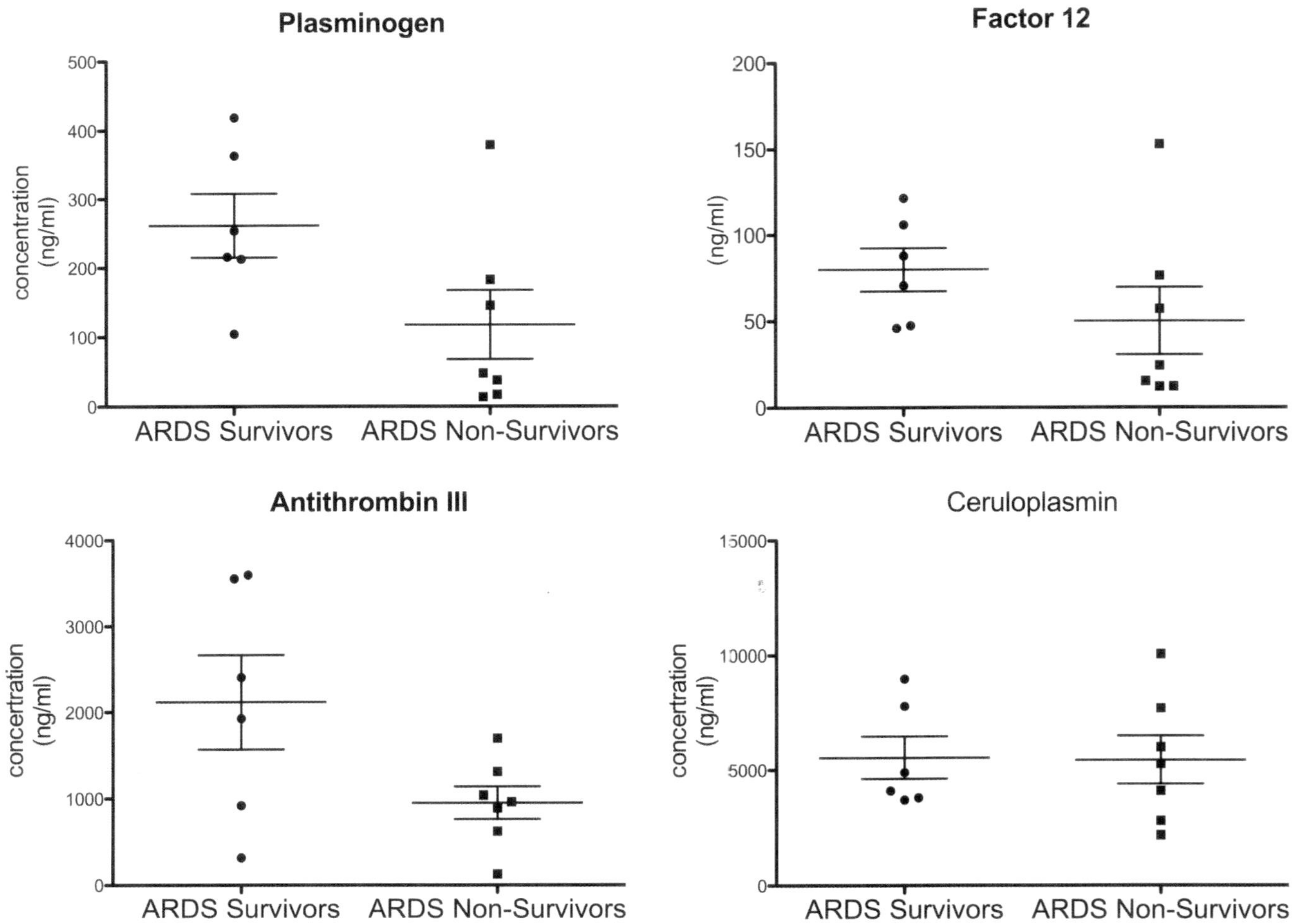

Figure 4. Protein levels of selected proteins that represent biological processes that are activated in early phase survivors (p-value plasminogen =0.06, antithrombin III=0.054, factor 12=0.2 and ceruloplasmin =0.9).

could be selected for testing in a separate cohort of well phenotyped patients. As the proteomic platform that we used only provides relative quantitation, complementary studies using multiplex ELISA or multiple reaction monitoring will be needed to measure absolute levels to select a limited number of proteins that could be further investigated. We used ELISA for measurement of protein levels for two main reasons. First, this provided validation that mass spectrometric measures of the protein amounts were

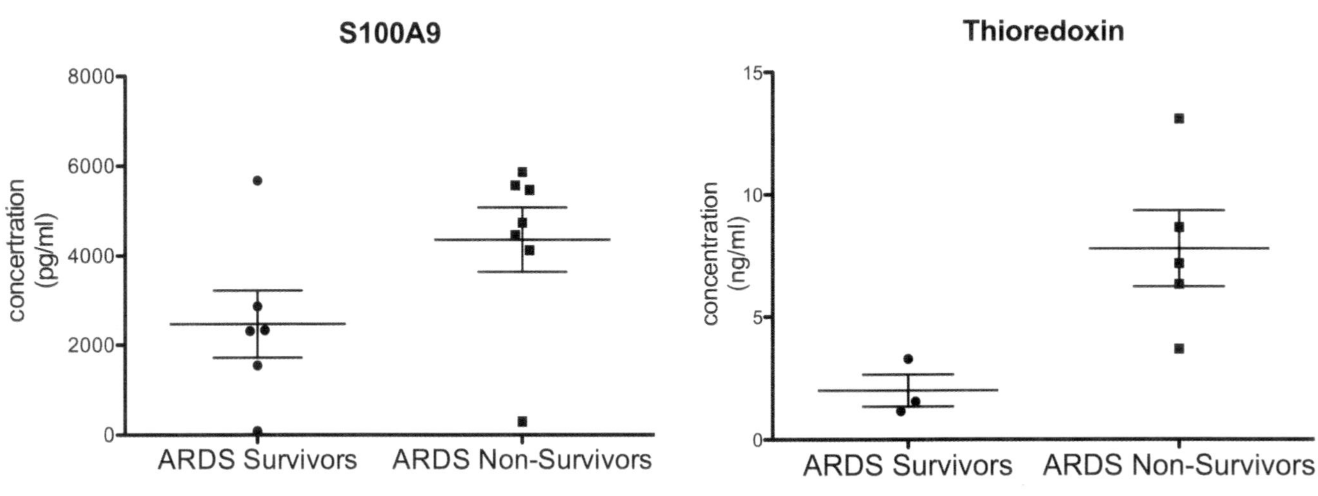

Figure 5. Protein levels of selected proteins that represented biological processes that are activated in early phase non-survivors. Thioredoxin was identified in only 3 survivors. (p-value <0.05 thioredoxin and <0.1 for S-100).

accurate. The fold change for CCSP (sp|P11684|UTER_HUMAN, Table S2, high in non-survivor tab, row 25) was 6.2 fold in the mass spectrometric studies. In line with these findings, the mean levels measured with ELISA demonstrated a >4.5 fold higher abundance in the protein level. Similarly, other proteins produced in the lung, Moesin, MMP9 and MUC5A, also demonstrated a trend toward higher levels in non-survivors by ELISA and mass spectrometry studies, whereas surfactant D did not demonstrate a significant change when measured in individual BALF samples. These proteins could represent epithelial damage and be candidate proteins to test in a larger cohort of well phenotyped subjects with ARDS.

CCSP is produced by small airway cells and has been implicated in regulating inflammatory responses in the lung. In patients with ventilator associated pneumonia, serum CCSP levels increased 2 days before the diagnosis of ARDS/ALI [51]. However, data regarding the utility of plasma CCSP levels is conflicting in small studies with one study demonstrating evidence in CCSP predicting mortality [52], while another study did not find any association of serum CCSP levels with mortality [53]. Our study suggests BALF CCSP levels alone or conjunction with other proteins could be marker of epithelial damage and could predict mortality in ARDS.

ERM (ezirin-radixin-moesin) proteins co-localize in cell matrix adhesion sites, filopodia, and membrane protrusions [54]. ERMs function by binding to and organizing the actin cytoskeleton [55] and in turn, stabilizing adherens junctions [56] and influencing cell migration [57,58]. In adult wild-type mice, moesin expression is limited to the alveolar epithelium of the distal lung. Moesin-deficient mice develop normally [59] demonstrate decreased moesin in the distal alveolar wall and have airspace enlargement. In response to bleomycin, moesin- deficient mice had lower survival [60], more inflammation, extensive alveolar destruction, hemorrhage and pulmonary edema, increased lung permeability, and a higher total BALF cell count. In moesin-deficient mice, fibrotic response to bleomycin was both earlier and more severe. This supports involvement of moesin in injury-repair response in the lung.

Matrix metalloproteinase (MMP) are proteases that are involved degradation of extracellular matrix. Type IV collagen is specific to the basement membrane and MMP-9 is a type IV collagenase. In ARDS, BALF MMP-9 levels were high compared to controls and correlated with degree of collagen breakdown as determined by measuring collagen breakdown products (7S collagen) [61]. Early elevations of MMP-9 levels have also been found to be associated with prolonged duration of mechanical ventilation in pediatric ARDS patients [62]. In our study, although we did not compare the BALF MMP-9 level in ARDS with controls, higher BALF MMP-9 were seen in patients who died. Though speculative, this could be a marker of worse epithelial damage in non-survivors. In addition we also measured MUC5A levels in the BALF by ELISA. MUC5A is a member of the mucins, large glycoproteins that form a protective biofilm covering the respiratory epithelial lining. MUC5AC is secreted mostly by the surface epithelial goblet cells [63]. MUC5AC transcript levels increase in airway epithelial cells upon cyclic stretch, in mice with ventilator induced lung injury and in humans with ARDS [63]. Though the proteins levels of MUC5AC in our studies did not differentiate survivors and non-survivors, this may have resulted from our relatively small sample.

In this study we also compared the BALF protein expression profiles of early- and late- phase survivors. This comparison highlights the dynamic changes in the airspace milieu during repair. Chang and colleagues [36] characterized BALF in ARDS patients on day 1, 3, and 7; their results demonstrated striking differences between normal controls and ARDS patients on day 1, but less dramatic changes between days 1, 3 and 7. The changes seen in their studies reflected alteration in the innate immune and oxidant pathways at day 3 and possibly lung regeneration at day 7. Similar to that study, we found that activation of the innate immune system and cation homeostasis were over-represented by proteins in early-phase survivors compared to late-phase survivors. However, in our late-phase survivors – whose samples were obtained 18 days after the onset of ARDS, much later than in previous studies – the ontologies were drastically different and included cell migration and actin cytoskeleton organization. Since all of these patients survived, these findings suggest a critical role of these processes during lung repair. The proteins that are represented in these ontologies could be potential targets to stimulate repair mechanisms as potential molecular targets for therapy in ARDS.

We acknowledge the limitations of our study. We were limited by the amount of available BALF therefore are the protein characterization was performed on pooled BALF samples. Pooled samples are subject to influence by a minority of outliers within the pool. We were limited to a single run for the mass-spectrometry. However, we demonstrate changes in protein levels using ELISA studies that were performed on individual subject samples. Another limitation is the study design, i.e. binary outcome that can be influenced by a number of confounders not controlled in our study. Our approach was to enrich the medium and low abundance protein fractions by depleting high abundance proteins. We chose depletion over alternative method to avoid an unwieldy dynamic range with a subsequent limited depth of proteome coverage. In addition, many of the abundant proteins that were eliminated are found in the plasma, which can leak into the alveolar space during lung injury. Another limitation is our relatively small number of subjects. Despite the small sample size, our sample preparation optimization methods enabled us to successfully identify a number of differentially expressed proteins. Our findings provide a starting point for subsequent studies characterizing BALF in individual patients for biomarker identification in ARDS.

Conclusion

This study illustrates a framework whereby protein profiling can be used to identify panels of proteins that parallel the pathophysiological changes occurring in ARDS. We demonstrate dynamic changes in BALF protein expression during the course of ARDS and also early divergence in the protein expression profile in ARDS. Differences in absolute levels of the proteins that represent divergent biological processes in survivors and non-survivors will facilitate identification of prognostic biomarkers in ARDS.

Supporting Information

Table S1 BALF proteins identified using iTRAQ MS/MS.

Table S2 Differentially expressed proteins between early phase survivors and non survivors.

Table S3 Differentially expressed proteins between early and late phase survivors.

Acknowledgments

The authors thank Dr. LeeAnn Higgins for acquisition of mass spectrometry data and Dr. Anne Marie Weber-Main for her critical review and editing of manuscript drafts. The mass spectrometry proteomics data have been deposited to the ProteomeXchange Consortium [32] via the PRIDE partner repository with the dataset identifier PXD001095.

Author Contributions

Conceived and designed the experiments: MB DHI PBB VK CHW PDJ. Performed the experiments: MB TLB KJV. Analyzed the data: MB BW SD MSS PDJ CHW. Contributed reagents/materials/analysis tools: MB DHI CHW. Wrote the paper: MB PDJ MSS PBB CHW.

References

1. Ashbaugh DG, Bigelow DB, Petty TL, Levine BE (1967) Acute respiratory distress in adults. Lancet 2: 319–323.
2. Suratt BT, Parsons PE (2006) Mechanisms of acute lung injury/acute respiratory distress syndrome. Clinics in chest medicine 27: 579–589; abstract viii.
3. Rubenfeld GD, Caldwell E, Peabody E, Weaver J, Martin DP, et al. (2005) Incidence and outcomes of acute lung injury. The New England journal of medicine 353: 1685–1693.
4. Rubenfeld GD, Herridge MS (2007) Epidemiology and outcomes of acute lung injury. Chest 131: 554–562.
5. Wiedemann HP, Wheeler AP, Bernard GR, Thompson BT, Hayden D, et al. (2006) Comparison of two fluid-management strategies in acute lung injury. The New England journal of medicine 354: 2564–2575.
6. Guerin C, Reignier J, Richard JC, Beuret P, Gacouin A, et al. (2013) Prone Positioning in Severe Acute Respiratory Distress Syndrome. The New England journal of medicine.
7. (2000) Ventilation with lower tidal volumes as compared with traditional tidal volumes for acute lung injury and the acute respiratory distress syndrome. The Acute Respiratory Distress Syndrome Network. The New England journal of medicine 342: 1301–1308.
8. Villar J, Blanco J, Anon JM, Santos-Bouza A, Blanch L, et al. (2011) The ALIEN study: incidence and outcome of acute respiratory distress syndrome in the era of lung protective ventilation. Intensive care medicine 37: 1932–1941.
9. Cohen MJ, Brohi K, Calfee CS, Rahn P, Chesebro BB, et al. (2009) Early release of high mobility group box nuclear protein 1 after severe trauma in humans: role of injury severity and tissue hypoperfusion. Critical care 13: R174.
10. Gallagher DC, Parikh SM, Balonov K, Miller A, Gautam S, et al. (2008) Circulating angiopoietin 2 correlates with mortality in a surgical population with acute lung injury/adult respiratory distress syndrome. Shock 29: 656–661.
11. Bersten AD, Hunt T, Nicholas TE, Doyle IR (2001) Elevated plasma surfactant protein-B predicts development of acute respiratory distress syndrome in patients with acute respiratory failure. American journal of respiratory and critical care medicine 164: 648–652.
12. Katayama M, Ishizaka A, Sakamoto M, Fujishima S, Sekiguchi K, et al. (2010) Laminin gamma2 fragments are increased in the circulation of patients with early phase acute lung injury. Intensive care medicine 36: 479–486.
13. Calfee CS, Gallagher D, Abbott J, Thompson BT, Matthay MA (2012) Plasma angiopoietin-2 in clinical acute lung injury: prognostic and pathogenetic significance. Critical care medicine 40: 1731–1737.
14. Fremont RD, Koyama T, Calfee CS, Wu W, Dossett LA, et al. (2010) Acute lung injury in patients with traumatic injuries: utility of a panel of biomarkers for diagnosis and pathogenesis. The Journal of trauma 68: 1121–1127.
15. Ware LB, Fremont RD, Bastarache JA, Calfee CS, Matthay MA (2010) Determining the aetiology of pulmonary oedema by the oedema fluid-to-plasma protein ratio. The European respiratory journal 35: 331–337.
16. Calfee CS, Ware LB, Eisner MD, Parsons PE, Thompson BT, et al. (2008) Plasma receptor for advanced glycation end products and clinical outcomes in acute lung injury. Thorax 63: 1083–1089.
17. Calfee CS, Ware LB, Glidden DV, Eisner MD, Parsons PE, et al. (2011) Use of risk reclassification with multiple biomarkers improves mortality prediction in acute lung injury. Critical care medicine 39: 711–717.
18. Suratt BT, Eisner MD, Calfee CS, Allard JB, Whittaker LA, et al. (2009) Plasma granulocyte colony-stimulating factor levels correlate with clinical outcomes in patients with acute lung injury. Critical care medicine 37: 1322–1328.
19. Eisner MD, Parsons P, Matthay MA, Ware L, Greene K (2003) Plasma surfactant protein levels and clinical outcomes in patients with acute lung injury. Thorax 58: 983–988.
20. McClintock DE, Starcher B, Eisner MD, Thompson BT, Hayden DL, et al. (2006) Higher urine desmosine levels are associated with mortality in patients with acute lung injury. American journal of physiology Lung cellular and molecular physiology 291: L566–571.
21. Calfee CS, Eisner MD, Parsons PE, Thompson BT, Conner ER, Jr., et al. (2009) Soluble intercellular adhesion molecule-1 and clinical outcomes in patients with acute lung injury. Intensive care medicine 35: 248–257.
22. Cheng IW, Ware LB, Greene KE, Nuckton TJ, Eisner MD, et al. (2003) Prognostic value of surfactant proteins A and D in patients with acute lung injury. Critical care medicine 31: 20–27.
23. Parsons PE, Eisner MD, Thompson BT, Matthay MA, Ancukiewicz M, et al. (2005) Lower tidal volume ventilation and plasma cytokine markers of inflammation in patients with acute lung injury. Critical care medicine 33: 1–6; discussion 230–232.
24. Parsons PE, Matthay MA, Ware LB, Eisner MD (2005) Elevated plasma levels of soluble TNF receptors are associated with morbidity and mortality in patients with acute lung injury. American journal of physiology Lung cellular and molecular physiology 288: L426–431.
25. Ware LB, Eisner MD, Thompson BT, Parsons PE, Matthay MA (2004) Significance of von Willebrand factor in septic and nonseptic patients with acute lung injury. American journal of respiratory and critical care medicine 170: 766–772.
26. Ware LB, Matthay MA, Parsons PE, Thompson BT, Januzzi JL, et al. (2007) Pathogenetic and prognostic significance of altered coagulation and fibrinolysis in acute lung injury/acute respiratory distress syndrome. Critical care medicine 35: 1821–1828.
27. Ware LB, Koyama T, Billheimer DD, Wu W, Bernard GR, et al. (2010) Prognostic and pathogenetic value of combining clinical and biochemical indices in patients with acute lung injury. Chest 137: 288–296.
28. Cribbs SK, Martin GS (2008) Biomarkers in acute lung injury: are we making progress? Critical care medicine 36: 2457–2459.
29. Knaus WA, Draper EA, Wagner DP, Zimmerman JE (1985) APACHE II: a severity of disease classification system. Crit Care Med 13: 818–829.
30. Zhang Y, Wroblewski M, Hertz MI, Wendt CH, Cervenka TM, et al. (2006) Analysis of chronic lung transplant rejection by MALDI-TOF profiles of bronchoalveolar lavage fluid. Proteomics 6: 1001–1010.
31. Griffin T, Chilton J, Johnson J, de Jong E, Onsongo G, et al. (2013) Galaxy-P: Transforming MS-based proteomic informatics via innovative workflow development, dissemination, standardization and transparency. American Society of Mass Spectrometry and Allied Topiecs. Minneapolis, USA.
32. Vizcaino JA, Deutsch EW, Wang R, Csordas A, Reisinger F, et al. (2014) ProteomeXchange provides globally coordinated proteomics data submission and dissemination. Nat Biotechnol 32: 223–226.
33. Storey JD (2002) A direct approach to false discovery rates. J R Statist Soc 64: 479–498.
34. Huang da W, Sherman BT, Lempicki RA (2009) Systematic and integrative analysis of large gene lists using DAVID bioinformatics resources. Nature protocols 4: 44–57.
35. Gharib SA, Nguyen E, Altemeier WA, Shaffer SA, Doneanu CE, et al. (2010) Of mice and men: comparative proteomics of bronchoalveolar fluid. The European respiratory journal 35: 1388–1395.
36. Chang DW, Hayashi S, Gharib SA, Vaisar T, King ST, et al. (2008) Proteomic and computational analysis of bronchoalveolar proteins during the course of the acute respiratory distress syndrome. American journal of respiratory and critical care medicine 178: 701–709.
37. Kosanam H, Sato M, Batruch I, Smith C, Keshavjee S, et al. (2012) Differential proteomic analysis of bronchoalveolar lavage fluid from lung transplant patients with and without chronic graft dysfunction. Clinical biochemistry 45: 223–230.
38. Magi B, Bini L, Perari MG, Fossi A, Sanchez JC, et al. (2002) Bronchoalveolar lavage fluid protein composition in patients with sarcoidosis and idiopathic pulmonary fibrosis: a two-dimensional electrophoretic study. Electrophoresis 23: 3434–3444.
39. Merkel D, Rist W, Seither P, Weith A, Lenter MC (2005) Proteomic study of human bronchoalveolar lavage fluids from smokers with chronic obstructive pulmonary disease by combining surface-enhanced laser desorption/ionization-mass spectrometry profiling with mass spectrometric protein identification. Proteomics 5: 2972–2980.
40. Wu J, Kobayashi M, Sousa EA, Liu W, Cai J, et al. (2005) Differential proteomic analysis of bronchoalveolar lavage fluid in asthmatics following segmental antigen challenge. Molecular & cellular proteomics: MCP 4: 1251–1264.
41. Farjanel J, Hartmann DJ, Guidet B, Luquel L, Offenstadt G (1993) Four markers of collagen metabolism as possible indicators of disease in the adult respiratory distress syndrome. The American review of respiratory disease 147: 1091–1099.
42. Clark JG, Milberg JA, Steinberg KP, Hudson LD (1995) Type III procollagen peptide in the adult respiratory distress syndrome. Association of increased peptide levels in bronchoalveolar lavage fluid with increased risk for death. Annals of internal medicine 122: 17–23.
43. Idell S, Koenig KB, Fair DS, Martin TR, McLarty J, et al. (1991) Serial abnormalities of fibrin turnover in evolving adult respiratory distress syndrome. The American journal of physiology 261: L240–248.
44. Ware LB, Fang X, Matthay MA (2003) Protein C and thrombomodulin in human acute lung injury. American journal of physiology Lung cellular and molecular physiology 285: L514–521.
45. Ware LB, Bastarache JA, Wang L (2005) Coagulation and fibrinolysis in human acute lung injury–new therapeutic targets? The Keio journal of medicine 54: 142–149.
46. Prabhakaran P, Ware LB, White KE, Cross MT, Matthay MA, et al. (2003) Elevated levels of plasminogen activator inhibitor-1 in pulmonary edema fluid

are associated with mortality in acute lung injury. American journal of physiology Lung cellular and molecular physiology 285: L20–28.
47. Quinlan GJ, Chen Y, Evans TW, Gutteridge JM (2001) Iron signalling regulated directly and through oxygen: implications for sepsis and the acute respiratory distress syndrome. Clinical science 100: 169–182.
48. Connelly KG, Moss M, Parsons PE, Moore EE, Moore FA, et al. (1997) Serum ferritin as a predictor of the acute respiratory distress syndrome. American journal of respiratory and critical care medicine 155: 21–25.
49. Ghio AJ, Carter JD, Richards JH, Richer LD, Grissom CK, et al. (2003) Iron and iron-related proteins in the lower respiratory tract of patients with acute respiratory distress syndrome. Critical care medicine 31: 395–400.
50. Lagan AL, Quinlan GJ, Mumby S, Melley DD, Goldstraw P, et al. (2008) Variation in iron homeostasis genes between patients with ARDS and healthy control subjects. Chest 133: 1302–1311.
51. Determann RM, Millo JL, Waddy S, Lutter R, Garrard CS, et al. (2009) Plasma CC16 levels are associated with development of ALI/ARDS in patients with ventilator-associated pneumonia: a retrospective observational study. BMC Pulm Med 9: 49.
52. Lesur O, Langevin S, Berthiaume Y, Legare M, Skrobik Y, et al. (2006) Outcome value of Clara cell protein in serum of patients with acute respiratory distress syndrome. Intensive Care Med 32: 1167–1174.
53. Kropski JA, Fremont RD, Calfee CS, Ware LB (2009) Clara cell protein (CC16), a marker of lung epithelial injury, is decreased in plasma and pulmonary edema fluid from patients with acute lung injury. Chest 135: 1440–1447.
54. Berryman M, Franck Z, Bretscher A (1993) Ezrin is concentrated in the apical microvilli of a wide variety of epithelial cells whereas moesin is found primarily in endothelial cells. J Cell Sci 105 (Pt 4): 1025–1043.
55. Niggli V, Rossy J (2008) Ezrin/radixin/moesin: versatile controllers of signaling molecules and of the cortical cytoskeleton. Int J Biochem Cell Biol 40: 344–349.
56. Mangeat P, Roy C, Martin M (1999) ERM proteins in cell adhesion and membrane dynamics. Trends Cell Biol 9: 187–192.
57. Arpin M, Chirivino D, Naba A, Zwaenepoel I (2011) Emerging role for ERM proteins in cell adhesion and migration. Cell Adh Migr 5: 199–206.
58. Okayama T, Kikuchi S, Ochiai T, Ikoma H, Kubota T, et al. (2008) Attenuated response to liver injury in moesin-deficient mice: impaired stellate cell migration and decreased fibrosis. Biochim Biophys Acta 1782: 542–548.
59. Doi Y, Itoh M, Yonemura S, Ishihara S, Takano H, et al. (1999) Normal development of mice and unimpaired cell adhesion/cell motility/actin-based cytoskeleton without compensatory up-regulation of ezrin or radixin in moesin gene knockout. J Biol Chem 274: 2315–2321.
60. Hashimoto S, Amaya F, Matsuyama H, Ueno H, Kikuchi S, et al. (2008) Dysregulation of lung injury and repair in moesin-deficient mice treated with intratracheal bleomycin. Am J Physiol Lung Cell Mol Physiol 295: L566–574.
61. Torii K, Iida K, Miyazaki Y, Saga S, Kondoh Y, et al. (1997) Higher concentrations of matrix metalloproteinases in bronchoalveolar lavage fluid of patients with adult respiratory distress syndrome. Am J Respir Crit Care Med 155: 43–46.
62. Kong MY, Li Y, Oster R, Gaggar A, Clancy JP (2011) Early elevation of matrix metalloproteinase-8 and -9 in pediatric ARDS is associated with an increased risk of prolonged mechanical ventilation. PLoS One 6: e22596.
63. Koeppen M, McNamee EN, Brodsky KS, Aherne CM, Faigle M, et al. (2013) Detrimental role of the airway mucin Muc5ac during ventilator-induced lung injury. Mucosal Immunol 6: 762–775.

Geographic Access to High Capability Severe Acute Respiratory Failure Centers

David J. Wallace[1,2]*, Derek C. Angus[1], Christopher W. Seymour[1,2], Donald M. Yealy[2], Brendan G. Carr[3], Kristen Kurland[4], Arthur Boujoukos[1], Jeremy M. Kahn[1]

1 Clinical Research, Investigation and Systems Modeling of Acute Illness (CRISMA) Center, Department of Critical Care Medicine, University of Pittsburgh School of Medicine, Pittsburgh, Pennsylvania, United States of America, **2** Department of Emergency Medicine, University of Pittsburgh School of Medicine, Pittsburgh, Pennsylvania, United States of America, **3** Department of Emergency Medicine, University of Pennsylvania Perelman School of Medicine, Philadelphia, Pennsylvania, United States of America, **4** Heinz College School of Public Policy and Management, Carnegie Mellon University, Pittsburgh, Pennsylvania, United States of America

Abstract

Objective: Optimal care of adults with severe acute respiratory failure requires specific resources and expertise. We sought to measure geographic access to these centers in the United States.

Design: Cross-sectional analysis of geographic access to high capability severe acute respiratory failure centers in the United States. We defined high capability centers using two criteria: (1) provision of adult extracorporeal membrane oxygenation (ECMO), based on either 2008–2013 Extracorporeal Life Support Organization reporting or provision of ECMO to 2010 Medicare beneficiaries; or (2) high annual hospital mechanical ventilation volume, based 2010 Medicare claims.

Setting: Nonfederal acute care hospitals in the United States.

Measurements and Main Results: We defined geographic access as the percentage of the state, region and national population with either direct or hospital-transferred access within one or two hours by air or ground transport. Of 4,822 acute care hospitals, 148 hospitals met our ECMO criteria and 447 hospitals met our mechanical ventilation criteria. Geographic access varied substantially across states and regions in the United States, depending on center criteria. Without interhospital transfer, an estimated 58.5% of the national adult population had geographic access to hospitals performing ECMO and 79.0% had geographic access to hospitals performing a high annual volume of mechanical ventilation. With interhospital transfer and under ideal circumstances, an estimated 96.4% of the national adult population had geographic access to hospitals performing ECMO and 98.6% had geographic access to hospitals performing a high annual volume of mechanical ventilation. However, this degree of geographic access required substantial interhospital transfer of patients, including up to two hours by air.

Conclusions: Geographic access to high capability severe acute respiratory failure centers varies widely across states and regions in the United States. Adequate referral center access in the case of disasters and pandemics will depend highly on local and regional care coordination across political boundaries.

Editor: Jorge I. F. Salluh, D'or Institute of Research and Education, Brazil

Funding: Grant support was received from the National Institutes of Health: K12-HL109068 (Wallace), K23-GM104022 (Seymour). The NIH had no role in study design, data collection, analysis, decision to publish, or preparation of the manuscript.

Competing Interests: The authors have declared that no competing interests exist.

* E-mail: wallacedj@upmc.edu

Introduction

An estimated 332,100 cases of severe respiratory from acute respiratory distress syndrome (ARDS) occur in the United States each year, resulting in approximately 133,500 deaths [1] as well as significant long-term morbidity [2,3]. Treatment for ARDS and other forms of severe acute respiratory failure is resource intensive and requires specialized care for optimal patient outcomes [4–7]. This level of care is typically not available at all hospitals, suggesting that patient outcomes may be improved by directing more seriously ill patients to high capability centers [8].

There are no established hospital criteria for high capability centers for severe acute respiratory failure; however, candidate criteria include high mechanical ventilation hospital volumes or the ability to perform extracorporeal membrane oxygenation (ECMO). A volume-outcome relationship exists for mechanically ventilated medical patients, with higher annual hospital volumes associated with improved patient outcomes [9]. Likewise, patients treated at hospitals with ECMO capability have improved outcomes with severe ARDS [8] and a more than two-fold mortality benefit with influenza H1N1-associated ARDS [10].

Quantifying geographic access to hospitals with these capabilities has great public health importance. Determining the number, location, distribution and bed counts of these centers in the United States will help inform public health planning efforts. In addition, quantifying geographic access is a first step towards identifying regions with potentially strained resources, which has implications for routine critical care delivery as well as for pandemic event planning [11]. Severe respiratory illnesses caused by Middle East Respiratory Syndrome Coronavirus [12], avian influenza A [13] or other respiratory pathogens may place abrupt demands on regional intensive care resources underscoring the importance of a geographic access evaluation. Finally, this evaluation could inform a larger discussion regarding the value of regionalized intensive care for more broadly defined severe critical illness.

We sought to evaluate geographic access to high capability severe acute respiratory failure centers in the United States using two candidate criteria: (1) reporting adult ECMO cases to the Extracorporeal Life Support Organization (ELSO) or in Medicare discharge claims, and (2) reporting a high annual volume of mechanical ventilation in Medicare discharge claims from medical patients. In contrast to other time-sensitive medical conditions [14–16], severe ARDS can develop over days, often after hospital admission [17,18]; therefore, we incorporated interhospital transfers into our geographic access calculations. We included long distance transits in our model as they are considered feasible and safe by ground [19] or air [8,20] in this patient population. We determined geographic access to high capability centers using national census, air medical transport and street network databases.

Methods

We performed a cross-sectional analysis of high capability severe acute respiratory failure center geographic access for the adult population based on previous resource allocation models [21,22]. As many patients with severe ARDS are initially treated at community hospitals [8], we created a two-level population geographic access model using high capability center locations and referring hospital locations. We defined geographic access as the percentage of the adult population living within a one-hour driving radius of a high capability center, plus the percentage of the adult population living within a one-hour driving radius of hospitals that may refer patients to these centers. We used a one-hour driving radius to liberally estimate the hospital catchment population, based on prior studies that show 95% of emergency department patients live within 12 miles of the hospital [23,24], but also expecting that patients with more severe symptoms will be willing to drive farther for emergency treatment [25]. For interhospital transport access, we performed separate analyses for both one-hour and two-hour transport intervals. We examined state-level, regional and national geographic access when patient transport between referring hospitals and high capability centers was conducted using ground or rotary air transportation.

High Capability Severe Acute Respiratory Failure Center Criteria

We defined high capability severe acute respiratory failure centers using two hospital criteria: (1) provision of adult ECMO, based on either ELSO reporting or provision of ECMO to 2010 Medicare beneficiaries; or (2) high hospital mechanical ventilation volume, based 2010 Medicare claims. We developed these criteria based on a conceptual model of high capability severe acute respiratory failure centers that recognizes the established volume-outcome relationships in mechanical ventilation and the frequent use of ECMO in severe influenza [26].

We used two data sources to identify high capability centers performing adult ECMO for respiratory failure. First, we used the ELSO website to identify hospitals performing adult ECMO [27]. ELSO maintains an on-line list of active adult ECMO centers that have submitted cases in the past five years. We excluded adult cases reported from children's hospitals, to identify hospitals that provide routine care of adult patients. Second, we used the 2010 Medicare Provider Analysis and Review (MedPAR) file to identify hospitals reporting ECMO in administrative claims. MedPAR includes the final action claims of all hospitalized fee-for-service Medicare beneficiaries and is the only national source of hospital claims data. We analyzed claims for patients 18 and older from the 50 United States and the District of Columbia. We identified ECMO using the International Classification of Diseases, 9th Revision, Clinical Modification (ICD-9-CM) procedure code 39.65 [28].

To identify high capability centers using high mechanical ventilation criteria, we also used the 2010 MedPAR file, identifying adult, non-surgical patients receiving mechanical ventilation using ICD-9-CM procedure codes 96.70, 96.71, 96.72 and a non-surgical diagnosis related group code [28]. We defined hospitals as having a high volume of mechanical ventilation if they reported more than 315 mechanical ventilation claims from adult Medicare patients in 2010. We used this threshold based on a prior volume-outcome study in medical patients receiving mechanical ventilation [9] and the age distribution of medical patients receiving mechanical ventilation in the United States [29]. The 315 threshold in Medicare estimates an all-payer hospital volume of approximately 600 mechanical ventilation cases per year, calculated using the proportion of medical patients in the United States who are aged 65 or older and are mechanically ventilated (52%) [29].

Other Data Sources

We used the 2009 American Hospital Association (AHA) Annual Survey to characterize hospitals, summarize ICU bed counts and obtain geographic coordinates [30]. We linked reporting hospitals with the AHA Annual Survey using the hospital Medicare Provider Identification number. We used the 2012 Atlas and Database of Air Medical Services (ADAMS) to identify hospitals that routinely receive rotatory air transfers of patients [31]. We calculated the population aged 18 and older using block group data from the 2010 United States Census [32].

Hospital Characteristics Analysis

We summarized hospital characteristics for each high capability center criteria and for all short term acute care hospitals in the United States. Variables of interested included the number of hospital beds, number of intensive care unit (ICU) beds, United States region, (Northeast, Midwest, South or West), urbanicity according to the metropolitan statistical area designation of the hospital ZIP code (division: more than 2.5 million persons; metropolitan: between fifty thousand and 2.5 million persons; micropolitan: ten to fifty thousand persons; or rural), teaching status according to each hospital's resident to bed ratio (non-teaching: 0; small teaching: >0 to 0.2; large teaching: >0.2) and ownership status (nonprofit, for profit or government).

Ground Transport Analysis

To identify hospitals potentially referring patients by ground, we analyzed road network and speed limit data from the ArcGIS StreetMap database using ArcInfo 10.1 (ESRI Corporation; Redlands, California) and the Network Analyst extension. All adult short term acute care hospitals located within one- and two-hour driving radii of high capability centers were considered referring hospitals.

Rotary Air Transport Analysis

We identified all high capability centers that routinely receive rotary air transports using the ADAMS database [31]. We then identified all adult short term acute care hospitals within a one hundred twenty (one-hour) and a two hundred forty (two-hour) mile geodesic radius of air-capable high capability centers. We used these distance based on the typical one- and two-hour flight characteristics of rotary aircraft reported to ADAMS.

Population Geographic Access

We compared state-level, regional and national geographic access using each high capability center criteria. Our analysis included all adult United States residents, excluding those living in United States territories. We used the geometric center of each United States Census block group to summarize the population with high capability center geographic access. We did not include day of week or time of day in our calculations based on prior work that showed these variables to have a negligible effect, on average, on transport time estimates for emergency medical transports [33].

We created maps of ground and rotary air coverage using ArcGIS version 10.1 software (ESRI, Redlands, CA). We created two types of geographic access maps: continuous Albers equal area projections and isodemographic cartograms using the Gastner-Newman method of spatial transformation [34]. In the isodemographic projections, state geometry is distorted proportionally to the state population.

We analyzed data analysis using STATA 12.1 (StataCorp, College Station, TX). This research received human subjects review approval by the University of Pittsburgh.

Results

In 2010, of 4,822 acute care hospitals, there were 498 (10.3%) high capability severe acute respiratory failure centers in the United States. We identified 148 hospitals meeting our ECMO criteria and 447 hospitals meeting our mechanical ventilation criteria. A minority of hospitals (n = 97/498, 19.5%) met our criteria for both ECMO and high annual volume of mechanical ventilation.

Both high capability center criteria identified hospitals with higher median numbers of hospital beds (501 for ECMO criteria and 489 for high volume mechanical ventilation criteria) and ICU beds (64 and 54, respectively) compared to all acute care hospitals in the United States (Table 1). The ECMO criteria identified a greater proportion of large teaching hospitals compared to the high volume mechanical ventilation criteria (49% and 33%, respectively). High capability centers were located predominantly in urban areas.

Direct High Capability Severe Acute Respiratory Failure Center Geographic Access

Direct high capability center geographic access was 58.5% for the ECMO criteria and 79.0% for the high volume mechanical ventilation criteria (Table 2). Regionally, direct high capability center geographic access ranged from 47.9% in the South for ECMO to 92.2% in the Northeast for high volume mechanical ventilation. Nine states had no direct geographic access to high capability centers using the ECMO criteria and three states by high mechanical ventilation criteria (Figures 1 & 2).

Indirect High Capability Severe Acute Respiratory Failure Center Geographic Access through Interhospital Transport

A total of 274 high capability centers reported helipads to ADAMS. Nationally, 87.5 and 96.5% of the adult population had geographic access to a high capability center with one-hour interhospital transport using ECMO and high volume mechanical ventilation criteria, respectively (Table 2). Geographic access increased to 96.4% and 98.6% with two-hour interhospital transport, respectively. High capability center geographic access varied by state and region, with Western states having the lowest regional and state-level geographic access (Figures 1 & 2).

Discussion

Geographic access to high capability severe acute respiratory failure centers varies substantially across states and regions in the United States. An estimated 58.5 to 79.0% of the population has direct geographic access to a high capability center. Geographic access increases to 96.4 to 98.6% when accounting for interhospital transport of up to two hours. This suggests the existing hospital infrastructure is geographically capable of reaching most Americans who develop severe acute respiratory failure; however, some states had no high capability centers, and many rural areas were without timely access using more restrictive interhospital transport assumptions.

Our analysis provides important preliminary insight into geographic access to high capability centers for severe acute respiratory failure in the United States. We defined geographic access using accessibility, which is the relationship between the location of patients and the location of health care resources. This is an important component of health care access [35]; however, true access to these centers involves more than just accessibility. Practically, access also requires complex coordination efforts across multiple hospitals and explicit regional planning to address other key access domains. These domains include capacity (e.g., the relationship between demand and ICU supply–including ICU beds and ICU personnel), accommodation (e.g., the relationship between the development of acute respiratory failure and the ability of the health care system to move the patient to a high capability center), affordability (e.g., the relationship between the cost of care and the patient's or insurer's ability to pay), and acceptability (e.g., the patient's or hospital's comfort with characteristics of client-provider relationship) [36]. All of these domains require further study as we attempt to organize the health system to best meet the needs of patients with severe acute respiratory failure.

The final domain, acceptability, includes both the hospital perspective and patient choice. While there may be survival benefits to moving the location of ICU care hundreds of miles to a regional center, a patient-centered approach optimally incorporates patient and family preferences. Our model defined transports up to two hours by helicopter to reach a high capability center as "available" – corresponding to approximately two hundred forty miles. A moderate additional travel burden for regional center care may be acceptable to some patients [37]; however, there is likely a threshold for others, beyond which they would prefer local hospital services [38]. The success of regionalized care will certainly depend on finding a balance between system capability and patient preferences.

We acknowledge that the criteria we used to identify high capability severe acute respiratory failure centers were proxies, and other elements of care are likely associated with high quality, beyond ECMO and high volumes. Other interventions associated

Table 1. High Capability Severe Acute Respiratory Failure Center Characteristics.

	ECMO Criteria[a] (n = 148)	High Volume Mechanical Ventilation Criteria[b] (n = 447)	All Acute Care Hospitals (n = 4822)
Number of hospital beds, median (IQR[c])	501 (336 to 740)	489 (380 to 652)	101 (36 to 227)
Number of ICU[d] beds, median (IQR)	64 (42 to 95)	54 (39 to 76)	8 (2 to 22)
Region, n (%)			
Northeast	37 (25)	109 (24)	600 (12)
Midwest	41 (28)	100 (22)	1423 (30)
South	44 (30)	175 (39)	1853 (38)
West	26 (18)	63 (14)	946 (20)
Urbancity, n (%)			
Division (>2.5 million persons)	40 (27)	131 (29)	687 (14)
Metropolitan (50K[e]–2.5 million)	106 (72)	309 (69)	2068 (43)
Micropolitan (10K–50K)	2 (1)	5 (1)	872 (18)
Rural (<10K)	0	2 (1)	1195 (24)
Teaching status, n (%)			
Large teaching	73 (49)	148 (33)	355 (7)
Small teaching	34 (23)	141 (32)	910 (19)
Non-teaching	41 (28)	158 (35)	3557 (74)
Financial status, n (%)			
Nonprofit	112 (76)	356 (80)	2745 (57)
For profit	11 (7)	41 (9)	784 (16)
Government	25 (17)	50 (11)	1293 (27)

[a]*Hospitals reporting extracorporeal membrane oxygenation cases to the Extracorporeal Life Support Organization or extracorporeal membrane oxygenation procedure codes in Medicare discharge claims;*
[b]*hospitals reporting more than 315 annual claims for medical mechanical ventilation,*
[c]*interquartile range,*
[d]*intensive care unit,*
[e]*thousand.*

with improved quality include the ability to use prone positioning [4], use of paralytic agents [5] or routinely applying low tidal volumes in ARDS [7]. However, in the absence of a consensus definition, the provision of ECMO or high annual volumes of mechanical ventilation may identify hospitals with these other capabilities. Indeed, it is notable that there are currently no standardized definitions for categorizing critical care resources. Such definitions are urgently needed to facilitate further evaluation

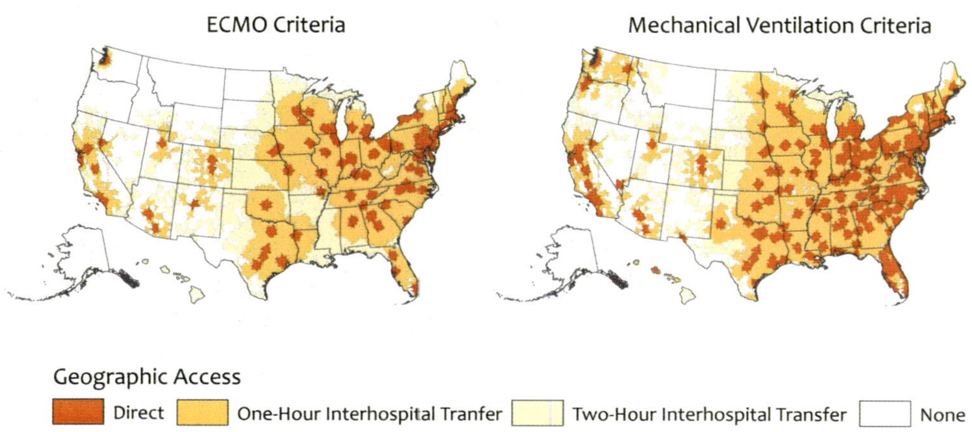

Figure 1. Continuous Albers equal area projections showing geographic access to high capability severe acute respiratory failure centers in the United States. Geographic access is defined using two separate hospital criteria: provision of ECMO or high annual volume of mechanical ventilation. The dark orange areas show regions with direct high capability severe acute respiratory failure center geographic access. Medium orange areas show regions with geographic access after a one-hour ground or air interhospital transfer. Light orange areas show regions with geographic access after a two-hour ground or air interhospital transfer. *ECMO: extracorporeal membrane oxygenation; MV: high annual volume of mechanical ventilation.*

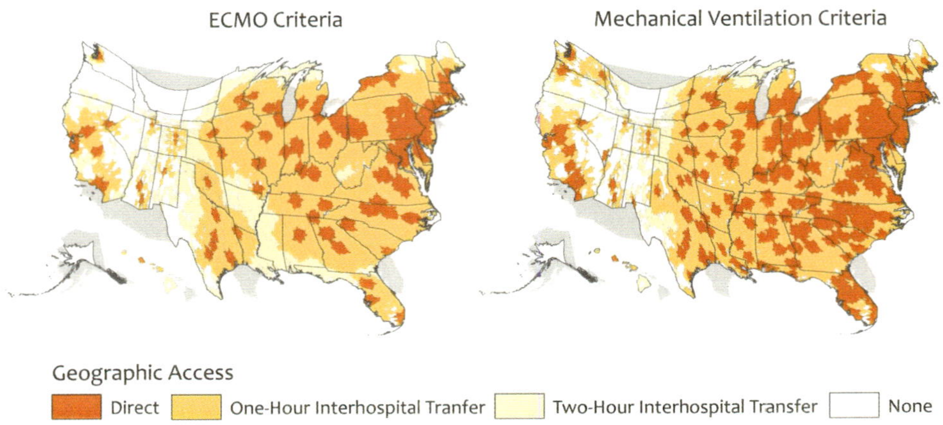

Figure 2. Gastner-Newman transformations of continuous Albers equal area projections of the United States showing geographic access to high capability severe acute respiratory failure centers in the United States. Geographic access is defined using two separate hospital criteria: provision of ECMO or high annual volume of mechanical ventilation. The dark orange areas show regions with direct high capability severe acute respiratory failure center geographic access. Medium orange areas show regions with geographic access after a one-hour ground or air interhospital transfer. Light orange areas show regions with geographic access after a two-hour ground or air interhospital transfer. *ECMO: extracorporeal membrane oxygenation; MV: high annual volume of mechanical ventilation.*

of regional critical care organization. We believe the criteria we examined are well supported by the available literature and thus have face validity for identifying high quality severe acute respiratory failure care.

In evaluating the validity of our definition, it is worth noting that high mechanical ventilation volume and ECMO identified 498 high capability centers in the United States, which is similar to the number of level 1 or 2 trauma system hospitals (n = 445) [21]. The annual number of severe ARDS cases is lower than the estimated 678,000 severely injured patients treated at trauma centers each year [39], though ICUs do not exclusively provide ARDS care. Similarly, in the United States there are 925 primary stroke centers [40] and as of 2008 there were 298 hospitals performing coronary artery bypass graft surgery [41]. This indicates that our criteria identified a similar proportion of centers to other formally and informally regionalized care systems.

Geographic access to hospitals meeting the ECMO criteria ranged form 58.5 to 96.4%, depending on interhospital transport assumptions. Quantifying geographic access to state and regional ECMO-capable hospitals is especially important for pandemic planning, as a subset of patients with severe acute respiratory failure may not improve with conventional ventilator support. ECMO infrastructure expansion will not be practical in all areas, therefore hospitals in geographic "white spaces" should consider developing regional transfer agreements in anticipation of these events as well as for the routine care of the most severely ill patients with acute respiratory failure.

Further study is required to measure other aspects of resource availability, including regional center staffing and measures of ICU capacity [42]. As stressed by the United States Department of Health and Human Services' Hospital Preparedness Program, regional capability should be viewed as a community attribute, rather than a facility one [43].

Our analysis has other limitations. We did not address redundant geographic access to high capability centers. Several regions had tightly clustered hospitals meeting our center criteria, raising the question if similar geographic access would be possible with fewer high capability centers. Furthermore, structure is not equivalent to organization. We specified transfer relationships between referring and receiving hospitals that may not occur in practice. Additionally, high capability centers may already be operating near or at capacity, making them unable to serve as referral centers. Coordination of regional critical care for severe acute respiratory failure will clearly require planning and protocols to achieve efficient and high quality regional care.

Our ECMO center criteria also had limitations. We identified patients who received ECMO through Medicare claims, rather than an all-payer database. We may have missed potential ECMO centers because they provide ECMO only to young patients or exclusively serve a Medicare Advantage population (who do not appear in fee-for-service Medicare claims). Further, the ELSO criterion only identified adult hospitals performing veno-venous ECMO. Finally, we did not include pediatric hospitals, though some may perform adult ECMO cannulation in nearby adult hospital centers.

Our modeling approach also included real-world simplifications. For example, we did not account for the effects of extreme winter weather or daily traffic patterns. Additionally, we used the geometric centroid of each census block group to calculate the catchment area population. As such, our estimates should be considered in a "best case scenario" context, and may overestimate true geographic access.

Despite these limitations, our findings have practical significance. First, we identified several states have no geographic access to high capability centers. These states should immediately consider the capabilities of their hospitals to transfer patients with severe acute respiratory failure to the closest high capability center. Second, we identified many states with incomplete geographic access. Further work is needed to evaluate the cost of infrastructure expansion against competing regionalization priorities, recognizing that geographic access to high capability severe acute respiratory failure centers may be implausible.

Our analysis provides a conceptual framework for evaluating intensive care infrastructure. Action is needed to focus attention on other domains of access by engaging stakeholders in a discussion of regionalized critical care. Important next steps include standardizing criteria for ICU levels of care, creating protocols for transferring patients with severe acute respiratory failure to high capability centers and developing regional systems of audit and feedback to promote a continuous improvement process. The alignment of health care systems with public health efforts has the potential to improve the routine care of patients with severe acute

Table 2. Geographic Access to High Capability Severe Acute Respiratory Failure Center in the United States.

	ECMO Critiera[a]			High Volume Mechanical Ventilation Criteria[b]		
	Direct	One-Hour Interhospital Transfer	Two-Hour Interhospital Transfer	Direct	One-Hour Interhospital Transfer	Two-Hour Interhospital Transfer
United States, %	58.5	87.5	96.4	79.0	96.5	98.6
Northeast, %	79.4	98.7	99.8	92.2	99.9	99.9
Connecticut	85.9	99.9	99.9	99.6	100	100
Maine	45.1	90.4	98.4	61.7	96.1	99.1
Massachusetts	81.7	99.8	99.8	95.9	99.9	99.9
New Hampshire	69.7	100	100	52.7	100	100
New Jersey	85.7	99.8	99.8	99.5	100	100
New York	78.2	98.8	99.8	91.9	99.9	99.9
Pennsylvania	84.1	100	100	92.0	100	100
Rhode Island	63.0	99.8	99.8	99.8	99.9	99.9
Vermont	0	45.7	100	61.0	100	100
Midwest, %	57.7	92.8	98.7	73.4	97.1	99.3
Illinois	75.9	100	100	80.1	100	100
Indiana	50.6	100	100	70.8	100	100
Iowa	18.9	99.1	100	42.6	100	100
Kansas	31.8	61.6	100	64.3	94.0	100
Michigan	65.1	93.2	99.5	83.0	96.1	99.5
Minnesota	63.7	89.0	99.0	73.8	97.7	99.4
Missouri	52.7	90.9	99.3	70.4	99.3	99.3
Nebraska	60.3	85.9	99.4	60.3	86.2	99.4
North Dakota	0	0	37.2	22.7	47.8	85.8
Ohio	59.6	100	100	89.5	100	100
South Dakota	0	7.1	68.9	28.2	60.2	75
Wisconsin	56.2	97.7	99.7	52.6	95.2	99.7
South, %	47.9	85.0	99.6	78.6	99.2	99.8
Alabama	23.7	79.5	99.9	71.6	100	100
Arkansas	0.4	20.8	99.6	39.4	99.6	99.6
Delaware	92.2	100	100	71.8	100	100
District of Columbia	100	100	100	100	100	100
Florida	47.2	88.0	99.4	93.7	99.6	99.8
Georgia	60.0	98.0	99.8	77.5	99.9	99.9
Kentucky	43.9	99.9	100	69.8	100	100
Louisiana	9.5	32.4	98.9	60.4	99.4	99.4
Maryland	87.2	99.8	99.8	89.5	99.9	99.9
Mississippi	0	16.6	99.9	47.9	99.9	99.9
North Carolina	41.1	99.7	99.8	84.0	99.8	99.8
Oklahoma	34.2	92.3	100	61.8	99.2	100
South Carolina	38.6	99.9	99.9	81.9	99.9	99.9
Tennessee	49.9	83.7	100	80.6	100	100
Texas	63.0	82.4	99.0	77.4	96.9	99.6
Virginia	52.8	99.8	99.9	86.5	99.9	99.9
West Virginia	7.1	90.2	99.9	53.3	99.9	99.9
West, %	59.4	77.6	86.6	74.3	88.8	95.1
Alaska	0	0	0	0	0	0
Arizona	77.3	87.4	97.0	78.4	91.9	97
California	71.7	97.2	99.5	85.3	98.8	99.5
Colorado	70.9	90.5	98.0	72.2	90.3	98

Table 2. Cont.

	ECMO Critiera[a]			High Volume Mechanical Ventilation Criteria[b]		
	Direct	One-Hour Interhospital Transfer	Two-Hour Interhospital Transfer	Direct	One-Hour Interhospital Transfer	Two-Hour Interhospital Transfer
Hawaii	68.7	69.6	69.6	69.1	85.1	97.7
Idaho	0	1.8	47.0	8.2	22.1	89.2
Montana	0	0	0	0	1.9	36.9
Nevada	19.5	22.9	96.5	89.6	94.2	96.5
New Mexico	42.4	57.9	94.1	8.3	16.1	51.3
Oregon	0	0	8.8	60.2	80.5	97.9
Utah	71.6	89.8	96.7	74.0	94.8	97.9
Washington	49.5	62.4	68.8	74.6	95.7	98.8
Wyoming	0	26.7	65.7	0	26.7	65.7

[a]*Hospitals reporting extracorporeal membrane oxygenation cases to the Extracorporeal Life Support Organization or extracorporeal membrane oxygenation procedure codes reported in Medicare discharge claims;*
[b]*hospitals reporting more than 315 annual claims for medical mechanical ventilation.*

respiratory failure, as well as to improve health system resilience during times of additional strain.

Conclusions

Geographic access to high capability severe acute respiratory failure centers varied substantially across states and regions in the United States, depending on center criteria. An estimated 96.4% and 98.6% of the national population had geographic access to a high capability center; however, this degree of access required substantial interhospital transfer of many patients, including up to two hours by rotatory air transport. Adequate referral center access in the case of disasters and pandemics will depend highly on local and regional care coordination across political boundaries.

Author Contributions

Conceived and designed the experiments: DJW DCA CWS BGC AB KK DMY JMK. Performed the experiments: DJW KK JMK. Analyzed the data: DJW DCA CWS BGC AB KK DMY JMK. Contributed reagents/materials/analysis tools: DJW KK JMK. Wrote the paper: DJW DCA CWS BGC AB KK DMY JMK.

References

1. Rubenfeld GD, Caldwell E, Peabody E, Weaver J, Martin DP, et al. (2005) Incidence and outcomes of acute lung injury. N Engl J Med 353: 1685–1693.
2. Dowdy DWD, Eid MPM, Dennison CRC, Mendez-Tellez PAP, Herridge MSM, et al. (2006) Quality of life after acute respiratory distress syndrome: a meta-analysis. Intensive Care Med 32: 1115–1124.
3. Herridge MS, Tansey CM, Matté A, Tomlinson G, Diaz-Granados N, et al. (2011) Functional disability 5 years after acute respiratory distress syndrome. N Engl J Med 364: 1293–1304.
4. Guérin C, Reignier J, Richard J-C, Beuret P, Gacouin A, et al. (2013) Prone Positioning in Severe Acute Respiratory Distress Syndrome. N Engl J Med 368: 2159–2168.
5. Papazian L, Forel J-M, Gacouin A, Penot-Ragon C, Perrin G, et al. (2010) Neuromuscular blockers in early acute respiratory distress syndrome. N Engl J Med 363: 1107–1116.
6. Kress JP, Pohlman AS, O'Connor MF, Hall JB (2000) Daily interruption of sedative infusions in critically ill patients undergoing mechanical ventilation. N Engl J Med 342: 1471–1477.
7. The Acute Respiratory Distress Syndrome Network (2000) Ventilation with lower tidal volumes as compared with traditional tidal volumes for acute lung injury and the acute respiratory distress syndrome. The Acute Respiratory Distress Syndrome Network. N Engl J Med 342: 1301–1308.
8. Peek G, Mugford M, Tiruvoipati R, Wilson A, Allen E, et al. (2009) Efficacy and economic assessment of conventional ventilatory support versus extracorporeal membrane oxygenation for severe adult respiratory failure (CESAR): a multicentre randomised controlled trial. The Lancet 374: 1351–1363.
9. Kahn JM, Goss CH, Heagerty PJ, Kramer AA, O'Brien CR, et al. (2006) Hospital volume and the outcomes of mechanical ventilation. N Engl J Med 355: 41–50.
10. Noah MA, Peek GJ, Finney SJ, Griffiths MJ, Harrison DA, et al. (2011) Referral to an Extracorporeal Membrane Oxygenation Center and Mortality Among Patients With Severe 2009 Influenza A (H1N1). JAMA: The Journal of the American Medical Association 306: 1659–1668.
11. Rubinson L, Mutter R, Viboud C, Hupert N, Uyeki T, et al. (2013) Impact of the Fall 2009 Influenza A(H1N1)pdm09 Pandemic on US Hospitals. Med Care 51: 259–265.
12. Centers for Disease Control and Prevention CDC (2013) Update: Recommendations for Middle East respiratory syndrome coronavirus (MERS-CoV). MMWR Morb Mortal Wkly Rep 62: 557.
13. Centers for Disease Control and Prevention CDC (2013) Emergence of avian influenza A(H7N9) virus causing severe human illness - China, February-April 2013. MMWR Morb Mortal Wkly Rep 62: 366–371.
14. Demetriades DD, Murray JJ, Charalambides KK, Alo KK, Velmahos GG, et al. (2004) Trauma fatalities - time and location of hospital deaths. J Am Coll Surg 198: 7–7.
15. The National Institute of Neurological Disorders and Stroke rt-PA Stroke Study Group (1995) Tissue Plasminogen Activator for Acute Ischemic Stroke. N Engl J Med 333: 1581–1588.
16. The GUSTO investigators (1993) An international randomized trial comparing four thrombolytic strategies for acute myocardial infarction. N Engl J Med 329: 673–682.
17. Valta PP, Uusaro AA, Nunes SS, Ruokonen EE, Takala JJ (1999) Acute respiratory distress syndrome: frequency, clinical course, and costs of care. Critical care medicine 27: 2367–2374.
18. Writing Committee of the WHO Consultation on Clinical Aspects of Pandemic H1N1 2009 Influenza, Bautista E, Chotpitayasunondh T, Gao Z, Harper SA, et al. (2010) Clinical aspects of pandemic 2009 influenza A (H1N1) virus infection. N Engl J Med 362: 1708–1719.
19. Uusaro A, Parviainen I, Takala J, Ruokonen E (2002) Safe long-distance interhospital ground transfer of critically ill patients with acute severe unstable respiratory and circulatory failure. Intensive Care Med 28: 1122–1125.
20. Seymour CW, Kahn JM, Schwab CW, Fuchs BD (2008) Adverse events during rotary-wing transport of mechanically ventilated patients: a retrospective cohort study. Crit Care 12: R71.
21. Branas CC, MacKenzie EJ, Williams JC, Schwab CW, Teter HM, et al. (2005) Access to trauma centers in the United States. JAMA: The Journal of the American Medical Association 293: 2626–2633.
22. Klein M, Kramer C, Nelson J, Rivara F, Gibran N, et al. (2009) Geographic access to burn center hospitals. JAMA: The Journal of the American Medical Association 302: 1774–1781.

23. Lerner EB, Billittier AJ, Sikora J, Moscati RM (1999) Use of a geographic information system to determine appropriate means of trauma patient transport. Academic Emergency Medicine 6: 1127–1133.
24. Carr BG, Branas CC, Metlay JP, Sullivan AF, Camargo CA (2009) Access to emergency care in the United States. Ann Emerg Med 54: 261–269.
25. Henneman PL, Garb JL, Capraro GA, Li H, Smithline HA, et al. (2011) Administration of Emergency Medicine. J Emerg Med 40: 333–339.
26. Adalja AA, Watson M, Waldhorn RE, Toner ES (2013) A conceptual approach to improving care in pandemics and beyond: severe lung injury centers. J Crit Care 28: 318.e9–.e15.
27. Extracorporeal Life Support Organization. Available: http://elsonet.org/. Accessed 10 May 2013.
28. Quan H, Parsons GA, Ghali WA (2004) Validity of procedure codes in International Classification of Diseases, 9th revision, clinical modification administrative data. Med Care 42: 801–809.
29. Wunsch H, Linde-Zwirble WT, Angus DC, Hartman ME, Milbrandt EB, et al. (2010) The epidemiology of mechanical ventilation use in the United States. Critical care medicine 38: 1947–1953.
30. American Hospital Association Annual Survey Database for Fiscal Year 2009 (2010).
31. Atlas and Database of Air Medical Services. Available: http://www.adamsairmed.org. Accessed 23 May 2013.
32. Minnesota Population Center (2011) National Historical Geographic Information System: Version 2.0. Minneapolis, MN: University of Minnesota.
33. Wallace DJ, Kahn JM, Angus DC, Martin-Gill C, Callaway CW, et al. (2014) Accuracy of Prehospital Transport Time Estimation. Academic Emergency Medicine 21: 9–16.
34. Gastner MT, Newman MEJ (2004) Diffusion-based method for producing density-equalizing maps. Proc Natl Acad Sci U S A 101: 7499–7504.
35. Penchansky R, Thomas JW (1981) The concept of access: definition and relationship to consumer satisfaction. Med Care 19: 127–140.
36. Kahn JM, Asch RJ, Iwashyna TJ, Rubenfeld GD, Angus DC, et al. (2008) Perceived barriers to the regionalization of adult critical care in the United States: a qualitative preliminary study. BMC Health Serv Res 8: 239.
37. Hagen H, Stene-Larsen G (1989) Attitudes of the population and patients to regionalization in Oslo. Journal of the Norwegian Medical Association 109: 607–609.
38. Finlayson SRS, Birkmeyer JDJ, Tosteson ANA, Nease RFR (1999) Patient preferences for location of care: implications for regionalization. Med Care 37: 204–209.
39. Nathens AB, Jurkovich GJ, MacKenzie EJ, Rivara FP (2004) A Resource-Based Assessment of Trauma Care in the United States. The Journal of Trauma: Injury, Infection, and Critical Care 56: 173–178.
40. Joint Commission: Accreditation, Health Care, Certification. Available: http://www.jointcommission.org/. Accessed 10 September 2013.
41. Horwitz JR, Nichols A, Nallamothu BK, Sasson C, Iwashyna TJ (2013) Expansion of Invasive Cardiac Services in the United States. Circulation 128: 803–810.
42. Halpern SD (2011) ICU capacity strain and the quality and allocation of critical care. Current Opinion in Critical Care 17: 648–657.
43. Office of Assistant Secretary for Preparedness and Response. From Hospitals to Healthcare Coalitions: Transforming Health Preparedness and Response in Our Communities. Available: http://www.phe.gov/Preparedness/planning/hpp/Documents/hpp-healthcare-coalitions.pdf.

Recombinant Human Activated Protein C in the Treatment of Acute Respiratory Distress Syndrome

Alexander D. Cornet[1,2,3]*, A. B. Johan Groeneveld[1,3,4], Jorrit J. Hofstra[5,6], Alexander P. Vlaar[5,6,7], Pieter R. Tuinman[5,6], Arthur van Lingen[8], Marcel Levi[7], Armand R. J. Girbes[1,3], Marcus J. Schultz[5,6], Albertus Beishuizen[1,3,9]

1 Department of Intensive Care, VU University Medical Center, Amsterdam, The Netherlands, **2** Department of Internal Medicine, VU University Medical Center, Amsterdam, The Netherlands, **3** Institute for Cardiovascular Research ICaR-VU, VU University Medical Center, Amsterdam, The Netherlands, **4** Department of Intensive Care, Erasmus Medical Center, Rotterdam, The Netherlands, **5** Department of Intensive Care, Academic Medical Center, Amsterdam, The Netherlands, **6** Laboratory of Experimental Intensive Care and Anesthesiology, Academic Medical Center, Amsterdam, The Netherlands, **7** Department of Internal Medicine, Academic Medical Center, Amsterdam, The Netherlands, **8** Department of Nuclear Medicine, VU University Medical Center, Amsterdam, The Netherlands, **9** Department of Intensive Care, Medisch Spectrum Twente, Enschede, The Netherlands

Abstract

Rationale: Pulmonary coagulopathy may play a pathogenetic role in acute respiratory distress syndrome (ARDS), by contributing to alveolocapillary inflammation and increased permeability. Recombinant human activated protein C (rh-APC) may inhibit this process and thereby improve patient outcome.

Methods: A prospective randomized, saline-controlled, single-blinded clinical trial was performed in the intensive care units of two university hospitals, and patients with ARDS were included within 24 h after meeting inclusion criteria.

Intervention: A 4-day course of intravenous rh-APC (24 mcg/kg/h) (n = 33) versus saline (n = 38).

Outcomes: The primary outcome parameter was the pulmonary leak index (PLI) of ^{67}Gallium-transferrin as a measure of alveolocapillary permeability and secondary outcomes were disease severity scores and ventilator-free days, among others.

Results: Baseline characteristics were similar; in 87% of patients the PLI was above normal and in 90% mechanical or non-invasive ventilation was instituted at a median lung injury score of 2.5. There was no evidence that Rh-APC treatment affected the PLI or attenuated lung injury and sequential organ failure assessment scores. Mean ventilator-free days amounted to 14 (rh-APC) and 12 days (saline, P = 0.35). 28-day mortality was 6% in rh-APC- and 18% in saline-treated patients (P = 0.12). There was no difference in bleeding events. The study was prematurely discontinued because rh-APC was withdrawn from the market.

Conclusion: There is no evidence that treatment with intravenous rh-APC during 4 days for infectious or inflammatory ARDS ameliorates increased alveolocapillary permeability or the clinical course of ARDS patients. We cannot exclude underpowering.

Editor: Matthias Briel, University Hospital Basel, Switzerland

Funding: This trial has been supported via an unrestricted research grant from Eli Lilly Inc. (Indianapolis, IN, USA). The funders had no role in study design, data collection and analysis, decision to publish, or preparation of the manuscript.

Competing Interests: The study received funding by Eli Lilly Inc. (Indianapolis, IN, USA).

* E-mail: cornet@vumc.nl

Introduction

Acute respiratory distress syndrome (ARDS), with its milder form formerly known as acute lung injury (ALI), occurs in 30 to 80 per 100,000 person-years and is a major cause of morbidity and mortality in the critically ill [1,2]. Treatment of ARDS is supportive since there are no routine drugs for treatment, other than treatment of the underlying disease [3]. A key factor in the pathogenesis of ARDS is alveolocapillary inflammation, leading to endothelial barrier dysfunction and increased permeability, that can be assessed at the bedside, with help of the non-invasively measured pulmonary leak index (PLI) of ^{67}Gallium (^{67}Ga)-transferrin [4–6]. In previous studies it was demonstrated that the PLI parallels the clinical severity and course of ARDS, for

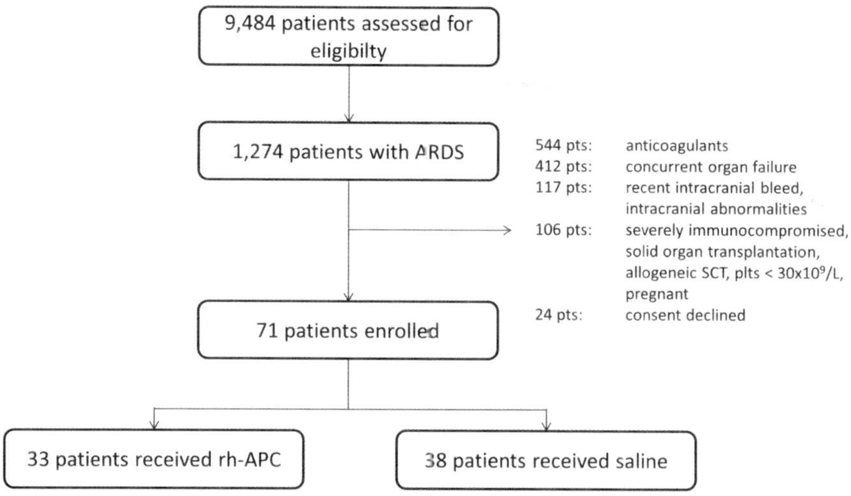

Figure 1. CONSORT diagram. ARDS, acute respiratory distress syndrome; SCT, stem cell transplantation; plts, platelet count.

instance expressed as changes in the lung injury score [5]. Furthermore, the PLI appeared to be more accurate in assessing the degree of permeability than extravascular lung water measurements [7].

There is an extensive crosstalk between inflammation, activated coagulation and depressed fibrinolysis, so that alveolar fibrin depositions and small vessel thrombi are thought to contribute and perpetuate alveolocapillary inflammation, pulmonary vascular injury and barrier dysfunction [3,8–11]. The alveolar and systemic levels of naturally occurring anticoagulants, such as activated protein C (APC), may be depressed because of consumption, impaired synthesis and degradation, and inhibitors of fibrinolysis may be increased, and both phenomena may be associated with pulmonary and remote organ dysfunction and mortality [8,9]. In healthy volunteers, infusion of rh–APC attenuated coagulopathy and neutrophils in the lungs after inhalation of endotoxin [12,13]. This is in line with beneficial effects of rh–APC infusion in models of sepsis and ARDS on pulmonary coagulopathy and consequently on alveolocapillary inflammation, as well as with directly ameliorating effects on endothelial barrier dysfunction via stimulation of protease-activated receptor-1 (PAR-1), protein C and sphingosine-1-phosphate (S1P) receptors in the endothelium [11,14,15]. The latter may downregulate, among others, pulmonary endothelial release of angiopoietin-2 that may play a direct role in the increased permeability in patients with ARDS, and may attenuate cytoskeletal rearrangement via Rho-associated kinase [11,14–17]. In patients with severe sepsis, often accompanied by ARDS, infusion of recombinant human (rh) APC reduced mortality by ameliorating organ dysfunction, including respiratory dysfunction as demonstrated in two multicenter trials (PROWESS, ENHANCE) [18,19,20]. Of note, infusion was particularly effective in patients who presented with lung infection, community–acquired pneumonia or need for mechanical ventilation [21,22]. In a recent large study in patients with septic shock (PROWESS SHOCK), rh-APC appeared of no benefit and was withdrawn from the market after publication, although two prior multicenter trials (ADDRESS, RESOLVE) already raised concerns regarding its efficacy [23–25]. About 43% had a pulmonary origin of sepsis in the PROWESS-SHOCK trial. In a recent meta-analysis, including the aforementioned negative trial [25], however, the drug was suggested to maintain effectiveness [26].

For the current study, performed before publication of the last multicenter study on APC [25], we hypothesized that infusion of rh–APC attenuates the increase in pulmonary vascular permeability and thereby benefits patients with ARDS as a single organ failure. We performed a single-blinded, randomized controlled multicenter trial of patients with ARDS comparing intravenous infusion of rh–APC with saline, studying the effect on the PLI as primary outcome measure [4–6]. Secondary outcomes included lung injury score (LIS) and sequential organ failures score (SOFA), duration on mechanical ventilation and ventilator-free days, and mortality. A substudy of our trial was recently published and suggested attenuated hypercoagulability, increased fibrinolysis and thereby less lung injury by rh-APC treatment [27].

Patients and Methods

Study design

This is a report of the infectious and inflammatory ALI/ARDS (INFALI) trial, a multicenter prospective, single-blinded, randomized, saline-controlled clinical trial in patients with ALI/ARDS (trial registration number ISRCTN 52566874). The patients were blinded for the allocated treatment. The Ethics Committee of the VU University Medical Center, Amsterdam, the Netherlands, approved the study protocol. Written informed consent was obtained from all patients or their next of kin before enrolment in the trial. All clinical investigations have been conducted according to the principles expressed in the Declaration of Helsinki. The protocol for this trial and supporting CONSORT checklist are available as supporting information; see Checklist S1 and Protocol S1.

Inclusion and exclusion criteria

Patients, over 18 years of age and admitted to the mixed medical–surgical intensive care units (ICU's) of two participating university medical centers in Amsterdam, were to be included because of respiratory insufficiency within 24 hours after diagnosis of ALI/ARDS, of any cause, including pneumonia, sepsis, aspiration according to standard clinical criteria, irrespective of the need for ventilatory support. The definition used to establish the diagnosis pneumonia was radiographic evidence of pulmonary consolidation in association with the production of purulent sputum with plus two positive SIRS criteria (1. core temperature of

Table 1. Baseline characteristics.

	rh-APC (n = 33)	saline (n = 38)	P-value
Age	62.2±14.4	60.6±17.7	0.940
Sex (male)	15 (45)	25 (66)	0.099
Height (cm)	168.5±8.7	172.8±9.6	0.097
Weight (kg)	73.9±14.9	71.6±16.3	0.518
Comorbidities			
Cardiovascular	15 (45)	21 (55)	0.479
Pulmonary	5 (15)	14 (37)	0.059
Renal	1 (3)	3 (8)	0.618
malignancy	4 (12)	6 (16)	0.739
Etiology of ARDS			
pneumonia	27 (82)	34 (89)	0.242
abdominal sepsis	3 (9)	1 (3)	
near-drowning	0	2 (5)	
smoke inhalation	2 (6)	0	
miscellaneous	1 (3)	1 (3)	
Severity of ARDS (Berlin criteria)			
mild	9 (27)	12 (32)	0.582
moderate	23 (70)	23 (61)	
severe	1 (3)	3 (7)	
Blood stream infection	6	10	0.459
Streptococcus pneumoniae	3	4	
Listeria monocytogenes	1	0	
Enterococcus faecium	0	1	
Coagulase-negative staphylococcus	2	5	
Tracheal aspirate			
Streptococcus pneumoniae	3	8	0.685
Beta-haemolytical streptococcus	1	-	
Staphylococcus aureus	2	6	
Enterococcus faecalis	1	-	
Listeria monocytogenes	1	-	
Escherichia coli	3	4	
Pseudomonas aeruginosa	4	1	
Proteus mirabilis	-	2	
Hafnia alveii	2	-	
Enterobacter cloacae	1	-	
Haemophilus influenzae	1	2	
Klebsiella oxytoca	1	-	
Klebsiella pneumoniae	-	3	
Aeromonas spp	-	1	
Pneumocystis jirovecii	1	-	
Aspergillus spp	2	1	
Candida spp	2	3	
Disease severity			
APACHE II	17.3±6.2	16.9±5.4	0.707
SAPS II	41.5±12.8	37.8±12.8	0.266
SOFA	7.3±2.3	7.0±2.0	0.867
Vital signs			
Temperature (°C)	36.6±1.4	36.5±1.7	0.703
Heart rate (/min)	101.0±32.2	112.3±27.8	0.121

Table 1. Cont.

	rh-APC (n = 33)	saline (n = 38)	P-value
MAP (mmHg)	69.9±11.7	69.0±16.2	0.503
Treatment			
Vasopressors	26 (79)	30 (79)	1.000
Corticosteroids	23 (70)	24 (63)	0.800
Duration between admission and start of study (days)	1.8±3.4	1.7±2.4	0.595

Mean/median ± standard deviation/interquartile range, respectively, or number (percentage), where appropriate. Rh-APC, recombinant human activated protein C; APACHE, acute physiology and chronic health evaluation; SAPS, simplified acute physiology score; SOFA, sequential organ failure assessment; MAP, mean arterial pressure.

≥38°C or ≤36°C; 2. heart rate of ≥90 beats/min; 3. respiratory rate ≥20 breaths/min or a $PaCO_2$ ≤32 mmHg or the use of mechanical ventilation for an acute respiratory process; 4. white cell count ≥12,000/mm^3 or ≤4,000/mm^3 or a differential count showing >10% immature neutrophils) [28]. This was adjudicated by ADC, JJH, MJS and AB. ALI/ARDS was diagnosed using the North American European Consensus Conference (NAECC) definition [29]. Although inclusion was on the basis of ALI/ARDS, we recoded conditions according to the current Berlin definition of ARDS, according to variables at enrollment [2].

Table 2. Pulmonary variables.

	Baseline)			Day 5			Day 15		
	rh-APC	saline	P	rh-APC	saline	P	rh-APC	saline	P
	(n = 33)	(n = 38)		(n = 33)	(n = 38)		(n = 19)	(n = 11)	
Gasometrics									
PaO_2, mmHg	88.0±21.5	88.9±23.0	0.921	88.8±19.2	90.7±27.7	0.756	89.7±17.8	84.8±7.7	0.713
F_IO_2, %	53.1±12.5	55.2±16.8	0.924	43.9±9.9	44.3±11.2	0.965	41.4±10.8	40.8±6.7	0.868
PaO_2/F_IO_2	175.1±48.6	170.7±53.8	0.624	220.2±72	217.7±95.4	0.732	227.7±69.8	213.8±41.3	0.483
$PaCO_2$, mmHg	45.7±12.5	47.2±11.6	0.604	43.3±9.7	45.6±9.3	0.393	45.2±11.91	44.4±5.3	0.867
pH	7.36±0.08	7.34±0.10	0.390	7.44±0.05	7.42±0.07	0.502	7.43±0.04	7.44±0.02	0.524
Ventilation									
Mode			0.551			0.551			0.702
Unassisted breathing	4 (12)	3 (8)		4 (12)	3 (8)		7 (37)	3 (27)	
Invasive ventilation	29 (88)	34 (89)		29 (88)	34 (89)		12 (63)	8 (73)	
Non-invasive ventilation	0	1 (3)		0	1 (3)		0	0	
Prone position	5 (15)	11 (29)	0.255	5 (15)	11 (29)	0.255	1 (5)	0	1.000
Respiratory rate (/min)	25.8±6.3	25.5±6.1	0.766	20.8±4.9	22.6±4.8	0.288	23.8±4.8	23.4±4.1	0.928
PIP (cm H_2O)	32.0±9.3	31.6±7.5	0.989	26.0±8.8	26.2±8.4	0.825	23.3±10.5	18.4±6.1	0.384
PEEP (cm H_2O)	12.3±4.6	12.8±4.3	0.819	11.0±4.3	10.7±4.2	0.839	9.8±3.8	8.5±2.8	0.482
Tidal volume (mL)	459±96	451±120	0.544	449±76	476±77	0.193	430±65	407±74	0.571
Tidal volume (mL/kg IBW)	7.5±1.8	6.8±2.0	0.091	7.4±1.4	7.3±1.9	0.628	7.4±1.1	6.3±1.9	0.135
Compliance (mL/cm H_2O)	24.5±7.8	24.3±6.5	0.843	33.5±13.4	32.9±11.7	0.944	40.8±23.1	50.8±29.6	0.343
Chest radiograph quadrants	2.2±0.9	1.9±0.7	0.249	1.7±0.8	1.6±0.8	0.851	1.0±1.1	1.5±1.2	0.245
Lung injury									
PLI ($x10^{-3}$/min)	33.8±20.7	31.2±20.6	0.335						
Lung injury score	2.5±0.7	2.5±0.6	0.862						

Mean or median ± standard deviation or interquartile range, respectively, or number (percentage), where appropriate. Rh-APC, recombinant human activated protein C; PaO_2, partial pressure of O_2; F_IO_2, inspiratory O_2 fraction; PIP, peak inspiratory pressure; PEEP, positive end-expiratory pressure; IBW, ideal body weight; PLI, pulmonary leak index; LIS, lung injury score (between 0 and 4).

Table 3. Primary and secondary outcome measures.

	rh-APC (n = 33)	saline (n = 38)	P-value
Primary outcome			
PLI day 5, $\times10^{-3}$/min	26.2±16.0	27.0±15.8	0.878
Decrease PLI day 1–5, $\times10^{-3}$/min	9.1±24.2	4.6±18.1	0.619
Secondary outcomes			
LIS day 5	1.8±0.9	1.9±1.0	0.654
LIS day 15	1.5±1.1	1.8±1.0	0.327
Ventilator-free days (days)	14.5±10.5	12.0±11.3	0.348
Duration of ventilation (days)	12.4±9.9	12.2±10.0	0.958
SOFA day 5	5.4±3.2	5.2±3.5	0.744
SOFA day 15	4.5±2.5	3.8±2.5	0.396
28-day mortality	2 (6)	7 (18)	0.157
ICU mortality	5 (15)	11 (29)	0.255
90-day mortality	6 (18)	11 (29)	0.404
Hospital mortality	7 (21)	12 (32)	0.423

Mean or median ± standard deviation or interquartile range, respectively, or number (percentage), where appropriate. Rh-APC, recombinant human activated protein C; PLI, pulmonary leak index; LIS, lung injury score; SOFA, sequential organ failure assessment; ICU, intensive care unit.

Patients were excluded if rh–APC treatment was indicated based on national guidelines at the time of the study (i.e., severe sepsis or septic shock, acute physiology, age and chronic health evaluation II score (APACHE II) score ≥25 and in the absence of informed consent [30]. Additional exclusion criteria were: platelet count $<30\times10^9$/L, any major surgery within 12 hours before inclusion, acute bleeding, severe head trauma, intracranial surgery or stroke within 3 months before inclusion, known intracranial abnormalities (e.g., malignancies or other tumors, arteriovenous malformation), known hypercoagulability (e.g., protein C resistance, hereditary deficiency of protein C, protein S or antithrombin, or anticardiolipin– or antiphospholipid–antibodies), congenital hemorrhagic diathesis, pregnancy or breast feeding, liver cirrhosis with portal hypertension and/or esophageal varices, presence of an epidural catheter; severely immune–compromised status (e.g., HIV–infected patients with CD4 count <50/mL, and patients treated with immunosuppressive medication following bone marrow or solid organ transplantation). The following concomitant medications were reasons for exclusion: heparin in therapeutic dose (within 8 hours of study entry), coumarin derivatives at any dose (within 7 days of study entry), acetylsalicylic acid at a dose >650 mg/day (within previous 3 days of study entry), thrombolytic therapy at any dose (within previous 3 days of study entry), glycoprotein IIb/IIIa inhibitors at any dose (within 7 days of study entry), antithrombin at any dose (within 3 days of study entry) and previous treatment with rh–APC (at any time within study entry). Prophylactic dose of low molecular weight heparin was allowed.

Treatment protocol

All patients were treated by the discretion of the supervising intensivists according to international guidelines. If needed, mechanical ventilation was performed after endotracheal intubation, in a pressure–controlled mode, aiming at a maximum airway pressures <35 cmH_2O, and tidal volumes ≤6 mL/kg predicted ideal body weight (Devine formula), with or without proning, when indicated on clinical grounds. Patients receiving mechanical ventilation after endotracheal intubation underwent selective decontamination of the digestive tract after collection of tracheal aspirate cultures, oropharyngeal and perineal swabs. Antibiotic therapy was guided by Gram–stains and cultures, according to local guidelines for antimicrobial therapy. Fluid therapy consisted of crystalloids, with or without gelatins and/or hydroxyethyl starches, in order to maintain arterial blood pressure (MAP >70 mmHg) and diuresis (>30 mL/h).

Study protocol

Patients were randomly assigned to infusion of rh–APC or a similar volume of normal saline. Prior to the start of the trial sealed opaque envelopes, containing the treatment assignment for each patient, were numbered through block randomization, with 6 blocks of patients, stratified per participating unit. Open label rh–APC (Eli Lilly, Indianapolis, IN, USA), at a dose of 24 mcg/kg/h, or saline was infused at a constant rate for a total of 96 hours, starting within 6 hours after randomization. Randomization was within 12 h after meeting above inclusion criteria. Infusion of rh–APC was interrupted 1 hour before any invasive percutaneous procedure or major surgery. When no bleeding complications occurred, infusion of rh–APC was resumed 1 hour after a percutaneous procedure, and 12 hours after major surgery, in line with international guidelines. All patients completed the 96-hour treatment. No patient met the criteria for APC administration according to the national guidelines prevailing at the time of the study.

PLI

The PLI was measured within 0–4 hours prior to the start of infusion of the study drug or saline, and repeated within 12 hours following the end of 96 hour infusion, according to published methods [4–6]. Transferrin was labeled in vivo, after intravenous injection of 4–5 MBq ^{67}Ga-citrate (physical half-life 78 hrs; Mallinckrodt Diagnostica, Petten, the Netherlands). Patients were in supine or prone position, and two scintillation probes (Eurorad C.T.T., Strasbourg, France) were placed over the left and right lung apices. Starting from the time of ^{67}Ga injection, radioactivity was measured for 30 minutes. The ^{67}Ga counts are corrected for background activity, physical half-life of ^{67}Ga and decay after injection, and expressed as counts per minute per lung. At 0, 5, 8, 12, 15, 20, 25 and 30 minutes, blood samples were taken. Each blood sample was weighed and radioactivity was measured with a single-well well-counter (LKB Wallac 1480 WIZARD, Perkin Elmer, Life Science, Zaventem, Belgium) taking background and physical half-life into account. Results are expressed as counts per minute per gram. For each blood sample, a time-matched counts per minute over each lung was taken. The radioactivity ratio was calculated as $(^{67}Ga_{lung})/(^{67}Ga_{blood})$ and plotted against time. The PLI was calculated from the slope of the increase of the radioactivity ratio, divided by the intercept, to correct for physical factors in radioactivity detection and pulmonary blood volume. The PLI thus represents the transport rate of ^{67}Ga-transferrin from the intravascular to the extravascular space of the lungs and is therefore a measure of pulmonary vascular permeability. The values for both lungs were averaged. The upper limit of normal for the PLI is 14.1×10^{-3}/min, and the measurement error (coeffecient of variation if measurement is repeated in the same patient) is approximately 10% [31].

Data collection

Upon enrolment, data on baseline demographics, comorbidity and reasons of admission to the intensive care unit (ICU), as well

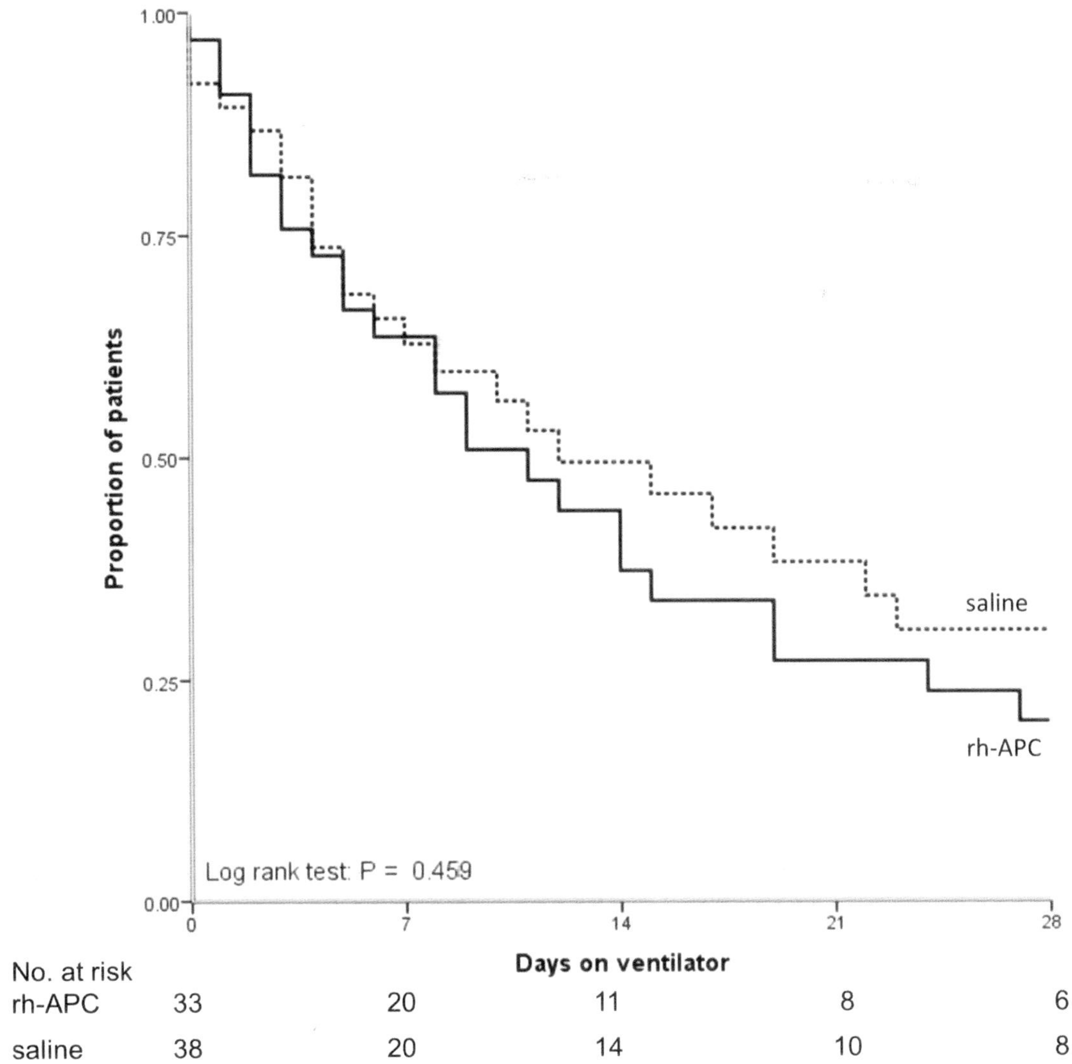

Figure 2. Probability of being alive and off the ventilator until day 28 in study groups.

as hemodynamic and respiratory parameters were collected. The APACHE II [30], the simplified acute physiology score (SAPS II)[32], the sequential organ failure assessment score (SOFA) [33] and the lung injury score (LIS) [34] were calculated from worst values in the 24 h preceding enrolment and, for SOFA and LIS, on day 5 and 15 after enrolment. For the LIS we evaluated daily chest radiographs and scored the number of consolidated quadrants. From the blood gas measurements, done for routine care, daily worst values were taken and also the worst ventilatory settings were taken from the patient data management system available in the units. Total respiratory dynamic compliance was calculated from tidal volume/(peak inspiratory pressure - positive end expiratory pressure), mL/cm H_2O. We estimated in patients not on mechanical ventilation the inspiratory O_2 fraction (F_IO_2) from liters of O_2 administered nasally or via non-rebreathing mask, varying between 1 and 15 L, yielding an estimated F_IO_2 from 23 to 70%, respectively. The number of ventilator-free days (VFD) was defined as the number of days with unassisted breathing (>24 h) from randomization to day 28 after enrolment. Patients who died before day 28 while receiving ventilator support, were assigned zero ventilator-free days [35]. Lengths of stay and mortality at day 28 and 90 were recorded, within or outside the ICU or the hospital.

Statistical analysis

The study was powered (at 80%) to include 96 patients to detect an anticipated difference in PLI of 20% at a standard deviation (SD) of 40% ($\alpha = 0.05$). The Kolmogorov-Smirnov test was used to check for normal data distribution (if $P>0.05$). Data were expressed as means ($\pm$ standard deviation) for normally distributed data, medians ($\pm$ interquartile range) for non-normally distributed data, or absolute numbers where appropriate. Nonparametric data were analyzed using Mann–Whitney U and categorical data by Fisher's exact test. The Spearman rank correlation was used to express relations. Kaplan-Meier plots were made and a log rank test performed for ventilatory independency and survival in time in the groups. A Cox proportional-hazards model was used to estimate the hazard ratio (HR) for death with the use of rh-APC versus saline in different posthoc defined subgroups (with 95% confidence intervals). A P value of <0.05 was considered statistically significant and exact values are given unless <0.001. Statistical analysis was performed using SPSS 19.0 (SPSS,

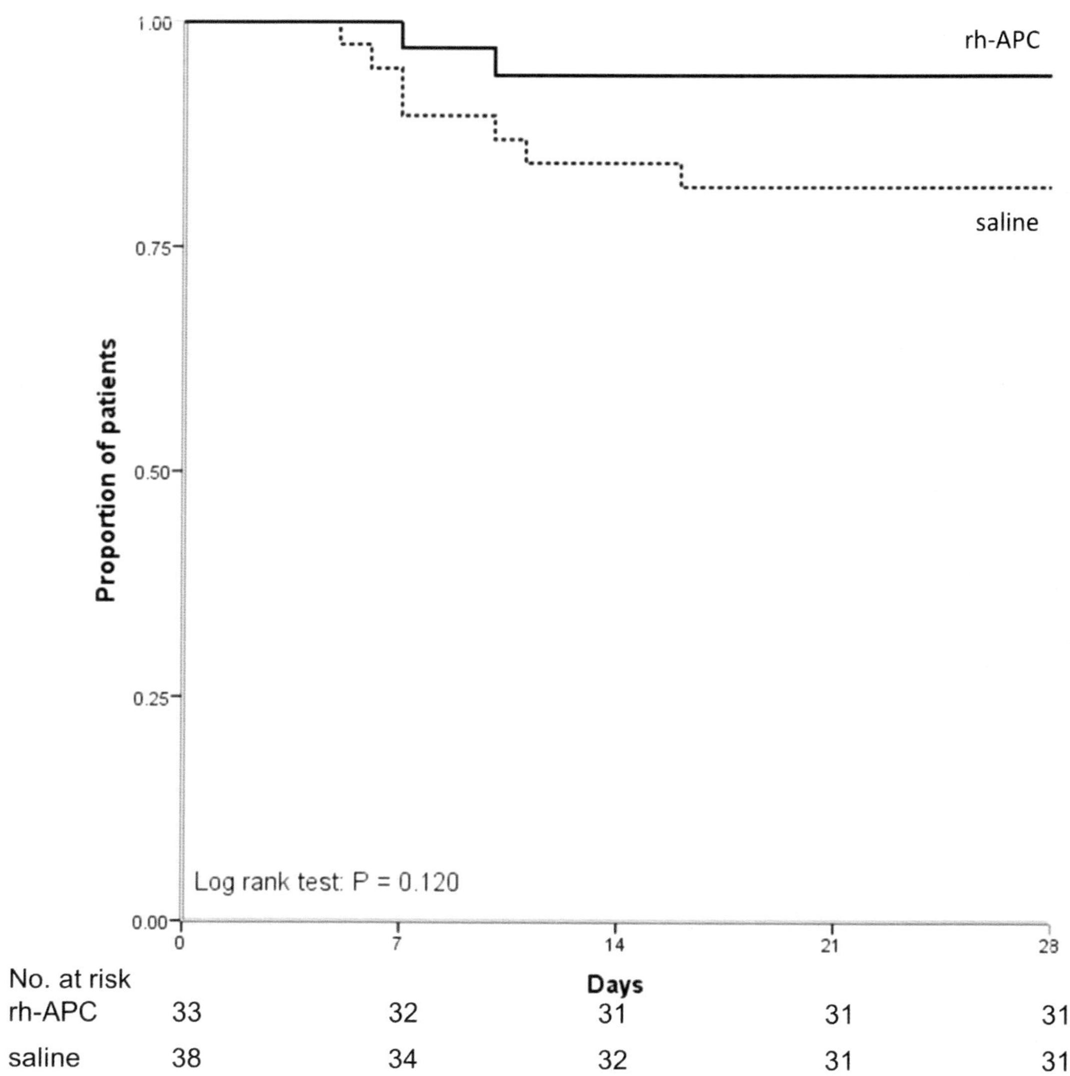

Figure 3. Probability of survival until day 28 in study groups.

Chicago, IL, USA) and Prism 5.0 (GraphPad Software, San Diego, CA, USA).

Results

Between 1 January 2007 and 1 May 2011 9,484 patients were assessed for eligibility (Fig. 1). Of these patients, 71 patients were enrolled in the study. Reasons for exclusion are given in Fig. 1. There were 33 patients assigned to rh-APC and 38 to saline. The study was prematurely discontinued because rh-APC was withdrawn form the market and no longer commercially available.

Baseline characteristics

Patient groups did not differ with regard to demographic and baseline parameters (Table 1). In 61 patients the reason for inclusion was pneumonia. There was a trend towards more pulmonary comorbidity in the saline-treated group. With regard to disease severity as expressed by APACHE II and SAPS II scores, groups did not differ. Furthermore, the frequency of treatment with vasopressors and steroids was similar. In the majority of patients (56/71) tracheal aspirate cultures were positive. In 14 patients (n = 5 rh-APC and n = 9 saline) multiple pathogens were isolated. *Streptococcus pneumoniae* was the most prevalent identified micro-organism, both in tracheal aspirate and in blood cultures. Ninety percent of the patients (64/71) needed invasive mechanical ventilation.

Pulmonary variables

At baseline, the PLI was increased as compared to normal values in 87% (62/71) of patients. The baseline PLI and LIS, which did not differ among groups, correlated at $R_s = 0.26$, $P = 0.030$ (Table 2). The baseline LIS was associated with the duration of mechanical ventilation ($R_s = 0.33$, $P = 0.005$). There were no differences between groups in the course of ventilator pressures, tidal volumes, gas exchange, and oxygen requirements.

Primary and secondary outcome measures

Table 3 shows that there is no difference in day 5 PLI between treatment groups, although the reduction in PLI was more pronounced in the rh-APC group, yet not reaching statistical significance. There was no effect of rh-APC on the general disease severity score (SOFA) nor the more lung-specific LIS and the number of ventilator-free days. Fig. 2 shows the lack of difference in ventilator-dependency in the groups until day 28 after

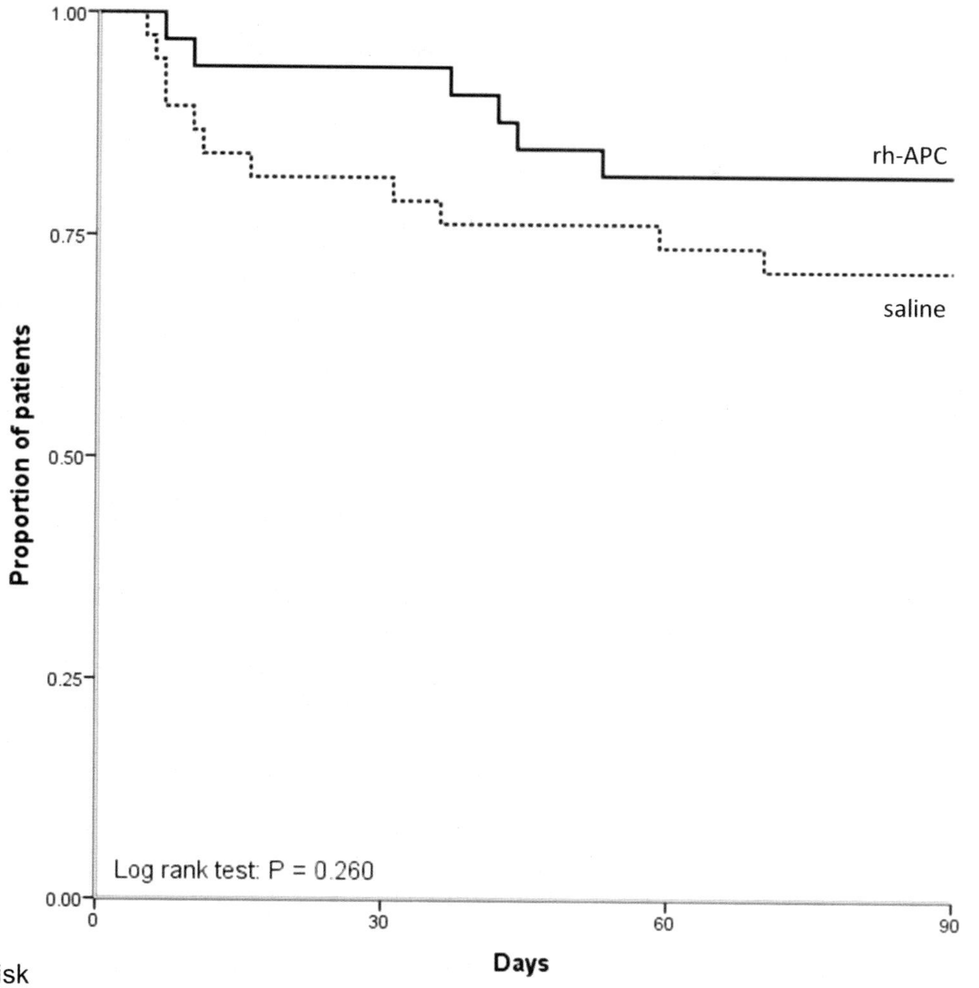

No. at risk				
rh-APC	33	31	27	27
saline	38	31	28	27

Figure 4. Probability of survival until day 90 in study groups.

randomization. The day 5 LIS score was associated with the duration of mechanical ventilation ($R_s = 0.58$, $P < 0.001$). With regard to mortality, no differences were found between treatment groups (Table 3 and Fig. 3 & 4).

Post-hoc subgroup analysis

Cox regression analysis did not identify any subgroup in which treatment with rh-APC resulted in a statistically significant survival benefit, even though all HR were below 1 (Table 4). In patients with pneumonia and supranormal PLI the P for 28-day survival with log-rank testing was 0.045 in favor of rh-APC.

Adverse events

Two pneumothoraces occurred during the study, one in each patient group. There were no bleeding complications.

Discussion

Our study suggests that a 4-day course of intravenous rh-APC does not ameliorate the increased permeability and clinical course of ARDS in critically ill patients. However, our study was underpowered.

The study was designed with the hypothesis that APC plays a role in the endothelial barrier function in the lung. The study was powered for a 20% change in PLI since increased alveolocapillary permeability was considered central in the pathogenesis and clinical presentation of ARDS [4–6]. We previously demonstrated that the PLI increases before ARDS becomes clinically manifest and declines when it resolves [4]. Our current study again documents that increased permeability is associated with the clinical manifestations of ARDS expressed as the LIS, as noted before [4–6], and that the latter is a determinant of duration of ventilatory support. Yet, in a substudy of this trial, we demonstrated that rh-APC infusion actually attenuates pulmonary coagulopathy [27]. Apparently, this effect on pulmonary coagulopathy does not result in a clinically significant enhancement of barrier function as expressed by the PLI. Therefore, we could not find evidence for the concept that rh-APC ameliorates endothelial barrier dysfunction and increased permeability and thereby attenuates the course of ARDS in man, as suggested by preclinical studies via a cytoprotective effect involving PAR-1 and S1P pathways, irrespective of anti-inflammatory effects [11,14,15]. In some animal studies (rats with pulmonary infection) intravenous

Table 4. Hazard ratios for death on day 28.

	No. of patients	No. of deaths (%) rh-APC	saline	HR (95% CI)
All patients	71	2 (6)	7 (18)	0.310 (0.064–1.492)
Etiology of ARDS				
pneumonia	61	1(4)	7 (20)	0.165 (0.020–1.342)
other	10	1 (17)	0	-
Berlin criteria for ARDS				
mild	21	0	2 (17)	-
moderate/severe	50	2 (8)	5 (19)	0.414 (0.080–2.136)
Pulmonary leak index				
above normal	60	2 (7)	7 (22)	0.304 (0.063–1.462)
≥2× upper limit of normal	32	1 (6)	4 (27)	0.208 (0.023–1.861)
<2× upper limit of normal	39	1 (7)	3 (13)	0.511 (0.053–4.917)
≥2.5× upper limit of normal	22	0	4 (36)	-
<2.5× upper limit of normal	49	2 (10)	3 (11)	0.865 (0.145–5.176)
Lung injury score				
≥2.5	39	2 (11)	4 (19)	0.577 (0.106–3.152)
<2.5	32	0	3 (18)	-
Sequential organ failure assessment				
≥7	48	2 (9)	6 (24)	0.334 (0.067–1.658)
<7	23	0	1 (8)	-
Baseline steroids				
Yes	47	2 (9)	6 (25)	0.320 (0.064–1.583)
no	24	0	1 (7)	-
C-reactive protein				
≥175 mg/L	32	1 (63)	4 (25)	0.233 (0.026–2.089)
<175 mg/L	37	1 (7)	3 (14)	0.461 (0.048–4.429)

ARDS, acute respiratory distress syndrome; HR, hazard ratio with 95% confidence intervals.

administration of rh-APC limited bronchoalveolar coagulation, whereas it did not exert anti-inflammatory effects [36,37].

The 28-day mortality rate of patients in our study was relatively low (13%), likely attributable to a lower overall disease severity, as severe sepsis, septic shock and APACHE II ≥25 were exclusion criteria, when compared with large international trials on ARDS that did not exclude the latter patients and reported mortality rates of 25 to 46% [38,39]. It was however comparable to the 60-day mortality rate of 13% in the trial of Liu et al., who applied similar inclusion criteria for the 75 patients in their study, of whom only 40% had pneumonia [35]. Additionally, our study is in line with the results from the ADDRESS (Administration of Drotrecogin Alfa (Activated) in Early Stage Severe Sepsis) trial, focusing on patients with relatively low disease severity (APACHE II <25 or single organ failure) suffering from severe sepsis in whom rh-APC administration did not show clinical benefits [23]. In the double-blind, phase III, RESOLVE (REsearching severe Sepsis and Organ dysfunction in children; a gLobal perspectiVE) trial, 477 children with severe sepsis were enrolled. Again, there was no difference between rh-APC and placebo with regard to the composite time to complete organ failure resolution score. Mortality at 28 days was 17.2% in the rh-APC group versus 17.5% in the placebo group [24].

The limitations of our study include its premature discontinuation because rh-APC was withdrawn from the market, as described before [25]. The stringent exclusion criteria that we applied in order to reduce bleeding risks, contributed to the small number of patients that were enrolled. As a result, our study is underpowered to demonstrate amelioration of increased permeability and clinical course of ARDS in critically ill patients by intravenous rh-APC, as well as to demonstrate an effect on mortality, particularly in pneumonia-induced ARDS with increased alveolocapillary permeability. The single prior study on human ALI (n = 75), which also proved negative [35], was underpowered as well. Their case mix was more heterogeneous than in our study (only 40% had pneumonia) [35], suggesting that, when even in a more homogeneous population a benefit cannot be demonstrated, the contributory role of APC in ARDS must indeed be low. Nevertheless, our post hoc analyses, which should be interpreted with caution, serve to suggest the validity of trial design. The tidal volumes delivered to the patients in our study were larger than the 6 mL/kg ideal body weight described in the treatment protocol. However, the tidal volumes were comparable in both treatment groups throughout the study period. Moreover, the mean tidal volumes were within the range of 6 to 8 mL/kg ideal body weight, which is in keeping with the suggested lung-protective mechanical ventilation strategies in the Surviving Sepsis Campaing Guidelines [40].

The external validity of our study is compromised, as it was performed in 2 centers. The possibility of recruiting more centers was deemed impossible, both practically and logistically. The PLI measurements require highly specialized, custom-made scintillation probes. Furthermore, since many hospitals do not have a department of nuclear medicine, the isotopes would have needed to be transported via public roads for which government permission would have been needed, as well as additional permission for transportation through the hospital and administration in the ICU. Then the radioactive blood samples would have been needed to be transported back to one of both academic centers to perform the radioactivity count.

Our study is a single-blinded study. As a part of standard care, APTT and PT are regularly monitored in both centers. As rh-APC prolongs APTT, a truly double-blinded study was not considered feasible.

Conclusion

In conclusion, this study suggests that treatment for 4 days with intravenous rh-APC for infectious or inflammatory ARDS does not ameliorate increased alveolocapillary permeability nor the clinical course of critically ill patients with ARDS as a single organ failure mostly caused by pneumonia.

Key messages

- Increased pulmonary vascular permeability is associated with the clinical manifestations of ARDS
- Intravenous rh-APC for 4 days does not ameliorate increased alveolocapillary permeability nor the clinical course of critically ill patients with infectious or inflammatory ARDS as a single organ failure

Acknowledgments

We thank Erna Albers, Ingrid van den Hul and the intensive care unit staff of VUmc and AMC for support in conducting this trial.

Author Contributions

Conceived and designed the experiments: ABG AB. Performed the experiments: ADC JJH APV PRT. Analyzed the data: ADC ABG AB ARG AL ML MJS. Wrote the paper: ADC ABG JJH APV PRT AL ML ARG MJS AB. Developed the radio-isotope measurement known as the pulmonary leak index: AL ABG.

References

1. Wind J, Versteegt J, Twisk J, van Bindels AJ, Spijkstra JJ, et al. (2007) Epidemiology of acute lung injury and acute respiratory distress syndrome in The Netherlands: a survey. Respir Med 101:2091–2098
2. Ranieri VM, Rubenfeld GD, Thompson BT, Ferguson ND, Caldwell E, et al. (2012) Acute respiratory distress syndrome: the Berlin definition. JAMA 307:2526–2533
3. Cepkova M, Matthay MA (2006) Pharmacotherapy of acute lung injury and the acute respiratory distress syndrome. J Intensive Care Med 21:119–143
4. Raijmakers PG, Groeneveld AB, Schneider AJ, Teule GJ, van Lingen A, et al. (1993) Transvascular transport of ^{67}Ga in the lungs after cardiopulmonary bypass surgery. Chest 104:1825–1832
5. Groeneveld AB, Raijmakers PG, Teule GJ, Thijs LG (1996) The ^{67}Gallium pulmonary leak index in assessing the severity and course of the adult respiratory distress syndrome. Crit Care Med 24:1467–1472
6. Verheij J, Raijmakers PG, van Lingen A, Groeneveld AB (2005) Simple versus complex radionuclide methods of assessing capillary protein permeability for diagnosing acute respiratory distress syndrome. J Crit Care 20:162–171
7. Groeneveld AB, Verheij J (2006) Extravascular lung water to blood volume ratios as measures of permeability in sepsis-induced in ALI/ARDS. Intensive Care Med 32:1315–1321
8. Groeneveld AB, Kindt I, Raijmakers PG, Hack CE, Thijs LG (1994) Systemic coagulation and fibrinolysis in patients with or at risk for the adult respiratory distress syndrome. Thromb Haemost 78:1444–1449
9. Schultz MJ, Haitsma JJ, Zhang H, Slutsky AS (2006) Pulmonary coagulopathy as a new target in therapeutic studies of acute lung injury or pneumonia – a review. Crit Care Med 34:871–877
10. Ware LB, Matthay MA, Parsons PE, Thompson BT, Januzzi JL, et al. (2007) Pathogenetic and prognostic significance of altered coagulation and fibrinolysis in acute lung injury/acute respiratory distress syndrome. Crit Care Med 35:1821–1828
11. Cornet AD, van Nieuw Amerongen GP, Beishuizen A, Schultz MJ, Girbes AR, et al. (2009) Activated protein C in the treatment of acute lung injury and acute respiratory distress syndrome. Exp Opin Drug Discovery 4:219–227
12. Nick JA, Coldren CD, Geraci MW, Poch KR, Fouty BW, et al. (2004) Recombinant human activated protein C reduces human endotoxin-induced pulmonary inflammation via inhibition of neutrophil chemotaxis. Blood 104:3878–3885
13. Van der Poll T, Levi M, Nick JA, Abraham E (2005) Activated protein C inhibits local coagulation after intrapulmonary delivery of endotoxin in humans. Am J Respir Crit Care Med 171:1125–1128
14. Finigan JH, Boueiz A, Wilkinson E, Damico R, Skirball J, et al. (2009) Activated protein C protects against ventilator-induced pulmonary capillary leak. Am J Physiol Lung Cell Mol Physiol 296:L1002–1011
15. Bir N, Lafarque M, Howard M, Goolaerts A, Roux J, et al. (2011) Cytoprotective-selective activated protein C attenuates Pseudomonas aeruginosa-induced lung injury in mice. Am J Respir Cell Mol Biol 45:632–641
16. Van der Heijden M, van Nieuw Amerongen GP, Koolwijk P, van Hinsbergh VW, Groeneveld AB (2008) Angiopoietin-2, permeability oedema, occurrence and severity of ALI/ARDS in septic and non-septic critically ill patients. Thorax 63:903–909
17. Bae J-S, Rezaie AR (2010) Thrombin upregulates the angiopoietin-Tie2 axis: endothelial protein C receptor occupancy prevents the thrombin mobilization of angiopoietin 2 and P-selectin from Weibel-Palade bodies. J Thromb Haemost 8:1107–1115
18. Bernard GR, Vincent JL, Laterre PF, LaRosa SP, Dhainaut JF, et al. (2001) Efficacy and safety of recombinant human activated protein C for severe sepsis. N Engl J Med 344:699–709
19. Vincent J-L, Angus DC, Artigas A, Kalil A, Basson BR, et al. (2003) Effects of drotrecogin alfa (activated) on organ dysfunction in the PROWESS trial. Crit Care Med 31:834–840
20. Vincent JL, Bernard GR, Beale R, Doig C, Putensen, et al. (2005) Drotrecogin alfa (activated) treatment in severe sepsis from the global open-label trial ENHANCE: further evidence for survival and safety and implications for early treatment. Crit Care Med 33:2266–2277
21. Ely W, Laterre P-F, Angus DC, Helterbrand JD, Levy H, et al. (2003) Drotrecogin alfa (activated) administration across clinically important subgroups of patients with severe sepsis. Crit Care Med 31:12–19
22. Laterre PF, Garber G, Levy H, Wunderink R, Kinasewitz GT, et al. (2005) Severe community-acquired pneumonia as a cause of severe sepsis: data from the PROWESS study. Crit Care Med 33:952–961
23. Abraham E, Laterre PF, Garg R, Levy H, Talwar D, et al. (2005) Drotrecogin alfa (activated) for adults with severe sepsis and low risk of death. N Engl J Med 353:1332–1341
24. Nadel S, Goldstein B, Williams MD, Dalton H, Peters M, et al. (2007) Drotrecogin alfa (activated) in children with severe sepsis: a multicentre phase III randomised controlled trial. Lancet 369:836–843
25. Ranieri VM, Thompson BT, Barie PS, Dhainaut JF, Douglas IS, et al. (2012) Drotrecogin alfa (activated) in adults with septic shock. N Engl J Med 366:2055–2064
26. Kalil AC, LaRosa SP (2012) Effectiveness and safety of drotrecogin alfa (activated) for severe sepsis: a meta-analysis and metaregression. Lancet Infect Dis 12:678–686
27. Cornet AD, Hofstra JJ, Vlaar AP, Tuinman PR, Levi M, et al. (2013) Activated protein C attenuates pulmonary coagulopathy in patients with acute respiratory distress syndrome. J Thromb Haemost 11:894–901
28. Levy MM, Fink MP, Marshall JC, Abraham E, Angus D, et al. (2003) SCCM/ESICM/ACCP/ATS/SIS international sepsis definitions conference. Crit Care Med 31:1250–1256
29. Bernard GR, Artigas A, Brigham KL, Carlet J, Falke K, et al. (1994) The American-European Consensus Conference on ARDS. Definitions, mechanisms, relevant outcomes, and clinical trial coordination. Am J Respir Crit Care Med 149:818–824

30. Knaus WA, Draper EA, Wagner DP, Zimmerman JE (1985) APACHEII: a severity of disease classification system. Crit Care Med 13:818–829
31. Raijmakers PG, Groeneveld AB, Teule GJ, Thijs LG (1996) Diagnostic value of the gallium-67 pulmonary leak index in pulmonary edema. J Nucl Med 37:1316–1322
32. Le Gall JR, Lemeshow S, Saulnier F (1993) A new Simplified Acute Physiology Score (SAPS II) based on a European/North American multicenter study. JAMA 270:2957–2963
33. Vincent JL, Moreno R, Takala J, Willatts S, de Mendonca MA, et al. (1996) The SOFA (sepsis-related organ failure assessment) score to describe organ dysfunction/failure. Intensive Care Med 22:707–710
34. Murray JF, Matthay MA, Luce JM, Flick MR (1988) An expanded definition of the adult respiratory distress syndrome. Am Rev Respir Dis 138:720–723
35. Liu KD, Levitt J, Zhuo H, Kallet RH, Brady S, et al. (2008) Randomized clinical trial of activated protein C for the treatment of acute lung injury. Am J Respir Crit Care Med 178:18–23
36. Choi G, Hofstra JJ, Roelofs JJ, Florquin S, Bresser P, et al. (2007) Recombinant human activated protein C inhibits local and systemic activation of coagulation without influencing inflammation during Pseudomonas aeruginosa pneumonia in rats. Crit Care Med 35:1362–1368
37. Hofstra JJ, Vlaar AP, Cornet AD, Dixon B, Roelofs JJ, et al. (2010) Nebulized anticoagulants limit pulmonary coagulopathy, but not inflammation in a model of experimental lung injury. J Aerosol Pulm Drug Deliv 23:105–111
38. Wiedemann HP, Wheeler AP, Bernard GR, Thompson BT, Hayden D, et al. (2006) Comparison of two fluid-management strategies in acute lung injury. N Engl J Med 354:2564–2575
39. Taccone P, Pesenti A, Latini R, Polli F, Vagginelli F, et al. (2009) Prone positioning in patients with moderate and severe acute respiratory distress syndrome: a randomized trial. JAMA 302:1977–1984
40. Dellinger RP, Levy MM, Rhodes A, Annane D, Gerlach H, et al. (2013) Surviving Sepsis Campaign: international guidelines for management of severe sepsis and septic shock: 2012. Intensive Care Med 39:165–228

Identification of Novel Single Nucleotide Polymorphisms Associated with Acute Respiratory Distress Syndrome by Exome-Seq

Katherine Shortt[1,2], Suman Chaudhary[1], Dmitry Grigoryev[1,2], Daniel P. Heruth[1], Lakshmi Venkitachalam[2], Li Q. Zhang[1], Shui Q. Ye[1,2*]

1 Department of Pediatrics, Division of Experimental and Translational Genetics, Children's Mercy Hospital, University of Missouri - Kansas City School of Medicine, Kansas City, Missouri, United States of America, **2** Department of Biomedical and Health Informatics, University of Missouri - Kansas City School of Medicine, Kansas City, Missouri, United States of America

Abstract

Acute respiratory distress syndrome (ARDS) is a lung condition characterized by impaired gas exchange with systemic release of inflammatory mediators, causing pulmonary inflammation, vascular leak and hypoxemia. Existing biomarkers have limited effectiveness as diagnostic and therapeutic targets. To identify disease-associating variants in ARDS patients, whole-exome sequencing was performed on 96 ARDS patients, detecting 1,382,399 SNPs. By comparing these exome data to those of the 1000 Genomes Project, we identified a number of single nucleotide polymorphisms (SNP) which are potentially associated with ARDS. 50,190SNPs were found in all case subgroups and controls, of which89 SNPs were associated with susceptibility. We validated three SNPs (rs78142040, rs9605146 and rs3848719) in additional ARDS patients to substantiate their associations with susceptibility, severity and outcome of ARDS. rs78142040 (C>T) occurs within a histone mark (intron 6) of the Arylsulfatase D gene. rs9605146 (G>A) causes a deleterious coding change (proline to leucine) in the XK, Kell blood group complex subunit-related family, member 3 gene. rs3848719 (G>A) is a synonymous SNP in the Zinc-Finger/Leucine-Zipper Co-Transducer NIF1 gene. rs78142040, rs9605146, and rs3848719 are associated significantly with susceptibility to ARDS. rs3848719 is associated with APACHE II score quartile. rs78142040 is associated with 60-day mortality in the overall ARDS patient population. Exome-seq is a powerful tool to identify potential new biomarkers for ARDS. We selectively validated three SNPs which have not been previously associated with ARDS and represent potential new genetic biomarkers for ARDS. Additional validation in larger patient populations and further exploration of underlying molecular mechanisms are warranted.

Editor: You-Yang Zhao, University of Illinois College of Medicine, United States of America

Funding: Funding was in part provided by NHLBI/NIH Grant (HL080042 & HL080042-S1, Ye, SQ), start-up fund and endowments of Children's Mercy Hospitals and Clinics, UMKC (Ye, SQ), and a Sarah Morrison Student Research Award of UMKC (Shortt, K). The funders had no role in study design, data collection and analysis, decision to publish, or preparation of the manuscript.

Competing Interests: The authors have declared that no competing interests exist.

* Email: sqye@cmh.edu

Introduction

Acute respiratory distress syndrome (ARDS), a severe form of acute lung injury, is characterized by the inflammation and fluid build-up in the alveoli of the lungs, which reduces the ability of oxygen to cross over into the blood stream [1,2]. ARDS has an extremely high mortality rate where over a third of sufferers die, and many of the survivors experience complications such as brain damage due to prolonged oxygen deprivation [3,4]. The mortality rate is even higher in cases with common comorbidities such as sepsis with suspected pulmonary source (40.6%) and witnessed aspiration (43.6%) [3]. ARDS is estimated to have an age-adjusted incidence of 86.2 new cases per 100,000 person-years in adults age 15 and older. The total number of cases estimated to occur yearly in the US is about 190,000 [3]. Pneumonia and sepsis are most common causes of ARDS, and Sepsis is the leading cause of ARDS. There is a paucity of effective and specific therapy to ARDS though low tidal volume ventilation has been demonstrated for some therapeutic utilities [5–8]. This is because the etiology and pathology of the disease are still not well understood and there remains a need for new specific and effective preventative measures and treatments.

The role of genetics in ARDS is increasingly recognized and it has recently been shown that complex diseases can be between 50 and 90% genetically determined [9]. Biomarkers that have been previously studied that are present in blood serum include surfactant-associated proteins (SP-A, B, and C), Mucin-associated antigens (KL-6 and MUC1), Cytokines (IL-1, 2, 6, 8, 10, and 15, TNFα), endothelium activation markers (E-selectin, L-selectin, I-CAM-1, V-CAM-1, and VWF), and neutrophil activation markers (MMP-9, LTB4, and Ferritin). Cytokine levels have been identified as a moderately effective measure of severity [10]. Additional biomarkers of ARDS severity have been obtained from breath analysis, including hydrogen peroxide levels and breath acidity [11]. Pre-B cell Colony Enhancing Factor (PBEF), also called nicotinamide phosphoribosyltransferase (NAMPT), was identified previously as a novel biomarker of ARDS by our group [12]. Analysis of two SNPs in the human PBEF promoter revealed an association with ARDS. The −1535T variant allele was associated with a decreased susceptibility to ALI/ARDS and a better outcome in septic patients in a Caucasian population when compared with patients without the variation. The −1001G variant allele was associated with increased susceptibility to acute lung injury and ARDS in African American and Caucasian populations. The −1001G variant was also associated with a higher ICU mortality rate in septic patients in a Caucasian population [6,13–15]. Despite the previous identification of several available biomarkers, their available data are inconsistent and clinical relevance has not yet been established.

With the development of next-generation sequencing technologies and improvements in data analysis capabilities, it is now feasible to sequence and analyze whole genomes within a couple of days [16]. However, the cost of whole genome sequencing is still a prohibitive factor for sequencing more samples. Whole exome sequencing (WES) is faster and less expensive than whole-genome sequencing, making it ideal for the study of variants that cause changes to the protein-coding regions of genes [17]. WES has been used to identify genetic risk factors for both Mendelian and complex diseases alike [17–19]. The purpose of this study was to

Table 1. Participant demographics and comorbidities for the ARDS cases.

Whole-exome Sequencing Sample group	**Participants***	**Gender (%male)**	**Age± SD**	**APACHEII score ±SD**	**Ventilator-free days per 28 days ±SD**	**60-day mortality (% dead at 60 days post-onset)**
ARDS total	96	46.9	50±14.6	97.2±30.4	12.6±10.2	29.4
Caucasian ARDS	70	44.3	50.7±13.8	94.5±30.2	13.6±10.0	23.9
African American ARDS	26	53.8	47.8±16.6	104.6±30.2	9.9±10.5	44
ARDS with Sepsis total	48	50	52.0±15.1	105.2±32.2	10.2±10.1	38.3
Caucasian ARDS with Sepsis	37	43.2	51.8±15.0	102.6±31.1	10.5±9.8	33.3
African American ARDS with Sepsis	11	72.7	52.9±16.1	113.6±35.8	9.3±11.7	54.5
ARDS with Pneumonia total	48	43.8	47.9±13.9	88.9±26.2	14.9±9.87	20
Caucasian ARDS with Pneumonia	33	45.5	49.5±12.4	85.0±26.6	17.0±9.2	12.9
African American ARDS with Pneumonia	15	40	44.1±16.6	97.6±24.0	10.3±10.0	35.7
TaqMan Genotyping Sample group	**Participants**	**Gender (%male)**	**Age± SD**	**APACHEII score ±SD**	**Ventilator-free days per 28 days ±SD**	**60-day mortality (% dead at 60 days post-onset)**
ARDS Total	117	46.2	50.8±16.6	105.1±32.7	12.0±10.5	31
Caucasian ARDs	75	40	52 1±15.4	104.3±31.4	11.8±10.5	29.2
African American ARDS	17	64.7	51 6±22.8	113.3±33.8	12.2±10.6	29.4
Other ancestry ARDS	25	52	46.4±15.3	101.8±36.2	12.6±10.7	37.5
ARDS with Sepsis total	59	52.5	51.5±17.3	112.9±31.5	11.3±11.0	37.9
Caucasian ARDS with Sepsis	34	50	51.1±15.6	113.6±29.7	10.9±11.1	33.3
African American ARDS with Sepsis	9	66.7	56.6±27.1	121.8±33.0	12.9±11.5	33.3
Other ancestry ARDS with Sepsis	16	50	49.6±14.8	106.4±34.7	11.4±11.0	50
ARDS with Pneumonia total	58	39.7	50.1±16.0	96.9±32.3	12.7±9.9	23.6
Caucasian ARDS with Pneumonia	41	31.7	52.9±15.3	96.4±31.0	12.6±10.0	25.6
African American ARDS with Pneumonia	8	62.5	46±16.9	103.8±34.3	11.4±10.2	25
Other ancestry ARDS with Pneumonia	9	55.6	46.8±15.2	92.4±39.7	14.9±10.3	12.5
Total ARDS	**Participants**	**Gender (%male)**	**Age± SD**	**APACHEII score ±SD**	**Ventilator-free days per 28 days ±SD**	**60-day mortality (% dead at 60 days post-onset)**
All ARDS patients	213	46.5	50.4±15.7	101.6±31.9	12.3±10.3	30.2

*, 8 samples, 4 exome sequenced and 4 TaqMan genotyped ARDS patients did not have these phenotypes available. An additional 2 exome sequenced ARDS patients did not have ventilator-free day's data. In addition to the 8 patients missing severity and mortality phenotype data, 2 patients were excluded from the regression because their phenotypes were thought to be missing until after the regressions were completed.

Table 2. Summary of the filtering applied to candidate SNPs.

Criteria for filtering	Number of remaining variants
SNPs detected in ARDS SNPs	1,382,399
matched in 1000 Genomes Project	169,376
common across 4 ARDS race and etiology groups*	50,190
χ^2 p-value <0.01 in top 5 ARDS groups**	99
χ^2 p-value $<2.95\times10^{-7}$ in at least 2/5 top 5 ARDS groups	76(in 65 genes)
coding variants	38(in 32 genes)
nonsynonymous	20
synonymous variants	18

*, African American with pneumonia, African American with sepsis, Caucasian with pneumonia, Caucasian with sepsis subgroups. Out of the 50,190 SNPs, 49,723 are bi-allelic. **, All ARDS, all pneumonia, all sepsis, all African American, all Caucasian groups.

discover new biomarkers for ARDS using WES. Exome sequencing of 96 ARDS patient DNA samples from the ARDSnet (www.ardsnet.org) and 48 race, gender and age matched normal healthy control subject DNAs from Coriell (www.coriell.org) was performed using Illumina's HiScanSQ system. By comparing SNP analysis of whole exome sequence data between the ARDS patient population (96 patients) and the normal healthy controls from Coriell (48 subjects) as well as the 1000 Genomes Project (440 total, 379 European Ancestry (EUR), 61 African Americans in the southwest (ASW), www.1000genomes.org) [20], we have identified a number of coding SNPs potentially associated with ARDS susceptibility. We also performed regression analyses within the

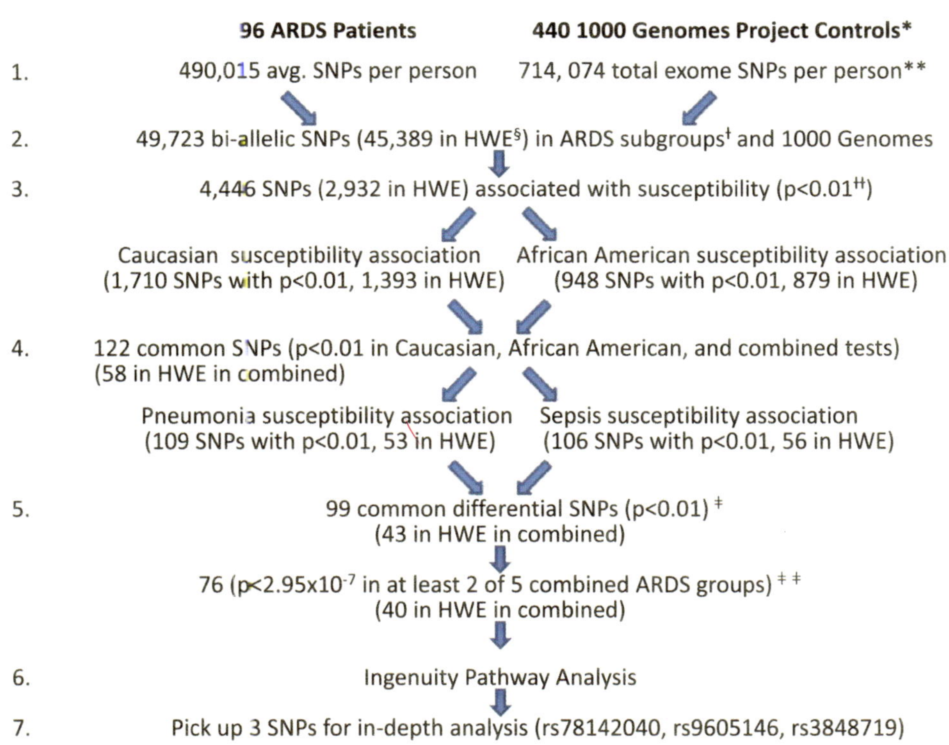

Figure 1. Pipeline of the exome-seq data analysis workflow. After processing the data using the GATK pipeline, this filtering workflow was derived to identify SNPs which were associated with measures of susceptibility across the racial and etiology groups of cases. SNPs were filtered based on strength of association, coding effect, and functional prediction prior to testing for association with other ARDS phenotypes. *, The sample contains African American and Caucasian patients, so the EUR and ASW healthy controls from 1000 Genomes were used for comparison; **, In the 1000 Genomes Project exome sequence, the same 714,074 SNPs are present for all 440 EUR and ASW; §, HWE = Hardy Weinberg Equilibrium, $p > 0.0001$; +, African American with pneumonia, African American with sepsis, Caucasian with pneumonia, Caucasian with sepsis; + +, χ^2 test of ARDS vs. respective 1000 Genomes Project control groups; ‡, SNPs with P-value <0.01 in the overall comparison, Caucasian ARDS comparison, and African American comparison with 1000 Genomes were filtered further by $p<0.01$ in the sepsis comparison and pneumonia comparison; ‡‡, All ARDS cases, all pneumonia cases, all sepsis cases, all African American cases, all Caucasian cases.

ARDS patient population to assess association of some newly identified SNPs with ARDS severity (APACHE II score) and outcome (60 day mortality). In addition, we validated three SNPs (rs78142040, rs9605146 and rs3848719) in an additional 117 ARDS patients for a total of 213 cases using TaqMan genotyping assays (Life Technologies) to substantiate their associations with the susceptibility, severity and outcome of ARDS.

Materials and Methods

ARDS patients and healthy control subjects

To perform this case-control study, we used 213 ARDS patient DNA samples from the ARDSnet (www.ardsnet.org) and 440 healthy control subjects (379 EUR and 61 ASW) from the 1000 Genomes Project (www.1000genomes.org). The African Ancestry 1000 Genomes Project panel used in our study is ASW (Americans of African Ancestry in Southwest USA). The European Ancestry 1000 Genomes Project panels used in our study include CEU (Utah residents with Northern and Western European ancestry), FIN (Finnish in Finland), GBR (British in England and Scotland), IBS (Iberian population in Spain), and TSI (Toscani in Italia). Clinical information for 213 ARDS cases was obtained from the NHLBI ARDS network 05: Fluid and Catheter Treatment Trial [21,22] as managed by the Biologic Specimen and Data Repository Information Coordinating Center (BioLINCC, http://biolincc.nhlbi.nih.gov.home). Limited demographic variables for normal control subjects were obtained from the 1000 Genomes Project (www.1000genomes.org).

Exome-seq and data analysis

Exome sequencing was performed on 96 ARDS cases using HiScanSQ (Illumina, CA, USA). Briefly, the libraries for exome sequencing were created using the TrueSeq Exome Enrichment Kit (http://www.illumina.com). Paired-end sequencing with 101 base pair read lengths was performed using Illumina's HiScanSQ, which provides a minimum average coverage depth of 50×. Consensus Assessment of Sequence And VAriations (CASAVA) software was used for the conversion of HiScanSQ reported.bcl files to.fastq format and for demultiplexing (http://www.illumina.com). The sequences were aligned to the hg19 human reference genome and variants alleles were called using the Genome Analysis Toolkit (GATK) (http://www.broadinstitute.org/gatk/). Sequencing data are submitted to the NCBI BioProject database (Accession ID: 262819, http://www.ncbi.nlm.nih.gov/bioproject/262819).

Both the lab-generated data for ARDS patient samples and the 1000 Genomes Project controls were processed using the GATK methodology [23]. GATK was also used to generate the list of SNPs from the sequence data. Sequencing data of the patient samples were considered to be high-confidence if the Phred-like quality was a minimum of 20 and there were at least 4× coverage depths. SNPs from the two data sources were merged by location from alpha ordered datasets and minor allele counts were determined from the merged data.

For the analysis of candidate SNPs associated with the ARDS susceptibility, the ARDS SNP data were compared with the 1000 Genomes Project SNP data. The total control sample size in the 1000 Genomes Project is 1092, and the data identifies about 15 million SNPs which underwent stringent quality control [20,24]. We studied the 440 ASW and EUR samples obtained from this dataset. In racially stratified analyses, the ASW population in the 1000 Genomes Project was used as a control population for the African American ARDS samples and the EUR population was used as a control for the Caucasian ARDS population (Table S1). SNPs in HWE in the cases with high data quality were selected for genotype validation. The detailed association analysis and Hardy-Weinberg equilibrium analysis are provided in Supporting Information S1 [25,26].

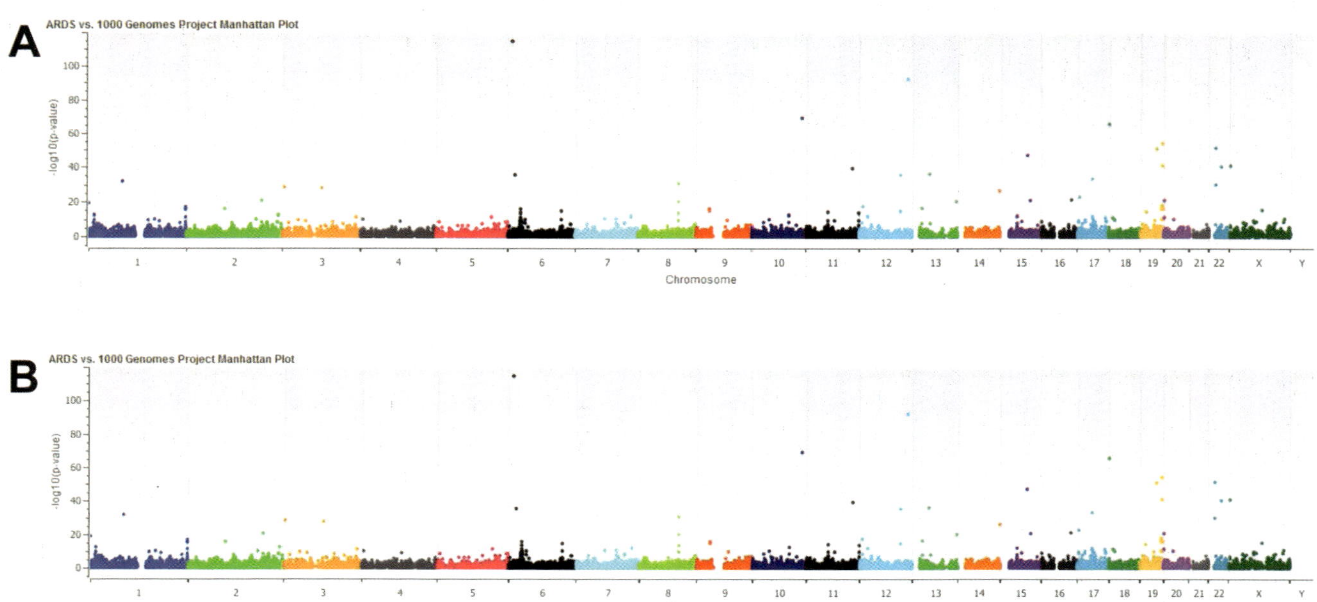

Figure 2. Manhattan plot of ARDS patients and 1000 genomes project controls. A number of strong associations with susceptibility to ARDS were observed using a χ^2 test. (**A**) A Manhattan plot of the whole exome sequence all ARDS cases vs. European Ancestry and ASW 1000 Genomes Project controls created using SVS v8.2.0. This is a graphic representation of the chromosome location (x axis) vs. the –log10 (χ^2 p-value) of the allele frequencies. SNPs whose chi-square tests yield a smaller p-value fall higher on the log scale are more significant [42]. (**B**) The same Manhattan plot with a zoomed Y-axis.

Table 3. Pathway analysis.

Top Canonical Pathways	p-value*	Ratio**	Molecules
Graft-versus-Host Disease Signaling	8.07×10^{-9}	6/48	KIR2DL1/KIR2DL3, HLA-DRB1, HLA-B, HLA-DQA1, HLA-DQB1, HLA-DRB5
Autoimmune Thyroid Disease Signaling	4.35×10^{-7}	5/49	HLA-DRB1, HLA-B, HLA-DQA1, HLA-DQB1, HLA-DRB5
Nur77 Signaling in T Lymphocytes	9.37×10^{-7}	5/57	HLA-DRB1, HLA-DQA1, HLA-DQB1, HLA-DRB5, SIN3A
Calcium-induced T Lymphocyte Apoptosis	1.68×10^{-6}	5/64	HLA-DRB1, HLA-DQA1, HLA-DQB1, ITPR1, HLA-DRB5
B Cell Development	3.75×10^{-6}	4/34	HLA-DRB1, HLA-DQA1, HLA-DQB1, HLA-DRB5

Top canonical pathways as predicted from the 65genes containing the76 SNPs that were identified using χ^2tests. Pathway predictions were done using the Core Analysis function of Ingenuity Pathway Analysis. *, P-Value of <0.05 indicates a non-random association between the genes and pathway; **, Ratio of the number of genes in the dataset involved in the pathway to the total number of genes in the pathway.

For the analysis of candidate SNPs associated with the ARDS severity, the correlation between SNPs and the APACHEII score (a measure of the severity of a disease in adult patients) as well as the number of ventilator-free days per 28 days (an indication of a patient's ability to breathe on their own) was conducted.

For the identification of candidate SNPs associated with the ARDS outcome, the logistic regression analysis between SNPs and 60 day mortality was performed.

Following the results of the genetic association study the data were further analyzed through the use of the Variant Analysis component of SNP & Variation Suite v8.2.0 (SVS v8.2.0, Golden Helix, Inc., Bozeman, MT, www.goldenhelix.com). This software ranked the SNPs in order of likely importance based on location, as well as amino acid change predictions. This information was joined with predictions of protein functional effect changes made by Sift and Provean (http://provean.jcvi.org/index.php) as well as Polyphen2 (http://genetics.bwh.harvard.edu/pph2/index.shtml). Ingenuity Pathway Analysis Software (www.ingenuity.com/) from Ingenuity Systems was used to screen for SNPs which are likely to alter the function of relevant biologic pathways. To accomplish this a list of the genes that contain SNPs with χ^2 p-value of< 2.95×10^{-7} in at least 2 of the 5 main susceptibility comparisons and a χ^2 p-value of <0.01 in all of the 5 main comparisons of exome sequence data (All ARDS vs. 1000 Genomes, All Sepsis vs. 1000 Genomes, All Pneumonia vs. 1000 Genomes, African American ARDS vs. ASW1000 Genomes, and Caucasian ARDS vs. EUR 1000 Genomes) was submitted to IPA. Additional information on the statistical methods preformed in this study can be found in Supporting Information S1, which contains descriptions of the principal component analysis and genomic inflation factor calculations [27–31].

Genotyping of Selected Candidate SNPs

Three selected SNPs (rs78142040; rs9605146, and rs3848719) in the additional 117 ARDS patient DNA samples from the NHLBI Ardent were genotyped using TaqMan human SNP genotyping assays on the ViiA 7 Real Time PCR System (Life Technologies, Grand Island, NY) according to the supplier's instruction. Genotyping accuracy was validated using 10 previously exome-sequenced samples in-lab. Genotyping data from the additional samples was combined with the existing 96 patient sample to increase sample size for the 3 SNPs and association tests were repeated using the total 213 patient population.

Results

Identification of novel coding SNPs associated with the ARDS susceptibility

In order to identify novel coding SNPs associated with the ARDS susceptibility, we performed the exome-seq of 96 ARDS patient DNAs. These patients consisted of 70 Caucasian and 26 African Americans (Table 1). In Caucasian patients, 37 cases were due to the initiating etiology of sepsis and 33 were due to pneumonia. In African American patients, 11 cases were due to the initiating etiology of sepsis and 15 were due to pneumonia. We detected 1,382,399 SNPs in 96 ARDS patients by exome-seq (Table 2) and 490,015 SNPs per person on average (Figure 1). Among them, 169,376 SNPs matched records from 625 healthy control subjects in the 1000 human genome project. From 169,376 SNPs, there are 49,723 bi-allelic SNPs out of 50,190 total SNPs in all ARDS patient subgroups based on race and initiating etiologies: Caucasian sepsis, Caucasian pneumonia, African-American sepsis and African American pneumonia. Of our 1,382,399 ARDS SNPs, 608,723 were common between the sepsis and pneumonia cases while 369,639 and 404,037 are non-overlapping SNPs, respectively. There are 442,235 common SNPs between our African American cases and Caucasian cases while 337,738 and 602,426 are non-overlapping SNPs, respectively. 87.8% of the 1,382,399 ARDS SNPs (i.e., 1,213,023 ARDS SNPs) are not found in the 1000 Genomes Project Exome, but 85.4% of the 1,213,023 ARDS SNPs (i.e., 1,035,921 SNPs) were assigned RS numbers, suggesting our data collection and processing are reliable. By comparing the frequencies of the minor alleles in those newly detected SNPs in 96 ARDS patients with those in 440 Caucasian and African-Americans from the Southwest healthy control subjects of the 1000 human genome project, we found that there are 3,867 differential SNPs ($p<0.01$) (Figure 2). In Caucasians, between ARDS patients and healthy controls, there are 788 differential SNPs ($p<0.01$). In African-Americans, between ARDS patients and healthy controls, there are 948 differential SNPs ($p<0.01$). There are 122 common differential SNPs ($p<0.01$) between either Caucasian or African American patients or healthy controls. When we examined sepsis- or pneumonia-initiated ARDS separately, we found that 106 and 109 differential SNPs ($p<0.01$), respectively. Between them, there are 99 common differential SNPs ($p<0.01$). When the Bonferroni correction ($p<2.95\times10^{-7}$) was applied, 76SNPs remains significantly different. These SNPs are potentially novel coding SNPs associated with the ARDS susceptibility.

Table 4. Profile of 3 SNPs.

	rs3848719	rs9605146	rs78142040
Location	20:44596545	22:17265194	X:2832771
Gene ID	ZNF335	XKR3	ARSD
Call Rate (Cases+Controls)	0.962	0.995	0.991
Call Rate (Cases)	0.883	0.986	0.972
HWE P-value (Cases)	2.86E-4	0.422	1.18E-3
HWE P-value (Controls)	0.887	3.72E-5	1
HWE P-value (Cases+Controls)	0.034	1.94E-12	0.471
Reference: Alternate Allele	G>A	G>A	C>T
Alt. Allele Freq. (Cases)	39.4%	38.6%	22.0%
Alt. Allele Freq. (Controls)	38.5%	4.0%	0%
Number AA (%) (Cases)	41 (21.8%)	34 (16.2%)	2 (1.0%)
Number AA (%) (Controls)	66(15.0%)	4(0.9%)	0(0%)
Number Ar (%) (Cases)	66 (35.1%)	94 (44.8%)	87 (42.0%)
Number Ar (%) (Controls)	207 (47.0%)	27 (6.1%)	0 (0%)
Number rr (%) (Cases)	81 (45.1%)	82 (39.1%)	118 (57.0%)
Number rr (%) (Controls)	339 (77.0%)	35 (8.0%)	0 (0%)
SNP classification	Coding	Coding	Intronic
Coding classification	Synonymous	Nonsynonymous	Intronic
Reference amino acid	S	P	NK
Alternate amino acid	S	L	NK
Provean prediction (cutoff = −25)[1]	Neutral	Deleterious	NK
Sift prediction (cutoff = 0.05)[1]	Tolerated	Tolerated	NK
Pph2 prediction[2]	NK	benign	NK

NK: Not known, HWE, Hardy-Weinberg equilibrium; AA, alternate genotype or homozygous minor genotype; Ar, heterozygous genotype; rr, reference genotype or homozygous major genotype; 1, http://provean.jcvi.org/genome_submit.php; 2, http://genetics.bwh.harvard.edu/pph2/.

Pathway Analysis

These 76 SNPs occur in 65 genes. To determine the functional consequences of these SNPs, Ingenuity Pathway Analysis was conducted on these 65 genes to identify biologic pathways in which these genes function. The top canonical pathway is *graft-versus-host disease signaling* and included 6 genes that contained associated SNPs, comprising 13% of the genes involved in the pathway ($p = 8.07 \times 10^{-9}$). The top 5 canonical pathways addi-

Table 5. Overall association summary.

	rs3848719	rs9605146	rs78142040
Susceptibility (cases vs. controls)			
Chi-squared p-value	0.780	1.68E-59	3.64E-47
Odds Ratio (95% CI)[1]	1.04(0.81–1.33)	15.16(10.25–22.41)	498.09 (30.83–8,047.51)
Severity (ventilator-free days/28 days)			
p-value	NS	NS	NS
Odds Ratio (95% CI)[2]	NS	NS	NS
Severity (APACHE II score)			
p-value	0.032	NS	0.061**
Odds Ratio (95% CI)[2]	0.55 (0.31–0.96)	NS	2.60(0.93–7.26)
Outcome (60-day mortality)			
p-value	NS*	NS	0.017
Odds Ratio (95% CI)[2]	NS	NS	2.04 (1.13–3.68)

NS, Not significant; *, significantly associated in genotyped Caucasian, pneumonia, and Caucasian pneumonia subgroups; **, for 117 genotyped samples only, not in total 213; 1, Odds ratio for alternate allele (allelic test); 2, additive genotypic model.

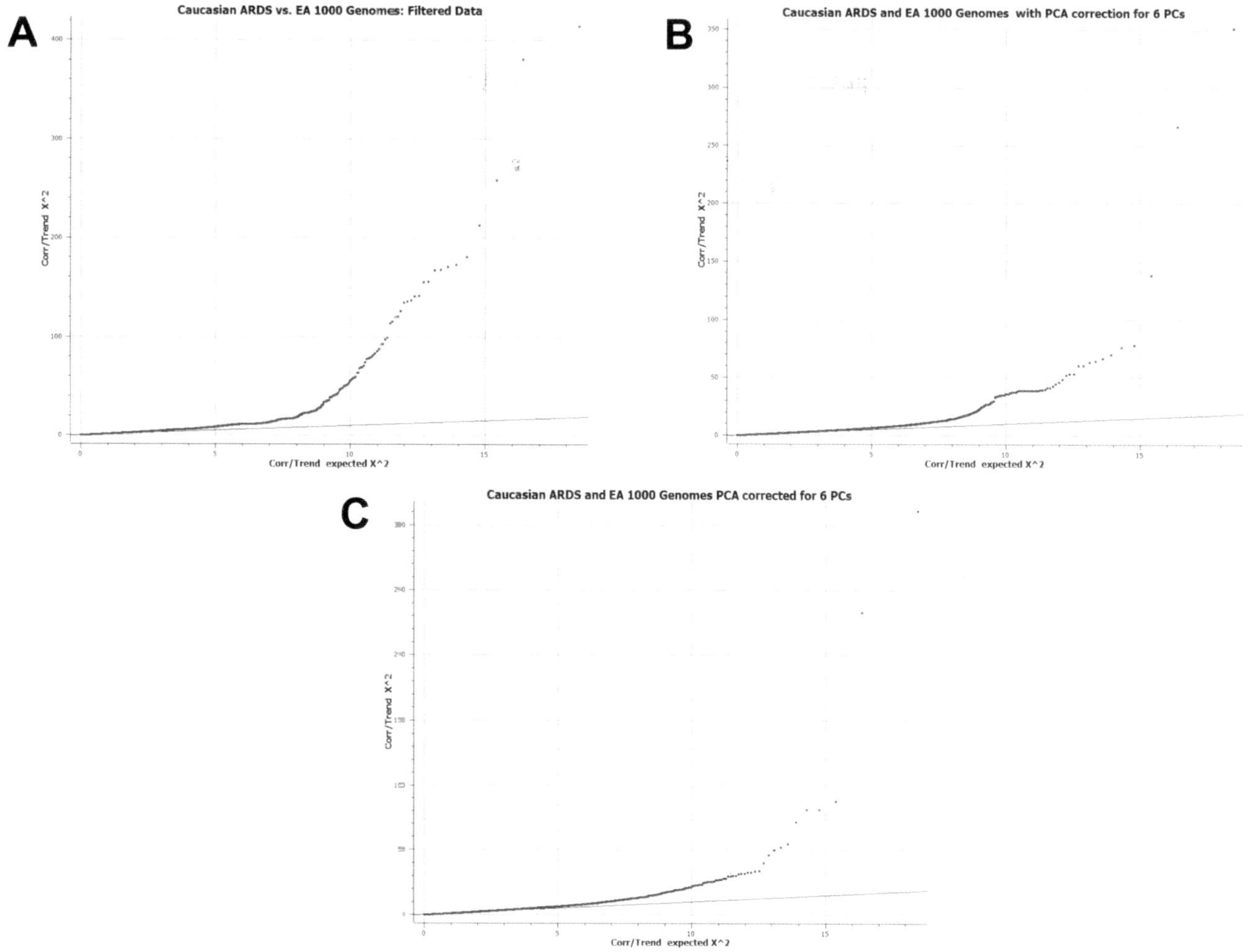

Figure 3. Quantile-quantile plots of Caucasian ARDS and EUR 1000 genomes. In the example of our Caucasian cases and EUR controls, we observe that correction for principal components improves the fit of our data with the expected distribution. (**A**) QQ plot of expected χ^2values versus the actual χ^2values for the genotypic trend test of case-control status. The data are filtered on HWE, LD, and SNP call rate but not PCA corrected. (**B**) QQ plot of expected χ^2values versus the actual χ^2values for the genotypic trend test of case-control status. The data have been filtered and corrected for 6 PCs. (**C**) QQ plot of expected χ^2values versus the actual χ^2values for the genotypic trend test of case-control status. The data have been filtered and corrected for 6 PCs and undergone sample outlier removal.

tionally include *autoimmune thyroid disease signaling*, *Nur77 signaling in T lymphocytes*, *calcium-induced T lymphocyte apoptosis*, and *B-cell development signaling* (Table 3). Among the 76 remaining significantly different SNPs after the Boneferroni correction (Figure 1), 38 SNPs are coding variants. Of these, 20 SNPs can cause nonsynonymous amino acid changes while 18 SNPs can cause synonymous amino acid changes (Table 2).

Selected validations of three SNPs (rs78142040, rs9605146 and rs3848719)in additional 117 ARDS patients

To validate the result of SNP identification by exome-seq, we selectively genotyped three SNPs (rs78142040, rs9605146 and rs3848719) in an additional 117 ARDS patients using the TaqMan genotype assay (Table 4). We then examined their association with the susceptibility, severity and outcome to ARDS in a combined 213 ARDS patients (96 by exome-seq +117 by TaqMan = 213) (Table 5, Table S2, Table S3, and Table S4).

rs78142040 has a major allele C and a minor allele T and is found on the X chromosome position X: 2832771 in the Arylsulfatase D gene (ARSD). The SNP was determined to lie within a histone mark of intron 6 using the UCSC Genome Browser (http://genome.ucsc.edu/) and could potentially play a role in regulation of expression. The ARSD was associated with bone and cartilage development and was identified previously as having involvement in sphingolipid metabolism and as a potential biomarker for chronic lymphocytic leukemia [32]. The SNP is in Hardy-Weinberg Equilibrium (HWE $p>1\times10^{-4}$) in the 1000 Genomes controls and the ARDS population and subgroups.

The SNP is associated significantly with susceptibility ($p< 2.95\times10$^-7) in the total 213 patient population (MAF = 0.22) and the subgroups when compared with those from the 1000 Genomes Project (MAF = 0.00) (Table 5, Additional file 6: Table S5). rs78142040 approaches association with APACHEII score when the score quartiles are compared for the genotyped ARDS patients (p = 0.061, OR = 2.603, 95% CI = 0.933–7.260) (Table 5, Table S4). rs78142040 is associated with the 60-day mortality in the total ARDS population (p = 0.017, OR = 2.039, 95%CI 1.130–3.681) (Table S3).

rs9605146 (also known as rs114989947) has a major allele G and minor allele A. It is a nonsynonymous SNP found within exon 4 of chromosome 22 (22:17265194) in the "XK, Kell blood group complex subunit-related family, member 3" gene (XKR3) and causes a predicted amino acid change from proline to leucine. The protein encoded by XKR3 is a homolog of XK, which is a putative membrane transporter [33]. XKR3 has not been previously associated with human disease. This amino acid change has a deleterious effect predicted by a Provean score of -5.494, where a score of maximum -2.5 is considered to be deleterious. The SNP is in HWE ($p>1\times10^{-4}$) in the EUR 1000 Genomes Project samples as well as in the ARDS population and subgroups. rs9605146 is associated with disease susceptibility ($p<2.95\times10^{-7}$) in the total ARDS population (MAF = 0.39) and subgroups when compared with the 1000 Genomes controls (MAF = 0.04) with the exception of the African Americans when the sepsis and pneumonia etiologies are analyzed individually (Table 5, Table S6). The SNP also approaches significant association with 60-day mortality in the exome-sequenced patients with pneumonia ($p = 0.080$).

rs3848719 has a major allele of G and a minor allele A. It is a synonymous SNP in the 5th exon of the Zinc-Finger/Leucine-Zipper Co-Transducer NIF1 gene in chromosome 20 (ZNF335, location 20:44596545). The ZNF335 gene is expected to play a role in transcription regulation and is involved in neural progenitor cell proliferation and self-renewal. It is associated with the disease microcephaly [34,35]. The SNP is in Hardy-Weinberg Equilibrium (HWE $p>1\times10^{-4}$) in the 1000 Genomes controls and the ARDS population and subgroups.

The SNP was not associated with susceptibility in the total ARDS population (MAF = 0.39) when compared with the 1000 Genomes controls (MAF = 0.385) (Table 5, Table S7), however rs3848719 is associated with APACHEII score when the score quartiles are compared for total ARDS patients ($p = 0.032$, OR = 0.549, 95%CI = 0.313–0.96). The SNP is associated with 60-day mortality in the TaqMan genotyped Caucasian ARDS ($p = 0.012$, OR = 2.753, 95% CI = 1.196–6.336), TaqMan genotyped pneumonia ($p = 0.032$, OR = 2.511, 95% CI = 1.053–5.984), and TaqMan genotyped Caucasians with pneumonia ($p = 0.012$, OR = 4.045, 95% CI = 1.219–13.433).

Discussion

Overview of WES Findings

Whole-exome sequencing (WES) had been performed in 96 ARDS patients from the ARDSnet with the intent of identifying coding SNPs whose minor allele frequencies are significantly different in ARDS than those of healthy controls and of identifying those novel SNPs who may be predictors of ARDS severity and outcome. In the overall ARDS population 1,382,399 SNPs were detected by exome-seq (Table 2) and 490,015 SNPs per person on average (Figure 1) compared to 714,074 SNPs per person from 625 healthy control subjects in the 1000 Genome Project. Among them, only 169,376 SNPs overlapped between two populations. The majority of un-overlapped SNPs in ARDS patients may represent ARDS specific SNPs barring the individual variability, sequencing error and data analysis discrepancy. From 169,376 SNPs, there are 49,789 bi-allelic SNPs in all ARDS patient subgroups based on race and initiating etiologies: Caucasian sepsis, Caucasian pneumonia, African-American sepsis and African American pneumonia. These SNPs may represent sepsis or pneumonia etiology specific SNPs of ARDS. The reason why we initially focused on the identification of novel coding SNPs associated with ARDS in sepsis and pneumonia origins was that in the original ARDS patient population, sepsis and pneumonia etiologies accounted for most cases [21,22]. We selectively genotyped and validated three SNPs (rs78142040, rs9605146 and rs3848719) in an additional 117 ARDS patients using the TaqMan genotype assay and performed in depth association analyses of these SNPs with the susceptibility, severity and outcome to ARDS in a combined 213 ARDS patients (96 by exome-seq +117 by TaqMan = 213). These validations lend a solid support to the validity and prowess of novel ARDS associated SNP identifications by exome-seq. This study provides a rich resource for further experimentation and replication to develop and establish new genetic biomarkers and therapeutic targets to ARDS.

Validation of selected three SNPs

Among three selectively validated SNPs (rs78142040, rs9605146 and rs3848719) in an additional 117 ARDS patients, rs78142040 in the ARSD gene is associated with increased ARDS susceptibility in the overall ARDS population (213 patients) as well as all racial and comorbidity subpopulations. It approaches significant association with an increase in APACHEII score ($p = 0.061$) when samples in the highest and lowest score quartiles are compared in ARDS patients. rs78142040 is associated significantly ($p<0.05$) with an increase in 60-day mortality in the total ARDS population ($p = 0.017$, OR = 2.039, 95%CI 1.130–3.681). The molecular mechanisms underlying these associations are presently unknown. The ARSD gene encodes a sulfatase that is associated with bone and cartilage development and has been identified previously as having involvement in sphingolipid metabolism (involved in signal transmission and cellular recognition) and as a potential biomarker for chronic lymphocytic leukemia [32]. ARSD protein isoforms have a highly conserved catalytic peptide domain when compared with other arylsulfatases [36,37]. ARSD is widely expressed and is suspected to play a role in housekeeping or multiple other processes, however specific substrates have not been identified [38]. It was reported that there were changes in activities of lung liposomal enzymes including sulfates during ARDS [39]. It may be interesting to explore whether rs78142040 causes the differential expression of the ARSD gene, thus sulfatase activity, which may link its role in the pathogenesis of ARDS.

rs9605146 in the XKR3 gene is associated with increased susceptibility in the ARDS population and all subgroups except the African American with sepsis etiology group and the African American with pneumonia etiology group when analyzed individually. XKR3 is a member of the XK/Kell complex in the Kell blood group system. XKR3 is a homolog of XK, which is a putative membrane transporter. XK is associated with McLeod syndrome (characterized by late-onset abnormalities in the central nervous system and neuromuscular system) and red cell acanthocytosis [33]. XKR3 has previously been indicated as a potential biomarker for blood transfusion compatibility [40]. While it is currently unknown what underlies the association of rs9605146 with susceptibility in ARDS, it causes a deleterious amino acid coding change from proline to leucine in the XKR3 gene as predicted by Provean (score = -5.494). These observations make rs9605146 a legitimate candidate for further study of its role in the pathogenesis of ARDS.

rs3848719 in the ZNF335 gene is not associated significantly with susceptibility, however the SNP is associated with a decreased APACHEII score when the highest and lowest score quartiles are compared in the total ARDS population ($p = 0.032$, OR = 0.55, 95%CI 1.27–2.05), and with an increased 60-day mortality in Caucasian and pneumonia groups ($p<0.05$). It is a synonymous

SNP in the 5th exon of the Zinc-Finger/Leucine-Zipper Co-Transducer NIF1 gene (ZNF335). ZNF335 gene is involved in neural progenitor cell proliferation and self-renewal as a component of the vertebrate-specific, trithorax H3K4-methylation complex. ZNF335 is associated with the disease microcephaly (a neurodevelopmental disorder), small somatic size and neonatal death. The gene is essential as homozygous knockout mouse models have a lethal effect [34,35]. The role of the gene in cellular differentiation and gene expression could implicate an effect on the fundamental physiology and neural signaling in the lungs, contributing to the pathogenesis of ARDS.

Limitations

Although we applied the Bonferroni correction ($p<2.95\times10^{-7}$) and several SNP filtering steps during our data analysis as well as validations of three selected candidate SNPs to ARDS, our data come with potential limitations. First, we only performed exome-seq of 96 ARDS samples. Although we would argue that this is a very reasonable sample size considering the restriction of high exome-seq cost per sample, even though the exome-seq cost per sample is cheaper than whole genome-seq per sample, the sample size is not large. Our 76 SNPs which are associated strongly with susceptibility are all present in an age and race matched 48 sample control set, which will be used to validate our findings in further studies (117,35 out of the 169,376 SNPs which are in the ARDS cases and 1000 Genomes Project are found in this control set). Confirmation of our findings in larger patient populations is warranted. Second, during analysis of SNP associations with ARDS susceptibility, we used the healthy control subjects from the 1000 Genome Project. Both ARDS patients and healthy control subjects do not derive from the same population. Since population admixture is assumed in the African American cases, we have elected to compare these cases with the ASW subset of the 1000 Genomes Project African Ancestry panel. We feel this is the best fitting control group due to the observed reduction in genomic inflation factor (inflation factor = 1.18 when compared with ASW, after filtering for informative markers based on HWE, call rate, number of alleles, and LD) compared to the total African Ancestry controls (inflation factor = 1.70), YRI alone (inflation factor = 1.59), or LWK alone (inflation factor = 1.98) [41]. An ancestry-informative SNP panel with good coverage of our dataset was not available. Although we have applied HWE, PCA analysis and Q–Q plot determination as well as race specific comparison to filter the identified SNPs, it may not totally correct the population admixtures (Figure 3, Figure S1, Figure S2, Table S8). Two of the SNPs (rs9605146, control MAF 4.0% and rs78142040, control MAF 0% respectively) have extremely minor allele frequencies which causes inflation of the type-1 error of the Goodness-of-fit test for HWE [26]. In this study, we explicitly searched for SNPs in which the MAF differed between cases and controls, so we expect that we might see some deviation where the minor alleles are rare in healthy controls. The observed associations with other disease phenotypes within our case cohort support our conclusion that variations at these loci contribute to disease. Replication of our findings in larger and different populations may strengthen and develop the candidate SNPs identified here as true genetic biomarkers of ARDS.

Conclusion

The primary focus of this study was to identify new and novel SNPs associated with ARDS susceptibility, severity and outcome using whole exome-sequencing. We have identified a number of potential ARDS associated SNPs, which has demonstrated that WES is a powerful tool to identify new biomarkers in ARDS. We selectively validated 3 SNPs that are associated with the susceptibility (rs78142040 and rs9605146), severity (rs3848719) and outcome (rs78142040 and rs3848719) of ARDS. More validations in larger and different patient populations as well as further investigation of the underlying molecular mechanisms are warranted to establish them as true new diagnostic and therapeutic targets for ARDS.

Supporting Information

Figure S1 The scree plots of the eigenvalues generated by principal component analysis. The largest eigenvalues are used in corrections for population structure. (**A**) The All ARDS and ASW+EUR 1000 Genomes population eigenvalues. 535 principal components were measured and the largest eigenvalue is 7.32. (**B**) The Caucasian ARDS and EUR ARDS population eigenvalues. 449 principal components were measured and the largest eigenvalue is 1.52. (**C**) The African American ARDS and ASW 1000 Genomes population eigenvalues. 86 principal components were measured and the largest eigenvalue is 0.94.

Figure S2 The quantile-quantile plots of genotypic trend test χ^2 values for the African American ARDS and ASW 1000 Genomes population were derived using SVS v8.2.0. The straight line on each plot represents $y = x$. (**A**) QQ plot of expected χ^2values versus the actual χ^2values for the genotypic trend test of case-control status. The data are filtered on HWE, LD, and SNP call rate but not PCA corrected. (**B**) QQ plot of expected χ^2values versus the actual χ^2values for the genotypic trend test of case-control status. The data are corrected for the 2 largest principal components. (**C**) QQ plot of expected χ^2values versus the actual $\chi^2$for the genotypic trend test of case-control status. The data have been filtered and corrected for 2 PCs and undergone sample outlier removal.

Table S1 A summary of the comparison groups used for the genetic association analysis. Association of the exome-seq SNPs with susceptibility was explored by comparing 96 ARDS patients to 440 controls from the 1000 Genomes Project. Analysis was stratified by race and etiology.

Table S2 A summary of the susceptibility χ^2 tests for the 3 SNPs. The allelic chi-square test p-values for the exome sequenced ARDS patients ARDS patients and subgroups compared with the 1000 Genomes Project participants and subgroups, TaqMan genotyped ARDS patients and subgroups compared with the 1000 Genomes Project participants and subgroups, and the total ARDS patient population and subgroups compared with the 1000 Genomes Project participants and subgroups. P-values were considered to be significant if they were smaller than the Bonferroni corrected p-value of 2.95×10^{-7}.

Table S3 Logistic regression with 60-day mortality from the day of diagnosis was used to assess SNP association with outcome. Included in this table are the p-values of the logistic regression of 60-day mortality against genotype using an additive model in the ARDS exome samples, TaqMan genotyped samples, and total ARDS samples. Associations were considered significant if $p<0.05$.

Table S4 Logistic regression with APACHE II score was used to assess SNP association with overall disease

severity. Included in this table are the p-values of the logistic regression of ARDS patient genotype and APACHEII score by quartile. The APACHEII scores are split into quartiles and the 1st and 4th quartiles are used in a logistic regression against genotype using an additive model in the ARDS exome samples, TaqMan genotyped samples, and total ARDS samples. Regressions were also run on the stratified sub-populations of the ARDS patients. Associations were considered to be significant if $P<0.05$.

Table S5 A summary of the descriptive statistics for SNP rs78142040 in the exome sequenced ARDS, TaqMan genotyped ARDS patients, and total ARDS patients, where the controls are 1000 Genomes Project participants. *, Chi-square tests were run on SNPs that were in both the controls and the cases; A, alternate allele; r, reference allele.

Table S6 A summary of the descriptive statistics for SNP rs9605146 in the exome sequenced ARDS, TaqMan genotyped ARDS patients, and total ARDS patients, where the controls are 1000 Genomes Project participants. *, Chi-square tests were run on SNPs that were in both the controls and the cases; A, alternate allele; r, reference allele.

Table S7 A summary of the descriptive statistics for SNP rs3848719 in the exome sequenced ARDS, TaqMan genotyped ARDS patients, and total ARDS patients, where the controls are 1000 Genomes Project participants. *, Chi-square tests were run on SNPs that were in both the controls and the cases; A, alternate allele; r, reference allele.

Table S8 A summary of the effect of the PCA adjustments on the genotypic trend test of the 3 SNPs. 2 of the 3 SNPs were present in the filtered Caucasian ARDS+EUR controls population. PCA, principal components analysis; PCs, principal components; AA, African American ARDS; ASW, African Americans in the southwest 1000 Genomes Project; EA, European Ancestry or Caucasian; corr/trend, trend association test.

Supporting Information S1 The Supporting Information contains a detailed description of statistical methods used in this study.

Acknowledgments

We would like to acknowledge the sponsorship of Roy G Brower, MD, Division of Pulmonary and Critical Care Medicine, Johns Hopkins University School of Medicine for our application to the ARDSnet to secure the ARDS patient DNA samples and the ARDSnet teams (www.ardsnet.org) for providing 213 ARDS patient DNA samples in this study.

Author Contributions

Conceived and designed the experiments: SQY LZ. Performed the experiments: KS SC. Analyzed the data: KS DG DPH. Contributed reagents/materials/analysis tools: SQY KS. Contributed to the writing of the manuscript: SQY LZ LV DPH DG KS.

References

1. Ashbaugh DG, Bigelow DB, Petty TL, Levine BE (1967) Acute respiratory distress in adults. Lancet 2: 319–323.
2. Bernard GR, Artigas A, Brigham KL, Carlet J, Falke K, et al. (1994) The American-European Consensus Conference on ARDS. Definitions, mechanisms, relevant outcomes, and clinical trial coordination. Am J Respir Crit Care Med 149: 818–824.
3. Rubenfeld GD, Caldwell E, Peabody E, Weaver J, Martin DP, et al. (2005) Incidence and outcomes of acute lung injury. N Engl J Med 353: 1685–1693.
4. Blank R, Napolitano LM (2011) Epidemiology of ARDS and ALI. Crit Care Clin 27: 439–458.
5. Flores C, Pino-Yanes MM, Casula M, Villar J (2010) Genetics of acute lung injury: past, present and future. Minerva Anestesiol 76: 860–864.
6. Garcia JG (2005) Searching for candidate genes in acute lung injury: SNPs, Chips and PBEF. Trans Am Clin Climatol Assoc 116: 205–219; discussion 220.
7. Gong MN (2006) Genetic epidemiology of acute respiratory distress syndrome: implications for future prevention and treatment. Clin Chest Med 27: 705–724; abstract x.
8. McGlothlin JR, Gao L, Lavoie T, Simon BA, Easley RB, et al. (2005) Molecular cloning and characterization of canine pre-B-cell colony-enhancing factor. Biochem Genet 43: 127–141.
9. Parks BW, Nam E, Org E, Kostem E, Norheim F, et al. (2013) Genetic control of obesity and gut microbiota composition in response to high-fat, high-sucrose diet in mice. Cell Metab 17: 141–152.
10. Tzouvelekis A, Pneumatikos I, Bouros D (2005) Serum biomarkers in acute respiratory distress syndrome an ailing prognosticator. Respir Res 6: 62.
11. Crader KM RJ, Repine JE (2012) Breath Biomarkers and the Acute Respiratory Distress Syndrome. J Pulmonar Respirat Med 2.
12. Ye SQ, Simon BA, Maloney JP, Zambelli-Weiner A, Gao L, et al. (2005) Pre-B-cell colony-enhancing factor as a potential novel biomarker in acute lung injury. Am J Respir Crit Care Med 171: 361–370.
13. Bajwa EK, Yu CL, Gong MN, Thompson BT, Christiani DC (2007) Pre-B-cell colony-enhancing factor gene polymorphisms and risk of acute respiratory distress syndrome. Crit Care Med 35: 1290–1295.
14. Lee KA, Gong MN (2011) Pre-B-cell colony-enhancing factor and its clinical correlates with acute lung injury and sepsis. Chest 140: 382–390.
15. Liu Y, Shao Y, Yu B, Sun L, Lv F (2012) Association of PBEF gene polymorphisms with acute lung injury, sepsis, and pneumonia in a northeastern Chinese population. Clin Chem Lab Med 50: 1917–1922.
16. Gullapalli RR, Desai KV, Santana-Santos L, Kant JA, Becich MJ (2012) Next generation sequencing in clinical medicine: Challenges and lessons for pathology and biomedical informatics. J Pathol Inform 3: 40.
17. Goh G, Choi M (2012) Application of whole exome sequencing to identify disease-causing variants in inherited human diseases. Genomics Inform 10: 214–219.
18. Takata A, Kato M, Nakamura M, Yoshikawa T, Kanba S, et al. (2011) Exome sequencing identifies a novel missense variant in RRM2B associated with autosomal recessive progressive external ophthalmoplegia. Genome Biol 12: R92.
19. Fang X, Bai C, Wang X (2012) Bioinformatics insights into acute lung injury/acute respiratory distress syndrome. Clin Transl Med 1: 9.
20. Abecasis GR, Altshuler D, Auton A, Brooks LD, Durbin RM, et al. (2010) A map of human genome variation from population-scale sequencing. Nature 467: 1061–1073.
21. Wheeler AP, Bernard GR, Thompson BT, Schoenfeld D, Wiedemann HP, et al. (2006) Pulmonary-artery versus central venous catheter to guide treatment of acute lung injury. N Engl J Med 354: 2213–2224.
22. Wiedemann HP, Wheeler AP, Bernard GR, Thompson BT, Hayden D, et al. (2006) Comparison of two fluid-management strategies in acute lung injury. N Engl J Med 354: 2564–2575.
23. McKenna A, Hanna M, Banks E, Sivachenko A, Cibulskis K, et al. (2010) The Genome Analysis Toolkit: a MapReduce framework for analyzing next-generation DNA sequencing data. Genome Res 20: 1297–1303.
24. Abecasis GR, Auton A, Brooks LD, DePristo MA, Durbin RM, et al. (2012) An integrated map of genetic variation from 1,092 human genomes. Nature 491: 56–65.
25. Melum E, Franke A, Schramm C, Weismuller TJ, Gotthardt DN, et al. (2011) Genome-wide association analysis in primary sclerosing cholangitis identifies two non-HLA susceptibility loci. Nat Genet 43: 17–19.
26. Lunetta KL (2008) Genetic association studies. Circulation 118: 96–101.
27. Pearson TA, Manolio TA (2008) How to interpret a genome-wide association study. Jama 299: 1335–1344.
28. Laurie CC, Doheny KF, Mirel DB, Pugh EW, Bierut LJ, et al. (2010) Quality control and quality assurance in genotypic data for genome-wide association studies. Genet Epidemiol 34: 591–602.
29. Price AL, Patterson NJ, Plenge RM, Weinblatt ME, Shadick NA, et al. (2006) Principal components analysis corrects for stratification in genome-wide association studies. Nat Genet 38: 904–909.
30. Hinrichs AL, Larkin EK, Suarez BK (2009) Population stratification and patterns of linkage disequilibrium. Genet Epidemiol 33 Suppl 1: S88–92.
31. Khrunin AV, Khokhrin DV, Filippova IN, Esko T, Nelis M, et al. (2013) A genome-wide analysis of populations from European Russia reveals a new pole of genetic diversity in northern Europe. PLoS One 8: e58552.

32. Trojani A, Di Camillo B, Tedeschi A, Lodola M, Montesano S, et al. (2011) Gene expression profiling identifies ARSD as a new marker of disease progression and the sphingolipid metabolism as a potential novel metabolism in chronic lymphocytic leukemia. Cancer Biomark 11: 15–28.
33. Calenda G, Peng J, Redman CM, Sha Q, Wu X, et al. (2006) Identification of two new members, XPLAC and XTES, of the XK family. Gene 370: 6–16.
34. Mahajan MA, Murray A, Samuels HH (2002) NRC-interacting factor 1 is a novel cotransducer that interacts with and regulates the activity of the nuclear hormone receptor coactivator NRC. Mol Cell Biol 22: 6883–6894.
35. Yang YJ, Baltus AE, Mathew RS, Murphy EA, Evrony GD, et al. (2012) Microcephaly gene links trithorax and REST/NRSF to control neural stem cell proliferation and differentiation. Cell 151: 1097–1112.
36. Franco B, Meroni G, Parenti G, Levilliers J, Bernard L, et al. (1995) A cluster of sulfatase genes on Xp22.3: mutations in chondrodysplasia punctata (CDPX) and implications for warfarin embryopathy. Cell 81: 15–25.
37. Urbitsch P, Salzer MJ, Hirschmann P, Vogt PH (2000) Arylsulfatase D gene in Xp22.3 encodes two protein isoforms. DNA Cell Biol 19: 765–773.
38. Dooley TP, Haldeman-Cahill R, Joiner J, Wilborn TW (2000) Expression profiling of human sulfotransferase and sulfatase gene superfamilies in epithelial tissues and cultured cells. Biochem Biophys Res Commun 277: 236–245.
39. Anasiewicz A, Maciejewski R, Juskiewicz W, Lakowska H, Madej B, et al. (1997) [Changes of lysosomal enzyme activity in the lungs during the course of acute pancreatitis]. Wiad Lek 50 Suppl 1 Pt 2: 96–100.
40. Le Goff GC, Bres JC, Rigal D, Blum LJ, Marquette CA (2010) Robust, high-throughput solution for blood group genotyping. Anal Chem 82: 6185–6192.
41. Devlin B, Roeder K (1999) Genomic control for association studies. Biometrics 55: 997–1004.
42. Robinson JT, Thorvaldsdottir H, Winckler W, Guttman M, Lander ES, et al. (2011) Integrative genomics viewer. Nat Biotechnol 29: 24–26.

Permissions

All chapters in this book were first published in PLOS ONE, by The Public Library of Science; hereby published with permission under the Creative Commons Attribution License or equivalent. Every chapter published in this book has been scrutinized by our experts. Their significance has been extensively debated. The topics covered herein carry significant findings which will fuel the growth of the discipline. They may even be implemented as practical applications or may be referred to as a beginning point for another development.

The contributors of this book come from diverse backgrounds, making this book a truly international effort. This book will bring forth new frontiers with its revolutionizing research information and detailed analysis of the nascent developments around the world.

We would like to thank all the contributing authors for lending their expertise to make the book truly unique. They have played a crucial role in the development of this book. Without their invaluable contributions this book wouldn't have been possible. They have made vital efforts to compile up to date information on the varied aspects of this subject to make this book a valuable addition to the collection of many professionals and students.

This book was conceptualized with the vision of imparting up-to-date information and advanced data in this field. To ensure the same, a matchless editorial board was set up. Every individual on the board went through rigorous rounds of assessment to prove their worth. After which they invested a large part of their time researching and compiling the most relevant data for our readers.

The editorial board has been involved in producing this book since its inception. They have spent rigorous hours researching and exploring the diverse topics which have resulted in the successful publishing of this book. They have passed on their knowledge of decades through this book. To expedite this challenging task, the publisher supported the team at every step. A small team of assistant editors was also appointed to further simplify the editing procedure and attain best results for the readers.

Apart from the editorial board, the designing team has also invested a significant amount of their time in understanding the subject and creating the most relevant covers. They scrutinized every image to scout for the most suitable representation of the subject and create an appropriate cover for the book.

The publishing team has been an ardent support to the editorial, designing and production team. Their endless efforts to recruit the best for this project, has resulted in the accomplishment of this book. They are a veteran in the field of academics and their pool of knowledge is as vast as their experience in printing. Their expertise and guidance has proved useful at every step. Their uncompromising quality standards have made this book an exceptional effort. Their encouragement from time to time has been an inspiration for everyone.

The publisher and the editorial board hope that this book will prove to be a valuable piece of knowledge for researchers, students, practitioners and scholars across the globe.

List of Contributors

Hung-Jen Tang
Department of Medicine, Chi Mei Medical Center, Tainan, Taiwan
Department of Health and Nutrition, Chia Nan University of Pharmacy and Science, Tainan, Taiwan

Wei-Lun Liu and Chih-Cheng Lai
Department of Intensive Care Medicine, Chi Mei Medical Center, Liouying, Tainan, Taiwan

Hsin-Lan Lin
Department of Nursing, Chi Mei Medical Center, Liouying, Tainan, Taiwan

Hyun-Woo Jeong and Young-Yun Kong
School of Biological Science, College of Natural Sciences, Seoul National University, Seoul, South Korea

Sun-Kyoung Im
School of Biological Science, College of Natural Sciences, Seoul National University, Seoul, South Korea
Department of Life Science, Division of Molecular and Life Science, POSTECH, Pohang, South Korea

Kyong-Tai Kim
Department of Life Science, Division of Molecular and Life Science, POSTECH, Pohang, South Korea

HyoBin Jeong and Daehee Hwang
School of Interdisciplinary Biosciences and Bioengineering, POSTECH, Pohang, South Korea

Machiko Ikegami
Division of Pulmonary Biology, Cincinnati Children's Hospital Medical Center and University of Cincinnati College of Medicine, Cincinnati, Ohio, United States of America

Silvana Gomes Benzecry
Universidade do Estado do Amazonas, Manaus, Amazonas, Brazil

Márcia Almeida Araújo Alexandre
Universidade do Estado do Amazonas, Manaus, Amazonas, Brazil
Fundação de Medicina Tropical Dr. Heitor Vieira Dourado, Manaus, Amazonas, Brazil
Universidade Nilton Lins, Manaus, Amazonas, Brazil

Marcus Vinícius Guimarães Lacerda
Universidade do Estado do Amazonas, Manaus, Amazonas, Brazil
Fundação de Medicina Tropical Dr. Heitor Vieira Dourado, Manaus, Amazonas, Brazil
Universidade Nilton Lins, Manaus, Amazonas, Brazil
National Institute of Science and Technology for Innovation in Neglected Diseases, Rio de Janeiro, Brazil

André Machado Siqueira
Universidade do Estado do Amazonas, Manaus, Amazonas, Brazil
Fundação de Medicina Tropical Dr. Heitor Vieira Dourado, Manaus, Amazonas, Brazil
National Institute of Science and Technology for Innovation in Neglected Diseases, Rio de Janeiro, Brazil

Belisa Maria Lopes Magalhães and Sheila Vitor-Silva
Universidade do Estado do Amazonas, Manaus, Amazonas, Brazil
National Institute of Science and Technology for Innovation in Neglected Diseases, Rio de Janeiro, Brazil

Ellen Fátima Caetano Lança
Universidade do Estado do Amazonas, Manaus, Amazonas, Brazil
Universidade Federal do Amazonas, Manaus, Amazonas, Brazil

Connor O'Brien
Columbia University Medical Center, New York, New York, United States of America

Quique Bassat
Centre de Recerca en Salut Internacional de Barcelona (CRESIB)/Hospital Clínic, Universitat de Barcelona, Barcelona, Spain

Heng-Chih Pan, Pei-Chun Fan and Chih-Hsiang Chang
Kidney Research Center, Department of Nephrology, Chang Gung Memorial Hospital, Taipei, Taiwan

Ming-Yang Chang, Ya-Chung Tian, Cheng-Chieh Hung, Ji-Tseng Fang, Chih-Wei Yang, Yung-Chang Chen and Chang-Chyi Jenq
Kidney Research Center, Department of Nephrology, Chang Gung Memorial Hospital, Taipei, Taiwan
Chang Gung University College of Medicine, Taoyuan, Taiwan

Ming-Hung Tsai
Division of Gastroenterology, Chang Gung Memorial Hospital, Taipei, Taiwan

Chang Gung University College of Medicine, Taoyuan, Taiwan

Renaud Tamisier, Sonia Dias-Domingos, Patrick Levy and Jean-Louis Pepin
INSERM U 1042, HP2 Laboratory, Université Joseph Fourier, Faculté de Médecine, Grenoble, France
CHU, Hôpital A. Michallon, Pôle Locomotion, Rééducation et Physiologie, Grenoble, France

Jean-Christian Borel
INSERM U 1042, HP2 Laboratory, Université Joseph Fourier, Faculté de Médecine, Grenoble, France
AGIRadom, Research and Development department, Meylan, France

Benoit Burel
CHU, Hôpital A. Michallon, Pôle Locomotion, Rééducation et Physiologie, Grenoble, France

Jean-Philippe Baguet
CHU, Hôpital A. Michallon, Département de cardiologie, Grenoble, France

Yi Zhang, Honglei Sun, Lihong Fan, Yuan Ma, Yipeng Sun, Juan Pu, Jun Yang and Jian Qiao
Key Laboratory of Animal Epidemiology and Zoonosis, College of Veterinary Medicine, China Agricultural University, Ministry of Agriculture, Beijing, China

Jinhua Liu
Key Laboratory of Animal Epidemiology and Zoonosis, College of Veterinary Medicine, China Agricultural University, Ministry of Agriculture, Beijing, China
Shandong Animal Disease Control Center, Shandong, China

Guangpeng Ma
China Rural Technology Development Center, Beijing, China

Amy M. Ahasic
Section of Pulmonary, Critical Care and Sleep Medicine, Department of Medicine, Yale School of Medicine, New Haven, Connecticut, United States of America

Yang Zhao
Department of Epidemiology and Biostatistics, School of Public Health, Nanjing Medical University, Nanjing, China

Li Su
Environmental and Occupational Medicine and Epidemiology Program, Department of Environmental Health, Harvard School of Public Health, Boston, Massachusetts, United States of America

David C. Christiani
Environmental and Occupational Medicine and Epidemiology Program, Department of Environmental Health, Harvard School of Public Health, Boston, Massachusetts, United States of America
Pulmonary and Critical Care Unit, Department of Medicine, Massachusetts General Hospital, Boston, Massachusetts, United States of America

Chau-Chyun Sheu
Division of Pulmonary and Critical Care Medicine, Kaohsiung Medical University Hospital, Kaohsiung Medical University, Kaohsiung, Taiwan

B. Taylor Thompson
Pulmonary and Critical Care Unit, Department of Medicine, Massachusetts General Hospital, Boston, Massachusetts, United States of America

D. Shane O'Mahony, Bradford J. Glavan, Tarah D. Holden and Christie Fong, Gail Rona and Mark M. Wurfel
Division of Pulmonary and Critical Care Medicine, Harborview Medical Center, University of Washington, Seattle, Washington, United States of America

Paula Tejera and David C. Christiani
Harvard School of Public Health, Harvard University, Boston, Massachusetts, United States of America

R. Anthony Black
Institute of Translational Health Sciences (ITHS), University of Washington, Seattle, Washington, United States of America

Hong Du, Jing Li, Wei Jiang, Haitao Yu, Ye Zhang, Junning Wang, Pingzhong Wang and Xuefan Bai
Center for Infectious Diseases, Tangdu Hospital, Fourth Military Medical University, Xi'an, Shaanxi, China

Shou-Hsuan Liu, Ja-Liang Lin, Cheng-Hao Weng, Huang-Yu Yang, Ching-Wei Hsu, Kuan-Hsing Chen, Wen-Hung Huang and Tzung-Hai Yen
Division of Clinical Toxicology, Department of Nephrology, Chang Gung Memorial Hospital and College of Medicine, Chang Gung University, Taipei, Taiwan

Krithika Lingappan, Weiwu Jiang, Lihua Wang, Xanthi I. Couroucli and Bhagavatula Moorthy
Department of Pediatrics, Section of Neonatology, Texas Children's Hospital, Baylor College of Medicine, Houston, Texas, United States of America

Chandra Srinivasan
Division of Pediatric Cardiology, Department of Pediatrics, University of Texas Medical School at Houston, Houston, Texas, United States of America

Airan Liu, Shixia Cai, Liang Dong, Le Liu, Yi Yang, Fengmei Guo, Xiaomin Lu, Hongli He, Qihong Chen, Shuling Hu and Haibo Qiu
Department of Critical Care Medicine, Zhongda Hospital, School of Medicine, Southeast University, Nanjing, P. R. China

Song Chen
State Key Laboratory of Natural Medicines, School of Life Science and Technology, China Pharmaceutical University, Nanjing, P. R. China

Jia-Yih Feng
Department of Chest Medicine, Taipei Veterans General Hospital, Taipei, Taiwan
Institute of Clinical Medicine; School of Medicine, National Yang-Ming University, Taipei, Taiwan

Wei-Juin Su and Kuang-Yao Yang
Department of Chest Medicine, Taipei Veterans General Hospital, Taipei, Taiwan
School of Medicine, National Yang-Ming University, Taipei, Taiwan

Wen-Feng Fang and Meng-Chih Lin
Division of Pulmonary and Critical Care Medicine and Department of Respiratory Therapy, Kaohsiung Chang Gung Memorial Hospital and Chang Gung University College of Medicine, Kaohsiung, Taiwan
Department of Respiratory Care, Chang Gung University of Science and Technology, Chiayi, Taiwan

Chieh-Liang Wu
Department of Internal Medicine, Chiayi Branch, Taichung Veterans General Hospital, Taichung, Taiwan
Department of Respiratory Therapy, College of Health Care, China Medical University, Taichung, Taiwan

Chong-Jen Yu
Department of Internal Medicine, National Taiwan University Hospital, Taipei, Taiwan
School of Medicine, National Taiwan University, Taipei, Taiwan

Shih-Chi Ku
Division of Pulmonary and Critical Care Medicine, Department of Internal Medicine, National Taiwan University Hospital, Taipei, Taiwan

Yu-Chun Chen
Department of Medical Research and Education, National Yang-Ming University Hospital, Yilan, Taiwan
School of Medicine, National Yang-Ming University, Taipei, Taiwan

Chang-Wen Chen
Medical Intensive Care Unit, Department of Internal Medicine, National Cheng-Kung University Hospital, Tainan, Taiwan

Chih-Yen Tu
Division of Pulmonary and Critical Care Medicine, Department of Internal Medicine, China Medical University Hospital, Taichung, Taiwan
School of Medicine, China Medical University, Taichung, Taiwan
Department of Life Science, National Chung Hsing University, Taichung, Taiwan

Yuanyuan Qi, Lijuan Liu, Panpan Wu and Libo Sun
Departments of Pediatrics, Children's Hospital of Fudan University, Shanghai, China

Liling Qian
Departments of Pediatrics, Children's Hospital of Fudan University, Shanghai, China
The Key Laboratory of Neonatal Disease, Ministry of Health, Shanghai, China

Bo Sun
Departments of Pediatrics, Children's Hospital of Fudan University, Shanghai, China
The Key Laboratory of Neonatal Disease, Ministry of Health, Shanghai, China
The Institutes of Biomedical Sciences of Fudan University, Shanghai, China

Sreedevi Avasarala, Fangfang Zhang, Guangliang Liu, Ruixue Wang, Steven D. London and Lucille London
Department of Oral Biology and Pathology, School of Dental Medicine, Stony Brook University, Stony Brook, New York, United States of America

Claudio Terzano, Fabio Di Stefano1, Vittoria Conti, Gregorino Paone, Angelo Petroianni and Alberto Ricci
Fondazione Eleonora Lorillard Spencer Cenci, Sapienza University of Rome, Rome, Italy

Marta Di Nicola
Laboratory of Biostatistics, Department of Biomedical Science, University "G.d'Annunzio" of Chieti-Pescara, Chieti, Italy

Wan-Jie Gu
Department of Anaesthesiology, the First Affiliated Hospital, Guangxi Medical University, Nanning, China
Department of Integrated Intensive Care Unit, the First Affiliated Hospital, Zhengzhou University, Zhengzhou, China

You-Dong Wan and Tong-Wen Sun
Department of Integrated Intensive Care Unit, the First Affiliated Hospital, Zhengzhou University, Zhengzhou, China

Hong-Tao Tie
The First College of Clinical Medicine, the First Affiliated Hospital, Chongqing Medical University, Chongqing, China

Quan-Cheng Kan
Pharmaceutical Department, the First Affiliated Hospital, Zhengzhou University, Zhengzhou, China

Allan J. Walkey
The Pulmonary Center, Boston University School of Medicine, Division of Pulmonary, Allergy and Critical Care Medicine, Boston Medical Center, Boston, Massachusetts, United States of America

Serkalem Demissie
Department of Biostatistics, Boston University School of Public Health, Boston, Massachusetts, United States of America

Dilip Shah, Freddy Romero, Leah Puklin and Ross S. Summer
Center for Translational Medicine and Korman Lung Center, Thomas Jefferson University, Philadelphia, Pennsylvania, United States of America

Min Yuan, Jie Shen, Yuxin Shi and Zhiyong Zhang
Department of Radiology, Shanghai Public Health Clinical Center, Fudan University, Shanghai, China

Yebin Jiang
Department of Radiology, Shanghai Public Health Clinical Center, Fudan University, Shanghai, China
Cancer Center, University of Michigan, Ann Arbor, Michigan, United States of America

Feng Feng
Department of Radiology, Shanghai Public Health Clinical Center, Fudan University, Shanghai, China
Department of Radiology, Nantong Tumor Hospital, Nantong University, Nantong, China

Huabin Yin
Department of Radiology, The Fifth People's Hospital of Shanghai, Fudan University, Shanghai, China

Daoying Geng
Department of Radiology, Huashan Hospital, Fudan University, Shanghai, China

Jianrong Xu
Department of Radiology, Renji Hospital, Shanghai Jiaotong University, Shanghai, China

Yanqing Hua
Department of Radiology, Huadong Hospital, Fudan University, Shanghai, China

Jingyun Shi
Department of Radiology, Shanghai Pulmonary Hospital, Tongji University, Shanghai, China

Xi Zheng, Yang Hu, Yong Yuan and Yong-Fan Zhao
Department of Thoracic Surgery, West China Hospital, Sichuan University, Chengdu, Sichuan Province, China

Jianfang Zhou and Bin Du
Medical ICU, Peking Union Medical College Hospital, Peking Union Medical College and Chinese Academy of Medical Sciences, Beijing, China

Chuanyun Qian
Department of Emergency Medicine and Medical ICU, The First Affiliated Hospital of Kunming Medical University, Kunming, China

Mingyan Zhao
Department of Critical Care Medicine, The First Affiliated Hospital of Harbin Medical University, Harbin, China

Xiangyou Yu
Department of Critical Care Medicine, First Affiliated Hospital, Xinjiang Medical University, Urumqi, China

Yan Kang
Department of Critical Care Medicine, West China Hospital, Sichuan University, Chengdu, China

Xiaochun Ma
Department of Critical Care Medicine, The First Affiliated Hospital of China Medical University, Shenyang, China

Yuhang Ai
Department of Critical Care Medicine, Xiangya Hospital, Central South University, Changsha, China

Yuan Xu
Department of Critical Care Medicine, Beijing Tongren Hospital, Capital Medical University, Beijing, China

Dexin Liu
Department of Critical Care Medicine, The Second Hospital of Jilin University, Changchun, China

Youzhong An
Department of Critical Care Medicine, Peking University People's Hospital, Beijing, China

Dawei Wu
Department of Critical Care Medicine, Qilu Hospital of Shandong University, Jinan, China

Renhua Sun
Department of Critical Care Medicine, Zhejiang Provincial People's Hospital, Hangzhou, China

Shusheng Li
Department of Critical Care Medicine, Tongji Hospital of Tongji Medical College, Huazhong University of Science and Technology, Wuhan, China

Zhenjie Hu
Department of Critical Care Medicine, Hebei Medical University Fourth Hospital, Shijiazhuang, China

Xiangyuan Cao
Department of Critical Care Medicine, General Hospital of Ningxia Medical University, Yinchuan, China

Fachun Zhou
Department of Emergency and Intensive Care Medicine, The First Affiliated Hospital of Chongqing Medical University, Chongqing, China

Li Jiang
Department of Critical Care Medicine, Fuxing Hospital, Capital Medical University, Beijing, China

Jiandong Lin
Department of Critical Care Medicine, The First Affiliated Hospital of Fujian Medical University, Fuzhou, China

Enqiang Mao
Emergency ICU, Ruijin Hospital, Shanghai Jiao Tong University, Shanghai, China

Tiehe Qin
Department of Critical Care Medicine, Guangdong General Hospital, Guangzhou, China

Zhenyang He
Department of Critical Care Medicine, Hainan Provincial People's Hospital, Haikou, China

Lihua Zhou
Department of Critical Care Medicine, The Affiliated Hospital of Inner Mongolia Medical University, Huhhot, China

Marcus J. Kitchen
School of Physics, Monash Institute of Medical Research, Clayton, Victoria, Australia

Melissa L. Siew, Megan J. Wallace and Stuart B. Hooper
The Ritchie Centre, Monash Institute of Medical Research, Clayton, Victoria, Australia

Arjan B. te Pas
Department of Pediatrics, Leiden University Medical Centre, Leiden, Netherlands

Andreas Fouras
Department of Mechanical and Aerospace Engineering, Monash University, Clayton, Victoria, Australia

Robert A. Lewis
Department of Medical Imaging and Radiation Science, Monash University, Clayton, Victoria, Australia
Biomedical Engineering, University of Saskatchewan, Saskatoon, Canada

Naoto Yagi and Kentaro Uesugi
SPring-8/Japan Synchrotron Radiation Research Institute, Sayo, Hyogo, Japan

Chih-Hsiang Chang, Pei-Chun Fan, Ming-Yang Chang, Ya-Chung Tian, Cheng-Chieh Hung, Ji-Tseng Fang, Chih-Wei Yang and Yung-Chang Chen
Kidney Research Center, Department of Nephrology, Chang Gung Memorial Hospital, Taipei, Taiwan
Chang Gung University College of Medicine, Taoyuan, Taiwan
Chang Gung University College of Medicine, Taoyuan, Taiwan

Wolfgang Huber, Josef Höllthaler, Andreas Umgelter, Michael Franzen, Bernd Saugel and Roland M. Schmid
II. Medizinische Klinik und Poliklinik, Klinikum rechts der Isar der Technischen Universität München, München, Germany

Tibor Schuster
Institut für Medizinische Epidemiologie und Statistik, Klinikum rechts der Isar der Technischen Universität München, Mu¨nchen, Germany

Colin Cordemans and Manu L. N. G. Malbrain
Department of Intensive Care, Ziekenhuis Netwerk Antwerpen, Antwerpen, Belgium

Maneesh Bhargava, Trisha L. Becker, Kevin J. Viken, Peter B. Bitterman and David H. Ingbar
Department of Medicine, University of Minnesota, Minneapolis, Minnesota, United States of America

Christine H. Wendt
Department of Medicine, University of Minnesota, Minneapolis, Minnesota, United States of America
Minneapolis VA Medical Center, University of Minnesota, Minneapolis, Minnesota, United States of America

Pratik D. Jagtap
Minnesota Supercomputer Institute, University of Minnesota, Minneapolis, Minnesota, United States of America

Sanjoy Dey, Michael S. Steinbach and Vipin Kumar
Department of Computer Science and Engineering, University of Minnesota, Minneapolis, Minnesota, United States of America

Baolin Wu
School of Public Health, University of Minnesota, Minneapolis, Minnesota, United States of America

Derek C. Angus, Arthur Boujoukos and Jeremy M. Kahn
Clinical Research, Investigation and Systems Modeling of Acute Illness (CRISMA) Center, Department of Critical Care Medicine, University of Pittsburgh School of Medicine, Pittsburgh, Pennsylvania, United States of America

David J. Wallace and Christopher W. Seymour
Clinical Research, Investigation and Systems Modeling of Acute Illness (CRISMA) Center, Department of Critical Care Medicine, University of Pittsburgh School of Medicine, Pittsburgh, Pennsylvania, United States of America
Department of Emergency Medicine, University of Pittsburgh School of Medicine, Pittsburgh, Pennsylvania, United States of America

Donald M. Yealy
Department of Emergency Medicine, University of Pittsburgh School of Medicine, Pittsburgh, Pennsylvania, United States of America

Brendan G. Carr
Department of Emergency Medicine, University of Pennsylvania Perelman School of Medicine, Philadelphia, Pennsylvania, United States of America

Kristen Kurland
Heinz College School of Public Policy and Management, Carnegie Mellon University, Pittsburgh, Pennsylvania, United States of America

Alexander D. Cornet
Department of Intensive Care, VU University Medical Center, Amsterdam, The Netherlands
Department of Internal Medicine, VU University Medical Center, Amsterdam, The Netherlands
Institute for Cardiovascular Research ICaR-VU, VU University Medical Center, Amsterdam, The Netherlands

Armand R. J. Girbes
Department of Intensive Care, VU University Medical Center, Amsterdam, The Netherlands
Institute for Cardiovascular Research ICaR-VU, VU University Medical Center, Amsterdam, The Netherlands

A. B. Johan Groeneveld
Department of Intensive Care, VU University Medical Center, Amsterdam, The Netherlands
Institute for Cardiovascular Research ICaR-VU, VU University Medical Center, Amsterdam, The Netherlands
Department of Intensive Care, Erasmus Medical Center, Rotterdam, The Netherlands

Albertus Beishuizen
Department of Intensive Care, VU University Medical Center, Amsterdam, The Netherlands
Institute for Cardiovascular Research ICaR-VU, VU University Medical Center, Amsterdam, The Netherlands
Department of Intensive Care, Medisch Spectrum Twente, Enschede, The Netherlands

Jorrit J. Hofstra and Pieter R. Tuinman and Marcus J. Schultz
Department of Intensive Care, Academic Medical Center, Amsterdam, The Netherlands
Laboratory of Experimental Intensive Care and Anesthesiology, Academic Medical Center, Amsterdam, The Netherlands

Alexander P. Vlaar
Department of Intensive Care, Academic Medical Center, Amsterdam, The Netherlands
Laboratory of Experimental Intensive Care and Anesthesiology, Academic Medical Center, Amsterdam, The Netherlands
Department of Internal Medicine, Academic Medical Center, Amsterdam, The Netherlands

Marcel Levi
Department of Internal Medicine, Academic Medical Center, Amsterdam, The Netherlands

Arthur van Lingen
Department of Nuclear Medicine, VU University Medical Center, Amsterdam, The Netherlands

Suman Chaudhary, Daniel P. Heruth and Li Q. Zhang
Department of Pediatrics, Division of Experimental and Translational Genetics, Children's Mercy Hospital, University of Missouri - Kansas City School of Medicine, Kansas City, Missouri, United States of America

Katherine Shortt, Dmitry Grigoryev and Shui Q. Ye
Department of Pediatrics, Division of Experimental and Translational Genetics, Children's Mercy Hospital, University of Missouri - Kansas City School of Medicine, Kansas City, Missouri, United States of America
Department of Biomedical and Health Informatics, University of Missouri - Kansas City School of Medicine, Kansas City, Missouri, United States of America

Lakshmi Venkitachalam
Department of Biomedical and Health Informatics, University of Missouri - Kansas City School of Medicine, Kansas City, Missouri, United States of America

Index